Gilles Walch • Pascal Boileau (Eds.)

Shoulder Arthroplasty

Springer-Verlag Berlin Heidelberg GmbH

Gilles Walch • Pascal Boileau (Eds.)

Shoulder Arthroplasty

Foreword from Norbert Gschwend
and Richard J. Hawkins

With 348 Figures (70 in Colour)
and 63 Tables

Springer

Gilles Walch, M.D.
Department of Orthopaedic Surgery
Clinique Emilie de Vialar - University of Lyon
116, Rue Antoine Charial
69003 Lyon, France

Pascal Boileau, M.D.
Department of Orthopaedic Surgery
Hôpital de L'Archet - University of Nice
151, Route de Saint-Antoine de Ginestière
06200 Nice, France

Library of Congress Cataloging-in-Publication Data
Shoulder Arthroplasty / G. Walch, P. Boileau (eds.)
Includes bibliographical references and index.
ISBN 978-3-642-63554-0 ISBN 978-3-642-58365-0 (eBook)
DOI 10.1007/978-3-642-58365-0
1. Shoulder Joint-Surgery. 2. Artificial shoulder joints.
I. Walch, G. (Gills), 1952 – . II. Boileau, P. (Pascal), 1956 – .
[DNLM: 1. Shoulder Joint-Surgery. 2. Joint Prosthesis-methods.
3. Arthroplasty-methods. WE 810 S558615 1999]
RD557.5.S543 1998
617.5'720592-dc21
DNLM/DLC
for Library of Congress

Originally published by Springer-Verlag Berlin Heidelberg New York in 1999
Softcover reprint of the hardcover 1st edition 1999

Production: PRO EDIT GmbH, D-69126 Heidelberg
Cover design: design & production GmbH, D-69121 Heidelberg
Typesetting: Hagedorn Kommunikation, D-68519 Viernheim

SPIN: 10780204 24/3111 – 5 4 3 2 1 – Printed on acid-free paper

To my wife Nicole and my children Arnaud, Matthieu, and Anne-Claire, who are the best part of my life.

G. Walch

To Dominique, Marie and Pierre; they made a dream come true, and to my parents for understanding and support through all the years.

P. Boileau

"Give me something different for there is a chance it might be better."

E. A. Codman, The Shoulder, 1934

"The tail is more important than the dog, but we shall have to have the dog to wag the tail!..."

Dr. Edward Martin, talking about the "end result idea" of Codman

Foreword

From Norbert Gschwend

Of all the medical specialities, orthopaedic surgery has become one of the most coveted by the public and tremendous advancement has been made in the last 20 years. To a great extent this can be attributed to the advent of artificial joint replacement. We are living in times in which many will enjoy a longer life, but, unfortunately, this is also accompanied by an increase of fear of sickness and invalidity. In such situations, those physicians who can offer a remedy for pain, and at the same time increase the quality of life, will be held in the highest regard by their patients. It was Sir John Charnley who, with the introduction of bone cement and the low friction principle of arthroplasty some 40 years ago, made the success of artificial joint replacement for the hip and later the knee joint possible. It then only became a question of time that other joints, such as the ones of the upper extremity, could also be replaced. Charles Neer II introduced a shoulder arthroplasty some 30 years ago for cases of posttraumatic destroyed shoulder joints. His technique became successful and generally accepted when it was possible to replace the humeral head as well as the glenoid surface despite poor bony conditions. So it was not surprising that speciality centers dealing with multiple joint disease in rheumatoid patients were at the forefront in developing total shoulder joint arthroplasty.

Pascal Boileau and Gilles Walch should be given great credit for having furthered our understanding of the functional anatomy of the glenohumeral joint as well as its relation to scapulo-thoracic motion. Based on their tremendous experience in the basic anatomy and its relation to function, they were able to develop a prosthetic device which could take into account individual anatomic variation in each patient, making the successful outcome of surgery much more predictable. Success in shoulder arthroplasty surgery is not necessarily dependent only on the principle of construction of a prosthetic device nor the way this devices is implanted or fixed to the bony interface, but more so by the understanding and handling of the soft tissues surrounding the articulation.

The book presented here by two outstanding young orthopaedic surgeons representing a new generation in the long tradition of French shoulder surgery not only informs the reader of the current state of the art in shoulder arthroplasty, but also enlightens him with an understanding of what advancements can be achieved with innovative thinking in this fascinating field of orthopaedic surgery.

Zürich,
Switzerland,
August, 1998

Professor Norbert Gschwend
(Founding Member
of the European Shoulder
and Elbow Society,
SECEC)

Foreword

From Richard J. Hawkins

It is indeed an honor and a pleasure to write a foreword for this outstanding book on shoulder arthroplasty by our friends Gilles Walch and Pascal Boileau. It provides a state-of-the-art overview of basic science research, including biomechanical design, to help us better understand and manage the different pathologies encountered requiring arthroplasty. Dr. Charles Neer, more than any other shoulder surgeon, has taught us that shoulder replacement is a highly successful operation. It has evolved from constrained to Neer's system to modular components and, finally, to humeral-glenoid mismatch, providing further improvements in outcome. This book and the proposed design changes take us to another level of shoulder arthroplasty.

Dr. Walch and Dr. Boileau are to be thanked for spear-heading and organizing a wonderful faculty to teach us about arthritis of the glenohumeral joint, bringing this book to a reality.

This is the most advanced and up-to-date discussion on arthritis and arthroplasty in the literature. The book addresses biomechanics, design, and many pathologies from osteoarthritis to fractures and massive cuff-tear arthropathy and includes surgical indications and techniques. It discusses the intricacies of avoiding and managing the many pitfalls that can occur during this challenging surgery.

The book allows the authors to introduce their concept of "prosthetic adaptability", based on careful analysis of proximal humeral anatomy. The major advantage is humeral component design changes that allow the prosthesis to be matched to the patient's anatomy, rather than matching the patient's anatomy to the prothesis. The adjustments allow individual accommodation of the patient's inclination, retroversion, and offsets. The glenoid component remains with a keel design, but the authors very carefully describe the necessary technique for its insertion. The humeral prosthesis is smooth and designed for cementing, something different for many North American surgeons who have found press-fitting to be successful. However, new design modification to allow press-fitting and other glenoid design options is ongoing.

The inventors have enlisted their friends in a multi-center trial and now report their highly successful outcomes. Arthritis and arthroplasty of the shoulder are growing in importance and deserve a comprehensive text that addresses all the related issues. This book is a must-read for any shoulder surgeon and will surely find its way onto our shelves as a reference.

Vail, Colorado,
August, 1998

Professor Richard J. Hawkins
(Founding Member and Former
President of the American
Shoulder and Elbow Surgeons)

Preface

This book is the result of three friendships: *The first close friendship* started in 1988, when the two of us met at the Orthopaedic Department of the University of Lyon, France. In our experience with shoulder arthroplasty we had both encountered consistent difficulties in recreating the normal anatomy and therefore we started working on the anatomy and kinematics of the normal shoulder and prostheses. We observed that the nonconstrained prostheses used at this time (monobloc, first generation prosthesis) rarely reproduced the normal kinematics of the shoulder. Using our anatomical studies and with the help of the engineers from Tornier, we designed a new type of humeral implant: this prosthesis was not only modular, to match the variations of dimension (second generation prosthesis), but also *adaptable*, to respect the individual shape of the proximal humerus of each patient. This third generation prosthesis was called Aequalis, because our goal was to equal the anatomy and kinematics of the normal shoulder. The first prostheses were inserted in 1991 by the two of us simultaneously in Lyon and in Nice. In the meantime, we tried to enhance the fixation of the glenoid component by designing an uncemented glenoid using a system of expanding screws and we developed instruments for the humeral component, the glenoid component and specific instruments for the fractures cases (the Aequalis Fracture Jig).

The second friendship started in 1992 when a group of 15 European surgeons agreed to use the Aequalis prosthesis with prospective assessment involving evaluation sheets and radiographs pre- and post-operatively. Although we had known many of those surgeons personally for a long time, we grew closer through the frequent contacts and meetings needed to evaluate our results, creating an "esprit de corps" where working and laughing could be present at the same time. This group of early users was called the Aequalis Group and has been working enthusiastically and in close cooperation since that time.

The third friendship is related to our close collaborators, rheumatologists, physiotherapists and radiologists who have been working with us for many years and who were willing to embark with us on the "adventure of shoulder arthroplasty". They agreed to share their knowledge and helped us to treat and rehabilitate our patients and finally to evaluate the results of both operative and nonoperative treatments.

In 1996 the time had come for us to analyze our results even though the follow-up was short. These results have been reported in a Symposium on Shoulder Arthroplasty, held in Nice on June 27, 28, 29th 1996. This book consists, in part, of the manuscripts based on presentations from this meeting and is the result of an intense and friendly collaboration of the entire "dream team"!

The objective of this book is fourfold:

- *First*, to expose the *concept of prosthetic adaptability* based on the basic research performed to improve the understanding of the three-dimensional geometry and kinematics of the shoulder.
- *Second* , to present the *early clinical and radiological results* of more than 400 patients operated on with the Aequalis prosthesis and prospectively followed since 1991; all the failures and complications as well as their management and the need for revision surgery are reported in detail and are closely analyzed for the various etiologies.
- *Third*, to expose the *improved understanding of the various disease processes* (osteoarthritis, rheumatoid arthritis, avascular necrosis, arthritis with massive cuff tear, acute fractures and fractures sequelae) *as well as their clinical and radiological presentation* which was gained from the large cohort of patients reviewed.
- *Fourth*, to give any *practical details that may help the surgeon and the physiotherapist* that we found to be important for an optimum result in shoulder arthroplasty.

It may be argued that a multicenter study and a short follow-up are useless for evaluating the results of prosthetic surgery. We disagree with this point of view for many reasons. First, we would have failed in our duty if we had not presented the early results of a new implant, based on a completely different concept. Secondly, the functional result for a prosthesis is established within 1 year. Thirdly, this series represents a unique experience of shoulder surgeons using the same prosthesis, inserted in a standard manner, which would naturally diminish the influence of technological elements on the results. Fourthly, the clinical results have been evaluated in a uniform manner in the different centers by using the Constant Score which has been recognized to be objective and interobserver reliable. Finally, these early results should serve as the foundation for the addition of the knowledge of tomorrow; they will not prevent us from continuing to follow our patients and to reevaluate carefully the results in the near future. We believe that our studies have already helped us to improve the quality of care provided to our patients.

We did take a different way. We would like to point it to others because it looks promising!...

Gilles Walch and Pascal Boileau

Lyon, Nice, August, 1998

Acknowledgments

It is a pleasure to acknowledge those who helped us develop the Aequalis project and who helped to write and edit this book.

We must first pay a tribute to our wives: they not only accepted that we spent so much time away from our families but also participated in the elaboration of this book and gave of their time with us to allow completion of the project: Nicole Walch has illustrated most of the articles while Dominique Boileau transcribed, typed and edited the text of this manuscript.

This book would not have been possible without the hard work and expertise of the contributing authors. We appreciate the time taken from their busy schedules and their families to help complete this project. We would like to express our gratitude to them. A special note of thanks to those who started with us fom the beginning because each of them has brought a stone to reinforce the edifice: Jean-Claude Scheffer and Maurice Basso for their team spirit, Jean-Pierre Franceschi for helping us "to brush away the ravens from our shoulders!", Dominique Gazielly for his enlarged view on shoulder arthroplasty, Peter Habermeyer for his initially open mind, Jean-Pierre Liotard for his refreshing aquatic contribution, Jean-Charles Le Huec for his creativity and enthusiasm, Luc Favard for his wisdom and rigor, Laurent Nové-Josserand and Christophe Lévigne for bringing the inheritance of Lyon's Orthopaedic School, Henri Mestdagh for his kindly support, Daniel Goutallier for his sharp (very sharp!) but progressive analyses, and Daniel Molé and Jean-François Kempf for their controversial but fruitful and friendly discussions.

We must pay a particular tribute to Christian Gerber. He "embarked on the boat" with us as soon as we got under way and always pointed us the right direction. We consider him a true friend. He remains for us an inspiration and a lasting example in teaching, research, and patient care.

When we decided to write this book we also decided to publish it in English, which is now internationally recognized as the language of science. However, it is a difficult task for people like us, whose native language is French, to write in Shakespeare's language. This is why we are forever grateful to Richard Sinnerton, Orthopaedic Surgeon, who spent a year with us as a fellow, and translated almost all the articles. Our friend Roger Emery Orthopedic Surgeon in London and mentor of Richard should be thanked for suggesting and encouraging him to come to Nice. Richard spoke not only fluent French but also worked with us daily in the anatomical laboratory, the operating room and the office and so was able to better understand our philosophy and the messages we wanted to deliver. This book would not exist without him and he should rank as co-editor.

Nataly Revel was responsible for the organization of the meeting in Nice and for the scientific coordination between the contributing authors. As ever, she did a great job, taking care of all details, even though she had to work outside the hospital (at home) every evening. For this, we are very grateful to her and to the secretaries who assisted and helped her: Françoise Gros, Mireille Kaufman, Sophie Plantier in Lyon and Muriel Houée, Muriel Cano and Carole Bolgari in Nice.

We are extremely grateful to the medical staff (anesthetists, nurses, and physiotherapists) who take care of the patients in the Orthopaedic Departments of Nice (Pr C. Argenson, Hôpital de l'Archet) and Lyon (Clinique Emilie de Vialar and Hôpital Lyon-Sud). We are specially grateful to Béatrice Cordéro for her rough but generous friendship. A special note of thanks to our residents and fellows as well as the many visitors from all countries who went to Lyon or Nice; they stimulated us with many questions that helped us to express more clearly our concepts and ideas.

In Europe it is not considered good form to acknowledge commercial undertakings, even though the work would not have been possible without their collaboration. However, we would like to truly thank the Tornier Company and especially Alain Tornier, who believed in us when others did not. He may be considered as "the spark which ignited the fire". His charisma and enthusiasm have been a great help in many difficult situations. We are also indebted to the team of engineers who helped us to find some of the technological innovations developed with the Aequalis prosthesis:

Frédéric Ducret, Denis Perret, and, more recently, Franck Bénis have worked over the years under the supervision of Yves-Alain Ratron. Many other people from Tornier should be thanked because of their participation, at one time or another, to the Aequalis project; we should mention Éric Beloux, Sylvie Humbert and Craig Jones and all the US team. We owe, above all, a debt of gratitude to Patricia Abraham: the immense amount of work she carried out over the last 5 years has stimulated us more than anything. She planned and took care of everything; she pushed us to our limits in such a way and with such a smile that we could not refuse.

We would also like to thank Ms. Gabriele M. Schröder, Ms. Judith Diemer and Ms. Sherryl Sundell, from the staff of Springer-Verlag, for their excellence in cooperation, for the quality of their work and for their patience in carrying the project to completion.

Finally, we would like to extend our gratitude to the hundreds of patients who returned for follow-up many years after arthroplasty of their arthritic or fractured shoulders. They taught us so much! ...

Contents

Section V: Advances in Glenoid Design and Surgical Technique

Section VI: Multicentre Studies

Section VII: Primary Osteoarthritis

Section VIII: Rheumatoid Arthritis

Section IX: Atraumatic Avascular Necrosis of the Humeral Head

Section X: Osteoarthritis with Massive Cuff-Tear

Section XI: Acute Fractures of the Proximal Humerus

Section XII: Sequelae of Proximal Humeral Fractures

Section XIII: Rehabilitation

Section XIV: Complications and Revision

Section XV: Synopsis

Contributors

ALISON, DANIEL, M.D.
Department of Radiology
Hôpital Trousseau
University of Tours
37044 Tours, France

ALLAIN, JÉROME, M.D.
Department of Orthopaedic Surgery
Hôpital Henri Mondor
University of Paris
51, Avenue du Marechal de Lattre de Tassigny
94010 Créteil, France

BADET, ROGER, M.D.
Department of Orthopaedic Surgery
University of Grenoble
38000 Grenoble, France

BANKES, MARCUS, F.R.C.S.
Department of Orthopaedics
Saint Mary's Hospital
Praed Street
London W2 1NY, England

BASSO, MAURICE, M.D.
Hôpital René Sabran
Bd. Edouard Herriot
83406 Hyères, France

BERNAGEAU, JACQUES, M.D.
Department of Radiology
Hôpital Henri Mondor
University of Paris
51, Avenue du Marechal de Lattre de Tassigny
94010 Créteil, France

BOILEAU, PASCAL, M.D.
Department of Orthopaedic Surgery
Hôpital de L'Archet
University of Nice
151, Route de Saint-Antoine de Ginestière
06200 Nice, France

BONNOMET, FRANÇOIS, M.D.
Department of Orthopaedic Surgery
Hôpital de Hautepierre
University of Strasbourg
Avenue Molière
67098 Strasbourg, France

BOULAHIA, AZIZ, M.D.
Department of Orthopaedic Surgery
Clinique Emilie de Vialar
116, Rue Antoine Charial
69003 Lyon, France

BOUTEMY, PATRICK, M.D.
Department of Orthopaedic Surgery
Hôpital de Haute Pierre
University of Strasbourg
Avenue Molière
67098 Strasbourg, France

BOUVIER, MAURICE, M.D.
Department of Rheumathology
Hôpital Lyon-Sud
University of Lyon
69003 Pierre Bénite, France

CALIGARIS-CORDERO, BÉATRICE, M.D.
Department of Rehabilitation
Centre Hélio-Marin de Vallauris
University of Nice
06000 Vallauris, France

CLÉMENT, PHILIPPE, M.D.
Department of Orthopaedic Surgery
Hôpital Trousseau
University of Tours
37044 Tours, France

COLIN, FRANÇOIS, M.D.
Department of Orthopaedic Surgery
Hôpital de Hautepierre
University of Strasbourg
Avenue Molière
67098 Strasbourg, France

Constantin, Adeline, M.D.
Department of Rheumatology
Hôpital Edouard Herriot
Place d'Arsonval
University of Lyon
69437 Lyon, France

Dehais, Joël, M.D.
Department of Rheumatology
Hôpital Pellegrin
University of Bordeaux
Place Raba Leon
33076 Bordeaux, France

Desperiez, Michel, M.D.
Department of Radiology
Hôpital Trousseau
University of Tours
37044 Tours, France

Dwyer, Sean, F.R.C.A.
Department of Anesthesia
Saint Mary's Hospital
Praed Street
London W21 NY, ENGLAND

Emery, Roger, F.R.C.S.
Department of Orthopaedic Surgery
Saint Mary's Hospital
Praed Street
London W2 1NY, England

Favard, Luc, M.D.
Department of Orthopaedic Surgery
Hôpital Trousseau
University of Tours
37044 Tours, France

Franceschi, Jean-Pierre, M.D.
Department of Orthopaedic Surgery
Centre Boreli - Mermoz
114, Rue Jean Mermoz
13008 Marseille, France

Gazielly, Dominique F., M.D.
Shoulder Unit
13, Place de l'Hôtel de Ville
42000 Saint-Étienne, France

Gerber, Christian, M.D.
Department of Orthopaedic Surgery
University of Zurich, Balgrist
Forchstrasse 340
8008 Zurich, Switzerland

Goutalier, Daniel, M.D.
Department of Orthopaedic Surgery
Hôpital Henri Mondor
University of Paris
51, Avenue du Marechal de Lattre de Tassigny
94010 Créteil, France

Grauer, Jean-Luc, M.D.
Department of Rheumatology
Hôpital Paul Cézanne
Avenue des Tamaris
13616 Aix-en-Provence, France

Habermeyer, Peter, M.D.
Sportklinik Stuttgart
Taubenheimstrasse 8
70372 Stuttgart, Germany

Hardy, Philippe, M.D.
Department of Orthopaedic Surgery
Hôpital Ambroise Parré
University of Paris
Avenue Charles De Gaulle
92104 Boulogne, France

Harrop-Griffiths, William, F.R.C.A.
Department of Anesthesia
Saint Mary's Hospital
Praed Street
London W2 1NY, England

Hovorka, Istvan, M.D.
Department of Orthopaedic Surgery
Hôpital de L'Archet
University of Nice
151, Route de Saint-Antoine de Ginestière
06200 Nice, France

Kelberine, François, M.D.
Department of Orthopaedic Surgery
Hôpital Paul Cézanne
Avenue des Tamaris
13616 Aix-en-Provence, France

Kempf, Jean-François, M.D.
Department of Orthopaedic Surgery
Hôpital de Hautepierre
University of Strasbourg
Avenue Molière
67098 Strasbourg, France

LACAZE, FANCK, M.D.
Department of Orthopaedic Surgery
Hôpital de Haute Pierre
University of Strasbourg
Avenue Molière
67098 Strasbourg, France

LAUTMANN, SABINE, M.D.
Department of Orthopaedic Surgery
Hôpital Trousseau
University of Tours
37044 Tours, France

LAVAU, LAURENT, M.D.
Department of Orthopaedic Surgery
Hôpital Henri Mondor
University of Paris
51, Avenue du Marechal de Lattre de Tassigny
94010 Créteil, France

LE HUEC, JEAN-CHARLES, M.D.
Department of Orthopaedic Surgery
Hôpital Pellegrin
University of Bordeaux
Place Raba Leon
33076 Bordeaux, France

LÉVIGNE, CHRISTOPHE, M.D.
Department of Orthopaedic Surgery
Clinique du Parc
86, Boulevard des Belges
69006 Lyon, France

LIOTARD, JEAN-PIERRE, M.D.
Department of Rehabilitation
Clinique Emilie de Vialar
116, Rue Antoine Charial
69003 Lyon, France

MESTDAGH, HENRI, M.D.
Department of Orthopaedic Surgery
Hôpital B, University of Lille
2, Avenue Oscar Lambret
59037 Lille, France

MEZZANA, MARC, M.D.
Department of Rehabilitation
Clinique des Fontaines
54, bd Aristide Briand
77007 Melun, France

MOLÉ, DANIEL, M.D.
Department of Orthopaedic Surgery
University of Nançy
49, Rue Hermine
54000 Nançy, France

NERISSON, DANIEL, M.D.
Department of Orthopaedic Surgery
Hôpital de Hautepierre
University of Strasbourg
Avenue Molière
67098 Strasbourg, France

NOËL, ERIC, M.D.
Department of Rheumatology
Hôpital Edouard Herriot
Place d'Arsonval
University of Lyon
69437 Lyon, France

NOVÉ-JOSSERAND, LAURENT, M.D.
Department of Orthopaedic Surgery
Clinique Saint-Charles
25, Rue Flesselle
69001 Lyon, France

OLLAGNIER, ERIC, M.D.
Department of Rheumatology
Hôpital Bellevue
University of Saint-Étienne
42000 Saint-Étienne, France

PAYEUR, FRÉDERIC, M.D.
Department of Rehabilitation
Centre Hélio-Marin de Vallauris
University of Nice
06000 Vallauris, France

POSTEL, JEAN MARIE, M.D.
Department of Orthopaedic Surgery
Hôpital Henri Mondor
University of Paris
51, Avenue du Maréchal de Lattre de Tassigny
94010 Créteil, France

POZZI, ISABEL, M.D.
Orthopaedic Surgeon
Rua Professor Duplan 72/02
Rio Brano, Porto Alegre
90420–030 R.S., Brasil

RIAND, NICOLAS, M.D.
Department of Orthopaedic Surgery
Hôpital Cantonal de Genève
24, Rue Micheli du Crest
1211 Genève, Switzerland

ROCHE, OLIVIER, M.D.
Department of Orthopaedic Surgery
University of Nançy
49, Rue Hermine
54000 Nançy, France

Romeo, Anthony, M.D.
Department of Orthopaedic Surgery
Hôpital de L'Archet
University of Nice
151, Route de Saint-Antoine de Ginestière
06200 Nice, France

Romero, José, M.D.
Department of Orthopaedic Surgery
University of Zurich, Balgrist
Forchstrasse 340
8008 Zurich, Switzerland

Scheffer, Jean-Claude, M.D.
Department of Orthopaedic Surgery
Clinique des Fontaines
54 bd Aristide Briand
77007 Melun, France

Shaeverbecke, Thierry, M.D.
Department of Rheumatology
Hôpital Pellegrin
University of Bordeaux
Place Raba Leon
33076 Bordeaux, France

Sinnerton, Richard, F.R.C.S.
Department of Orthopaedics
Ashford Hospital
London Road
Ashford
Middlesex TW15 3AA, England

Tebib, Jacques-Guy, M.D.
Department of Rheumathology
Hôpital Lyon-Sud
University of Lyon
69003 Pierre Bénite, France

Thomas, Thierry, M.D.
Department of Rheumatology
Hôpital Bellevue
University of Saint-Étienne
42000 Saint-Étienne, France

Tinsi, Laurent, M.D.
Department of Orthopaedic Surgery
Hôpital de L'Archet
University of Nice
151, Route de Saint-Antoine de Ginestière
06200 Nice, France

Trojani, Christophe, M.D.
Department of Orthopaedic Surgery
Hôpital de L'Archet
University of Nice
151, Route de Saint-Antoine de Ginestière
06200 Nice, France

Veneau, Benjamin
Department of Orthopaedic Surgery
Hôpital de L'Archet
University of Nice
151, Route de Saint-Antoine de Ginestière
06200 Nice, France

Walch, Gilles, M.D.
Department of Orthopaedic Surgery
Clinique Emilie de Vialar
116, Rue Antoine Charial
69003 Lyon, France

Section I:
History

Shoulder Replacement: Historical Perspectives

R. Emery and M. Bankes

Summary

The first modern shoulder arthroplasty with an anatomic shape was implanted by Krueger in 1950. The modern era of shoulder replacement dawned with the pioneering work of Neer, who in 1953 laid the foundations for our current knowledge of the indications, surgical technique, rehabilitation and results of shoulder replacement. During this time a number of designs emerged in both Europe and the United States addressing the problem of the absent rotator cuff by replacing the complete articulation with a linked prosthesis. The disappointing results of these designs led to a generally held view of the lack of success of shoulder replacement and rekindled an interest in alternative methods of treatment. An enormous number of designs, sometimes radically different from one another, have appeared, such as bipolar prostheses, surface replacements, and components made from other biomaterials. However, the recent development of modular components has rekindled the possibility of a prosthesis of truly anatomical design as envisaged by Krueger 45 years ago.

Péan's classic description of the first metallic prosthetic replacement, performed on 11 March 1893 at the Hôpital International in Paris, cites Themistocles Gluck four times [1]. Gluck made great contributions to many branches of experimental surgery at the end of the nineteenth century, including organ transplantation and fracture surgery. However, in the field of shoulder replacement his contribution is understated if not completely overlooked. He was without doubt the pioneer of joint replacement and devised prostheses for many joints including the shoulder.

Born at Jassy in Romania in 1853, Gluck was the son of the attending physician to the royal family and later studied medicine himself in Leipzig and Berlin. His teachers included Virchow, His and von Langenbeck [2]. After animal trials with various materials, including wood, glass, aluminium, and nickel plated steel, Gluck opted for cadaveric bone and ivory for his prostheses (Fig. 1). He had shown that these were integrated in recipients and claimed there was no difficulty disinfecting it. He also experimented with methods of fixing his prostheses to the skeleton and used a variety of substances as cement, including copper amalgam, plaster of Paris, and stone putty although his personal preference was for cementless osseointegration [3, 4]. Gluck was keen that his designs could be used in all age groups and so designed prostheses with interchangeable ivory ends, thereby producing the first modular prostheses [5]. This work culminated in 1890 with the insertion of a hinged ivory prosthesis into the tuberculous knee of a 17-year-old woman, and Gluck went on to insert a total of 14 arthroplasties, although only five, all tuberculous joints, were reported in detail: three knees, one wrist and one elbow [3]. The initial results were spectacular and Gluck used these to justify their continued use although he appreciated at an early stage that his implants would inevitably fail in the presence of infection.

His designs for shoulder replacements included a simple prosthesis consisting of an ivory humeral component inserted down the medullary canal which articulated by hooking on to an ivory eye screwed into the glenoid. He also developed more complex hinge and ball and socket joints using ivory and cadaveric bone. The method of fixation was osseointegration [2]. Although he described their insertion in his definitive article from this period published in 1891, he did not describe the results or state definitively that they were performed in living humans.

In 1890 Gluck planned to present his work on arthroplasty to the 10th International Surgical Congress in Berlin and, in order to allow his ideas to be visualised, used the combined expertise of a medical instrument company and the royal furniture craftsmen to fit a human skeleton with his shoulder, elbow, wrist, knee and ankle joint replacements [6]. Gluck was forced to abandon his presentation and his "Skeleton of Paris" was never presented to the Congress. The German surgical establishment fiercely opposed Gluck's work, believing it would publicly disgrace German science. In the climate of such hostility Gluck stopped his work on joint replacement permanently in 1891. The Skeleton of Paris was displayed around Europe until World War Two,

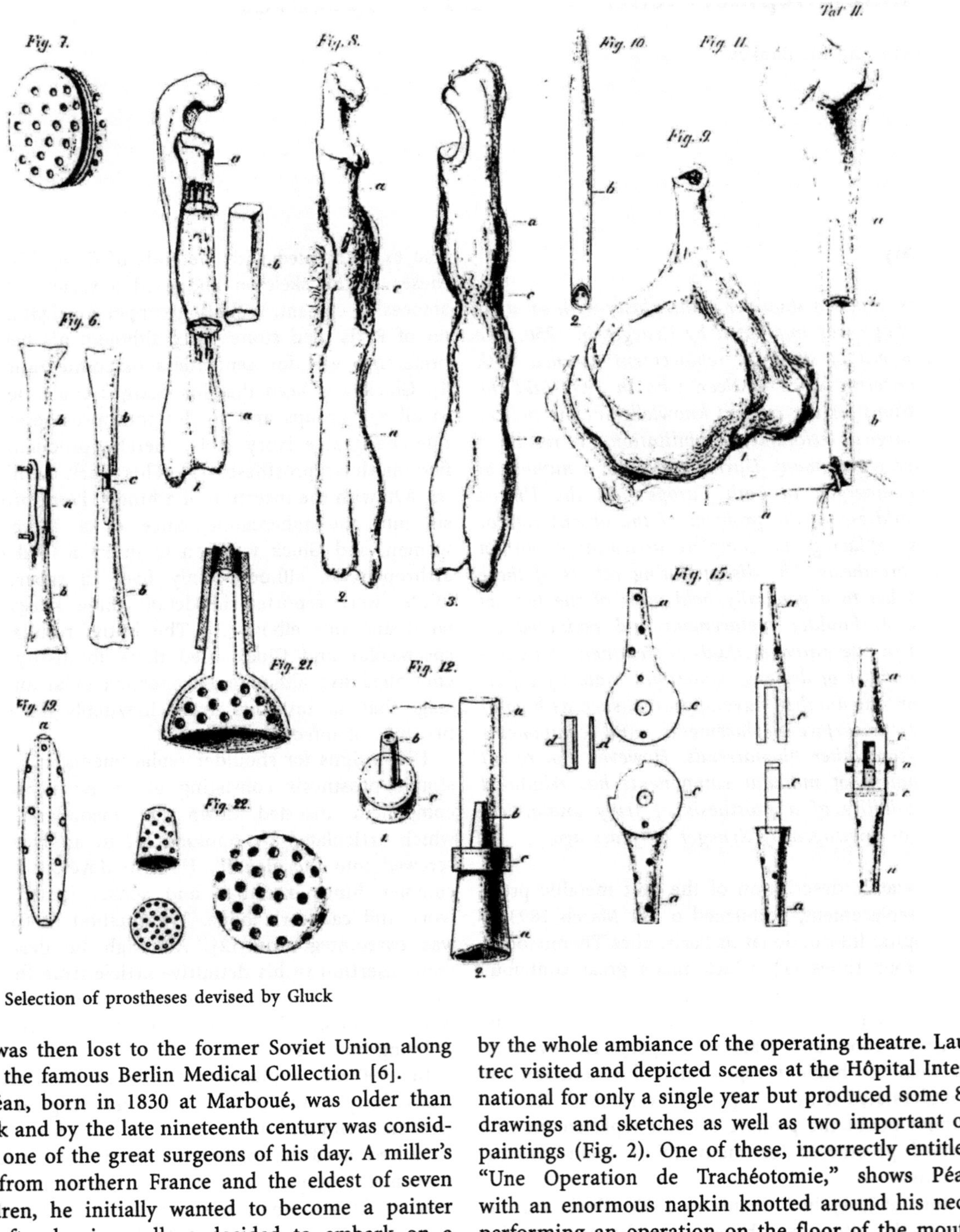

Fig. 1. Selection of prostheses devised by Gluck

but was then lost to the former Soviet Union along with the famous Berlin Medical Collection [6].

Péan, born in 1830 at Marboué, was older than Gluck and by the late nineteenth century was considered one of the great surgeons of his day. A miller's son from northern France and the eldest of seven children, he initially wanted to become a painter but after leaving college decided to embark on a medical career in Paris. He was not only a dextrous operator and inspirational teacher but also a great performer, enlivening his demonstrations in front of the gallery of students with witty repartee. In 1891, Gabriel Tapié de Céleyran, the cousin and constant companion of the celebrated French painter Toulouse-Lautrec, became one of Péan's interns. Through this connection Lautrec obtained permission to watch Péan operate and became enchanted by the whole ambiance of the operating theatre. Lautrec visited and depicted scenes at the Hôpital International for only a single year but produced some 80 drawings and sketches as well as two important oil paintings (Fig. 2). One of these, incorrectly entitled "Une Operation de Trachéotomie," shows Péan with an enormous napkin knotted around his neck performing an operation on the floor of the mouth as the patient is anaesthetised by a chloroform-soaked pad held over the nose [7].

Péan's case report concerns a 37-year-old baker dying from tuberculosis of the proximal humerus and shoulder joint [1, 8], complicated by the formation of a vast abscess beneath the proximal upper limb musculature. At operation, using an anterior approach, Péan encountered a glenohumeral joint lined by thickened spongiform synovium and full of pus. With a view to insertion of a prosthesis Péan subsequently resected the proximal half of the humerus back down to healthy bone and removed other infected tissue.

The patient had refused amputation and so Péan was left only with the possibility of excising the infected tissue and inserting a prosthesis. He rejected one of Gluck's ivory prostheses on the grounds that it was not strong enough and so ordered the design of another. The prosthesis was designed and constructed with some speed by J. Porter Michaels, a Parisian dentist who had previously made a maxillary implant for Péan. The shaft component was made of a platinum cylinder with two ridges and several holes for attachment of the periosteum and muscles. There were screw holes at the distal end for attachment to the bone stump. The head consisted of a ball of rubber previously hardened by boiling in paraffin for 24 h. The rubber ball contained two equatorial grooves arranged at right angles, each of which contained a metal loop, one of which was attached to the glenoid and the other to the proximal end of the shaft component. It was felt that this prosthesis provided ample strength combined with freedom of movement [8, 9].

The prosthesis was inserted at a second operation with the periosteum and articular capsule attached around it to completely enclose the shaft. The initial postoperative results were excellent, with the patient's fever subsiding and appetite returning within the first 12 days, and the patient being allowed home after 3 weeks. After a few months the patient had gained 35 lb and the strength and range of movement of the affected limb had greatly improved. The success of the operation was marred a year later by a recurrent abscess just above the epicondyle that required drainage on four separate occasions. The patient returned 2 years after his shoulder replacement with a sinus that had formed along the surgical scar. He was investigated with one of the first X-ray machines and the radiographs were presented at a meeting of the Académie de Médecine. It transpired that a long and resistant osseous shell had formed around the prosthesis, and Péan was subsequently forced to remove it at a further operation. A few days later the fistula had closed and the patient gradually resumed his daily activities but with his arm now somewhat shortened.

The prosthesis itself came into the possession of Edward Augustus Bogue, an American dentist acquainted with both Péan and Michaels. Bogue returned to the United States and donated the prosthesis to the Armed Forces Institute of Pathology in 1916. It is now on display in The Smithsonian Institution in Washington, DC [9].

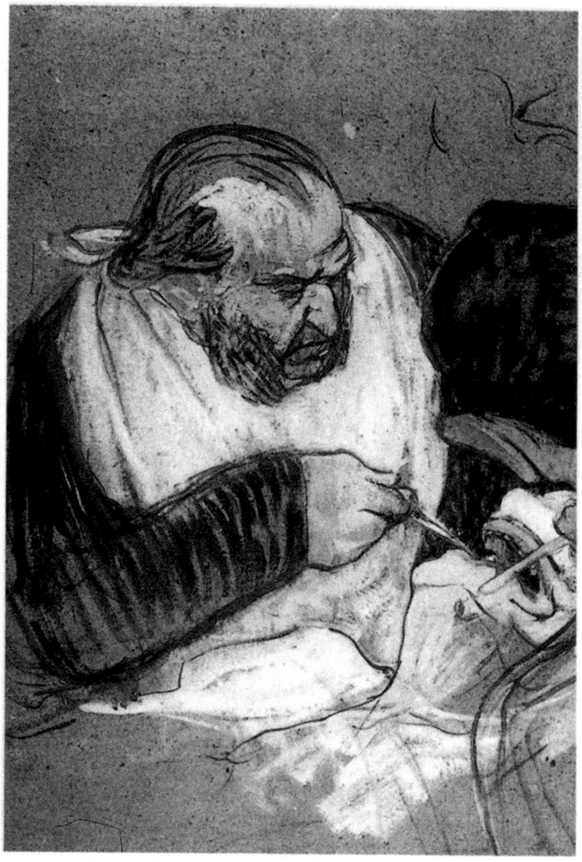

Fig. 2. Jules Emile Péan

It is interesting to reflect upon the fact that Péan certainly did not originate the concept of arthroplasty, nor did he design any prostheses. Péan was fortunate that he was the first to clearly document the successful application of Gluck's ideas of arthroplasty to the shoulder. Furthermore Péan would probably never have considered a prosthesis had it not been for the patient's refusal of amputation. It would be interesting to consider whether Gluck's contribution would have been overlooked. The skeleton of Paris had been lost in Russia and Péan's prosthesis is now on display in the smithsonian Institution [10]. There was no development of this prosthesis and for almost 60 years the only other documented prosthetic shoulder replacement was another attempt to use ivory by König in 1914 [11] (Fig. 3).

The failure of these early experiments was due to infection resulting in rapid loosening. Developments continued at a very slow rate due to the additional limitations of biomaterials and poor fixation methods. An acrylic prosthesis, modified from a Judet hip prosthesis, was described by Boron and Sevin in 1951 [12] (Fig. 4). Judet described the use of acrylic implants to replace the proximal part of the

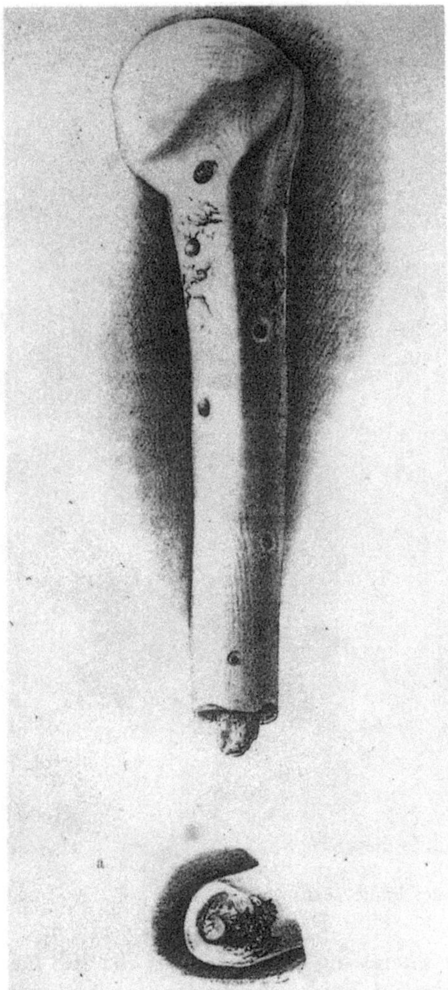

Fig. 3. Konig ivory humeral replacement

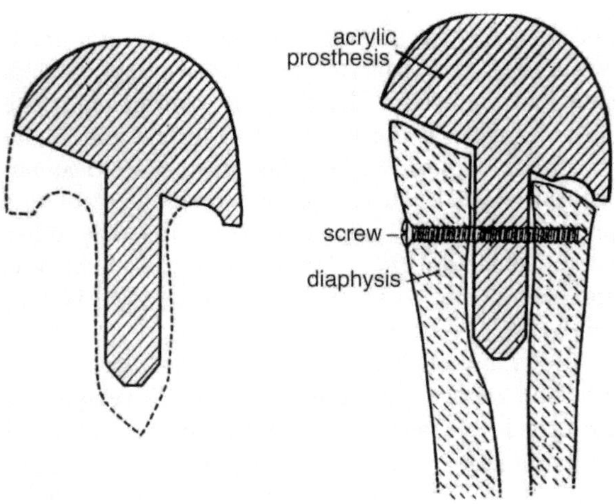

Fig. 4. Fracture prosthesis devised by Boron and Sevin. **Left,** frontal section. The **dotted line** indicates the femoral head; **hatched area,** humeral head. **Right,** placement on the diaphysis

humerus in fracture dislocation in 1952 [13]. Their modes of failure are well described in case reports by De Anquin and De Anquin in 1953 [14], Lynn et al. in 1965 [15] and Monteleone in 1969 [16]. Similar designs appeared in metal which became the forerunners of stemless surface replacements.

The first modern shoulder arthroplasty with an anatomic shape, including medial and posterior offset, was implanted by Frederick Krueger on 12th December 1950 [17]. His stemmed design was made from vitallium with fenestrations for bone intrusion (Fig. 5). He attempted to reproduce the human anatomy by making acrylic replicas of caderveric proximal humeri. The prosthesis was implanted in a young sailor with aseptic necrosis and achieved a "well functioning and painless shoulder".

The modern era of shoulder replacement dawns with the pioneering work of Dr. Charles S. Neer II. In 1953, probably due to the success of hemiarthroplasty for hip fracture, he devised a hemiarthroplasty for fractures of the neck of the humerus with dislocation of the head fragment which would have previously been treated by simple excision [18]. Two years later some modifications were made including nonanatomical flattening of the humeral head to permit seating in to the greater tuberosity and characteristic holes which not only allow permeation of bone but also the reattachment of tuberosities to each other, demonstrating its origins as a solution for fracture fixation (Fig. 6). The first series of 12 cases were performed during 1953 and early 1954 [19]. By 1964 Neer had applied his technique to 54 patients [20]. It is interesting to note that 20 years elapsed before the series of 48 replacement arthroplasties for glenohumeral arthritis were reported in 1974 [21]. This and the subsequent work by Neer laid the foundations for our current knowledge of the indications, surgical technique, rehabilitation and results of shoulder replacement.

During this time a number of designs emerged in both Europe and the United States addressing the problem of the absent rotator cuff by replacing the complete articulation with a linked prosthesis. It is interesting to observe that the need for such a prosthesis was also recognised by Neer, who designed two types of fixed fulcrum device, both of which failed and were subsequently abandoned (Fig. 7). These prostheses had a similar fate, usually as a consequence of aseptic loosening, such as the Stanmore total shoulder replacement introduced in 1969 [22]. In 1982 Lettin et al. reported 44 % loosening with 10 of 50 cases requiring revision, results which led to it being discontinued [23]. Similar results with the Liverpool prosthesis were obtained with 4 of 13 prostheses loose at short-term review [24]. In

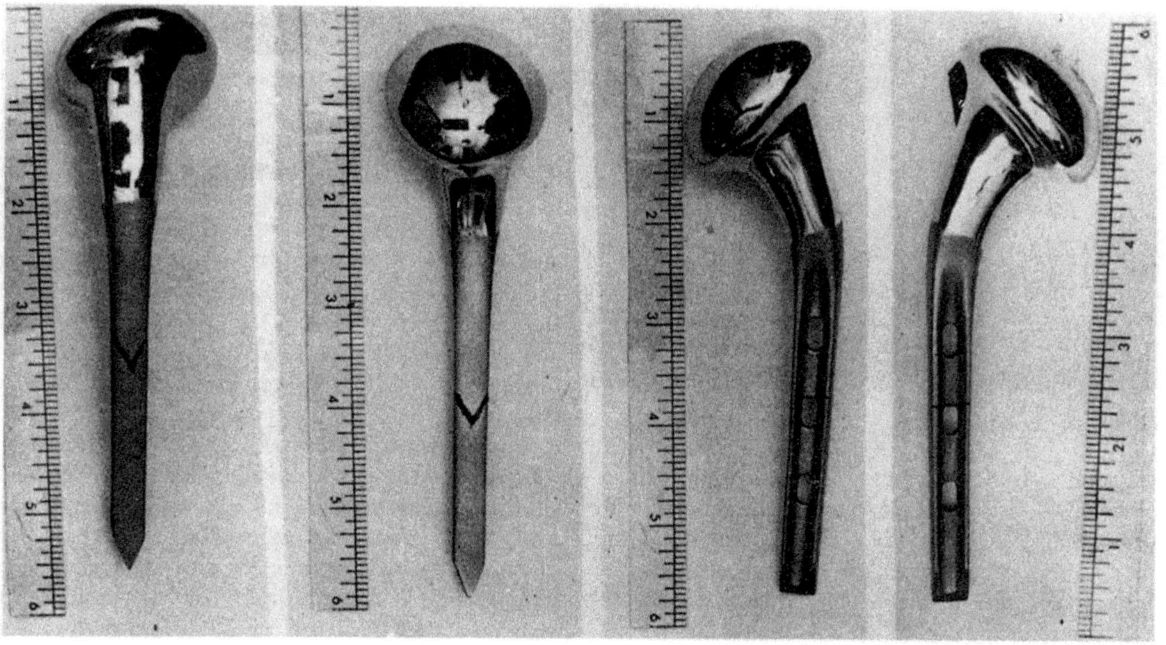

Fig. 5. Krueger's prosthesis showing medial and posterior offset

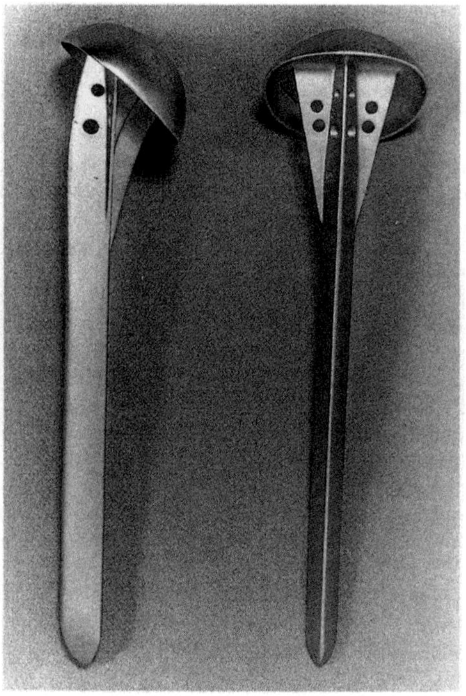

Fig. 6. Neer I Prosthesis

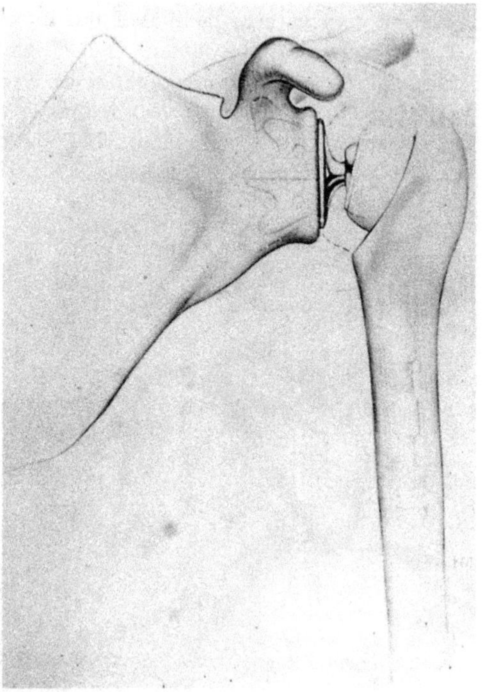

Fig. 7. Neer III Constrained prosthesis

the United States the Bickel design reported a reoperation rate of 50% at 5 years [25]. Similar poor loosening rates were obtained from the Michael Reese prosthesis. Even after a number of modifications the rate still remained at 30% [26]. In addition to the problems of scapular fixation (Fig. 8), the constrained configuration of prosthesis had difficulty in maximising range of motion without a small head and therefore a higher risk of dislocation.

The disappointing results of these designs led to a generally held view of the lack of success of shoulder replacement and rekindled an interest in alternative methods of treatment. Papers appeared on osteotomies by Benjamin [27], glenoid osteotomy and

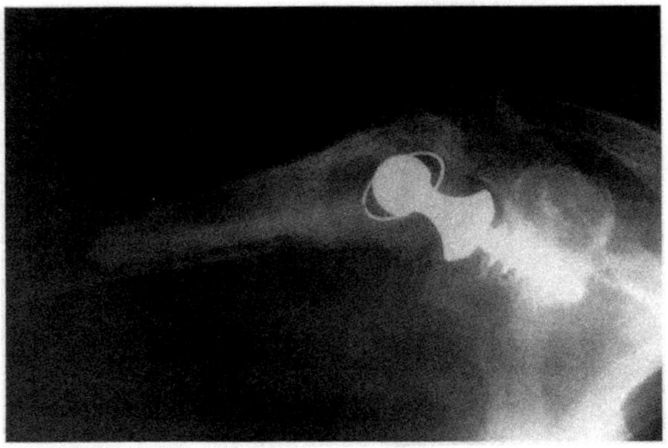

Fig. 8. Kessel constrained prosthesis

reshaping by Engelbrecht [28], resection arthroplasty [29], glenoidectomy [30] and cheilotomy by Bateman [31]. Fortunately, Neer's untiring work steered the development away from the constrained and towards the unconstrained type with increasingly impressive results.

Constrained designs were largely made possible by the introduction of methylmethacrylate cement by Sir John Charnley. This development and the use of acrylic cement also facilitated the introduction of high-density polyethylene (HDP) glenoid which was first reproduced in a paper of Neer in 1974 [21] (Fig. 9). In the same year Kenmore et al. reported on the development of an HDP liner for use with the Neer humeral replacement [32]. Many experimental glenoids were in use by 1982, when Neer reported on five different types, excluding the versions with an angled keel or asymmetrical thickness [33]. In 12 of 273 cases he used 200% and 600% oversized glenoids, i.e. semi-constrained components. These designs aimed to provide a fulcrum by preventing upward subluxation in the cuff deficient shoulder; the 600% Neer prosthesis even precluded reattachment of the supraspinatus tendon. Numerous other hooded designs for example the DANA [34], St. Georg [28], English-McNab [35] and Mazas [38]. The failure rates were high; for the DANA, which rests on the acromion, 20% of only 16 cases needed early revision.

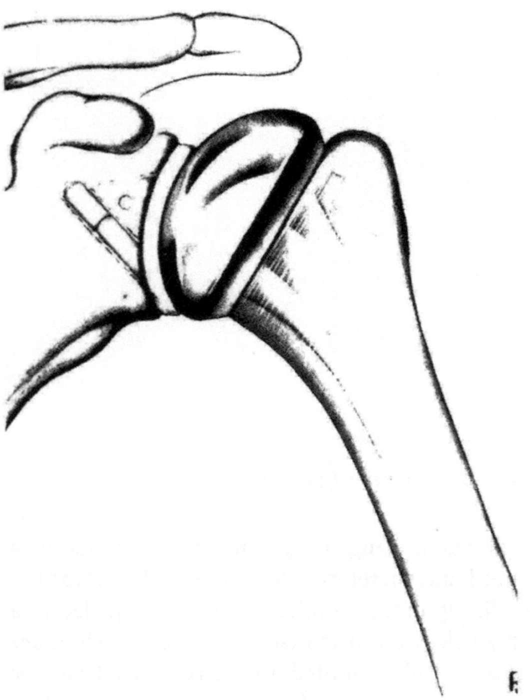

Fig. 9. First illustration of a glenoid component reproduced in Dr. Neer's paper (1974)

An enormous number of designs, sometimes radically different from one another, have appeared, such as bipolar prostheses, surface replacements, and components made from other biomaterials. However, in recent the development of modular components has rekindled the possibility of a prosthesis of truly anatomical design as envisaged by Krueger 45 years ago.

References

1. Péan JE (1884) Des moyens prosthetiques destinés à obtenir la réparation de parties osseuses. Gaz Hop Paris 67:291
2. Muster D (1990) Themistocles Gluck, Berlin 1890: A pioneer of multidisciplinary applied research in biomaterials for endoprostheses. Bull History Dent 38:3–6
3. Wessinghage D (1991) Themistocles Gluck: 100 Jahre kuntstlicher Gelenkersatz. Z Orthop 129:383–388
4. Eynon-Lewis NJ, Ferry D, Pearse MF (1992) Themistocles Gluck: an Unrecognised Genius. BMJ 305:1534–1536
5. Gluck T (1891) Referat über die durch das moderne chirurgische Experiment gewonnenen positiven Resultate, betreffend die Naht und den Ersatz von Defecten hoherer Gewebe, sowie über die Verwerthung resorbirbarer und lebendiger Tampons in der Chirurgie. Arch Klin Chir 41:187–239
6. Zippel J, Meyer-Ralfs M (1975) Themistocles Gluck (1853–1942): Wegbereiter der Endoprothetik. Z Orthop 113:134–139
7. Mack G (1989) Toulouse-Lautrec. Paragon, New York, pp 234–235
8. Lugli T (1978) Artificial shoulder joint by Pean (1893). Clin Orthop Rel Res 133:215–218
9. Pean JE (1973) On prosthetic methods intended to repair bone fragments. Clin Orthop Rel Res 94:4–7
10. Bankes M, Emery RJH (1995) Pioneers of shoulder replacement: Themistocles Gluck and Jules Emile Péan. J Shoulder Elbow Surg 4:259–262
11. König F (1913) Ueber die Implantation von Elfenbein zum Erstatz von Knochen und Gelenkenden Beittr Klin Chir 85:91–114
12. Boron R, Sevin L (1951) Prothèse Acrylique de l'épaule. Presse Med 59:1480

13. Richard A, Judet R, Rene L (1952) Acrylic prosthetic reconstruction of the upper end of the humerus for fracture-luxations. J Chir 68:537–547
14. De Anquin CA, De Anquin CE (1982) Prosthetic replacement in the treatment of serious fractures of the proximal humerus. In: Bayley I, Kessel L (eds) Shoulder surgery. Springer, Berlin Heidelberg New York, pp 207–215
15. Lynn TA, Alexakis PG, Bechtol CO (1965) Stem prosthesis to replace lost proximal humerus Clin Orthop 43:245–247
16. Monteleone M (1969) L'Endoprotesi sostitutiva mella terapia delle fratture-lussazioni dell'estremita superiore dell'omero. Chir Organ Mov 57:404
17. Krueger FJ (1951) A vitallium replica arthroplasty on the shoulder: A case report of aseptic necrosis of the proximal end of the humerus. Surgery 30:1005–1011
18. Neer CS, Brown TH, McLaughlin HL (1953) Fracture of the neck of the humerus with dislocation of the head fragment. Am J Surg 85:252–258
19. Neer CS (1955) Articular replacement for the humeral head. J Bone Joint Surg 37A 37:215–228
20. Neer CS (1964) Followup notes on articles previously published in the journal. Articular replacement for the humeral head. J Bone Joint Surg 46A 46:1607–1610
21. Neer CS (1974) Replacement arthroplasty for glenohumeral osteoarthritis. J Bone Joint Surg Am 56:1–13
22. Lettin AWF, Scales JT (1972) Total replacement of the shoulder joint (two cases). Proc R Soc Med 65:373–374
23. Lettin AWF, Copeland SA, Scales JT (1982) The Stanmore total shoulder replacement. J Bone Joint Surg 64B 64:47–51
24. Beddow FH, Elloy MA (1982) Clinical experience with the Liverpool shoulder replacement. In: Bayley I, Kessel L (eds) Shoulder surgery. Springer, Berlin Heidelberg New York, pp 164–167
25. Cofield RH, Stauffer RN (1977) The Bickel glenohumeral glenohumeral arthroplasty. In: Joint replacement in the upper limb. Institution of Mechanical Engineers, London, pp 15–19
26. Post M (1987) Constrained arthroplasty of the shoulder. Orthop Clin North Am 18:455–462
27. Benjamin A, Hirschowitz D, Arden GP, Blackburn N (1982) Double osteotomy of the shoulder. In: Bayley I, Kessel L (eds) Shoulder surgery. Springer, Berlin Heidelberg New York, pp 170–175
28. Engelbrecht E, Heinert K (1987) More than ten year's experience with unconstrained shoulder replacement. In: Kolbel R, Helbig B, Blauth W (eds) Shoulder replacement. Springer, Berlin Heidelberg New York, pp 234–239
29. Tillman K, Braatz D (1987) Results of resection arthroplasty and the Benjamin double osteotomy resection arthroplasty. In: Kolbel R, Helbig B, Blauth W (ed) Shoulder replacement. Springer, Berlin Heidelberg New York, pp 47–50
30. Gariepy R (1977) Glenoidectomy in the repair of the rheumatoid shoulder. J Bone Joint Surg 59B 59:122
31. Bateman JE (1978) Arthritis of the glenohumeral joint. In: Bateman (ed) The shoulder and neck. Saunders, Philadelphia, pp 343–362
32. Kenmore PI, MacCartee C, Vitek B (1974) A simple shoulder replacement. J Biomed Mater Res 329–330
33. Neer CS, Watson KC, Stanton FJ (1982) Recent experience in total shoulder replacement. J Bone Joint Surg Am 64:319–337
34. Ellman H, Jinnah R, Amstutz HC (1986) Experience with the DANA hooded component for cuff deficient shoulder arthroplasty. Orthop Trans 10:217
35. McElwain JP, English E (1987) The early results of porous-coated total shoulder. Clin Orthop 218:2317–224
36. Gagey O, Mazas F (1990) A new total shoulder prosthesis with acromial fixation. In: Post M, Morrey BF, Hawkins RJ (eds) Surgery of the shoulder. Mosby-Year Book, St. Louis, pp 282–284

Section II:

Kinematics and Biomechanics

Biomechanics of the Shoulder

J.F. Kempf, F. Lacaze, D. Nerisson, and F. Bonnomet

Summary

The complex biomechanics of the shoulder can be very difficult to unravel. The predominant importance of the capsulo-ligamentous and muscular structures over the osteo-articular components increases the mechanical refinement of this balance. During compressive movements of the shoulder almost full body weight passes through the joint, and about half body weight occurs in shearing movements. Because of the very small area of contact between the head and the glenoid during movement (1–5 cm², for abduction in the scapular plane) and their orientation, the soft tissues play a primary role (active and passive) in stabilising the whole ensemble. The total shoulder arthroplasty can only be an unconstrained prosthesis which matches the bony anatomy, in order to reproduce the normal kinematics and stability of the joint.

Introduction

In this chapter we discuss the major fundamental ideas of the anatomy, kinematics, stabilising factors and finally the forces which act at this level. These should present a detailed list of the elements which must be considered by any arthroplasty designed to replace this joint in order to assure a satisfactory function for the patient and longevity of the implant. We do not discuss here the characteristic anatomical features of the glenoid, scapula and proximal humerus, a knowledge of which is extremely important and should be reproduced in any future prosthetic design, as these are detailed in another chapter (see Boileau and Walch pp 127 ff this volume). We detail the analysis of the relationships between the two surfaces of the gleno-humeral joint.

Anatomy

The humeral head is part of a sphere with an arc which is variable, covered with cartilage and looking upwards (Fig. 1). This articular surface is only partially covered by the articular surface of the glenoid for about 25%–30%, which confers on this joint a limited intrinsic stability. The intrinsic stability is furthermore dependent on the surface contact between the glenoid and humeral cartilage (Fig. 2). This contact surface depends in turn on the congruency between the two surfaces, i.e. their radii of curvature.

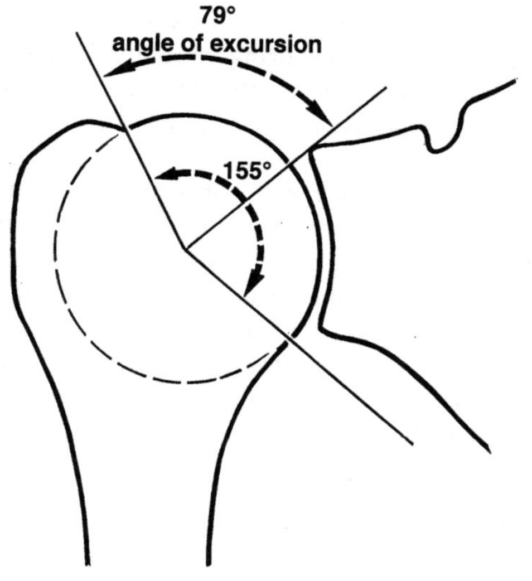

Fig. 1. Covering of the humeral head

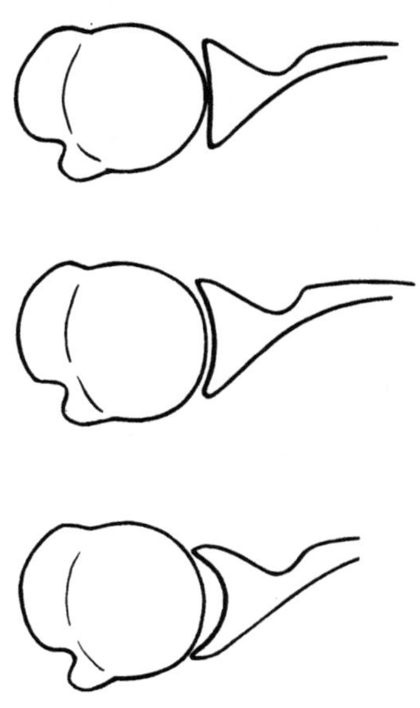

Fig. 2. Glenohumeral congruency

If the radii of curvature are the same, congruency is optimal, with ratio of 1. The surface contact is also maximised, and the division of the forces is be favoured and the intrinsic stability at its highest. This favourable anatomical configuration only exists in 9 % of cases, according to MacPherson and Friedman [8]. In fact, the humeral head has a radius of curvature less than that of the glenoid with ratio of less than 1, and this is the situation found most frequently in about 90 %. This configuration has the advantage of favouring mobility because it is less constrained but at the cost of stability. The forces acting across the joint also act over a smaller area.

It is much more rare to observe a humeral head which has a radius of curvature greater then the glenoid. In this configuration contact is only made at the periphery of the glenoid and not centrally as in the other two scenarios. This is a situation which can arise after inserting a hemi-arthroplasty with a large head as advised by some authors when there is a massive cuff tear.

Stability

The gleno-humeral joint is responsible for 50 % of the mobility and the main stability of the shoulder. It must be both strong and mobile. In spite of its lack of constraint the shoulder maintains the humeral head in a precise position within a 1- to 3-mm margin of the centre of the glenoid cavity throughout most of its range of movement. In fact, it is clear that this articulation, to all appearances unstable, is capable of assuring exact centralisation of the humeral head; resisting the force of gravity for long periods; carrying out slow, powerful movements such as lifting a heavy weight; and carrying out rapid movements such as throwing a baseball at 150 km/h [19].

Gleno-humeral stability comes from a hierarchy of mechanisms consisting of passive and active mechanisms. *Passive mechanisms*, which do not require the expenditure of muscular energy, are provided by bony elements, the capsulo-labral structures and the articular surface (i.e. the viscoelastic piston model) and the ligamentous structures. *Active mechanisms* of muscular origin are provided by the rotator cuff muscles and the peripheral muscles of the shoulder girdle which together assure the dynamic, rotatory three-dimensional recentering described by Bonnel [1].

The Passive Elements in Gleno-humeral Stability

It is now well established that muscular activity is not necessary to ensure shoulder stability. In fact an intact, fresh cadaveric shoulder or a shoulder in an anaesthetically paralysed subject neither dislocates nor subluxes in the rest position.

The Bony Elements

Glenoid version is usually nil: an antetorsion of 10° and a retroversion of 10° can be considered as normal values (Fig. 3a). Hyper-anteversion of the glenoid has been proposed by Saha [22] as a factor favouring recurrence of instability. This is currently contradicted by many authors. Increased glenoid retroversion (superior to 25°) is found in some cases of osteoarthritis.

The role of *humeral head retroversion* in shoulder stability is still controversial. Boileau et al. [3] have established that the average value is 17.9° but with very variable extremes from −6.5° to 47.5°. Other authors [22] consider that insufficient humeral retroversion is a factor in anterior instability and propose a corrective humeral osteotomy if the angle is less than 20°. In other studies [9] there has been no evidence of a difference in humeral retroversion in the populations with and without anterior instability.

Scapular inclination may influence the stability of the glenohumeral joint (Fig. 3b). In a recent study Itoi stated that the rotation of the scapular in the frontal plane around a sagittal axis (abduction or

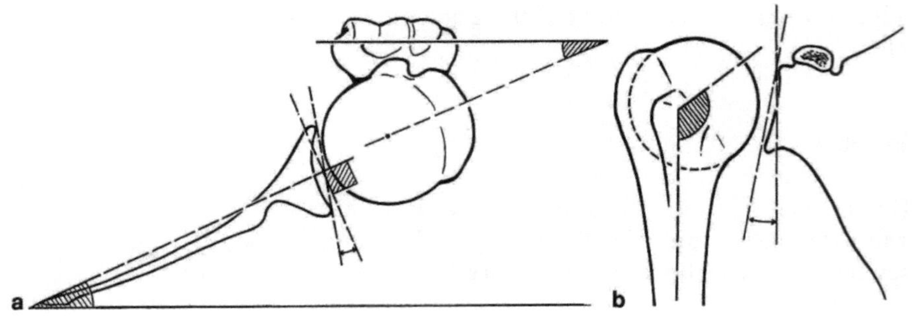

Fig. 3. Retroversion (**a**) and inclination (**b**) of the humeral head and glenoid articular surface

adduction) makes a significant contribution to inferior instability of the humeral head by way of a cam effect on the inferior glenoid border combined with tension in the upper ligaments – superior gleno-humeral and coracohumeral [13].

Labrum, Capsule and Articular Surface: The Viscoelastic Piston Model

The whole articular cavity functions as a sealed, fixed volume containing a fluid with a high viscous coefficient and a small volume. The sum of two physical models can basically explain the cohesion of the gleno-humeral joint without recourse to ligaments or muscles: the mechanism of a piston in a vacuum and the capillary adhesive mechanism of the two congruent articular surfaces. These two models acting together give the joint the capacity to develop a ventouse effect.

The principle of a piston in a vacuum (barometric hypopressure) is well known from the work of the Weber brothers [26] in 1837 and Fick in 1911. These authors have observed that all joints and in particular the shoulder, may be compared to a piston in a vacuum in which the arm acts as the piston and the labrum as the valve (Fig. 4). Habermeyer [10] has measured intra-articular pressures within the loaded gleno-humeral joint in cadavers and anaesthetised subjects. He concluded that the intra-articular pressure is –32 mmHg at rest, and that axial traction reduces it further while the presence of an anterior labral lesion or a clinical instability removes the possibility of creating a negative intra-articular pressure, which then remains zero. The ability of the gleno-humeral joint to develop a negative pressure under traction explains in part its stability. This is larger when the articular surface is more widespread, the labrum is intact, the capsule is not too lax and particularly not torn, the shoulder is in the neutral position, and the traction is applied perpendicularly in the glenoid plane.

Capillary attraction between two congruent surfaces is also a well-known physical model. This is the model of two wet glass surfaces where capillary adhesive force (surface tension of the liquid) allows the model to be very resistant to perpendicular forces but with little resistance to shear forces applied to the glass sheets. The gleno-humeral articular surfaces are lubricated by the articular fluid which has a high viscosity and acts in a similar manner giving high resistance to perpendicular forces but little resistance to shearing forces. This capillary effect is dependent on the viscous coefficient and volume of the fluid which may be altered during a synovial reaction (hydarthosis) or haemorrhage into the joint (hemarthosis). The nature of the contact surfaces also modifies the capillary attraction: the biological fluid has a higher viscosity when in contact with articular cartilage and reduced in contact with polyethylene or metal, as in a shoulder arthroplasty.

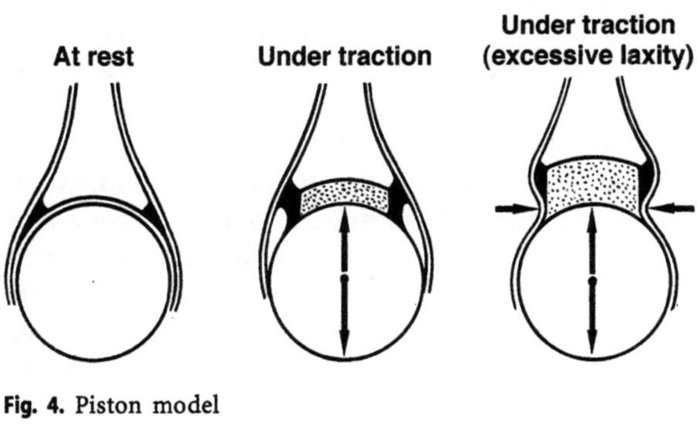

Fig. 4. Piston model

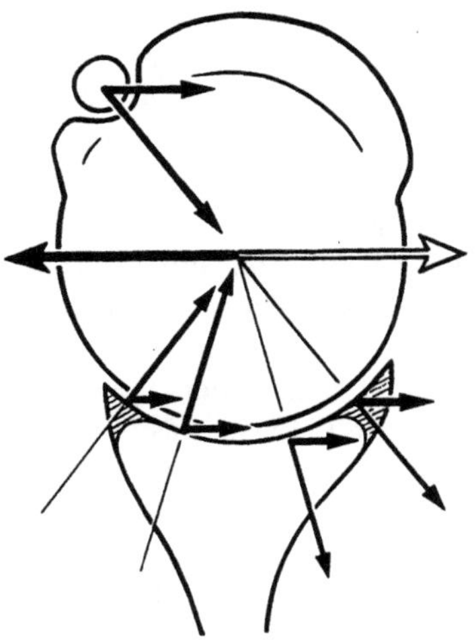

Fig. 5. Anteroposterior shearing forces

Shear forces remain a problem and may lead to instability. Although the viscoelastic piston model offers significant resistance to perpendicular traction forces, it is much less effective against shearing forces which can destabilise the shoulder in the anterior, posterior, superior and inferior planes (Fig. 5). There is, however, a non-insignificant resistance to these forces which comes from the concave shape of the glenoid augmented by the labrum which provides resistance to traction forces when shear forces are applied to the humeral head. The shear forces have been measured by Poppen and Walker as being 42% of body weight at 60° of abduction in the scapular plane [20].

The Reinforcing Ligamentous Structures

The gleno-humeral capsulo-ligamentous structures are lax but solid to allow the large degree of movement which characterises this joint. The first functional anatomical study of the gleno-humeral ligaments is credited to Turckel [24]. In neutral rotation with the arm alongside the body (position of rest) the ligamentous structures are relaxed. Throughout their anatomical range the ligaments tighten in external rotation and external rotation plus abduction adds a helicoidal tightening element. These ligaments only constitute a restraining sling on the humeral head when they are under tension. They complete the viscoelastic restraint from the articular surfaces, capsule and labrum and always have three actions which act to hold the head in the glenoid: (a) limitation of rotation (axial and shearing forces); (b) limitation of perpendicular traction on the glenoid (axial tension); (c) limitation of traction parallel to the glenoid (shearing forces) where they act as a mechanical block.

The inferior gleno-humeral ligament acts as a "hamac" for the humeral head The anterior fibres are tensioned from 45° of abduction and/or external rotation such that: they limit external rotation and abduction (with the posterior fibres), and they are the principle block to antero-inferior subluxation. On the other hand, the posterior fibres come under tension after 45° of abduction and/or internal rotation such that: they limit internal rotation and abduction (with the anterior fibres), they counter posterior subluxation, and they counter inferior subluxation. The ligamentous structure consisting of the anterior and posterior fibres and the axillary recess acts to limit abduction of the humerus and helps to place the humerus in the scapular plane allowing the joint to achieve its privileged position: controls rolling-sliding of the head in the hammock of the ligament complex and counters inferior subluxation in all degrees of abduction.

The middle gleno-humeral ligament is an inconstant structure. It is tensioned in external rotation and abduction and adduction up to 60° such that limits external rotation when abduction is less than 60° and is the principle barrier against anterior dislocation when the arm is in neutral rotation whatever the abduction (helped by the superior gleno-humeral ligament) and external rotation if abduction is less than 60° (maximal at 45°). It is a secondary barrier with the inferior ligament against antero-internal dislocation when the arm is in external rotation and abduction greater than 60° and has no role beyond 90° (sliding upwards) and is a secondary barrier with the superior ligament against inferior subluxation in adduction and external rotation.

The superior gleno-humeral ligament and the coracohumeral ligament are tensioned in adduction, extension and flexion with neutral rotation and especially in flexion and external rotation. These hold the tendon of the long head of biceps and the exit of the bicipital groove where it passes between the greater and lesser tuberosity attachments of the coracohumeral ligament.

The Dynamic Elements in Gleno-humeral Stability

One of the ways in which the shoulder muscles contribute to the stability of the joint is by applying compression of the humeral head into the gleno-labral socket. This action occurs rapidly and with force. Because of their peri-articular position and contact with the humeral head, the rotator cuff muscles are perfectly adapted to this function and are the first line and most important of the dynamic elements. They may be less important than some of the large peripheral muscles in certain physiological or pathological conditions.

The Stabilising Action of the Rotator Cuff

This is of primary importance. The four muscles (supraspinatus, subscapularis, infraspinatus and teres minor) making up this group have a similar anatomical topography which makes their role as coaptors of the humeral head more important that their isolated function as rotators. The tendon of the long head of biceps acts in concert but in a different manner. They all have a muscle belly originating from the scapular and terminate with a fairly long tendon crossing the glenohumeral joint and merging with the capsule distally.

Morrey [18] and Matsen [17] suggest that the cuff muscles act in three different ways (Fig. 6). (a) Due to their distal fusion with the capsule they adjust the tension on these structures so producing dynamic ligaments. (b) Acting as couples they hold the humeral head into the glenoid socket. This is the principle of stability from concavity compression. The compressive load leads to an increase in resistance to inferior subluxation by 67 % and to antero-inferior subluxation by 46 %. Resection of the labrum reduces this compression stability by 20 %. (c) By selective contraction the cuff muscles can resist displacement forces generated by contraction of the main peripheral shoulder muscles.

Apart form their main action (e.g. abduction, internal rotation) the peripheral muscles have a stabilising role on the humeral head: statically they emphatically block the shoulder in any given position, while dynamically they can complement or sometimes supplant the cuff muscles when they are weakened or damaged.

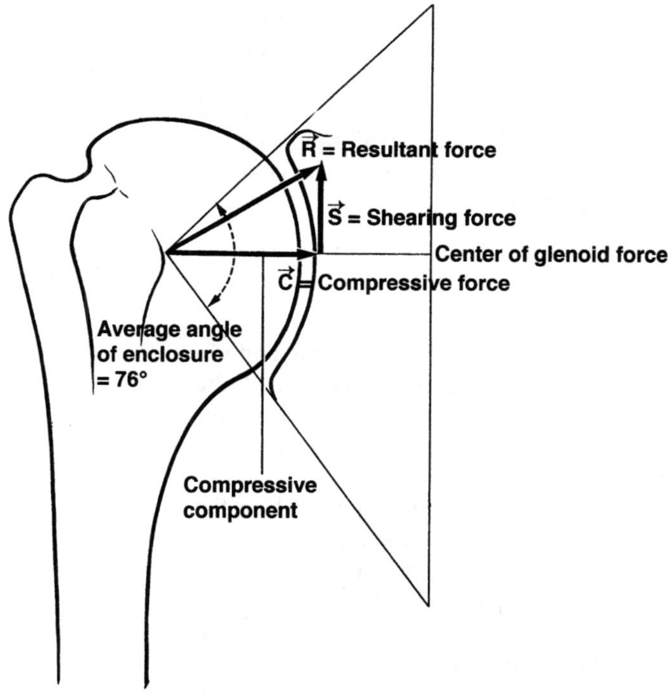

Fig. 6. The forces at the glenohumeral joint (adapted from Friedman [8])

The Overall Function of the Dynamic Stabilisers

Dynamic stabilisation of the gleno-humeral joint cannot be conceived without understanding the overall stability of all the shoulder joints, i.e. the scapulo-clavicular on one hand and the humeral on the other. Bonnel [1] describes this global function as obeying the law of "three-dimensional, dynamic rotatory recentering". The muscle groups of the shoulder must move and stabilise the scapulo-clavicular and humeral joints with the aid of rotatory couples in three planes: frontal (abduction - adduction); sagittal (flexion - extension) and horizontal (internal-external rotation).

Abduction is an extremely complex phenomenon in which no one muscle actually just abducts. There are three stages: (a) scapulo-humeral rotation allows for 90° of abduction by the combined action of the deltoid, the superior stabilisers (supraspinatus, long head of biceps) and the lateral stabilisers (depressors) (subscapularis, infraspinatus, pectoralis major and latissimus dorsi. (b) Rotation and scapular tilt gives a supplementary curve of 60° allowing to 150° by the muscles of serratus anterior and superior trapezius orientating the glenoid upwards, backwards and outwards. (c) Contralateral inclination of the spine from 150° to 180°.

Adduction occurs passively under the action of gravity in day-to-day life, but real adduction occurs in climbing and involves two steps: firstly, the scapulo-humeral is locked by the teres major and triceps; then, the scapulo-thoracic is hoisted by rhomboids and latissimus dorsi. This action is carried out by the contraction of two muscle groups: rhomboids–teres major, latissimus dorsi–triceps.

Flexion occurs in three steps:

- From 0° to 60° by scapulo-humeral flexion using anterior deltoid, upper pectoralis major and coracobrachialis. stabilised by teres minor, teres major and infraspinatus.
- From 60° to 120° by scapulo-thoracic antepulsion using trapezius and stabilised by latissimus dorsi and the lower pectoralis major.
- From 120° to 180° by spinal extension.

Extension occurs in two steps: by scapulo-humeral extension using teres major and minor, posterior deltoid and latissimus dorsi, then scapular retropulsion using rhomboids, middle part of trapezius and latissimus dorsi.

Internal rotation is a powerful action to lift weight and occurs in two steps. Firstly, there is scapulo-humeral rotation from latissimus dorsi, teres major, subscapularis and pectoralis major; then, scapular internal rotation and abduction using serratus anterior and pectoralis minor. The stabilisation comes from the antagonist.

External rotation is a weaker action used to support fine movements of the hand and occurs in two steps. First, there is scapulo-humeral rotation using infraspinatus and teres minor; then, scapular external rotation and adduction using rhomboids and trapezius. Again, the stabilisation is obtained from the antagonists.

In summary, as mentioned by Bonnel et al. [1], the shoulder muscles are organised into 25 couples for three-dimensional dynamic rotatory stability. The coracoid process acts as the combined central nucleus for static and dynamic stabilisation of the shoulder complex. Any asynchronicity in contraction can cause instability.

Mobility

The shoulder is the most mobile joint in the body in particular allowing complete circumduction of the upper limb. This is possible only due to the combined action of the gleno-humeral and scapula-thoracic joints.

An analysis of elevation of the upper limb in the plane of the scapula is usually agreed as involving a ratio of gleno-humeral to scapulo-thoracic movement of 2:1. For complete elevation about 120° comes from the gleno-humeral joint and 60° from the scapulo-thoracic. Poppen [20] and Freedman [5] have confirmed these figures but have shown that over the first 30° of elevation it is gleno-humeral dominant followed by an equal contribution from the two joints between 30° and 90°. Beyond that there is again a predominance from the gleno-humeral joint. The overall ratio however remains at about 2:1.

Gleno-humeral Movement

Three elemental movements are possible (Fig. 7): (a) sliding which can be compared to a wheel which skates across a slippery surface with a fixed centre of rotation at the level of the humeral head, (b) translation where the centre of rotation of the articulation is displaced, and (c) rolling of the humeral head on the glenoid leading also to a displacement of the centre of rotation of the joint.

In the vertical plane, it has been shown by Walker that the instantaneous centre of rotation remain very close to the centre of the humeral head [25]. The combination of these three basic movements explain all the displacements that are observed, but in practice it is the rotation-sliding and to a lesser extent translation which characterise the movements seen.

The author has observed on cineradiography that during elevation there is an upward translation of 3 mm over the first 30° before the rotation-sliding movement occurs.

In the horizontal plane, Howell has shown that overall the head remains central, i.e. the principle basic movement is also rotation-sliding although it may produce a translation essentially towards the rear, for example, in extension and external rotation of the arm [11]. The movement of translation can, however, be more important and occur in other directions if there is a deficiency in the capsulo-ligamentous structures as in anterior shoulder instability where there is only limited gleno-humeral congruency or in cases of rotator cuff muscle deficiency which, it should be recalled, act to centralise the head.

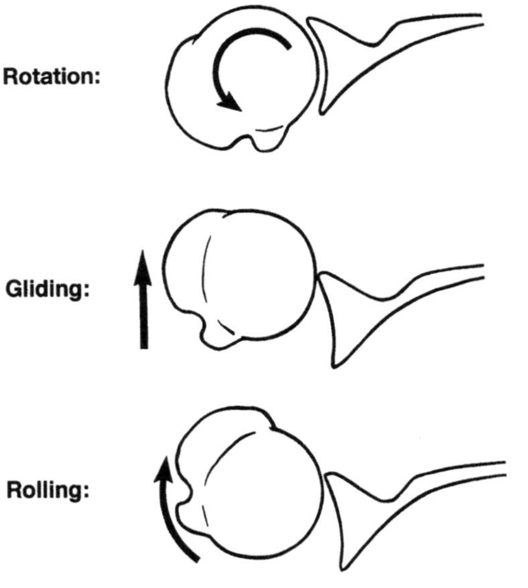

Fig. 7. The three elementary glenohumeral movements

Scapulo-thoracic Movement

The well-known swinging movement of the scapular on the thorax during abduction or elevation in the scapular plane is explained essentially by rotation but this occurs around many centres of rotation:

- From 0° to 60° of elevation the centre of rotation is close to the glenoid and occurs mainly due to movement at the acromio-clavicular joint
- From 60° to 120° the centre of rotation is closer to the base of the spine of the scapula, and here it is the sterno-clavicular joint which is mostly involved.

Then the centre of rotation of the scapula is displaced upwards and laterally towards the base of the coracoid process, and again it is the acromio-clavicular joint which is involved in the tilting movement of the scapula between 120 and 180° of elevation.

Forces Observed at the Gleno-humeral Joint

It is important to know about these forces as they are the ones which play a damaging role on the implants and their fixation.

It should be recalled that any muscular contraction at the level of the shoulder causes a compressive force on the glenoid (S) and another force producing shearing parallel to the joint line. These two forces give a resultant R whose intensity and direction depends (Fig. 6) on:

- The position of the upper limb including rotation.
- The weight of the upper limb in addition to any object being lifted and the lever arm used, depending particularly on whether or not the elbow is flexed.
- The contraction force developed by the different peri-articular muscles which depends largely on their volume.

Although this is not a weight-bearing joint, significant forces can still be generated across it. For example, elevation to 90° results in a force equal to body weight. If a 5 kg weight is lifted with a straight arm, this force increases to 2.5 times body weight. We therefore find values close to those seen in the hip with a contact surface area much smaller.

The Position of the Upper Limb

The vector R has a very variable direction during abduction or elevation. Therefore in neutral rotation the vector may be: directed downwards when the arm is alongside the body, from 0° to 60° the vector R is directed upwards and medially (Fig. 8) because the shearing forces are predominant but the vector remains inside the area of contact between the two articular surfaces and at 90° compression forces predominate and the vector R approaches the perpendicular to the glenoid which is a mechanically favourable position.

During these movements the position of rotation is very important: When the arm is in external rotation, the vector R keeps a direction similar to that described above but with a greater value particularly because of the compressive force developed by the deltoid. When the arm is in internal rotation, then the vector R has a more upward direction because of the predominance of the shearing forces developed by the anterior and middle deltoid.

This phenomenon can be easily demonstrated by asking the patient to hold both arms in abduction at 90° with one in internal rotation and the other in external. That in internal rotation becomes tired and painful more quickly than that in external rotation.

Any muscle imbalance and in particular any deficiency in one or other of the cuff muscles alters the direction and value of the vector R towards that of an increased shearing force, which means a resultant vector more upward and medial. This force can even pass beyond the area of contact of the gleno-humeral joint which inevitably leads to an upward migration of the head.

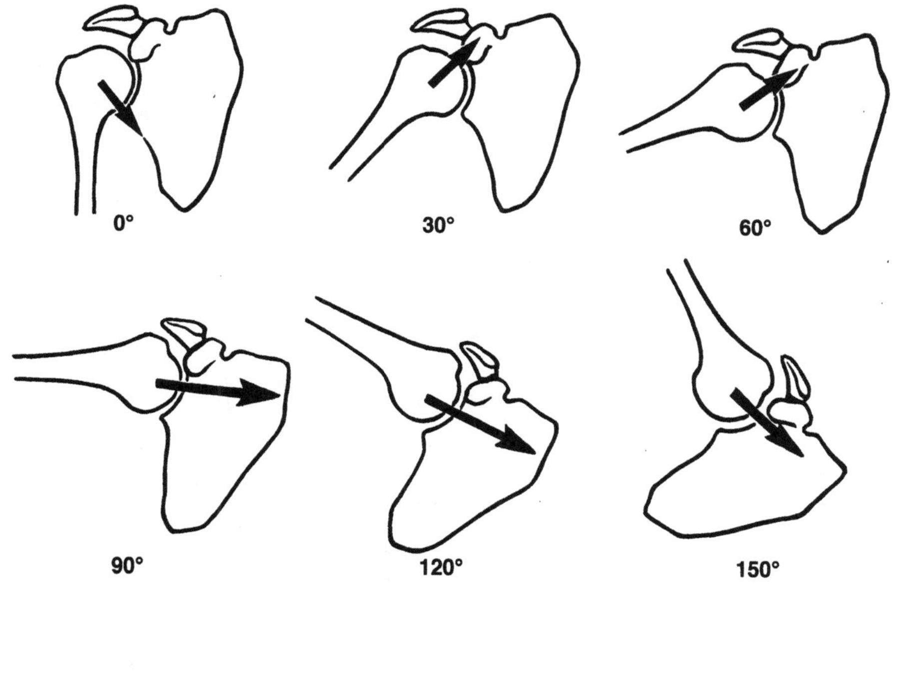

Fig. 8. Direction of the forces in relation to abduction of the arm (adapted from Friedman [8])

The Role of the Lever Arm

The resulting force depends on the lever arm action developed. That of the upper limb in extension varies with the position of the arm and also on whether the elbow is flexed or not.

The Force Developed by the Muscles

The deltoid is the most powerful muscle and can generate 6 times the weight of the upper limb. The supraspinatus develops 2.5 times upper limb weight. The infraspinatus and teres minor develop 5 times body weight. The direction and amplitude of the resultant vector R, as we have seen, depends on the position of the arm, but it also changes in degree and direction depending on the function of the muscles acting. The deltoid (Fig. 9a) has a more important shear force component, which explains why the resultant force is ascendant.

On the other hand, the supraspinatus (Fig. 9b) studied in isolation basically develops compression forces which explains why the force R in all positions remains close to the perpendicular of the glenoid surface. A study of their combined analysis gives a more favourable vector. It is well known that the absence of supraspinatus favours proximal migration of the humeral head by the deltoid and especially if the infraspinatus and subscapularis are damaged and cannot play their part as head depressors (Fig. 9 c,d).

The Specification for Non-constrained Shoulder Prostheses

The total shoulder arthroplasty can only be an unconstrained prosthesis which best reproduces the normal articulation and matches the anatomy, kinematics and stability of the joint. It should be able to resist the forces which act on it.

Restoration of Bony Anatomy

Humeral head retroversion, inclination and medial and posterior offset should all be matched by the implant, which therefore needs to be both modular and *adaptable*, following this example comes the Aequalis prosthesis [3].

With regard to the glenoid implant most have a radius of curvature identical to that of the humeral head. This gives the prosthesis a certain intrinsic

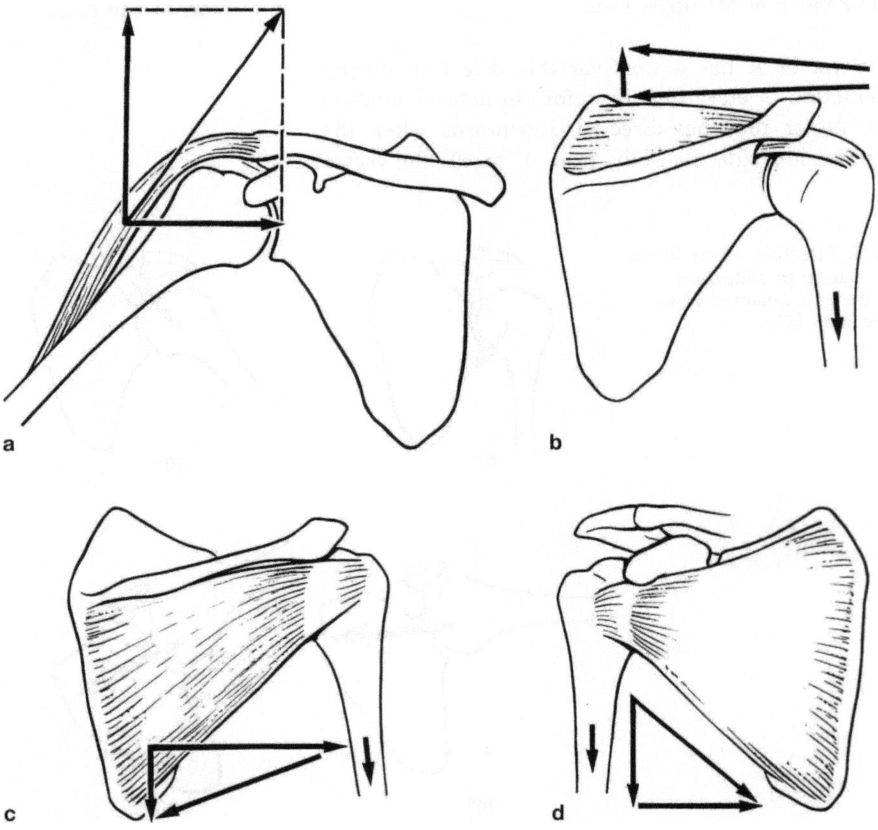

Fig. 9. Direction of the resulting force of the deltoid (**a**), the supraspinatus (**b**), the infraspinatus (**c**) and the subscapularis (**d**)

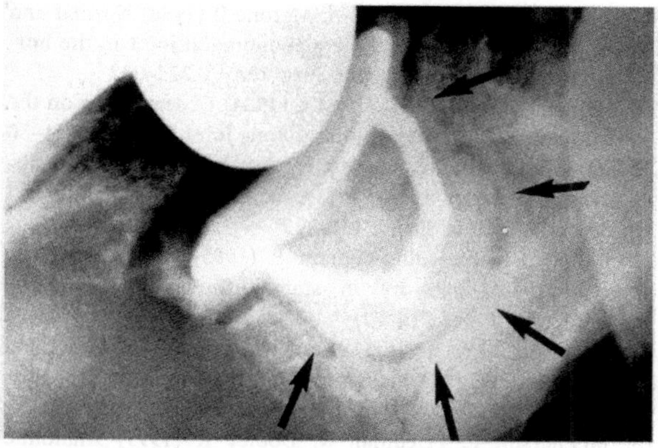

Fig. 10. The vertical "rocking horse effect" on the glenoid: ascendant shearing forces leading to loosening of the glenoid component (arrows)

stability by increasing surface contact area. Theoretically, this conformity reduces the risk of polyethylene wear. However, if translation movements forwards, backwards or upwards occur, the contact surface area is considerably reduced, and the humeral head applies increased, eccentric forces on it (Fig. 10). This mechanism has been compared by Matsen [17] to that of a "rocking horse" leading to loosening of the glenoid which lifts up on the side opposite to where the force is applied. It is this mechanism, which probably explains the frequency of loosening seen at the glenoid, when there is a massive cuff tear which, as we have seen, produces an inevitable translation of the humeral head upwards.

Perfect conformity between the glenoid and the humeral head does not have only advantages, nor does it reproduce the normal anatomy. It is for this reason that that several systems including the Aequalis [3] have a glenoid with a radius of curvature greater and thus flatter which does diminish the surface contact area but may increase polyethylene wear. On the other hand, the mobility is closer to physiological and the small translation movements are not damaging.

It is difficult to reproduce the position of the gleno-humeral joint line because of the thickness of the glenoid implant especially if this has a metal back. A degree of lateralisation of the joint-line so produced risks leading to a tighter shoulder than normal which in turn leads to a loss of mobility and an increase in force across the joint.

Restoration of Stability

The anterior capsulo-ligamentous structures are usually freed when inserting a prosthesis, but other factors which can lead to instability must be considered. Avoiding damage to the muscular envelope, correctly orientating the components and good conformity between the two implants are all of benefit.

Restoration of Mobility

The normal shoulder kinematics is very difficult to reproduce, and many studies have shown that as a general rule the kinematics is disrupted. Boileau [2] has shown that although the normal scapulo-humeral rhythm can be conserved, this only happens infrequently (20%). In 21 Neer total shoulder arthroplasties he recorded only 4 cases of normal scapulo-humeral rhythm and these in cases of minimally evolved pathology. The largest group of 10 cases presented with an upward excursion of the humeral implant without true gleno-humeral movement, which was explained by major muscle damage. A third group of 7 cases presented with an inverse scapulo-humeral rhythm where the scapulo-thoracic mobility was normal while the gleno-humeral was diminished. Friedman [5] also found that there was usually about a 50% reduction in the gleno-humeral component. He blamed this particularly on the fact that the implants used had a higher degree of conformity than seen in the normal anatomy.

Forces Applied on Prosthetic Components

The forces applied at the humeral level should not pose any particular problem to the metal implant, which has a large contact surface thanks to the stem. However, uncemented humeral component may migrate distally because of the shearing forces.

On the glenoid side, the resultant vector of all the forces acting on it may be in an unfavourable direction, with significant shearing forces applied depending partly on the integrity of the cuff muscles and partly on the position of the arm. These loosening forces need to be countered by a fixation system, but an ideal one has yet to be found. A separate chapter in this volume discusses the current situation with regard to cemented and uncemented implants, and it is at the level of glenoid implant fixation that progress remains to be made.

With regard to implant wear we have seen the advantages of using a glenoid which conforms to the humeral head, but we have also discussed its disadvantages. A compromise must be reached between the necessity for stability and the fight against wear by increasing the contact surface and, on the other hand, the need for mobility and reduction in forces acting on the bone-prosthesis interface. The best compromise is probably to use a glenoid whose radius of curvature is slightly greater than that of the humeral head.

Conclusion

It is essential to have a good understanding of the basic biomechanics of the shoulder both when designing a new prosthesis and for inserting it in the most efficient manner. The three essential elements are to use a prosthesis which restores normal anatomy, to respect the muscular envelope and to have high quality component fixation.

References

1. Bonnel F (1988) L'épaule: articulation à recentrage rotatoire tridimensionnel. In: L'épaule douloureuse chirurgicale. M. Mansat (ed) Cahiers d'Enseignement de la SOFCOT, no 33. Expansion Scientifique Française, Paris, pp 1–12
2. Boileau P, Walch G, Liotard JP (1992) Etude radio-cinématographique de l'élévation active de l'épaule prothésée. Rev Chir Orthop 78:355–364
3. Boileau P, Walch G (1995) Adaptabilité et modularité au cours des prothèses d'épaule. Acta Orthopedica Belgica 61 [Suppl 1]:49–61
4. Codman E (1934) The shoulder. Todd, Boston
5. Freedmann L, Munro R (1666) Abduction of the arm in the scapular plane: scapular and glenohumeral movements. J Bone Joint Surg 48A 48:1503–1510
6. Friedman R, Laberge EM, Dooley R, O'Hara A (1992) Finite element modeling of the glenoid component: effect of design parameters on stress distribution. J Shoulder Elbow Surg 1:261–270
7. Friedman R, Brookings G, Dooley R (1990) Finite element analysis of glenoid component design. Orthop Trans 14:253
8. Friedman RJ (1994) Biomechanics and design of shoulder arthroplasties. In: Friedman (ed) Arthroplasty of the shoulder. Thieme, Stuttgart, pp 27–40
9. Gerber C (1988) Les instabilités de l'épaule. In: L'épaule douloureuse chirurgicale. M. Mansat (ed) Cahiers d'Enseignement de la SOFCOT, no 33. Expansion Scientifique Française, Paris, pp 51–74
10. Habermeyer P, Schuller U (1989) Die Bedeutung des Labrum glenoidale für die Stabilität des Glenohumeralgelenkes. Unfallchirurg 92:1
11. Howell S, Galina B, Renzi A, Marone P (1988) Normal and abnormal mechanics of the glenohumeral joint in the horizontal plane. J Bone Joint Surg 70A 70:227–232
12. Inman V, Saunders M, Abbot L (1944) Observations on the function of the shoulder joint. J Bone Joint Surg Am 26:1–30
13. Itoi E, Motzkin NE, Morrey BF, Kai-Nan AN (1992) Scapular inclination and inferior stability of the shoulder. J Shoulder Elbow Surg 1:131–139
14. Kumar VP, Balasubramaniam P (1985) The role of the atmospheric pressure in stabilizing shoulder. J Bone Joint Surg Br 67:719–721
15. de Luca C, Forrest W (1973) Force analysis of individual muscles acting simultaneoulsly on the shoulder joint during isometric abduction. J Biomech 6:385–393
16. McPherson E, Friedman R, Dooley R (1993) Anatomic basis of total shoulder design. J Shoulder Elbow Surg 2:528
17. Matsen FA, Harrymann DT, Sidles JA (1991) Mechanics of glenohumeral instability. Clin. Sports Med 10(4) 783–788
18. Morrey BF, An KN (1990) Biomechanics of the shoulder. In: Rockwood CR, Matsen FA (ed) The shoulder. Saunders, Philadelphia, pp 208–245
19. Perry J (1988) Biomechanics of the shoulder. In: Carter R, Rowe (eds) The shoulder. Churchill-Linvingstone Inc, 1988, pp 1–15
20. Poppen N, Walker P (1976) Normal and abnormal motion of the shoulder. J Bone Joint Surg 58A 58:195–201
21. Rietveld A, Daanen H, Rozing P, Obermann W (1988) The lever arm in gleno-humeral abduction after hemiarthroplasty. J Bone Joint Surg 70B 70: 561–565
22. Saha AK (1971) Dynamic stability of the glenohumeral joint. Acta Orthop Scand 42:491–505
23. Snyder SJ, Rames RD, Morgan CD (1991) Anatomical variations of the glenohumeral ligaments. Arthroscopy 7 (3):328
24. Turckel SJ, Pannios MW, Marshall JL, Girgis FG (1981) Stabilizing mechanisms preventing anterior dislocation of the glenohumeral joint J Bone Joint Surg Am 63:1208–1217
25. Walker P (1977) Human Joints and their artificial replacements. Thomas, Springfield
26. Weber BG, Simpson A, Hardegger F (1984) Rotational osteotomy for recurrent anterior dislocation of the shoulder assiociated with large Hill-Sachs lesion. J Bone Joint Surg Am 66:1443
27. Zuckermann JD, Matsen FA (1988) Biomecanics of the shoulder, 2nd edn. In: Nordin and Frankel (eds) Basic biomecanics of the muskuloskeletal system. Lea & Febiger, London

Kinematics of Anterior Elevation in the Normal Shoulder

L. Favard, M. Desperiez, and D. Alison

Summary

Digitalised X-rays applied to the mechanics of the shoulder joint allows physiological movement to be studied and, especially, allows easy sorting of the images to make measurements. The goal of this study was to analyse active elevation of the shoulder using this technique in healthy volonteers. The measurements carried out on each one of the sequences were: the angle between the diaphyseal axis of the humerus and the vertical, the angle between the line of the glenoid and the vertical, the angle between the diaphyseal axis of the humerus and the line of the glenoid and the excursion of the humeral head on the glenoid. Moreover, for each of the selected intervals, the instantaneous centres of rotation were defined. The results of this study confirm that scapulo-humeral rhythm is 2/3 (two degrees for the scapulo-thoracic and three degrees for the gleno-humeral). Translation of the humeral head on the glenoid changes direction when elevation is above 60. This change must correspond to where different muscle 'couples' come into play. The head appears to be permanently, dynamically recentred because any excursion from its geometric centre is corrected by a displacement inverse to the instantaneous centre of rotation.

Introduction

In order to be able to assess the kinematics of a prosthetic shoulder it is essential to have an understanding of those of the normal shoulder in which the kinematics of anterior elevation are complex and involve several joints. Several techniques have already been used to look at this movement: cadaveric studies [2, 3, 5, 6], radiographs taken at regular intervals throughout elevation [4, 9] and cine-radiography [1]. Each of these systems has its faults, whether it be their static nature where the patient is required to hold the arm immobile for the time needed to take a radiograph, or the difficulty in interpreting the images produced. Digilatised radiography has the benefits of allowing the study of physiological movements as well as providing images that can be easily stored, retrieved and subjected to analysis. The goals of this study, based on an analysis of active anterior elevation of the healthy shoulder using this technique, were threefold: (a) to verify normal scapulo-thoracic rhythm under examination conditions; (b) to assess any vertical translation of the head on the glenoid during active elevation and (c) to define any concentrations of instantaneous centres of rotation.

Material and Methods

The study was carried out on six men and six women who had an average age of 33 years (28–48), and who had no previous shoulder problems. The dominant shoulder was used, and uninterrupted active anterior elevation in the scapular plane was analysed from a starting position with the arm alongside the body to a finish in maximal elevation. This movement was chosen as being the most physiological and causing the least torsion in the muscles or capsule [4, 8, 10]. The preliminary setup ensured that the gleno-humeral joint was correctly aligned. Images were recorded at a rate of six per second and those selected for measurement were taken at 0°, 30°, 45°, 60°, 90°, 120° and 150° and at maximal elevation and were developed onto radiographic film (Fig. 1). The recording was done using a Siemens Polydos 80 machine with an Elenna angioscope and the images were treated using a Digitron programme.

The measurements made on each of the images were (Fig. 2):

- The angle between the humeral diaphyseal axis and the vertical (AGB), representing the elevation angle.
- The angle between the surface line of the glenoid and the vertical (AST), representing scapulo-thoracic movement.
- The angle between the diaphyseal humeral axis and the surface line of the glenoid (AGH), representing scapulo-humeral movement.

The position of the geometric centre of the humeral head on the glenoid during movement was cal-

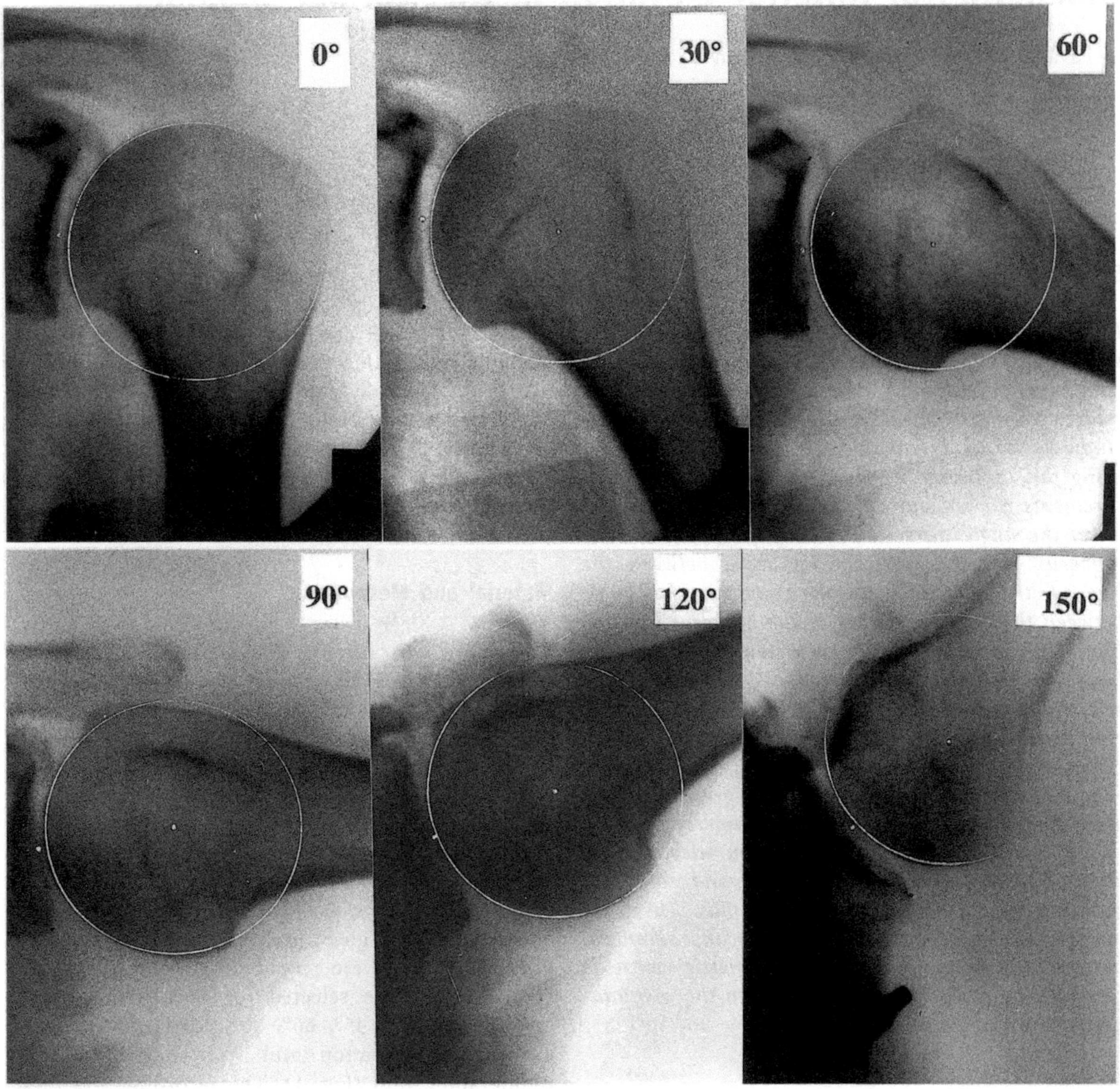

Fig. 1. An example of a sequence showing elevation from 0° to 150° where the arcs were selected from 30° to 30°. The gleno-humeral joint line must always be visible in order to have reliable measurements

culated. This represents any excursion of the humeral head on the glenoid (Fig. 3). Also for each of the selected intervals, the instantaneous centre of rotation (ICR) was recorded using the technique of Poppen and Walker [8], and these were then collated into a dispersion circle whose radii and centre were then calculated and recorded in relation to the geometric centre of the humeral head.

Results

Scapulo-thoracic Rhythm. At rest, with the arm alongside the body, the positions of the humeral head and the glenoid varied so greatly between subjects that over the first 30° of elevation there is no typical scapulo-thoracic rhythm (Fig. 4). However, after 30° it can be analysed, and from then the ratio of movements coming from the gleno-humeral and the scapulo-thoracic joints corresponds to an average of 2.1, of which there are 2° of scapulo-thoracic movement for each 4° of gleno-humeral movement.

Humeral Head Excursion. From 0° to 60° of elevation the head moves upwards for an average distance of 1.73 mm, i.e. the head translates superiorly at the

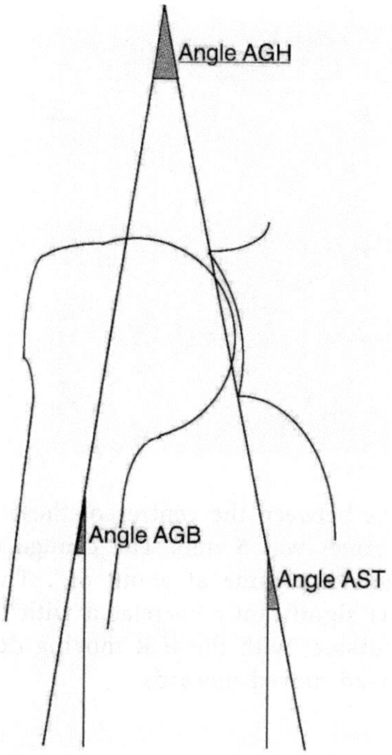

Fig. 2. Diagrams of the angles measured to determine the rhythm of scapulo-humeral movement. *AGB*, the angle between the humeral diaphyseal axis and the vertical. This equates to overall elevation; *AST*, the angle between the line of the glenoid and the vertical. This equates to scapulo-thoracic movement; *AGH*, the angle between the line of the glenoid and the humeral diaphyseal axis. This equates to gleno-humeral movement

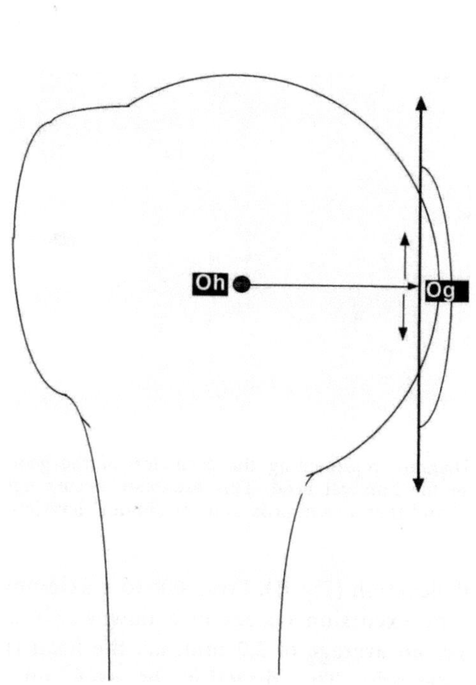

Fig. 3. Measurement of humeral head excursion on the glenoid. This excursion corresponds to the movement (*Og*) of the point Oh (geometric centre of the humeral head) on the line of the glenoid during elevation

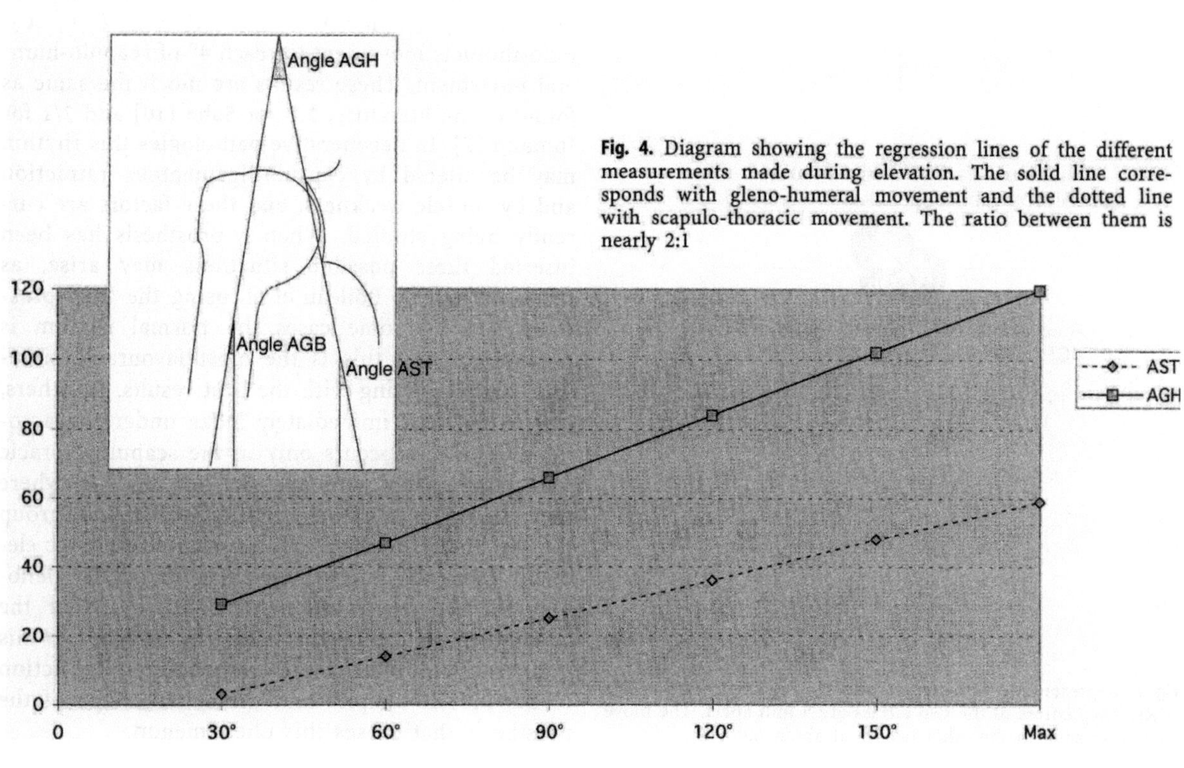

Fig. 4. Diagram showing the regression lines of the different measurements made during elevation. The solid line corresponds with gleno-humeral movement and the dotted line with scapulo-thoracic movement. The ratio between them is nearly 2:1

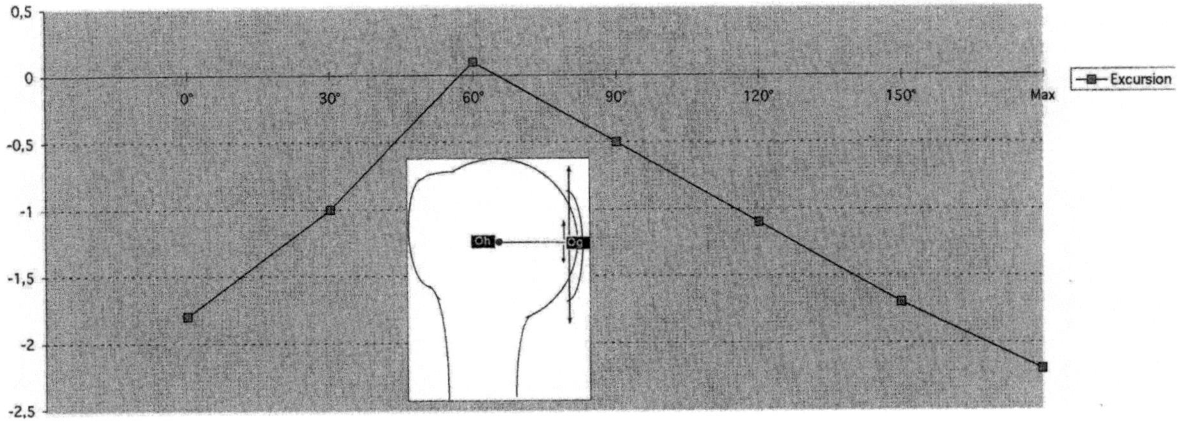

Fig. 5. Diagram representing the excursion of the geometric centre of the humeral head. This excursion occurs upwards until 60° and then downwards until maximum elevation

start of elevation (Fig. 5). From 60° to maximum elevation the excursion occurs in a downwards direction over an average of 2.2 mm, i.e. the head translates inferiorly. The direction of excursion was significantly correlated to the angle of elevation ($p<0.001$).

Instantaneous Centres of Rotation. A plot of the instantaneous centres of rotation showed two individual zones of concentration: one corresponded to the ICRs between 0° and 60° and the second to those between 60° and maximum elevation (Fig. 6).

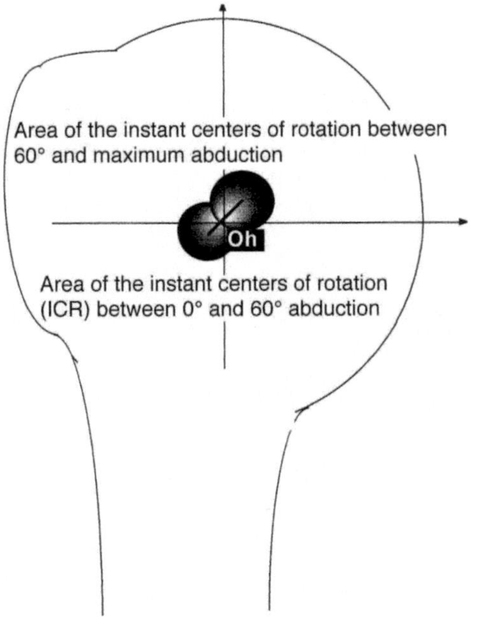

Fig. 6. Representation of the two zones of concentration of the ICRs. The centres of the two circles are 5 mm apart. The move from one zone to the other occurs at about 60°

The distance between the centres of these two concentration zones was 5 mm. The change from one zone to the other came at about 60°. The change in zone was significantly correlated with the direction of excursion, with the ICR moving downwards when the head moved upwards.

Discussion

By using a technique in which elevation can be continuously analysed by stopping the image rather than stopping the movement, so that all of the muscular, bony and articular elements involved are included.

The results of this study show that the scapulohumeral rhythm had a ratio of 2:1 with 2° of scapulo-thoracic movement for each 4° of scapulo-humeral movement. These results are much the same as found in the literature; 2/3 for Saha [10] and 2/1 for Inmann [7]. In degenerative pathologies this rhythm may be altered by capsulo-ligamentous retraction and by muscle weakness, and these factors are currently being studied. When a prosthesis has been inserted three possible situations may arise, as demonstrated by Boileau et al. using the Neer prosthesis [1]. In some cases the normal rhythm is maintained, and this is the most favourable situation, corresponding with the best results. In others, where the head immediately locks under the acromion, elevation occurs only in the scapulo-thoracic joint, as happens with massive cuff tears or where there is major bony destruction. In the final group the rhythm is reversed with the scapulo-thoracic element becoming more important than the glenohumeral. No significant abnormality in either the anatomical or technical aspects was observed in this group so that it must be the combination of the action of the muscle couples and the actual shape of the prosthesis that causes this phenomenon.

Translation of the humeral head on the glenoid has been little studied in the literature and usually in a passive manner [2, 5, 6]. In our analysis it changed direction when elevation passed 60°. This amplitude also corresponds to the change in the dispersions of the ICRs. This confirms the conclusions made by Fischer et al. [3] who found two zones of concentration of the ICRs. This change may correspond to muscle couples coming into play and having different effects. The head seems to be permanently, dynamically recentred as each excursion of the geometric centre of the head is corrected by an inverse displacement of the ICR. In practice, this means that there is a rolling and sliding movement of the head on the glenoid. This type of movement perhaps explains why at arthroscopy there is always a worn area seen in the middle of the glenoid. These results suggest that restoration of the bony anatomy should always be taken into account when selecting a prosthesis. If the curved surfaces are congruent, the head cannot move in excursion and the forces acting on the glenoid fixation are increased. However, if the glenoid is flat, the movement of translation causes wear by repeated movement of the head on the glenoid.

Conclusion

This study on healthy shoulders serves as a reference for the analysis of the behaviour of prosthetic shoulders in order to help to understand and, hopefully, correct any faults.

References

1. Boileau P, Walch G, Liotard JP (1992) Etude radio-cinématographique de l'élévation active de l'épaule prothésée. Rev Chir Orthop 6:115–119
2. Castaing J, Gouaze A, Soutoul JH, Plisson JL (1965) Les contacts tête-glène dans les différentes positions de l'articulation scapulo-humérale. CR Assoc Anat 1:259–264
3. Fischer LP, Carret JP, Gonon GP (1977) Etude cinématographique des mouvements de l'articulation scapulo-humérale. Rev Chir Orthop [Supp II]:108–112
4. Freedman L, Munro RR (1966) Abduction of the arm in the scapular plane: scapular and gleno-humeral movements. A roentgenographic study. J Bone Joint Surg Am 48:1506–1510
5. Friedman RJ (1990) Biomechanics of the shoulder following total shoulder replacement. In: Post M, Morrey BF, Hawkins RJ (eds) Surgery of the shoulder. Mosby-Year Book, St. Louis, pp 263–266
6. Harryman DT, Sidles JA, Clark JM, McQuade KJ, Gibb TD, Matsen FA (1990) Translation of the humeral head on the glenoid with passive glenohumeral motion. J Bone Joint Surg Am 72:1334–1343
7. Inman VT, Saunders SM, Abotti LC (1962) Observations on the fonction of the shoulder joint. J Bone Joint Surg Am 42:1–30
8. Johnston TB (1937) The movements of the shoulder joint. A plea for the use of the scapular as the plane of reference for movements of the humero-scapular joint. Br J Surg 25:252–260
9. Poppen NK, Walker P (1976) Normal and abnormal motion of the shoulder. J Bone Joint Surg Am 58:195–201
10. Saha AK (1950) Mechanism of shoulder movements and a plea for the recognition of "zeroposition" of glenohumeral joint. Indian J Surg 2:153–165

Kinematics of Shoulder Replacement

P. Boileau, G. Walch, and J.P. Liotard

Summary

A cineradiographic study of unconstrained Neer-type shoulder prosthesis during active anterior elevation has shown that the kinematics of the prosthetic components is rarely normal and is often limited or nil. Whilst physiological active elevation is possible in certain selected cases of shoulder replacement, the scapulo-humeral rhythm is often abnormal or reversed. An approach to the kinematics of the shoulder using an unconstrained prosthesis remains limited by: (a) the initial pathology, (b) the difficulties in operative technique and (c) the limited possibilities offered by the design of the prosthesis itself. Displacement of the centers of rotation, because of the relatively fixed geometry of this first generation of shoulder prosthesis, probably limits the possibilities to reproduce the normal kinematics of the gleno-humeral joint. These results had suggested us the need for research to improve the design and the technological possibilities of unconstrained shoulder prosthesis.

Introduction

During the past 10 years unconstrained shoulder arthroplasty has become the procedure of choice in the treatment of conditions such as osteoarthritis, rheumatoid arthritis, osteonecrosis or malunions of fractures of the upper end of the humerus. The Neer prosthesis can be considered as one of the first and most popular unconstrained shoulder prosthesis [15]. Clinical studies have shown that the first generation of "monobloc" unconstrained prostheses effectively relieve pain and restore satisfactory function in pathological lesions of the shoulder joint [3, 10, 15]. However, these studies showed that, whilst the clinical results appear to be satisfactory, the functional results often remain incomplete and do not always allow recovery of full active elevation.

Are these incomplete results seen after shoulder arthroplasty related to any changes in the kinematics of shoulder elevation after prosthetic replacement? In other words, do unconstrained prostheses of the Neer type allow physiological elevation? No work has been dedicated to the study of the kinematics of the shoulders after arthroplasty apart form that recently made by Friedman [7] and Itamura [12].

The aim of the present study was to analyse the dynamic behaviour of unconstrained prostheses during anterior elevation by observation with cineradioscopy and sequential radiographs. The relative contribution of gleno-humeral and scapulo-thoracic movements in the course of anterior elevation was assessed. Correlation with the aetiology, the condition of the humeral head and the rotator cuff, the size of the implant and possible technical errors were also investigated.

Methods and Materials

Patients

Between January 1985 and March 1989, 85 shoulder prostheses of Neer type were inserted in our Orthopedic Department. Of these, 21 prosthesis in 19 patients chosen at random have been reviewed, with a minimum follow-up of 1 year, and a cineradiographic study of active anterior elevation using fluoroscopic control has been done. Among the 19 patients there were 15 women and 4 men with an average age of 60 years at the time of operation and a range of 27–77 years. The average follow-up was 17 months, with range of 1–4 years.

Six patients were diagnosed as suffering from osteoarthritis, 4 from a cuff tear arthritis, 4 from rheumatoid arthritis, 2 of which were bilateral (6 shoulders), 3 from a malunited fracture of the humeral head, 2 from an osteonecrosis. In 10 cases the lesions affected the dominant shoulder. Two patients have already been operated on: the first had had a simple humeral prosthesis inserted for a fracture of the upper of the humerus but developed secondary loosening leading to the need for revision. The second had initially a biopsy with a secondary infection resulting in necrosis on the humeral head which had healed and was sterile at the time of the arthroplasty.

In 4 cases of cuff tear arthropathy, 3 of rheumatoid arthritis, 2 of traumatic arthritis and 1 of osteonecrosis, total shoulder replacement was indicated even though there was a major destruction of the rotator cuff and/or of bone. The patients were warned that they would not recover function except for a painless or almost painless shoulder. It was matter of prostheses with a "limited goal" as defined by Neer et al. [15, 17].

Surgical Technique

The surgical technique used was that recommended by Neer et al. without release of the anterior part of deltoid origin. The prosthesis used was an unconstrained type I (2 cases) or type II (19 cases) Neer prosthesis usually cemented except in 3 cases. A small prosthetic head (15 mm) was used in 16 cases and a large head (22 mm) in 5. The glenoid component was cemented in every case using either a polyethylene (12 cases) or a metal-backed component (9 cases). No semi-constrained glenoid implants were used in the series.

There was a rupture of the rotator cuff in 8 cases. In one case there was a partial rupture of the deep face of the supraspinatus discovered preoperatively by arthrography, but it did not require surgical treatment. In one case there was a large rupture affecting the supraspinatus which was able to be repaired satisfactorily after transosseous reinsertion into the greater tuberosity. Among the 6 massive rotator cuff lesions affecting 2 or 3 tendons with diminution of the acromio-humeral space one was able to be repaired by transfer of the supraspinatus and teres minor posteriorly and the subscapularis anteriorly. In the malunions of the proximal humerus (3 cases) the tuberosities after osteotomy were reattached with nonabsorbable sutures to avoid any risk of impingement and taking care not to lead to a malunion by inadequate displacement of the greater tuberosity. No reoperation, infection or nerve lesion and no component loosening occurred. *Physiotherapy* was given in 3 phases as recommended by Neer et al. [15], starting the day after operation. All the patients were kept in a rehabilitation centre and were looked after by the same physician and physiotherapists.

Cineradiographic Study of Active Anterior Elevation

A video-fluoroscopic record was made of movements of prosthetic shoulder under radioscopy. *The cineradioscopic study* concerned only active anterior elevation in the plane of scapula. The patients were standing, and care was taken to put the scapular plane parallel to the film and to direct the beam at right angles to and centered on the gleno-humeral joint. The shoulder region was visualized on the screen and the arm elevated in the plane of the scapula for a period of 5–10 s. The arm was then lowered to its original position along the side of the body for the same period of 5–10 s. This study was done at least 3 times for each patient so as to ensure good recordings. The images were recorded on videotape before being stored for analysis later in slow motion. A metal stem was attached in the posterior plane to indicate the vertical axis.

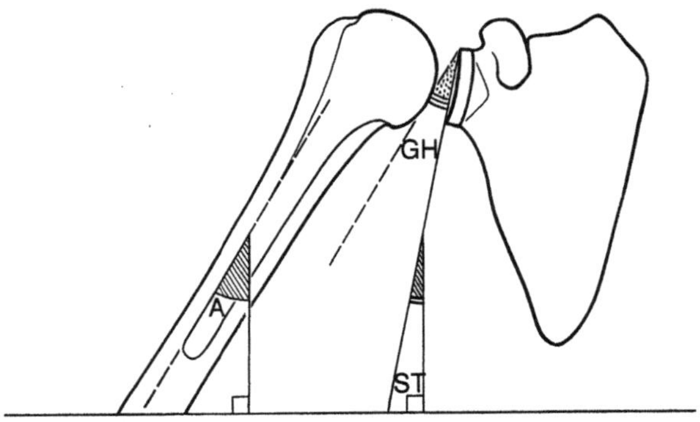

Fig. 1. The angle between the longitudinal axis of the glenoid component and the vertical (*ST*); the arm angle between the longitudinal axis of the humeral component and the vertical (*A*); the gleno-humeral angle between the humeral prosthetic component and the glenoid prosthetic component (*GH*) (A=GH+ST)

Scapulo-thoracic, gleno-humeral and overall movements were assessed by the measurement at three angles on the radiographs in maximal elevation (Fig. 1). *The scapulo-thoracic angle* (ST) consisted of the angle between the glenoid component and the vertical axis; *the arm angle* (A) consisted of the angle between longitudinal axis of the humeral prosthetic component and the vertical axis; and the *gleno-humeral angle* (GH) consisted to the angle between the humeral prosthetic component and the glenoid prosthetic component (A=GH+ST). We were thus able to asses the relationship between gleno-humeral movement (GH) and scapulo-thoracic (ST) movement (GH/ST).

Results

The recording of active anterior elevation on radioscopy and the calculation of gleno-humeral movement and scapulo-thoracic movement allowed three types of biomechanical behaviour after total arthroplasty to be defined:

A first group of prostheses (4 cases) showed biomechanical behaviour which was *almost normal.* Schematically, we found three essential periods (Fig. 2). In the first period gleno-humeral movement

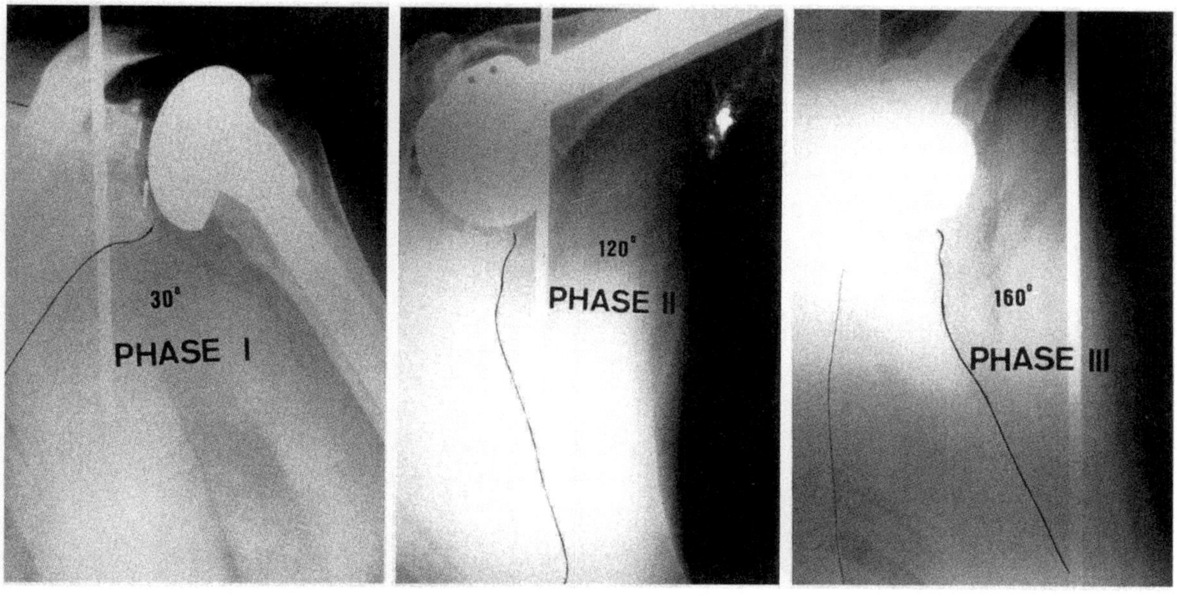

Fig. 2. Example of normal kinematics after total shoulder prosthesis (group I, 4 prostheses). Active anterior elevation (AAE) is 160°. Note the progressive rotation of the scapula. Gleno-humeral movement (GH) is normal and remains considerably greater than scapulo-thoracic movement (ST); the scapulo-humeral rhythm is preserved and is equal to 3/2 (GH/ST=3/2)

predominated; the rolling and gliding movement of the gleno-humeral joint allowed the scapulo-humeral compass to open up to 40°–50° of elevation. In the second period scapulo-thoracic movement predominated and made it possible to reach 100°–120° of elevation. In the third period gleno-humeral movement predominated once more, allowing 140°–160° to be achieved. Scapulo-humeral rhythm was normal: the relationship between gleno-humeral and scapulo-thoracic movement was approximately equal to 1.5 (GH/ST=3/2). A study of correlation with anatomical and clinical findings (Table 1) showed that these were patients whose shoulders presented no lesion of the rotator cuff. Only one patient showed a small rupture of the deep surface of supraspinatus on preoperative arthrography. Bone stock was preserved except in one case where glenoid wear was qualified as significant. Finally, no technical error was noted.

A second group of prostheses (10 cases) showed a totally *abnormal biomechanical behaviour.* The movements observed did not have much in common with a normal shoulder. It was found that the prosthetic head showed an upward movement and came to be embedded beneath the acromial arch and allowed elevation limited to only 60–80°, taking place mainly at the scapulo-thoracic joint (Fig. 3). The scapulo-humeral rhythm was completely abnormal, active anterior elevation of the upper limb being allowed only by scapulo-thoracic motion. A study of correlation with anatomical and clinical findings (Table 1) showed that these were shoulders whose major bony or muscular destruction did not allow normal anatomy to be reestablished. These were cases of prostheses with "limited goals": cuff tear arthropathy, advanced rheumatoid arthritis, old trauma and sequelae of osteomyelitis. In 6 cases, there was a massive rupture of the rotator cuff affecting 3 tendons (supraspinatus, infraspinatus and teres minor or long head of biceps) which was irreparable. In 5 cases bony destruction was noted to be significant with major erosion of the glenoid.

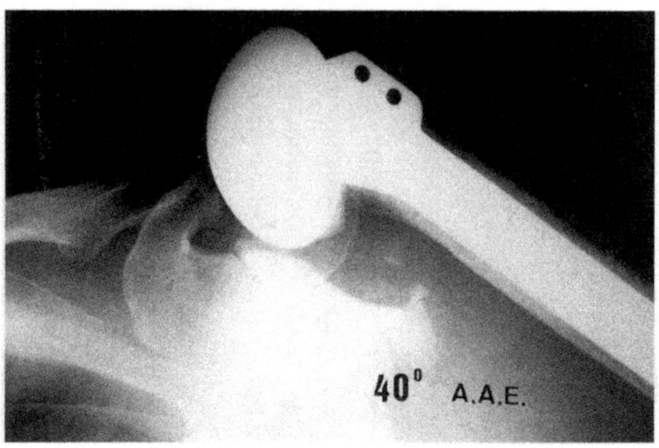

Fig. 3. Example of abnormal kinematics after total shoulder arthroplasty (group II, 10 prostheses). Active anterior elevation (AAE) is very limited (40°) and is made possible only by scapulo-thoracic movement. There is an upward excursion of the humeral component which is no longer opposite to the glenoid. The presence of an irreparable massive rupture of the cuff ("limited goal" prosthesis) is sufficient to explain the abnormal biomechanical behaviour

Table 1. Analysis of shoulder replacements: with normal scapulo-humeral rhythm (group I, n=4), with abnormal scapulo-humeral rhythm (group II, n=10), and with reversed scapulo-humeral rhythm (group III, n=7)

Pat. no.	Active anterior elevation				Aetiology	State of rotator cuff	Bone stock	Size of implant (prosthetic head)	Technical errors
	A	ST	GH	GH/ST					
Group I									
1	170°	66°	104°	1.57	Stage III necrosis	Intact	Preserved	22 mm	0
2	160°	48°	112°	2.3	Osteoarthritis	Intact (tenodesis long head biceps)	Preserved	22 mm	0
3	160°	64°	96°	1.5	Osteoarthritis		Significant wear	22 mm	0
4	145°	65°	80°	1.2	Osteoarthritis	Partial deep tear of supraspinatus	Preserved	15 mm	0
Group II									
1	90°	70°	20°	0.28	Cuff tear arthritis	Irreparable massive rupture	Destroyed glenoid	15 mm	Prosthesis too proud
2	50°	50°	0°	0	Cuff tear arthritis	Irreparable massive rupture (3 tendons)	Preserved	15 mm	–
3	30°	30°	0°	0	Cuff tear arthritis	Irreparable massive rupture (3 tendons)	Preserved	22 mm	–
4	80°	62°	18°	0.29	Cuff tear arthritis	Irreparable massive rupture (3 tendons + dis. long head biceps)	Preserved	15 mm	–
5	80°	60°	20°	0.26	Rhumatoid arthritis	Not known	Significant glenoid wear	15 mm	Prosthesis too low
6	60°	45°	15°	0.33	Rhumatoid arthritis	Initially intact but rupture at 3 years	Preserved	15 mm	–
7	90°	75°	15°	0.20	Rhumatoid arthritis	Major rupture (2 tendons): repaired	Wear 2/3 upper glenoid	15 mm	Head too small
8	40°	40°	0°	0	Malunion	Irreparable massive rupture (3 tendons)	Preserved	15 mm	–
9	40°	40°	0°	0	Malunion (ant. disloc.)	Intact	Glenoid destroyed	15 mm	–
10	30°	30°	0°	0	(Necrosis stage IV)	Irreparable massive rupture	Glenoid destroyed	15 mm	–
Group III									
1	120°	65°	55°	0.83	Osteoarthritis	Intact	Preserved	15 mm	0
2	110°	48°	62°	0.77	Osteoarthritis	Intact	Preserved	15 mm	0
3	170°	68°	102°	1.5	Osteoarthritis	Intact	Preserved	22 mm	0
4	120°	70°	50°	0.71	Rhumatoid arthritis	Intact but thin	Preserved	15 mm	0
5	120°	74°	66°	0.88	Rhumatoid arthritis	Intact but thin	Not known	15 mm	0
6	90°	72°	18°	0. 25	Rhumatoid arthritis	Intact but thin	Moderate erosion of glenoid	15 mm	0
7	90°	58°	32°	0.53	Posttraumatic arthritis	Intact	Preserved	15 mm	0

A, Angle of upper limb in maximal elevation; ST, scapulo-thoracic angle; GH, gleno-humeral angle.

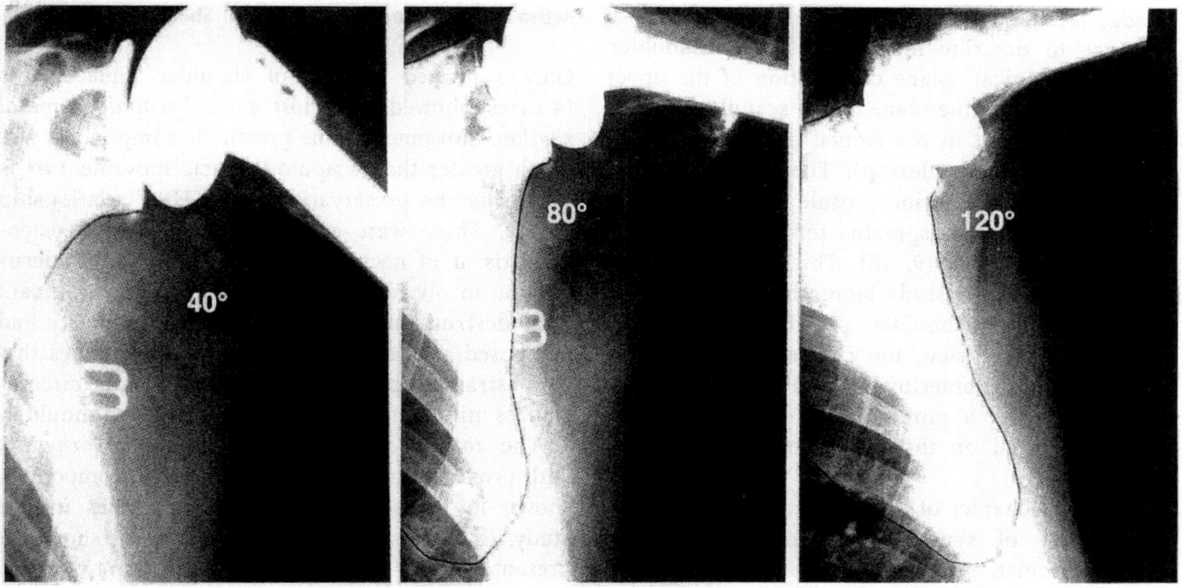

Fig. 4. Example of modified kinematics after total shoulder prosthesis (group III, 7 prosthesis). Active anterior elevation is incomplete (120°). There is a diminution of gleno-humeral movement (GH) between the prosthetic components without diminution of scapulo-thoracic movement (ST). The reversed scapulo-humeral rhythm poses the problem of biomechanical disturbance due to the design of the prosthesis itself

Finally, in between those two groups there was an intermediate group (7 cases) which showed *altered biomechanical behaviour.* Abduction was not full and reached 90–120°. Here there was diminished movement of the gleno-humeral joint without any change in scapulo-thoracic movement (Fig. 4). It seemed that the humeral prosthesis came rapidly to wedge itself against the glenoid so that scapulo-thoracic movement was the important movement. These prostheses functioned with a *reversed scapulo-humeral rhythm*, the GH/ST relationship being between 0.25 and 0.83. A study of anatomical and clinical correlation (Table 1) showed that 4 cases these were arthroplasties for gleno-humeral osteoarthritis or traumatic arthritis with no detectable technical errors. The rotator cuff and bone stock appeared to have been preserved preoperatively and at the review. In 3 cases there was a rheumatoid arthritis where the operative findings mentioned the existence of a thinning of the tendons of rotator cuff. These abnormal results were found in patients who were considered as good clinical results with significant improvement as regards pain, movement and function.

Discussion

Our intention was to verify whether total shoulder prostheses allow physiological anterior elevation. A radioscopic study of total shoulder prostheses during active anterior elevation has shown that three types of scapulo-humeral rhythm exist after arthrosplasty: normal, totally abnormal or reversed (Table 2). While it may be argued that this is a retrospective study on a small number of cases with various aetiologies, the important point that remains is that there is often a change in the kinematics of the shoulder after unconstrained prosthetic replacement. Movement between the prosthetic components can be nil or diminished whilst scapulo-thoracic movement remains unchanged. Reversed scapulo-humeral rhythm after total arthroplasty, present in 30 % of cases in this study, can explain certain imperfect functional results in clinical practice and poses the problem of biomechanical disturbances due to the design of the prosthesis itself.

Table 2. The three types of kinematics after unconstrained shoulder arthroplasty: mobility between the prosthetic components can be normal, decreased, or nil

Kinematics of shoulder replacement	Gleno-humeral motion	Scapulo-thoracic
Normal	+	+
Abnormal	±	+
Reverse	–	+

Anterior Elevation of the Shoulder and Scapulohumeral Rhythm

The problem of the plane of reference movements has been pointed out for a long time. Johnston [13] in 1930 and Saha [22] in 1950 had already pleaded for the choice of the scapula as the plane of reference to describe movements of the shoulder. The "physiological" plane of elevation of the upper limb is situated in the plane of the scapula (anterior elevation) and not in the frontal plane (abduction) or in sagittal plane (flexion). There is an absence of torsion of the inferior capsule an alignment of the deltoid and supraspinatus for elevation in the plane of the scapula [9, 18]. This is why we have chosen this plane to study biomechanical behaviour of unconstrained shoulder prostheses. From the practical point of view, the choice of plane of the scapula to study anterior elevation had the merit of only allowing a minimum of distortion of the angles measured on the screen and in the radiographs.

The biomechanics of the shoulder involve a complex variety of synchronous movements of the sterno-clavicular, scapulo-thoracic and gleno-humeral joints. Anterior elevation at the gleno-humeral joint is about 120° provided that is combined with lateral rotation of the humerus [1, 2, 5]. So that the arm can achieve full elevation (180°) a supplementary curve of 60° is needed and is possible because of rotation of the scapula [2, 14, 24]. The perfect synchronization which exists between movements of the gleno-humeral joints (GH) and that of the scapulo-thoracic joint (ST) was defined by Codman [2] as the "scapulo-humeral rhythm". Imman et al. [11] in 1944 showed that in the course of abduction the increase in the angle of oration of the scapula, and the gleno-humeral angle takes place in a conjoint manner in the course of almost the hole of the movement. More precisely, they showed that:

- In the course of the first 30° of abduction, there is great variability in the scapulo-thoracic movements, with the scapula seeking stability by rotating laterally, medially, in both directions or not at all in the course of what is called "the setting phase".
- Between 30° and 170° of abduction, gleno-humeral movement is twice that of the scapulo-thoracic joint with a constant ratio of 2 (GH/ST=2/1). Subsequent studies by Freedman and Munro [7] showed that there are 3° of gleno-humeral movement for 2° of scapulo-thoracic movement (GH/ST=3/2) whilst Poppen and Walker [18, 19] considered that there were 5° of gleno-humeral movement fir 4° of scapulo-thoracic movement (GH/ST=5/4). These contradictory findings could be due to differences in the planes chosen (abduction for Imman) and to considerable number of individual variations as was shown by the confidence interval carried out by Freedman and Munro [7].

Active Anterior Elevation After Total Shoulder Arthroplasty

Only a limited number of shoulder replacements (4 cases) showed an *almost normal scapulo-humeral rhythm*. Movement in the prosthetic components was much greater than scapulo-thoracic movement as is shown by the preservation of a GH/ST relationship of 3/2. These were cases of gleno-humeral osteoarthritis or of necrosis of the head of the humerus without involvement of the rotator cuff or significant bone destruction and in which the arthroplasty had not posed any technical problems. This implies that unconstrained prostheses can in certain circumstances mimic the normal kinematics of the shoulder.

The *totally abnormal scapulo-humeral rhythm*, with proximal migration of the humeral component, shown in the second group of prostheses in our study, is not surprising since these were shoulders presenting with major muscle and/or bone damage. The insertion of an unconstrained prosthesis without repairing the rotator cuff or with excessive bone wear constitutes a palliative solution. Although it is not very satisfactory from the biomechanical point of view, the solution, initially recommended by Neer et al. [15, 17], is acceptable from the clinical point of view ("limited goal prosthesis"). Antero-superior instability of the humeral component is related to superior translation because of predominant shear forces. This superior instability remains limited by the fulcrum provided by the acromial arch, if it has been conserved. However, insertion of a glenoid component is contraindicated in these cases because of the high shearing eccentric forces which increase the risk of glenoid loosening ("rocking horse effect"), as shown by Franklin et al. [6].

The possibility of *reversed scapulo-humeral rhythm after total shoulder arthroplasty* in the third group (7 cases of 21) is the most interesting result of our study. It shows that the movement between the prosthetic components is less than the normal gleno-humeral movement but that the scapulo-thoracic movement remains unchanged. Friedman considered that this reversal of scapulo-humeral rhythm was almost constant after total shoulder arthroplasty in a series of 15 patients studies by sequential radiographs [8]. This diminution of movement between the prosthetic components without diminished scapulo-thoracic movement poses questions as to its cause.

Factors Associated with Abnormal or Reversed Kinematics After Shoulder Arthroplasty

Three factors seem to be responsible for abnormal or reversed kinematics after shoulder replacement:

The *initial pathology* is certainly partly responsible for the abnormal movements observed. Whilst the bone stock was completely satisfactory, and there were no rotator cuff lesions, it is certain that the trophic quality of he cuff was not the same in the 7 cases of our series. The thinning of the cuff noted in the rheumatoid arthritis cases as well as the contractured cuff noted in one old traumatic case, without doubt, constitute factors which affect the gleno-humeral mobility. A more complete investigation of the trophic changes in the cuff by supplementary means (ultrasound, arthrography, computed tomography) would be desirable to verify this hypothesis but they were not made.

The *operative technique* constitutes another possible factor capable of disturbing the biomechanics of active anterior elevation after total arthroplasty. Complete restoration of external rotation is indispensable to the recovery of complete elevation. Relaising and lengthening the subscapularis is necessary in case of internal rotation contracture and was performed in all our patients ("soft tissue balancing"). The precise positioning of the prosthetic components in all spatial planes remains another difficult factor to control at operation because of the pathological changes encountered. Studies by Rietveld et al. [29] and Figgie et al. [4] have shown that any error in positioning of the prosthetic components in the vertical and/or the horizontal plane results in changes in the lever arm and/or in the positioning of the joint line which may be responsible for disturbed biomechanics of the shoulder.

Finally, the *prosthesis* itself, because of its fixed design and its technical limitations, is surely partly responsible for the reversed scapulo-humeral rhythm observed. Firstly, one must call to mind, as did Friedman [8], the much greater degree of conformity and stability between the prosthetic components compared with a normal gleno-humeral joint. The radius of curvature of the glenoid component suggested by Neer is identical with that of the humeral component, increasing the stresses on it and diminishing its movements. Secondly, one must consider the difficulties in adapting to geometrical variations of the proximal humerus when performing a shoulder arthroplasty. The choice of a prosthetic head adapted to the space available, for example, is essential to provide correct tension in the cuff muscles and to reestablish normal biomechanical behaviour. Currently we use two thickness of prosthetic head: 15 and 22 mm and one of diameter 44 mm. In an anthropometrical study of the proximal humerus we verified that there are significant variations in the dimensions as regards the diameter and thickness of the articular surface [23]. Moreover, our study has demonstrated that the shape of the proximal humerus is highly variable because of variations in inclination and retroversion as well as variations in posterior and medial offset of the articular surface. Thus trying to reproduce the variable three dimensional geometry of the proximal humerus with a fixed monobloc (first generation) or modular (second generation) humeral component can only be a compromise. For these reasons surgeons should not be surprised that kinematics of shoulder replacement may also be a compromise, sometimes altering the functional results.

Conclusion

Whilst physiological active elevation is possible in certain selected cases of unconstrained shoulder prostheses, the gleno-humeral mobility between the prosthetic components is often decreased or nil. An approach to the kinematics of the shoulder using an unconstrained prosthesis remains limited by the possibilities offered by the design of the prosthesis itself. Our study suggests that the relatively fixed geometry of the design of most shoulder prosthesis currently available, limits the possibilities to reproduce the normal kinematics of the gleno-humeral joint. These results had suggested to us the need for research to improve the design and the technical possibilities of unconstrained shoulder prostheses [23].

References

1. Boileau P, Walch G, Liotard JP (1992) Cineradiographic study of active elevation of the prosthetic shoulder. J Orthop Surg 6:351–359
2. Codman EA (1934) The shoulder. Rupture of supraspinatus tendon and other lesions in or about the subacromial bursa. Todd, Boston.
3. Cofield RH (1984) Total shoulder arthroplasty with Neer total prosthesis. J Bone Joint Surg Am 66:899–906
4. Figgie HE, Inglis AE, Golberg VM, Ranawat CS, Figgie MP, Wile JM (1988) An analysis of factors affecting the long term results of total shoulder arthroplasty in inflammatory arthritis. Arthroplasty 3:123–130
5. Fisher LP, Carret JP, Gonon GP et al (1977) Etude cinématique des mouvements de l'articulation scapulo-humérale. Rev Chir. Orthop 63 [Suppl II]:108–112
6. Franklin JL, Barrett WP, Jackins SE, Matsen FA III (1988) Glenoid loosening in total shoulder arthroplasty: association with rotator cuff deficiency. J Arthropl 3:39–46

7. Freedman L, Munro RR (1966) Abduction of the arm in the scapular plane: scapular and gleno-humeral movements. A roetgenographic study. J Bone Joint Surg Am 48:1506- 510
8. Friedman RJ (1990) Biomechanics of the shoulder following total shoulder replacement. In: Post M, Morrey BF, Hawkins RJ (eds) Surgery of the shoulder. Mosby-Year Book, St. Louis, pp 263–266
9. Gagey O, Bonfait H, Gillot C, Hureau J, Mazas F (1987) Bases anatomiques du contrôle ligamentaire de l'épaule (Position de référence de l'articulation scapulo-humérale) Surg Radiol Anat 9:19–26
10. Hawkins RJ, Bell RH, Jallay B (1989) Total shoulder arthroplasty. Clin Orthop 242:188–194
11. Inman VT, Saunders JB, Abbott LC (1944) Observations on the function of the shoulder joint. j bone Joint Surg Am 26:1–30
12. Itamura JM, Schmotzer HC, Chon JH, Mirzayan R, Vangness CT (1996) Kinematics of glenohumeral arthroplasty in abduction. Presented at the American Academy of Orthopaedics Surgeons. Atlanta, February, p 166
13. Johnston TB (1937) The movements of the shoulder Joint. A plea for the use of the "plane of scapula" as the plane reference for movements occuring at the humeral-scapular Joint. Br J Surg 25:252–260
14. Kondo M, Tazoe S, Yamada M (1984) Changes of tilting angle of the scapula following elevation of the arm. In: Batman JE, Welsh RP (eds) Surgery of the shoulder. Mosby, St. Louis, pp 12–16
15. Neer CS, Watson KC, Stanton FJ (1982) Recent experience in total shoulder replacement. J Bone Joint Surg Am 64:319–337
16. Neer CS, Kirby R (1982) Revision of humeral head and total shoulder arthroplasties. Clin Orthop 170:189–195
17. Neer CS, Craig EV, Fukuda H (1983) Cuff tear arthropathy. J Bone Joint Surg Am 65:1232–1244
18. Poppen NK, Walker PS (1976) Normal and abnormal motion of the shoulder. J Bone Joint Surg Am 58:195–201
19. Poppen NK, Walker PS (1978) Forces at the gleno-humeral joint in abduction. Clin Orthop 135:165–170
20. Rietveld ABM, Daanen HAM, Rzing PM, Obermann WR (1988) The lever arm in gleno-humeral abduction after hemi-arthroplasty. J Bone Joint Surg Br 70:561–565
21. Roberts SNJ, Foley APJ, Swallow HM, Wallace WA, Coughlan DP (1991) The geometry of humeral head and the design of prosthesis. J Bone Joint Surg Br 73:647–650
22. Saha AK (1950) Mechanism of shoulder mevements and a plea for the recognition of "zero position" of gleno-humeral joint. Indian J Surg 12:153–165
23. Walch G, Boileau P (1992) Morphological study of the humeral proximal epiphysis. J Bone Joint Surg Br 74:14
24. Wallace WA (1982) The dynamic study of shoulder movement. In: Bayley I, Kessel L (eds) Shoulder surgery. Springer, Berlin Heidelberg New York, pp 139–143
25. Wuelker N, Schmotzer H, Thren K, Korell M (1994) Translation of the glenohumeral joint with simulated active elevaton. Clin Orthop 309:193–200

Section III:

Preoperative Conditionning

Clinical Evaluation Prior to Shoulder Arthroplasty

D.F. Gazielly

Summary

The preoperative clinical evaluation of a patient presenting with shoulder pathology which might be treated by an arthroplasty consists of three equally important elements: the history, giving information about any relevant medical conditions, the clinical examination, and the standard radiological investigations, which often give information as to the aetiology of the diseased joint. The clinical examination must be bilateral and involve the whole upper limb. It allows the patient's morphotype to be assessed as well as the active and passive range of movement in the shoulder. The goal is for the surgeon to be aware of any elements which might alter the indications for surgery or have a direct influence on the technicalities of the operation and the postoperative functional prognosis. The clinical examination allows a preoperative functional evaluation to be determined which serves as a reference level for the follow-up period. Finally, it establishes a relationship of trust between the surgeon and the patient thanks to the information given about the role and duration of rehabilitation and on the functional result that can be expected after shoulder arthroplasty depending on the age of the patient and the aetiology of his diseased shoulder.

Introduction

A prosthetic arthroplasty should have beneficial effects on pain and function if a number of conditions can be combined to guarantee the successful outcome of the procedure. These conditions are partly technical and partly psychological. The insertion of a shoulder prosthesis requires good quality humeral and glenoid bone stock as well as a functional rotator cuff and adequate muscular strength. A deficit in one of these elements may represent a contraindication to arthroplasty. The psychological element is equally important. The patient should want to undergo the operation and be motivated to carry out the postoperative rehabilitation which plays a vital part in guaranteeing the optimal functional result. It is of primary importance that the patient has been informed about the way the prosthesis works, the likely outcome that he can expect after the surgery, particularly depending on the aetiology, and details of the methods used in the rehabilitation and the imposition that this will cause on his daily life. The preoperative clinical evaluation is usually carried out in two stages and is based on the patient's history, giving information about any antecedents as well as the current situation; on a structured and comparable clinical examination; on a detailed haemobiochemical investigation and on specific radiographic views. These allow the indications for arthroplasty to be adjusted depending on certain important parameters and for a relationship of trust to be established with the patient.

History

The circumstances very depending on whether there has been recent trauma, and whether the patient presents with a chronic complaint.

When the patient is seen following trauma, the therapeutic indications depend on the type of fracture as shown on the radiographs [1] and on the patient's age. Any preexisting medical history which might be a contraindication to urgent reconstruction of the proximal humerus using a prosthesis, for example, metabolic, cardiac, should be determined. When the patient is seen with a chronic problem, there is no such urgency involved, and the objective here is to gain accurate information about his medical and surgical history, what his actual complaints are of, and his degree of motivation in order to decide whether a prosthesis is a medical possibility, and whether his psychological profile would meet the demands of this sort of surgery. The interview should detail the patient's age, dominant side, family and professional situation, whether he are working, retired or on invalidity and the types of activities commonly pursued.

It is important to know straightaway whether he is being followed up for any metabolic or rheumatological conditions such as rheumatoid arthritis, and whether he are on steroid treatment, at what dose and for how long. In the case of the rheumatoid arthritic the surgeon should determine whether other joints are affected and have been or should be operated on before programming a logical, chronological sequence of treatment as it might be necessary to operate on a hip or an elbow as well as the ipsi- or contralateral shoulder.

Are there any preexisting neurological or neuromuscular diseases? Should EMGs be carried out? Has he already had surgery on the same shoulder and, if so, what operation and when? Is there any history of infection?

The patient may have referred himself because of pain or functional impairment, or he may have been referred by a general practitioner or another specialist for an opinion on a shoulder arthroplasty. The degree of pain and the functional handicap must be asked about and quantified on a functional evaluation score sheet which allows a preoperative reference score to be established. Many scoring systems are available. Our preference is to use the Constant score [2, 3] as employed by the European Society for Shoulder and Elbow Surgery. Pain is scored out of 15 points and the handicap in activities of daily living out of 20 points (Fig. 1). Details of the pain including its duration, site, what causes it, whether it is worse at night, its intensity and whether it has recently become worse, should all be recorded. The functional handicap and its effect on professional and pastime activities should be detailed at the same time as his level of work. All these responses are quantified on the Constant score (Fig. 1).

Any previous treatment is detailed: has he been prescribed medications, and if so what type, for how long and did they improve the pain? Has he had any infiltrations? Has he undergone any physiotherapy and what type?

Finally, an attempt should be made to understand the psychological profile of the patient: is he anxious or not, motivated or undemanding? These enquiries determine how well the postoperative period will run.

Overall, after this first interview, the surgeon should know why the patient has been referred, his medical and surgical history and have an idea of his motivation. Of course, these elements may not amount to a definite indication for arthroplasty, but certain parameters may appear as relative contraindications, especially a long medical history, neurological or muscular diseases or infection.

Physical Examination

The clinical examination must be bilateral and comparative and involve the shoulder girdle as well as the whole upper limb including the elbow and wrist. Polyarticular involvement in the upper limb in osteoarthritis or rheumatoid arthritis may effect the postoperative rehabilitation after shoulder arthroplasty. Clinical examination of the shoulder girdle should be carried out with a thought at the back of the surgeon's mind about the technical possibilities of inserting a shoulder prosthesis and the functional prognosis. It should begin with a systematic search for ligamentous hyperlaxity, on a patient stripped to the wrist, first standing and then lying supine. It is our usual practice to start with an examination of the thoracic and cervical spine, then the supra- and infraspinatus fossae to detect any atrophy. The patient's morphotype is noted because implanting a shoulder prosthesis, especially when the glenoid is also being replaced, is more difficult to do in a short, barrel-chested patient with a thoracic kyphosis than in a tall, thin patient.

The examination continues with the surgeon face on to the patient noting the appearance of his skin and his muscularity, especially of the deltoids. At the same time a neuro-vascular examination is carried out checking the radial pulse, motor function in the fingers and sensation around the shoulder. The passive movement of the damaged shoulder is compared to the healthy shoulder in anterior elevation, in external rotation with the elbow at the side and in 90° of abduction and in internal rotation with the hand behind the back. Active mobility is then tested in the same planes. The bilateral active and passive movements are accurately measured using a goniometer and are recorded on the examination sheet. Pain-free active movement is scored out of the 40 points used in the Constant system (Fig. 1). A reduction in certain planes found during the examination of mobility may have a direct effect on the operative technique employed or the functional prognosis: external rotation elbow at the side of zero or less forewarns of the need to carry out an elongation of the subscapularis tendon; active anterior elevation limited to less than 90° means that incomplete recovery of this movement after surgery can be predicted.

After the examination of active mobility and while the patient remains standing, certain specific tests can be carried out to assess the state of the tendons of the rotator cuff: resisted anterior elevation with the arm in internal rotation in the scapular plane (supraspinatus); resisted external rotation elbow at the side (infraspinatus) and the lift-off test of Gerber (subscapularis). However, these specific tests are often impaired by the patient's pain and limited range of movement. While the patient is standing, it is possible to measure muscular force

Fig. 1. Functional Constant Score

		RIGHT SHOULDER	LEFT SHOULDER
SUBJECTIVE 35 points/100	**PAIN: 15 points/100** NONE MILD MODERATE SEVERE 15 10 5 0		
	ACTIVITIES OF DAILY LIVING: 20 points/100 – PROFESSIONAL HANDICAP (0 to 4 points) 0 point: severe handicap, 4 points: Full work – RECREATIONAL HANDICAP (0 to 4 points) – SLEEP (0 to 2 points) AFFECTED SLEEP: 0 point, UNAFFECTED SLEEP: 2 points – LEVEL OF USE OF HANDS (10 points) WAIST XIPHOID NECK TOP OF HEAD ABOUT HEAD 2 points 4 points 6 points 8 points 10 points		
	Sub-total/35 points		
OBJECTIVE 65 points/100	**PAINLESS ACTIVE MOBILITY – 40 points/100** **FORWARD ELEVATION** 0–30 / 30–60 / 60–90 / 90–120 / 120–150 / 150–180 0 points 2 points 4 points 6 points 8 points 10 points **LATERAL ELEVATION** 0–30 / 30–60 / 60–90 / 90–120 / 120–150 / 150–180 0 points 2 points 4 points 6 points 8 points 10 points **EXTERNAL ROTATION** – hand behind head with elbow held forward 2 points – hand behind head with elbow held back 2 points – hand on top of head with elbow held forward 2 points – hand on top of head with elbow held back 2 points – full elevation from on top of head 2 points **INTERNAL ROTATION: DORSUM OF HAND TO** thigh buttock sacrum L3 Th 12 Th 7 0 points 2 points 4 points 6 points 8 points 10 points		
	POWER 25 points/100 MEASURED IN 90° ABDUCTION IN SCAPULA PLANE USING A DYNAMOMETER		
	Sub-total/65 points		
	TOTAL/100 points		

as detailed in the Constant system, using a dynamometer; the examiner imparts a down force on the patient's arm which must be maintained horizontally in the scapula plane. Muscular force is measured out of 25 points. At the end of the examination a Constant score can be established with a maximum value of 100 points. This score can be either an absolute value or a value relative to the unaffected shoulder or normalised for age and sex using Constant's standardised scale [2, 3].

At the same time as carrying out the clinical examination of the shoulder the examiner can ask about the level of impairment in the following movements used in everyday life (scored: normal=5, fair=4, difficult=3, assisted=2, impossible=1):

- Use back pocket
- Wash opposite underarm
- Comb hair
- Carry 4–6 kg, arm at side
- Use arm at should level

- Use arm above shoulder level
- Dress
- Eat with utensil
- Sleep on shoulder
- Reach behind back, fasten brassiere.

Should a prosthesis be inserted, this preoperative functional evaluation serves as the reference for the patient's follow-up consultations at 6 months and at 1, 2 and 5 years postoperatively. Finally, the passive range of motion must be measured with the patient supine, recording external rotation elbow at the side and particularly anterior elevation as this may increase in comparison to the passive range found when standing [1].

Overall, the clinical examination gives an idea of the general morphotype of the patient, his muscularity and his shoulder mobility in which a marked reduction would be a factor limiting the expected functional result with regard to recovery of range of movement. The state of the rotator cuff can be assessed using specific tests, but this may be difficult to carry out due to pain. Audible cracking, supra- and infraspinatus atrophy or a history of dislocation in a patient over 50 years old are all factors which would suggest damage to the rotator cuff and this can be confirmed by the radiographic and computed tomographic arthrogram, investigations which are systematically carried out preoperatively when an arthroplasty is suggested.

Preoperative Imaging

The history and clinical examination of the patient are inseparable from the imaging investigations, which are carried out in two stages. At the first consultation the patient is seen with an up-to-date set of five standard radiographs: three AP views (in neutral, external and internal rotation), a scapular view and an axillary view. Studying these radiographs gives an idea of the degree of humeral head and glenoid destruction, the level of glenohumeral joint space impingement, the existence of a varying volume of osteophyte at the inferior pole of the humeral head and the glenoid, the presence of any loose bodies, the presence of an anterior acromial beak and any upward migration of the head indicative of a rotator cuff lesion which may be great enough to be the cause of a postero-superior or antero-superior eccentricity of the head.

An assessment of the humeral and glenoid bone stock and any eccentricity of the humeral head should give an immediate idea as to whether the insertion of a prosthesis is technically possible, and whether it would be a hemi- or a total shoulder replacement. A second advantage in having a set of recent radiographs, especially if these can be compared to older ones, is that they help in making the diagnosis of the disease process by its evolution: primary osteoarthritis, rheumatoid arthritis, osteonecrosis, posttraumatic arthritis, cuff tear arthropathy, recent four-part fracture or the sequalae of anterior surgical intervention (Fig. 2). It is essential to have this radiographic information at the end of the first consultation when the time will have come to discuss with the patient whether he needs a shoulder replacement, whether this should be a total or a hemireplacement, and the functional prognosis that the operation should afford the patient.

If arthroplasty is proposed, standard radiographic views should be supplemented by a computed tomographic arthrogram (Fig. 3) which is preferred to an

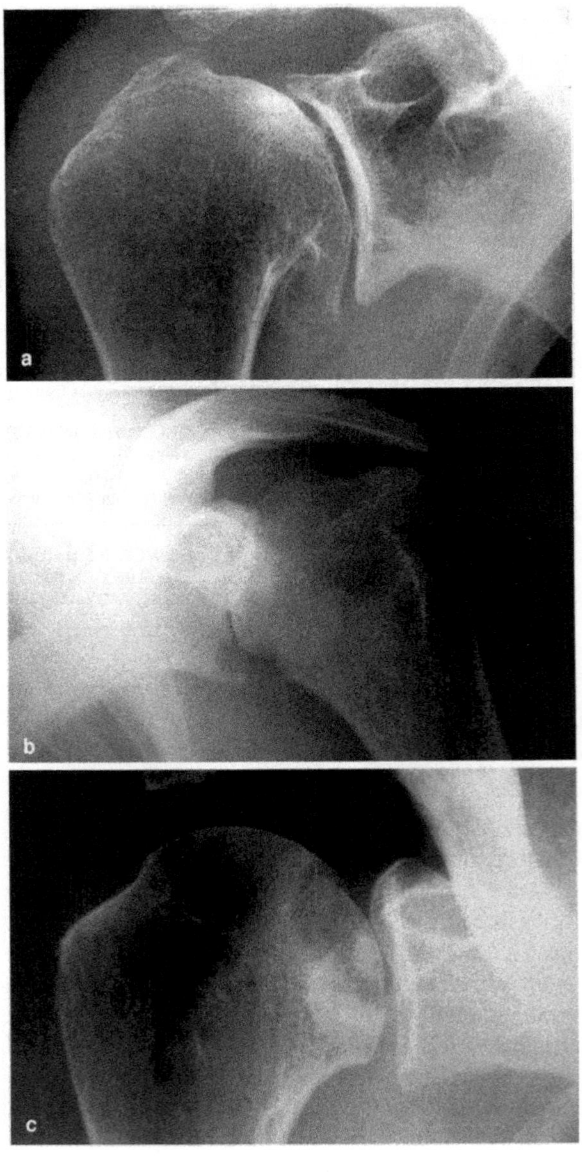

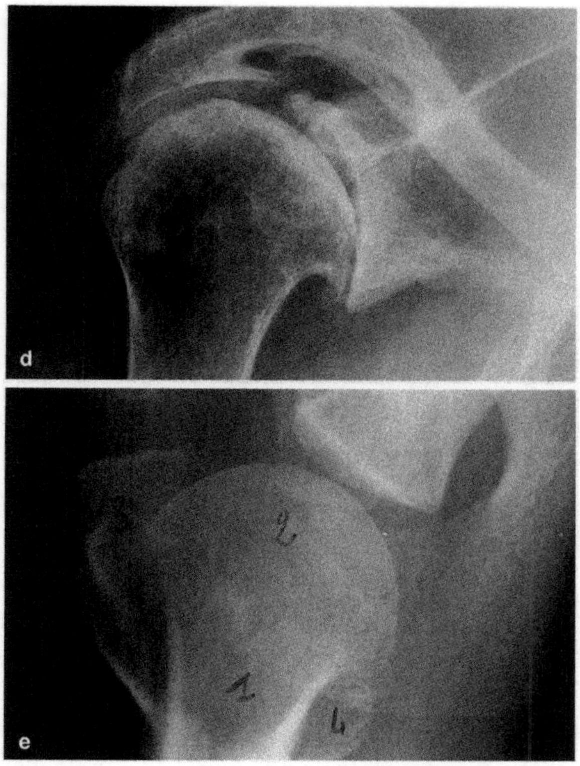

Fig. 2 a–e. Examples of various pathologies that may be treated with a shoulder arthroplasty. **a** Osteoarthritis. **b** Rheumatoid arthritis. **c** Avascular necrosis. **d** Cuff tear arthritis. **e** Four-part fracture

magnetic resonance imaging [4]. This complimentary imaging is essential and should be analysed during the second consultation where, with the information it gives on the state of the cuff and any glenoid erosion, it helps confirm the indications for arthroplasty and decides whether it will be a hemi- or a total replacement.

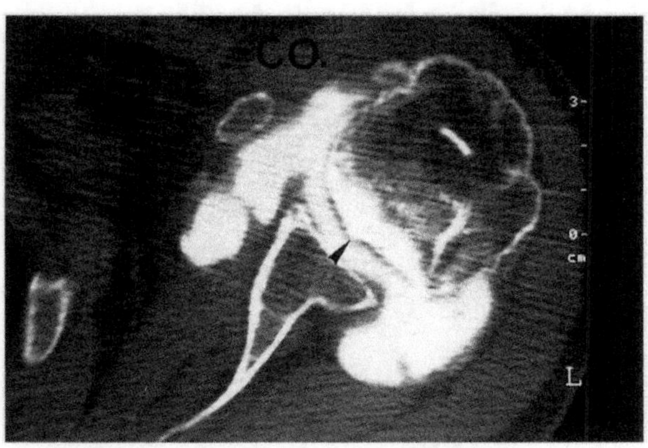

Fig. 3. Computed tomography required before total shoulder arthroplasty, allowing the glenoid wear and the degeneration of the cuff to be evaluated

Discussion with the Patient

After taking a history of the patient's (shoulder problem and any other medical conditions) and having carried out a complete clinical examination and review of the standard and complimentary images, the interview with the patient should have the goal of answering any questions that he may want to ask: if a shoulder prosthesis is indicated, what is the likely result in terms of pain and function that can be expected for his aetiology? What is the postoperative course and is he aware that he must take on the responsibility of 6–12 months rehabilitation which is essential in achieving a good functional result?

This information phase is very important in reassuring the patient because the public, and indeed general practitioners and rheumatologists, still know very little about shoulder arthroplasty. At this stage it is necessary to explain to the patient how the operation is carried out, and how it works due to the tendons of the rotator cuff and the muscles of the shoulder girdle and allows the surgeon to lay great emphasis on the importance of the postoperative rehabilitation.

The expected outcome depends on the aetiology, and this should be explained to the patient. *Osteoarthritis* is a good indication for shoulder replacement because in 90 % the rotator cuff is intact and one can promise the patient a good result in terms of pain reduction and recovery of active mobility (Fig. 4). In *rheumatoid arthritis* the result in terms of pain, which is often severe, is usually very satisfying, but the functional outcome depends on the duration of the disease, the degree of soft tissue damage and the severity of bony erosion, particularly in the glenoid, where implanting a replacement component may be impossible because of bony destruction and the risk of loosening. Disease in the ipsilateral elbow or the contralateral upper limb may impede rehabilitation. *Avascular necrosis* of the humeral head may give excellent results with regard to reducing the often severe pain and for active mobility which is conserved in the majority of stage 3 cases and reduced in stage 4.

In posttraumatic arthritis, the results which are good in terms of pain, depend in mobility on whether or not there is malunion of the tuberosities. The functional prognosis is reduced when the patient has already undergone one or more interventions. This is difficult surgery, and the result depends on the state of the soft tissues and the effectiveness of the postoperative rehabilitation. *Cuff tear arthropathy* is often associated with a supraspinatus tendon rupture retracted to the level of the glenoid and here the indication for a prosthesis is severe

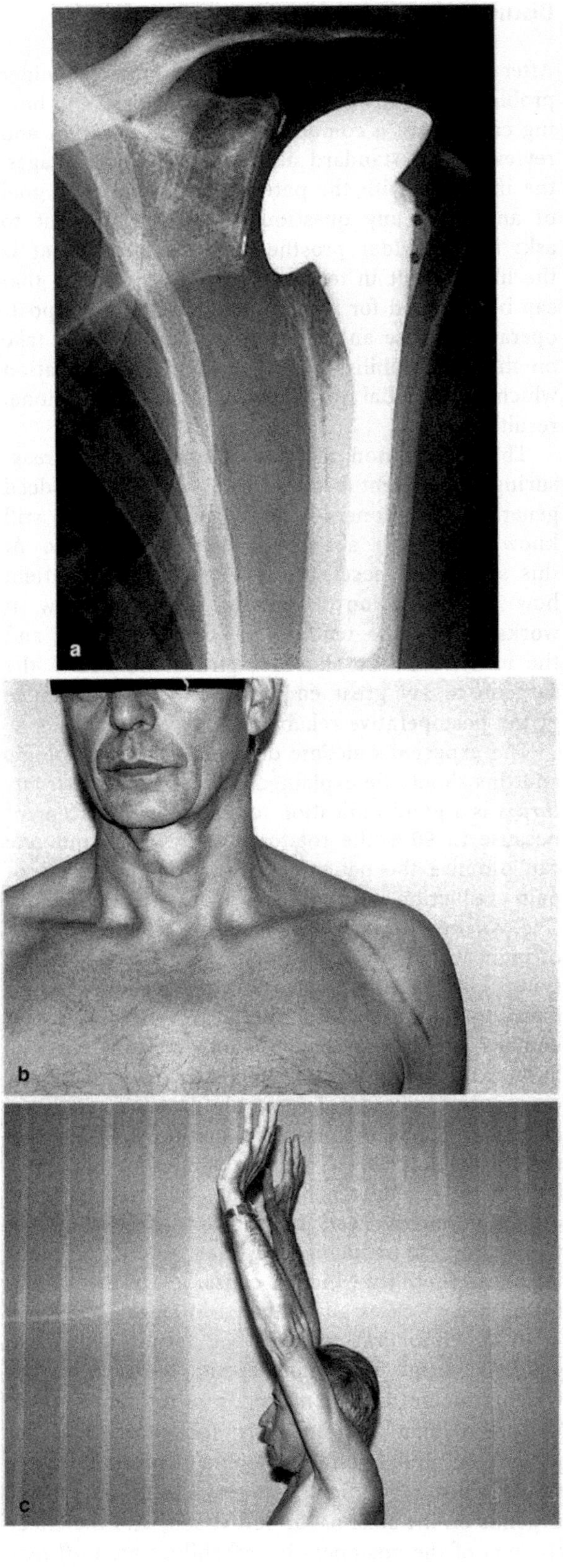

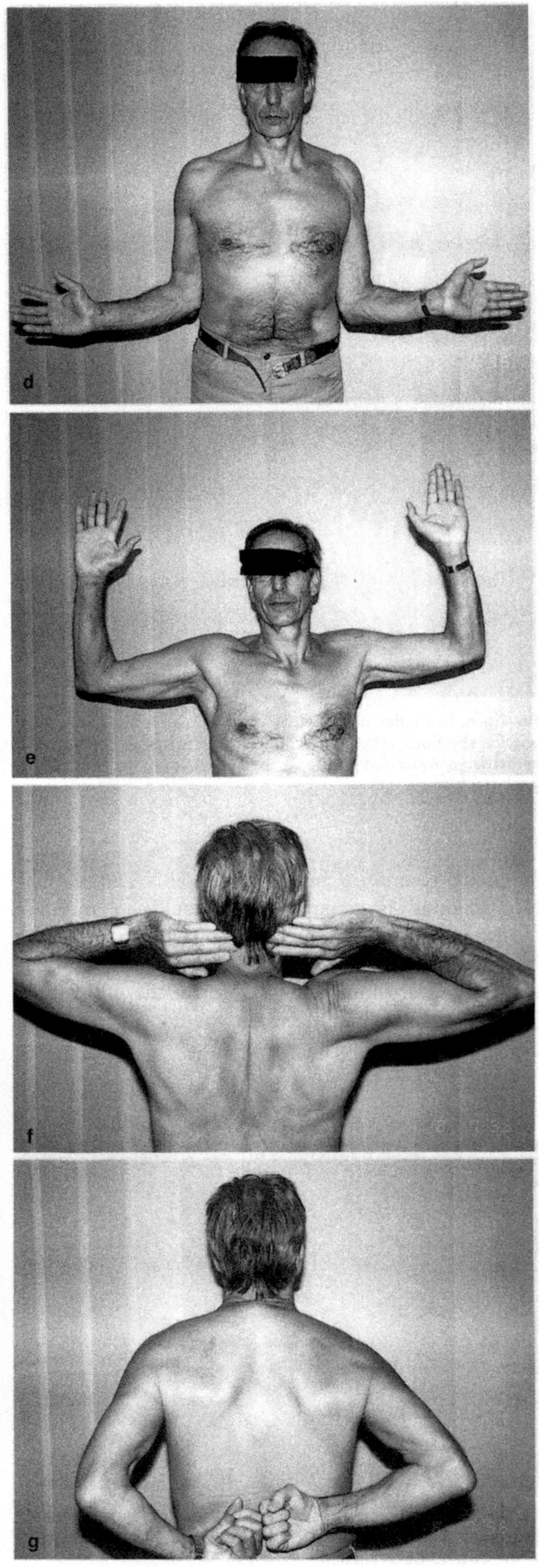

Fig. 4 a–g. Excellent functional result in a 57-year-old man with osteoarthritis, 3 months postoperatively pain, resistant to medical treatment (Fig. 5). With Neer [1], we prefer to insert a prosthesis with a large humeral head and without a glenoid component because there is a risk of glenoid loosening due to the "rocking horse effect". The results in terms of pain and function may make this worthwhile for a very handicapped and demanding patient. Lastly, the result of reconstructing *4-part fractures* around a humeral prosthesis depends on the quality of the tuberosity fixation, the age of the patient and the rehabilitation.

Finally, it is important to inform the patient about the methods that will be used in his rehabilitation, and that this can last for more than 6 months. We feel that immediate postoperative passive movement is essential to avoid stiffness, and that self-rehabilitation should be the dominant element taking the form of multiple daily sessions which may be carried out in outpatient physiotherapy or as an inpatient in a specialist rehabilitation centre. The rehabilitation will be much more effective if the patient has already been informed about the different phases in his rehabilitation, perhaps having been shown them on video, and has had some preoperative sessions with the physiotherapists. During these preoperative sessions the patient can familiarise himself with the simple exercises that he will be carrying out postoperatively both himself and under the guidance of the same physiotherapist (Fig. 6).

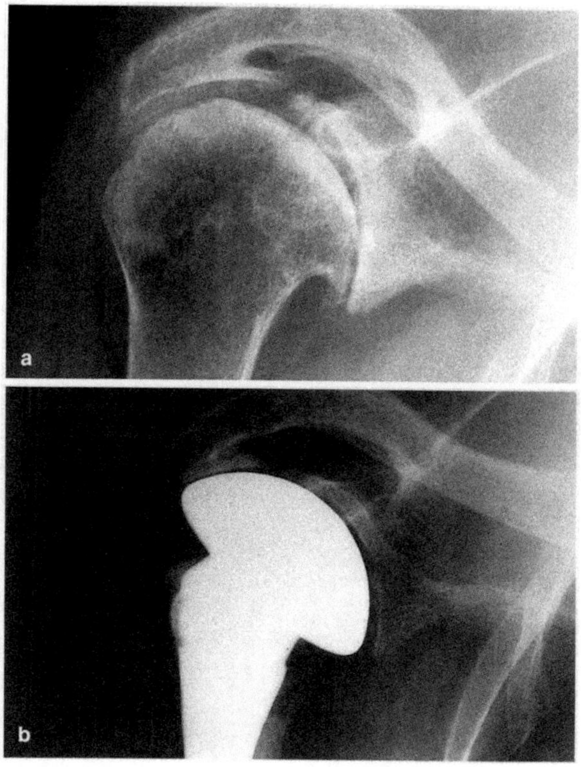

Fig. 5 a,b. Shoulder arthroplasty in a cuff tear arthritis

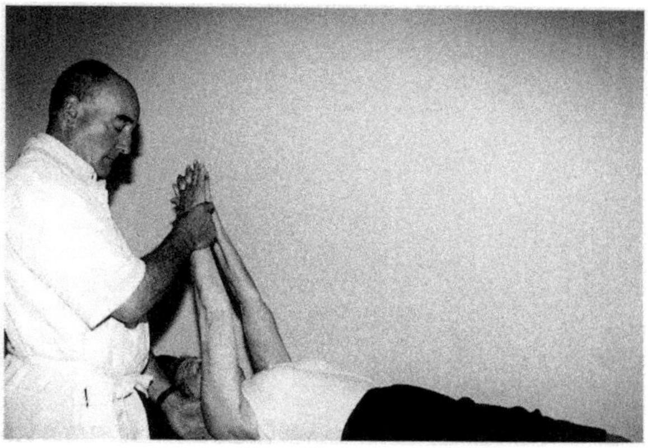

Fig. 6. Preoperative rehabilitation

Conclusion

The preoperative clinical evaluation of a patient in whom an arthroplasty may be indicated should set the scene for the surgeon providing him with an accurate idea of the current situation as well as preparing him for any potential per or postoperative problems. It establishes a relationship of trust between the patient and his surgeon which is essential in achieving good results in an operation which is heavily dependent on postoperative rehabilitation.

References

1. Neer CS (1990) Glenohumeral arthroplasty. In: Neer CS (ed) Shoulder reconstruction. Saunders, Philadelphia, pp 143–271
2. Constant CR, Murley AHG (1987) A clinical method of functional assessment of the shoulder. Clin Orthop 214(1):160–164
3. Constant CR (1997) Assessment of shoulder function. In: Gazielly DF, Gleyze P, Thomas T (eds) The cuff. Elsevier International, Paris, pp 39–44
4. Post M, Grinblat E (1994) Preoperative clinical evaluation. In: Friedman RJ (ed) Arthroplasty of the shoulder. Thieme Medical, New York, pp 41–52

Imaging Prior to Shoulder Arthroplasty

D. Goutallier, J. Alain, L. Lavau, and J. Bernageau

Summary

Imaging prior to shoulder arthroplasty allows accurate preoperative planning by evaluation of the bone stock and assessment of the musculo-tendinous status of the shoulder. Routine preoperative evaluation should consist of conventional radiology and modern imaging methods. The means for making this assessment are: (a) standard radiographs, particularly an anteroposterior view in neutral rotation, axillary view and lateral (outlet) view, (b) computed tomography scan with bony and soft tissue cuts, (c) computed tomographic arthrography. The latter two methods will no doubt be replaced by magnetic resonance imaging in the near future.

Preoperative imaging prior to a shoulder prosthesis plays an important role in confirming that gleno-humeral joint damage is present and in helping to determine its aetiology. It allows the differentiation between osteoarthritis and cuff tear arthritis, localises osteophytes and loose bodies in the joint or the bursae, defines the anatomy and shape of the proximal humerus and the glenoid, and assesses the state of the rotator cuff. It also gives information about the other joints of the shoulder such as the acromio-clavicular and sternoclavicular joints.

To provide this degree of information, imaging must include conventional radiography, computed tomography (CT) with bony and soft tissue settings, CT arthrography and or MRI.

Conventional Radiography

Routine preoperative evaluation should consist of at least an anteroposterior (AP) view in neutral rotation, an axillary view and a lateral (outlet) view. These allow the diagnosis of a gleno-humeral arthropathy and show the damage within the joint [1, 2, 3, 7, 11]. Damage to only one surface of the articulation favours a necrotic process whereas damage to both surfaces with narrowing of the joint space suggests rheumatoid or osteoarthritis. The arthritis is termed 'osteoarthritis' (Fig. 1) if the humeral head is normally situated in relation to the glenoid on both the AP and axillary radiographs.

In the frontal plane the humeral head is described as 'eccentric' if the acromio-humeral distance is less

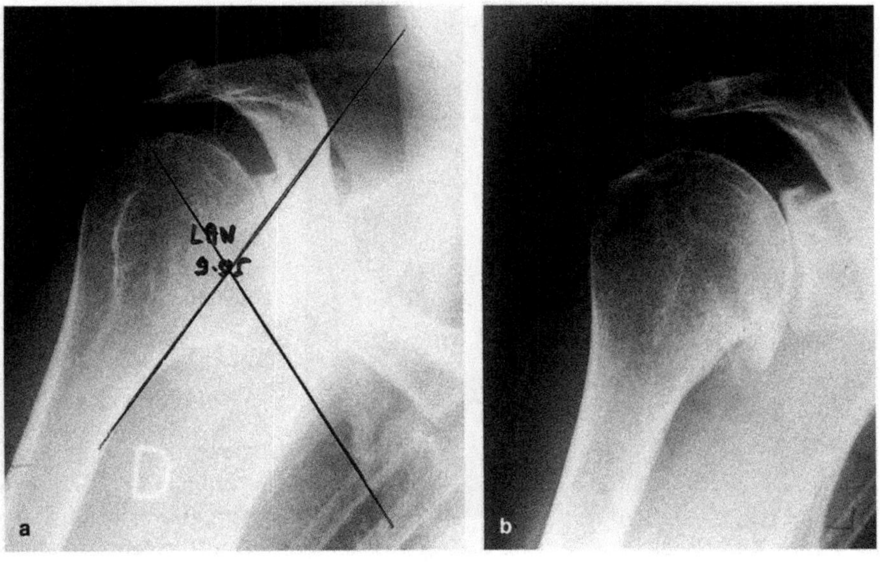

Fig. 1. AP view of gleno-humeral osteoarthritis.
a Poor technique does not allow a correct diagnosis.
b True AP view shows gleno-humeral cartilage space narrowing, inferior humeral osteophytes and a normal acromio-humeral distance

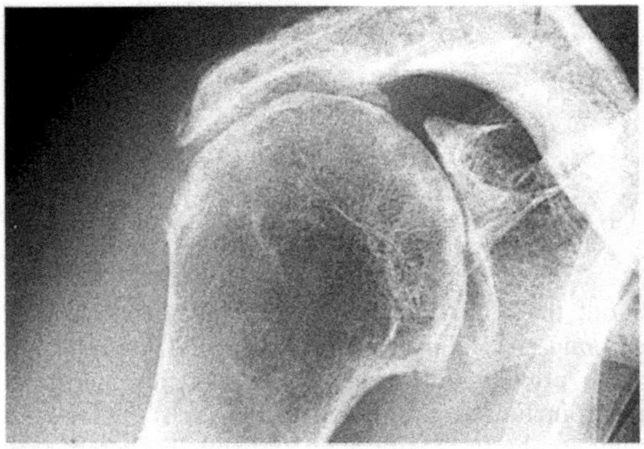

Fig. 2. Cuff tear arthritis: eccentricity of the humeral head in the frontal plane with narrowing of the gleno-humeral joint and narrowing of the acromio-humeral distance

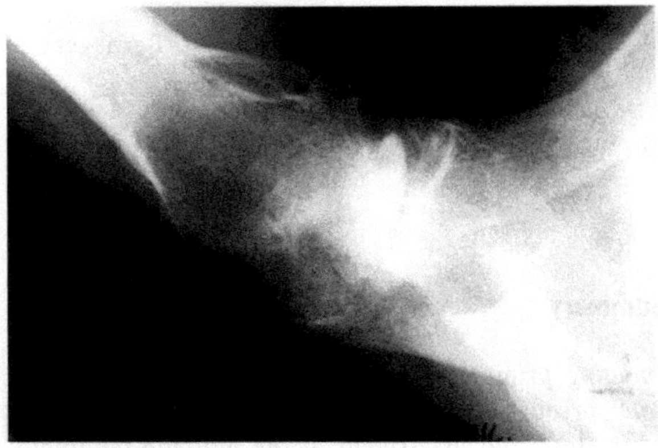

Fig. 4. Gleno-humeral osteoarthritis with posterior eccentricity of the humeral head as seen on the axillary view

than 5 mm on the AP neutral radiograph (Fig. 2). Such eccentricity, because of proximal migration of the humerus, almost always indicates a massive cuff tear [9]. However, a normally centred head may also coexist with a massive cuff tear. Wear of the inferior surface of the acromion is often found when the acromio-tuberosity distance is reduced but it can also be seen when this distance appears to be normal (>7 mm) and can be explained by a dynamic eccentricity of the humeral head which also accompanies a massive cuff tear. The humeral head is said to be in anterior or posterior eccentricity when the contact point between the head, and the glenoid is no longer central but has been displaced either towards the front or the rear.

Anterior eccentricity of more than 5 mm (Fig. 3) usually indicates a rupture of the subscapularis while posterior eccentricity (Fig. 4) indicates a rupture of the infraspinatus. However, recent ruptures of these tendons are not accompanied by such horizontal head eccentricity.

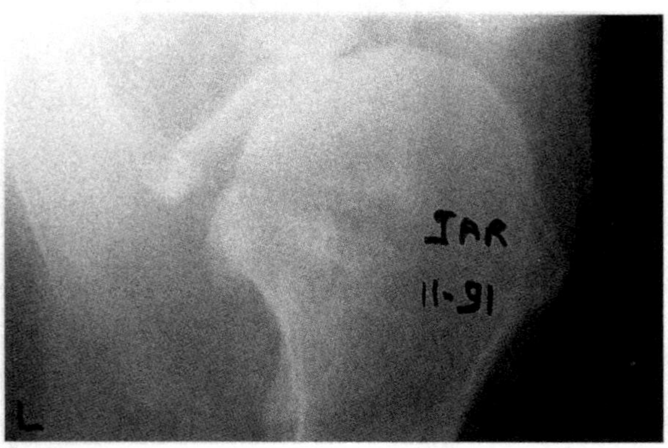

Fig. 3. Gleno-humeral osteoarthritis with anterior eccentricity of the humeral head as seen on the axillary view

The standard radiographs also demonstrate any loose bodies and their position within the joint or the bursae as well as showing osteophytes particularly of the inferior aspect of the humeral head or glenoid. The diameter of the humeral canal can be measured, and the shape and present position of the tuberosities can be seen. Analysis of the glenoid, however, is less accurate on these views [8].

CT Scan Bone Settings

These are essential to appreciate any congenital or acquired abnormalities in the orientation in the horizontal plane of the humeral and glenoid articular surfaces [4, 9]. The bone-setting views also show the site and size of any anterior or posterior osteophytes of the humerus or glenoid (Fig. 5) which need to be resected to allow the prosthesis to be properly inserted.

Only CT images demonstrate bone loss (Fig. 6) or changes in the glenoid (Fig. 7). This examination therefore determines whether it is possible to insert a glenoid component and forewarns of any potential peroperative difficulties.

As the scan is carried out with the patient supine, an anterior eccentricity which been seen on the axillary view is not demonstrated, and this indicates a non-fixed eccentricity. Similarly, the supine position may allow a non-fixed posterior subluxation of the humeral head to reduce.

Arthrography

Arthrography with images taken in the AP and in various rotations and in axillary and scapular views diagnose full and partial thickness cuff tears

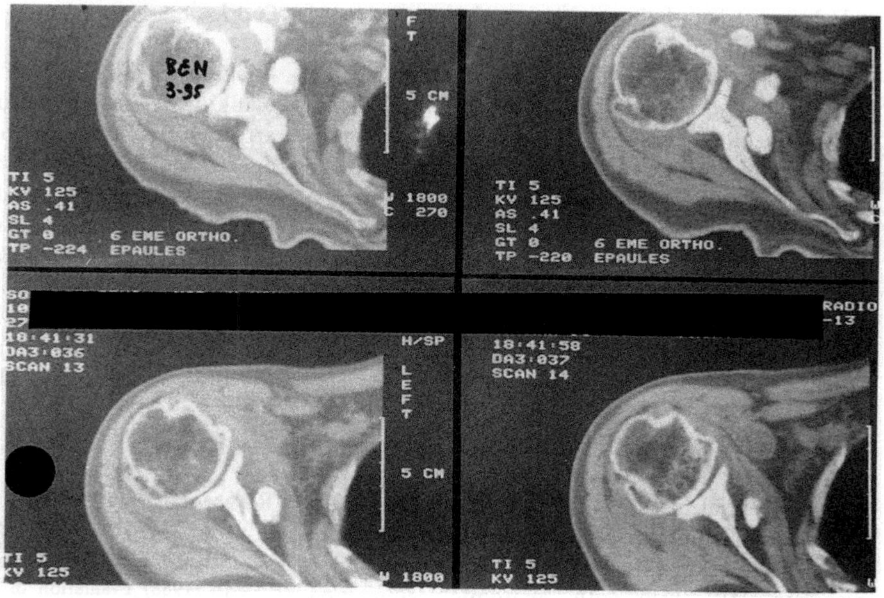

Fig. 5. CT appearance of an anterior glenoid osteophyte and anterior and posterior humeral osteophytes (note the large foreign body in the bursa)

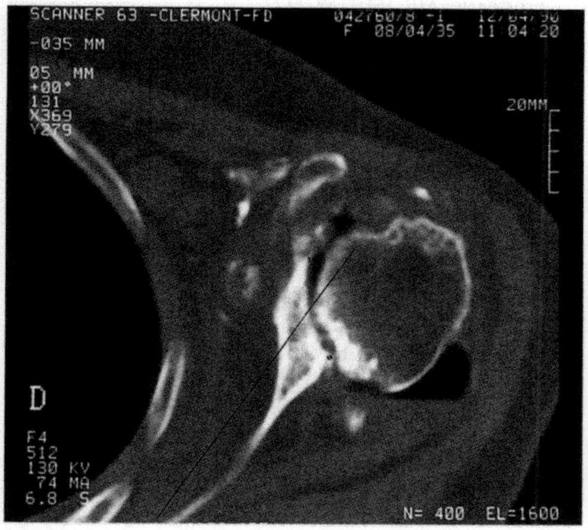

Fig. 6. CT appearance of predominantly posterior bone loss in the glenoid which is accentuated due to the increased glenoid retroversion. Note the posterior subluxation of the humeral head

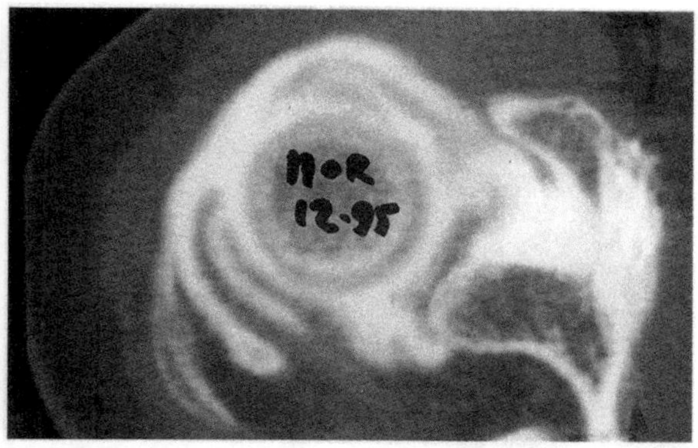

Fig. 8. View of a supraspinatus rupture combined with a cleavage in the infraspinatus tendon on the CT arthrogram

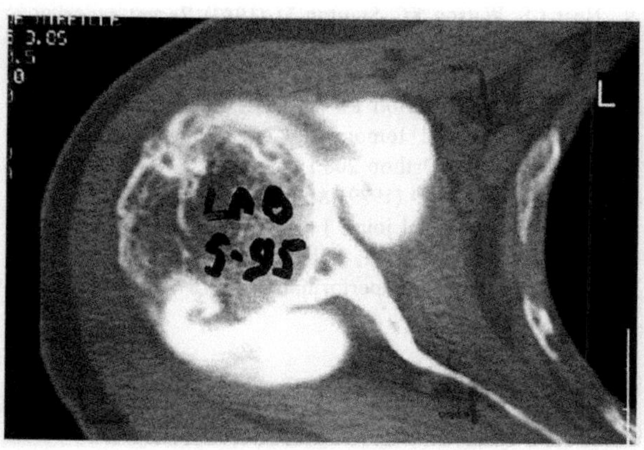

Fig. 7. CT appearance of concentric glenoid erosion with glenoid sclerosis in a patient with acromegaly

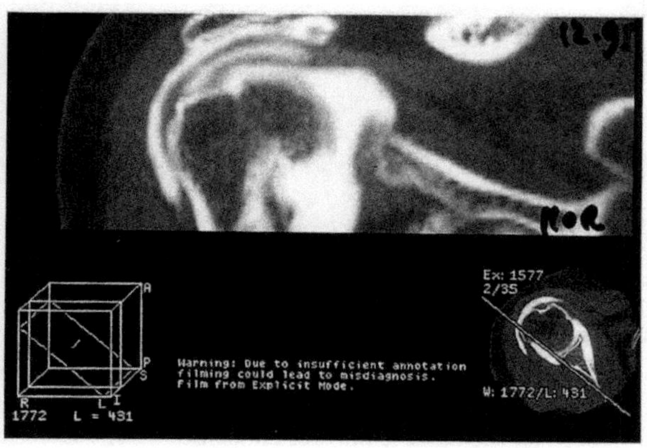

Fig. 9. Posterior cleavage of supraspinatus on CT reconstructed in the AP view

and demonstrate their position and the degree of musculo-tendinous retraction of supraspinatus [1]. The CT arthrogram with the images reconstructed in various planes, as possible with the new generation of machines, is a very powerful tool. It can precisely localise cuff tears and show their size and the degree of retraction of all the tendons not just supraspinatus. It can also show the intratendinous cleavages found with full and partial thickness tears (Figs. 8, 9) of the cuff [6]. In France CT arthrography provides better information than MRI, especially in analysing the subscapularis [1, 2, 6, 12].

CT Scan Soft-Tissue Settings

This is essential to assess the degree of fatty degeneration of the muscles of the cuff which determine muscular function [5]. It is much more powerful at this than MRI even with 'anatomic' sequencing. The scan allows the muscle degeneration to be classified into one of the five stages described (Fig. 10). It is important to realise that a gleno-humeral arthropathy without a cuff rupture may still be accompanied by fatty muscular degeneration although this is rarely greater than stage 2.

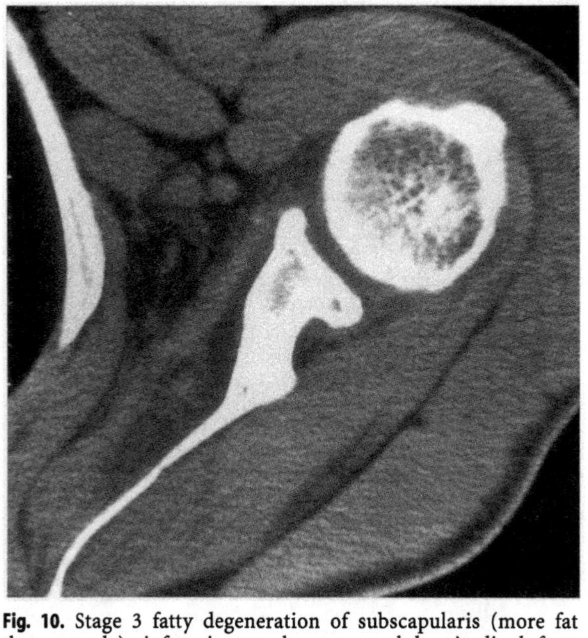

Fig. 10. Stage 3 fatty degeneration of subscapularis (more fat than muscle); infraspinatus shows several longitudinal fatty streaks (stage 1)

Conclusion

Imaging investigation of the shoulder when one is planning to insert a prosthesis allows the type of arthroplasty (hemi- or total), the implant sizes, peroperative difficulties and the quality of the postoperative functional result to be predicted. The preoperative imaging examination may also sometimes encourage quicker surgical intervention if the conditions for inserting a prosthesis already seem limited. On the other hand, in the case of a very damaged shoulder with poor bone stock and soft tissues, the investigations may also help decide against surgery.

References

1. Aliabadi P, Weissman BN, Thornhill T, Nikpoor N, Sosman JL (1988) Evaluation of a nonconstrained total shoulder prosthesis. AJR 151:1169–1172
2. Bernageau J, Goutallier D (1994) L'examen radiologique de la coiffe des rotateurs. In: Leprane M, Maldague B, Morvan G (eds) L'évaluation de l'imagerie de l'appareil moteur. Sauramps Médical, Paris, pp 329–343
3. DeKorvon LB, Ghossein IA, Kadouch R, Duvauferrier R (1989) Value of modern imaging in the anatomical study of the shoulder. Ann Radiol 32:234–243
4. Friedman RJ, Hawthorne KB, Genez BM (1992) The use of computerized tomography in the measurement of glenoid version. J Bone Joint Surg Am 74:1032–1037
5. Goutallier D, Postel JM, Bernageau J, Lavau L, Voisin (1995) Fatty degeneration in cuff ruptures pre and postoperative evaluation by CT-scan. Clin Orthop 304:78–83
6. Goutallier D, Postel JM, Lavau L, Bernageau J (1996) Clivage des tendons de la coiffe. In: Laredo JD, Bard H (eds) La coiffe des rotateurs et son environnement. Sauramps Médical, Paris, pp-45–49
7. Keer R, Resnick D, Pineda C, Haghighi P (1985) Osteoarthritis of the glenohumeral joint: a radiologic-pathologic study. AJR 144:967–972
8. Mallon WJ, Brown HR, Vogler JB, Martinez S (1992) Radiographic and geometric anatomy of the scapula. Clin Orthop 277:142–154
9. Neer CS, Watson KC, Stanton FJ (1982) Recent experience in total shoulder replacement. J Bone Joint Surg Am 64:319–337
10. Randelli M, Gambrioli PL (1986) Glenohumeral osteometry by computed tomography in normal and unstable shoulders. Clin Orthop 208:151–156
11. Silvka J, Resnick D (1979) An improved radiographic view of the genohumeral joint. J Can Assoc Radiol 30:83–85
12. Zlatkin MB, Iannotti JP, Roberts MC et al (1989) Rotator cuff tears: diagnostic performance of MR imaging. Radiology 172:223–229

Anaesthesia and Analgesia for Shoulder Arthroplasty

W. Harrop-Griffiths and S. Dwyer

Summary

The two techniques of anesthesia for shoulder arthroplasty (general anaesthesia and regional anaesthesia) are not mutually exclusive and can be usefully combined. Advantages, disadvantages and complications of general and regional anaesthesia, used alone or in combination, should be known and are reported in details. Furthermore, the anaesthetist should be aware of adverse cardiovascular effects related to the fact that shoulder replacement is performed in the beach chair position. Shoulder arthroplasty is associated with significant postoperative pain and all the options for analgesia should be familiar to the anaesthetist. Pain management techniques, including brachial plexus blockade, patient-controlled analgesia and brachial plexus catheterisation are also detailed.

Introduction

It would be easy to dismiss the subject of anaesthesia for shoulder arthroplasty as being so similar to that for other orthopaedic disciplines that it does not warrant separate discussion. However, anaesthesia for shoulder arthroplasty provides a variety of challenges that are seldom found in combination in other orthopaedic disciplines. The aim of this chapter is not to provide an exhaustive treatise on orthopaedic anaesthesia as a whole but to highlight those areas of anaesthesia and analgesia that are worthy of particular consideration with respect to the management of patients undergoing shoulder arthroplasty.

Joint replacement surgery is commonplace, and the overwhelming majority of anaesthetists are familiar with the principles and practice of anaesthesia for such procedures. However, joint replacement in the beach-chair, i.e. semi-recumbent position provides further physiological challenges of which the anaesthetist needs to be aware. The performance of brachial plexus nerve blocks to provide regional anaesthesia or analgesia requires additional knowledge, training and skill and carries with it a number of potentially hazardous complications. Shoulder arthroplasty is associated with significant postoperative pain, and the anaesthetist should therefore be familiar with a range of pain management techniques, including brachial plexus blockade, patient-controlled analgesia and brachial plexus catheterisation.

Preoperative Preparation

Assessment

The majority of patients scheduled to undergo emergency or elective shoulder arthroplasty are middle-aged or elderly. Many of the pathological processes responsible for postoperative morbidity and mortality are age related, and the anaesthetist therefore needs to perform a scrupulous preoperative assessment. In the course of this evaluation the anaesthetist should pay particular attention to the respiratory and cardiovascular systems. Although it is rarely necessary to cancel a patient's operation as a result of respiratory or cardiovascular disorders, it is often necessary to postpone surgery so that optimisation of these systems can be undertaken before surgery is performed. The anaesthetist should have a low threshold for referral of the patient to a physician of the appropriate speciality.

The common association between the need for shoulder arthroplasty and the existence of longstanding osteo-arthritis or rheumatoid arthritis should prompt the anaesthetist to explore the impact of these disorders on the patient. Difficulties in positioning the patient on the operating table may result from fixed flexion deformities. Limitation of neck movement in both osteo-arthritis and rheumatoid arthritis may produce difficulties in airway management and tracheal intubation. Rheumatoid arthritis may cause limited mouth opening as a result of its effects on the tempero-mandibular joints. Rheumatoid arthritis may lead to cervical spine instability, and lateral cervical spine X-rays should therefore be performed before surgery and the opinion of a radiologist should be sought on whether the patient's neck is unstable, and if so, whether neck extension may pose a threat to the patient's spinal cord during intubation, anaesthesia and surgery. If there is any suspicion of significant cervical spine instability that is not amenable to treatment, appropriate steps should be taken to ensure that the patient's neck is maintained in a safe position throughout anaesthesia and surgery. Rheumatoid arthritis is also associated with significant cardiac, pulmonary and renal pathology.

Chronic drug therapy for arthritis may include steroid therapy and treatment with non-steroidal anti-inflammatory drugs (NSAIDs). If the patient is on regular steroid therapy, replacement therapy must be instituted to minimise the possibility of an acute Addisonian crisis. Long-term NSAID therapy may be associated with anaemia as a result of adverse gastro-intestinal effects and with impaired renal function. Platelet dysfunction and hence marked haemorrhage during and after surgery may occur in patients taking NSAIDs.

After the performance of a full clinical history and examination, appropriate investigations should be conducted. Blood loss during shoulder arthroplasty can be significant and haemoglobin concentration should be measured. Many anaesthetists choose to cross-match blood for shoulder arthroplasty although it is rarely necessary to give a blood transfusion.

Informing the Patient

The options for both anaesthesia and analgesia should be discussed with the patient. The anaesthetist should ensure that the patient has as full an appreciation of the likely occurrences during and after surgery as is possible and appropriate. The complications of the techniques to be used should be discussed with the patient. The mode of anaesthesia and of analgesia should be a decision that is taken jointly by the patient, anaesthetist and surgeon.

Premedication

There is no one premedication that offers particular advantages to the patient about to undergo shoulder arthroplasty. The decision of whether to administer a premedication and, if so, which one to give should be left to the patient and the individual anaesthetist.

Choice of Anaesthetic Technique

The choice of anaesthetic technique is of course guided by the patient's general medical condition and the preferences expressed by anaesthetist, patient and surgeon. There is a long-running debate about whether regional anaesthesia is safer than general anaesthesia. Anaesthetists participating in shoulder surgery are likely to be biased towards regional anaesthesia as a fondness for loco-regional anaesthesia may have drawn them towards this speciality. However, many anaesthetists rely on a body of literature suggesting that regional anaesthesia offers little in terms of decreased risk when compared with general anaesthesia. Similarly, regional anaesthesia enthusiasts can cite an equally large body of literature supporting their view. It has been argued that "regional anesthesia is inherently safer because the risk of adverse respiratory events associated with general anesthesia are avoided" [48]. However, as is seen below, regional anaesthesia for shoulder arthroplasty is not free from adverse respiratory effects. Familiarity with the various techniques and scrupulous attention to detail is probably more important than the choice of technique itself in managing the vast majority of patients.

Although the choice of technique for shoulder arthroplasty lies simplistically between general anaesthesia and regional anaesthesia, the anaesthetist should avoid the temptation to become dogmatic in his or her choice. The two techniques are not mutually exclusive and can be usefully combined. Therefore the full range of choices includes: general anaesthesia alone, regional anaesthesia alone, regional anaesthesia with sedation and combined regional and general anaesthesia.

General Anaesthesia

Advantages of General Anaesthesia

General anaesthesia offers the patient a guarantee of unconsciousness during, and amnesia for, the surgical procedure and guarantees the surgeon a completely immobile patient throughout the course of surgery. All anaesthetists are familiar with the administration of a general anaesthetic. General anaesthesia is usually quick to administer and has a nearly 100 % success rate. Although only moderate muscle relaxation is provided by general anaesthetics, this is usually adequate for shoulder arthroplasty. If necessary, neuromuscular blocking drugs can be given during general anaesthesia to ensure total muscle paralysis.

Disadvantages of General Anaesthesia

Against the above advantages of general anaesthesia must be set its disadvantages. Foremost amongst these are physiological effects on the respiratory and cardiovascular systems which, although they may have few adverse effects on fit individuals, may have a significant impact on patients with impaired respiratory or cardiovascular function.

General anaesthesia has adverse pulmonary effects. Mucociliary function is impaired, and even subclinical amounts of general anaesthetic impair ventilatory responses to hypoxia and hypercarbia. General anaesthesia is associated with a decrease in functional residual capacity (FRC), i.e. the lung volume at the end of a normal expiration. If FRC falls below closing capacity (the lung volume at which small airways collapse begins), gas exchange is impaired, and hypoxia or relative hypoxia can occur. This effect is small in fit patients and is readily overcome by an increase in inspired oxygen concentration during and after anaesthesia. However, the impact on patients with pulmonary disease can be significant and as a result many anaesthetists would wish to avoid general anaesthesia in these patients. Some patients with severe chronic lung disease may become ventilator-dependent for a period of time after general anaesthesia, although this is a rare occurrence. Unfortunately, regional anaesthesia for shoulder arthroplasty is associated with impairment of ventilatory function as a result of phrenic nerve paralysis, which occurs in 100% of patients undergoing interscalene brachial plexus block [67].

The question of whether general anaesthesia or regional anaesthesia should be chosen for patients with significant lung disease remains unanswered. In the authors' experience, it is possible to perform shoulder arthroplasty under interscalene brachial plexus blockade alone in patients with severe chronic obstructive airways disease without any noticeable clinical deterioration in pulmonary function. The authors attribute this to the fact that diaphragmatic function is impaired in these patients as a result of lung over-expansion, and that therefore it is likely that the work of the diaphragm adds little to the patients' ventilatory capacity.

General anaesthesia has a significant impact on cardiovascular function. General anaesthetic agents are associated with decreased systemic vascular resistance and decreased myocardial contractility. A decrease in arterial blood pressure is therefore almost universal during general anaesthesia. Again, these effects are unlikely to have a significant impact on fit patients. However, changes in blood pressure are more marked in hypertensive patients and may produce myocardial ischaemia in those patients suffering from ischaemic heart disease. The vasodilation that accompanies general anaesthesia may prove very dangerous in patients with stenotic heart valve disease. Another important cardiovascular effect of general anaesthesia is its propensity to blunt or abolish cardiovascular homeostatic responses. In the unanaesthetised individual, hypotension leads to an increased sympathetic tone via a reflex mediated by baroreceptors. General anaesthesia impairs this reflex response. It is also worthy of note that there is evidence that even in healthy persons autonomic impairment inevitably begins in middle age and increases with advancing age.

Careful anaesthetic management can minimise the occurrence of hypotension as well as its extent and impact. However, the adoption of the beach-chair position for shoulder arthroplasty causes pooling of the blood in the dependent venous circulation and can further aggravate hypotension by reducing venous return. Therefore even in healthy patients the adoption of the beach-chair position under general anaesthesia can result in significant hypotension. This problem can, of course, be prevented, ameliorated or resolved with the use of intravenous fluids and vasoconstrictor agents. However, for the above reasons many anaesthetists prefer to avoid general anaesthesia in patients with significant cardiovascular disease.

General anaesthesia is occasionally the only option when the anaesthetist determines that there is an absolute contra-indication to regional anaesthesia. This situation may occur if the patient is suffering from a significant coagulopathy, generalised sepsis or sepsis localised to the area through which the brachial plexus block is placed. If the patient refuses to consider regional anaesthesia, general anaesthesia is also indicated.

Technique of General Anaesthesia

There is no one technique of general anaesthesia that is specifically indicated for shoulder arthroplasty. The technique used should be one with which the anaesthetist is familiar. Although many anaesthetists choose to intubate the patient's trachea for surgery in the beach-chair position, airway maintenance with a laryngeal mask airway (LMA) is often appropriate. The use of the LMA avoids many of the potential complications associated with tracheal intubation and is being increasingly favoured by anaesthetists for procedures of intermediate or long duration where spontaneous ventilation is feasible and safe. One disadvantage of the use of the LMA is that if its position alters during the operation, and the airway is compromised as a result, it may not be easy to gain rapid access to the patient's head if it is covered, and the patient is in the beach-chair position. LMA should not be used in patients at risk of regurgitation.

Routine monitoring for patients undergoing shoulder arthroplasty under general anaesthesia should include: ECG, non-invasive blood pressure, pulse oximetry and capnography. Further monitoring devices may be added to this list at the anaesthetist's discretion. Institution of this monitoring before adoption of the beach-chair position is advised because of the possibility of acute hypotension as described above. Capnography is of particular use as air embolism is a possibility because the operation site is above the level of the heart. The development of hypothermia is possible in long operations involving significant blood loss. Many anaesthetists therefore choose to use a heating blanket of some form. If external heating is used, the monitoring of patient temperature is advised. The intravenous cannula should be placed in the arm that is not the subject of the surgeon's attention. Two approaches can be adopted to avoid "back-tracking" of blood back up the intravenous infusion line. Either the blood pressure cuff can be placed on one of the patient's legs or a one way (anti-reflux) valve can be placed in the infusion line. Care should be exercised to ensure that the size of the blood pressure cuff is appropriate for the part of the leg to be used. The placement of an arterial line is seldom necessary.

If general anaesthesia alone is to be used for shoulder arthroplasty, the anaesthetist should ensure that adequate analgesia is given during the operation to guarantee that the patient does not awake to significant pain.

Regional Anaesthesia

Regional Anaesthesia Techniques for Shoulder Arthroplasty

It is a source of joy to all regional anaesthetists that the nerves to almost all of the upper limb are conveniently packaged within a fascial sheath that extends from the cervical vertebrae to mid-way down the upper arm (Fig. 1). It is therefore possible to produce local anaesthesia of the nerves supplying the upper limb with a single injection of local anaesthetic that then spreads within and is contained by the fascial sheath. However, the extent of the effects of local anaesthetic injection within the sheath varies with the exact location of the injection and the volume and concentration of local anaesthetic agent used.

The brachial plexus is formed from the anterior rami of the fifth cervical root to the first thoracic root, with variable contributions from the fourth cervical root and the second thoracic root. The distribution of the nerve supply is such that the shoulder and upper outer arm are supplied by the upper roots of the plexus, and the hand and the inner arm are supplied by the lower roots. Logic therefore dictates that the upper roots of the brachial plexus should be blocked to provide adequate anaesthesia for operations on the shoulder. As the nerves supplying the shoulder joint and the skin over it (the suprascapular and axillary nerves) leave the brachial plexus above the clavicle, it is again reasonable to assert that the approach used to the brachial plexus should be above the clavicle. Although it is certainly possible to block the nerves to the shoulder using infraclavicular approaches (i.e. the infraclavicular approach and the axillary approach), large volumes of local anaesthetic would be needed to guarantee an adequate spread of anaesthesia. Spread of local anaesthesia within the brachial plexus is largely determined by volume – the greater the volume the greater the spread. For direct local anaesthetic placement around the upper roots of the plexus, the interscalene approach first described by Winnie [72] has much to commend it.

An interscalene brachial plexus block can be performed as follows: intravenous access is placed, appropriate monitoring is attached and the patient lies supine with the head turned away from the shoulder to be anaesthetised. The patient is asked to tense the muscles of the neck as if he or she were about to lift his or her head off the pillow. This causes contraction and thus easy identification of the sternocleidomastoid muscle. The anaesthetist's index finger is placed on the muscle at the level of the cricoid cartilage (i.e. at the level of the sixth cervical vertebra) and is moved to the lateral

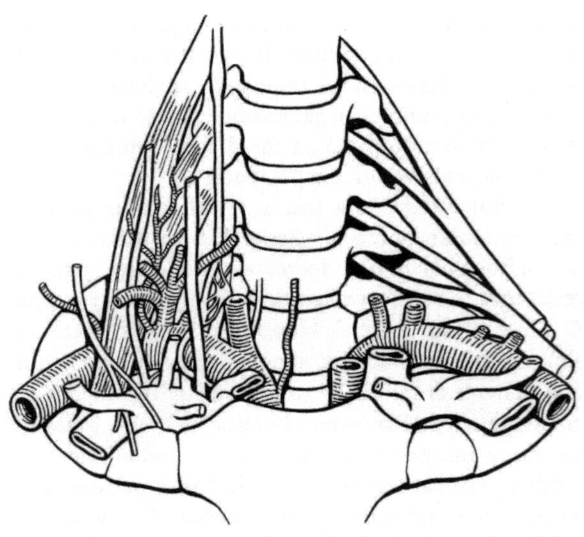

Fig. 1. The upper roots of the brachial plexus should be blocked to provide adequate anaesthesia for operations on the shoulder. The approach used to the brachial plexus should be above the clavicle

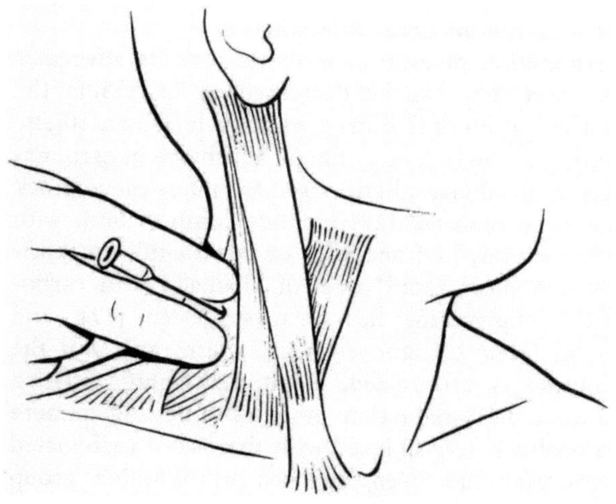

Fig. 2. Palpation of the groove between the anterior and middle scalene muscles, i.e. the interscalene groove, behind the sternocleidomastoid muscle, allows the needle to be passed at right angles to the skin, i.e. posteriorly, medially and inferiorly

border. The patient is asked to relax his or her neck. The anaesthetist's finger should now move slightly medially so that the fingernail on the palpating finger almost disappears behind the sternocleidomastoid muscle. The index finger should now lie on the belly of the anterior scalene muscle. Moving the finger laterally allows palpation of the groove between the anterior and middle scalene muscles, i.e. the interscalene groove. This is the point of insertion of the needle (Fig. 2). If the interscalene groove is not easily palpable, as may occur with obese, short-necked patients, a useful observation made by Winnie [73] is that "the external jugular vein, when visible, crosses the interscalene groove virtually 100 % of the time". Having identified the correct position, a needle is passed at right angles to the skin, i.e. posteriorly, medially and inferiorly. Confirmation of correct placement can be sought either by a report of paraesthesiae in the distribution of the brachial plexus or with the use of a nerve stimulator.

Use of Nerve Stimulators

Whenever two or more regional anaesthetists are gathered together in one place, they are likely at some point to discuss the advantages and disadvantages of the use of a nerve stimulator to identify nerves and nerve plexuses. There is a substantial number of anaesthetists who claim that a nerve stimulator is not needed – a paraesthesia evoked by a needle is all that is needed, and once this is produced, correct placement is assured and injection can be performed. Their axiom is: "no paraesthesia, no anaesthesia". They claim that knowledge of anatomy, scrupulous attention to detail and a target of a proximal paraesthesia is all that is to required to produce a near 100 % success rate in the performance of an interscalene brachial plexus block [45]. Anaesthetists who oppose this view claim that the production of a paraesthesia implies ipso facto nerve trauma and hence the possibility of persisting nerve damage. As prolonged neurological problems are known to be a complication, albeit rare, of regional anaesthesia, this camp adopt the axiom: "no paraesthesia, no dysaesthesia". The truth, as ever, lies somewhere in between. It matters not how one identifies the brachial plexus; it matters only that one does identify it and places the appropriate amount of local anaesthetic within the fascial sheath at the appropriate level while avoiding significant direct nerve damage and intraneural injection. It is becoming evident that the number of anaesthetists using nerve stimulators for plexus location is increasing, and that they now outnumber those who rely upon paraesthesiae alone.

Another factor of importance is that paraesthesiae can be sought only in the awake and co-operative patient whereas nerve location with a nerve stimulator can be performed on awake, heavily sedated or anaesthetised patients. However, to avoid intraneural injection (see below) many anaesthetists choose to perform regional blocks on awake or lightly sedated patients, regardless of whether they use a nerve stimulator.

Needle Tip Design

The shape of the tip of the needle to be used for regional anaesthesia is also a topic of debate. Most anaesthetists now prefer short-bevel needles to long bevel needles as these are felt to be less likely to transect nerve fibres if they enter a nerve and they give a more positive feeling of entry into the plexus sheath. Those still in favour of long-bevelled needles argue that if the very tip of a long-bevel needle enters a nerve, a paraesthesia is produced, but the injection is not placed directly into the nerve.

After their success in reducing postdural puncture headache in obstetric anaesthetic practice, pencil-point needles are making an impact on regional anaesthesia. Their extreme bluntness certainly gives an excellent indication of when the fascial sheath is penetrated; however, there is currently little convincing evidence to support their universal use [42]. There is an argument for a relationship between needle tip design and iatrogenic nerve damage [7, 31, 50], but the issue is not resolved. A relationship between tip design and nerve damage is supported by some basic science research [43, 44, 51]. A study specifically addressing the impact of needle tip design and orientation which included an assessment of a pencil point needle and both long and short bevelled needles concluded that the pencil point needle is likely to be associated with the lowest incidence of nerve damage and that short or long bevel needles cause less damage when the bevel is aligned parallel to the nerve fibres [23]. The authors find the arguments in favour of the use of pencil point needles to be convincing, and it is their current practice to use them for all interscalene brachial plexus blocks. It should be noted that pencil point needles can be extremely difficult to pass through skin without the assistance of a small hole made with a lancet or long bevel hypodermic needle.

Drugs for Interscalene Brachial Plexus Blocks

Local Anaesthetics

There are reports of most local currently available anaesthetics being used for interscalene brachial plexus blockade, including bupivacaine, lignocaine, etidocaine, prilocaine and mepivacaine. Each anaesthetist has his or her favoured drug or drugs and there seems little reason to choose between these, although lignocaine and bupivacaine (or a combination of the two) seem popular. Drug choice of course affects the onset time and duration of the block. If anaesthesia rather than analgesia is planned, drug concentrations towards the higher end of the scale for each local anaesthetic should be used to provide a pain free procedure with adequate motor block and hence muscle relaxation.

As suggested before, local anaesthetic volume is important. Using the interscalene approach, 20 ml should be considered a minimum volume. Most regional anaesthetists favour local anaesthetic volumes between 30 and 40 ml for shoulder arthroplasty. Attention must be paid to ensuring that the dose of local anaesthetic does not exceed the maximum acceptable dose in order to avoid local anaesthetic toxicity. Not surprisingly, there appears to be an inverse correlation between the weight of the patient and the maximum plasma concentration of the local anaesthetic after the performance of a brachial plexus block, although this relationship is not always reliable [39]. Adrenaline may be added to the solution to decrease the rate of systemic local anaesthetic absorption and to prolong the block. The addition of adrenaline may also increase motor blockade. Concentrations of adrenaline between 1:200 000 and 1:400 000 are popular.

Carbonation of Local Anaesthetics

Carbonation of local anaesthetics has its advocates as onset time can be decreased by increasing the concentration of free drug within a local anaesthetic solution. The lack of a clinical advantage in carbonation of local anaesthetics used for interscalene block has been reported [20] but this conflicts both with other studies [59] and with our own clinical experience. A more rapid onset of blockade with carbonated bupivacaine has been suggested [17], and blood levels of lignocaine rise more rapidly if the solution is carbonated, albeit not significantly so [55]. A 38 % reduction in onset time and a more extensive block achieved with the use of carbonated lignocaine has been reported by Winnie's group [54]. On balance, it seems highly likely that the carbonation of local anaesthetic solutions increases the speed of onset of interscalene blocks for shoulder surgery.

Addition of Opiate Drugs

The addition of opiate drugs to local anaesthetic solutions for brachial plexus anaesthesia is also an area of controversy. There is evidence that peripheral nerves, which do not normally express opioid receptors, may express these when there is tissue damage within their area of distribution. Butorphanol placed in the brachial plexus has been reported to provide superior analgesia to butorphanol given intravenously [69], and the addition of butorphanol to mepivacaine for postoperative axillary brachial plexus catheter infusion improves analgesic efficacy [70]. However, the lack of additional analgesic effect of the addition of morphine to bupivacaine for brachial plexus block for shoulder surgery has been demonstrated [13]. Anecdotal reports exist that the addition of fentanyl to local anaesthetic brachial plexus infusions can improve the quality of postoperative analgesia [26, 33]. Although the benefits of opiate administration to the brachial plexus await substantive proof, it is the authors' belief that formal studies will confirm the efficacy of this technique. Pethidine alone has been given by the interscalene route as a sole agent for shoulder surgery [10].

Ropivacaine

Ropivacaine, a recently (at the time of writing) introduced amide local anaesthetic, offers potential benefits in its use for brachial plexus blockade for both surgery and postoperative analgesia. Ropivacaine appears to have a lower capacity to block motor nerves than bupivacaine [28] and is thought to have a lower potential for cardiac toxicity. Its potential for producing this problem is between that of bupivacaine and that of lignocaine [29]. Clinical and pharmacokinetic properties similar to those of bupivacaine have been shown in axillary plexus block [68] and subclavian perivascular block [21, 22]. The addition of adrenaline does not appear to affect ropivacaine's pharmacokinetic [18] or clinical properties [20] when used for brachial plexus block.

The authors currently favour the following drug combination for interscalene brachial plexus blocks for shoulder arthroplasty in a healthy adult weighing about 70 kg: a mixture of: lignocaine 2% 20 ml, bupivacaine 0.5% 20 ml, adrenaline 100 µg, fentanyl 80 µg, and sodium bicarbonate 8.4% 4.4 ml.

Complications of Interscalene Blocks

Interscalene blocks are not without their side effects, and it is the potential severity of these that leads some anaesthetists to eschew them.

Nerve Damage

Brachial plexus damage during shoulder arthroplasty is not uncommonly the responsibility of the surgeon. However, it can„ on occasion„ occur after interscalene block. Barutell has reported permanent neurological damage to the motor outflow of at least two of the C7, C8 and T1 motor nerve roots [1]. It is likely that one possible cause of iatrogenic nerve damage is inadvertent intraneural injection. The hallmarks of intraneural injection are said to be:

- Pain and paraesthesia on needle placement.
- No diminution of muscle twitch amplitude on decreasing nerve stimulator current.
- Ability to produce muscle twitches at very low current, i.e. less than 0.25 mA.
- Extreme pain on injection.
- No disappearance of muscle twitches evoked by the stimulator on initiating local anaesthetic injection.

The performance of a brachial plexus block on a patient who is anaesthetised or so generously sedated that he or she is unable to report pain on injection removes from the anaesthetist the sign that some would consider to be the most reliable in the above list, i.e. severe pain on injection. It is therefore common practice to perform all blocks on the awake or only lightly sedated patient. However, there is also a significant body of responsible regional anaesthetic opinion that feels it entirely reasonable to perform a plexus block on an anaesthetised patient with a nerve stimulator, and that this is particularly desirable when surgery is related to trauma as it eliminates the pain which would be caused by movement of the shoulder or arm.

Accidental Intravascular Injection

The following blood vessels are in the vicinity of the interscalene portion of the brachial plexus: carotid artery, vertebral artery, internal jugular vein and external jugular vein. Injection of a significant amount of local anaesthetic into any of these vessels initially produces light-headedness, dizziness, tinnitus and peri-oral paraesthesiae followed by convulsions and cardiac arrest. Injection of local anaesthetic into the vertebral artery via a brachial plexus catheter has been reported [64].

Accidental Subarachnoid Injection

It is possible to deliver the local anaesthetic solution into the subarachnoid space if the dura is inadvertently punctured. If this happens, a "total spinal" block is likely to ensue [11]. The patient rapidly becomes profoundly hypotensive, loses consciousness, and stops breathing. Immediate support of both ventilation and circulation is mandatory. A case has been reported [34] of accidental subarachnoid injection followed by permanent neurological deficit (damage to the posterior spinal cord and the nerve to infraspinatus). Accidental subdural anesthesia producing apnoea and both high motor and sensory block has been reported [58].

Accidental Epidural Injection

Similarly, the epidural space can be accessed by accident during an interscalene block [25, 49]. It is interesting to note that Kumar's report was the second publication ever produced on interscalene block – the first one being Winnie's original description of the technique 1 year earlier. Small volumes of local anaesthetic given into the epidural space produces a sensory and then motor nerve block of the upper limbs. Larger volumes produce hypotension and difficulty in breathing as the phrenic nerves become blocked. Ventilation and circulation must be actively supported in this situation.

Pneumothorax

The dome of the pleura extends behind and above the clavicle in the posterior triangle of the neck. Although the production of a pneumothorax during an interscalene block is unlikely provided that the needle entry point is not positioned too caudally and the needle itself is not directed too caudally, it is a recognised complication. It is of interest that much of the popularity of the interscalene brachial plexus block for upper limb procedures derives from the low incidence of pneumothorax that it enjoys compared with the previously popular supraclavicular approach. If the pneumothorax is large or produces symptoms, it should be treated along conventional management lines with a chest drain.

Cervical Sympathectomy

This is such a frequent and benign accompaniment of interscalene brachial plexus block that it barely justifies the term "complication". The fibres of the cervical sympathetic chain lie in front of the brachial plexus at this level and can readily be blocked by local anaesthetic leaking out of the plexus sheath, even after a correctly placed interscalene block. A classical case of Horner's syndrome is produced, i.e. ptosis, meiosis, enophthalmos and anhydrosis. No action need be taken, although it is wise to warn the patient during the preoperative visit of its likely occurrence and persistence for about 1–2 h after the block is placed. A persistent Horner's syndrome has been reported [56].

Recurrent Laryngeal Nerve Palsy

Another nerve which lies in close proximity to the brachial plexus at this level is the recurrent laryngeal nerve. Blockade of this nerve causes brief ipsilateral vocal cord paralysis and results in a hoarse voice and difficulty in coughing effectively. If a recurrent laryngeal nerve palsy is produced, it is wise to advise the patient not to eat or drink until the voice has returned to normal as there is a theoretical risk of aspiration.

Phrenic Nerve Palsy

It has been shown that the incidence of phrenic nerve palsy after interscalene brachial plexus block approaches 100% [67]. An approx. 25% in forced vital capacity (FVC) and forced expiratory volume in 1 s (FEV_1), along with significantly decreased peak expiratory flow rate (PEFR) and maximum mid-expiratory flow rate have been demonstrated [38, 66]. The decrease in FVC is not affected by injection volume [65]. Reduction of bupivacaine concentration from 0.5% to 0.125% does not affect the changes in pulmonary function [36]. In healthy, awake patients minute volume is maintained by an increase both in respiratory frequency and in the rib cage contribution to tidal volume [14]. The arterial partial pressure may decrease, presumably as a result of ventilation perfusion mismatch [14]. There is a report of a persistent phrenic nerve paresis after interscalene block [2].

Bronchospasm

This has been reported on one occasion [60].

Hearing Impairment

Interscalene brachial plexus block can be associated with hearing impairment [47]. In the authors' experience this is rarely perceived by the patient, although there are some individuals who complain of altered hearing. The deficit resolves after a short period.

"The Wobble"

Another complication of shoulder surgery under interscalene block is the "wobble". About 15% of patients undergoing shoulder surgery under interscalene brachial block alone experience bradycardia and hypotension some 45–60 min after the block has been inserted. The first report of this occurrence came from Sharrock [52] who quoted an onset time 69+28 min after the institution of the block. A later analysis of the problem [9] ascribed the event to activation of the Bezold-Jarisch reflex, an arcane phenomenon occasionally used by cardiologists to stimulate syncope in patients by administering isoprenaline. In this study the odds for a complication related to blood catecholamine levels were stacked in the authors' favour by the addition of adrenaline to the local anaesthetic for both the brachial plexus block and port-site infiltration and to the joint irrigation fluid. The wobble, which occurred in 20 of 116 patients studied, occurred 61+18 min after the insertion of the block. The authors note that those patients who were given beta-adrenergic blocking drugs for hypertension and tachycardia tended not to wobble, hence their invocation of the Bezold-Jarisch reflex. They sought further support for their hypothesis by referring to two studies of plasma bupivacaine concentrations that they claim demonstrate that the peak level occurs some 30 min after interscalene block, and that therefore the wobble could not be related to high plasma bupivacaine levels.

Unfortunately, a close reading of those two references does not bear out their interpretation. In the first [46], although the *mean* level measured at 30 min was higher than that measured at 60 min, the possibility of the actual peak mean occurring in between these two times in the individual patient was considered, and the authors state that the maximum plasma level occurred after 30 or 60 minutes in most patients (of which there were 12 in all). Further, these investigators used bupivacaine 0.75%. The increase in plasma bupivacaine levels using this concentration might reasonably be expected to be greater than for the more commonly used 0.5% solution. The second paper [39] demonstrated a median time to peak level of 29.6 min using plain bupivacaine rather than that to which adrenaline had been added. In summary, it is not possible to categorically say that the wobble does not occur synchronously with peak plasma bupivacaine levels.

D'Alessio et al. [9] recommend the administration of intravenous fluids, anti-cholinergic agents and beta-blockers to prevent the wobble. It is not possible to argue against the use of anti-cholinergic agents, and the author employs this approach routinely. Intravenous fluids are unlikely to be absolutely necessary but are equally unlikely to be dangerous. However, the administration of beta-blockers to prevent bradycardia and hypotension is a practice that some consider to be intuitively incorrect.

The common observation that the wobble rarely occurs during general anaesthesia and in the generously sedated patient argues against the Bezold-Jarisch reflex as the sole originator of the wobble, although it could be argued that both general anaesthesia and sedation decrease the levels of endogenous catecholamines. The authors believe that it will prove to be a result of the combination of anxiety, the sitting position and high plasma levels of bupivacaine. Perhaps the most convincing refutal of the Bezold-Jarisch reflex lies in the wobble's successful treatment by ephedrine – a drug which owes part of its effect to the stimulation of endogenous catecholamine release. Perhaps some investigators will have the courage to treat the bradycardia and hypotension with small doses of adrenaline. If this reverses the bradycardia and hypotension, the Bezold-Jarisch reflex can be rejected. If it worsens it, it must be accepted.

Advantages and Disadvantages of Regional Anaesthesia

Regional anaesthesia can provide excellent anaesthesia and prolonged postoperative analgesia for patients undergoing shoulder arthroplasty. The use of moderate to high concentrations of local anaesthetic agents is associated with good muscle relaxation. General anaesthesia is avoided, and the incidence of the complications and side effects related to general anaesthesia are substantially reduced or eliminated. The stress response to surgery is commonly reduced significantly by regional anaesthesia but not by general anaesthesia alone. It has been suggested that interscalene brachial plexus blockade can reduce blood loss in shoulder surgery [57].

On the down side, the serious complications of interscalene brachial plexus blockade, although rare, can be life threatening. It is therefore mandatory that the block not be performed by an individual untrained in resuscitation and anaesthesia. Pulmonary function can be affected by interscalene brachial plexus block. Regional anaesthesia can take time to establish, and if the facilities are not available to establish the block safely in one patient while the previous patient's surgery is being conducted, the duration of operating lists can be prolonged. Regional anaesthetic techniques should not be undertaken in the presence of coagulopathy or sepsis. Many patients may be reluctant to undergo major surgery without the guarantee of unconsciousness.

General anaesthesia has, as mentioned above, an almost 100 % success rate. Few anaesthetists would in all honesty claim that their success rate for interscalene brachial plexus anaesthesia matches the 100 % *claimed* by Roch [45], however, success rates should exceed 95 % with practice. This statement accepts that occasionally the block produced is not adequate on its own for comfortable surgery. In this situation, sedation can be added or general anaesthesia can be used.

Sedation for Regional Anaesthesia

Although some patients opt to be fully conscious during surgery, the majority of patients electing to undergo shoulder arthroplasty under regional anaesthesia are happy to accept some form of sedation. The choice of sedation is not critical but care should, as ever, be taken not to be over-generous. If the patient is in the beach-chair position, airway manipulation may prove difficult, and it is therefore wise not to sedate the patient to the point that they need airway support.

A benzodiazepine of some sort is convenient and simple and provides excellent amnesia. A careful infusion of propofol is favoured by many. More intricate forms of propofol sedation are being introduced: patient-controlled sedation, target-controlled infusion and patient-controlled target infusion. If the anaesthetist has the time, hardware and enthusiasm, there seems little to criticise about these complex techniques.

Combined Regional and General Anaesthesia

On the face of it, combining general and regional anaesthesia may expose the patient to the complications of both techniques and may therefore seem illogical. However, the alternative view can be taken that it can provide the patient with the *benefits* of both techniques for the patient. Although many anaesthetists argue that the regional anaesthetic should be performed before inducing anaesthesia in order to minimise the chance of intraneural injection, it is acceptable to perform regional anaesthesia after induction of general anaesthesia. Indeed, there are potential advantages other than patient comfort for this approach. The analgesic effect of a single-shot interscalene block using bupivacaine is in the order of 10–20 h. If the operation is likely to be long, as a result of complex surgery or a slow surgeon, the duration of postoperative analgesia may be compromised if the block is performed at the beginning of anaesthesia. It is therefore not uncommon practice to perform the regional anaesthetic block at the end of surgery in order to maximise the period of postoperative analgesia.

The advantages of combined regional and general anaesthesia include:

- Decreased anaesthetic requirement, with more rapid emergence and a reduced incidence of side effects such as nausea and vomiting in the postoperative period.
- Obviation of the need for neuromuscular blocking drugs as the muscle relaxation can be provided by the brachial plexus block.
- Prolonged effective analgesia and the avoidance of the use of opioid analgesic agents.
- Patient unconsciousness, which may be viewed as an advantage by patient, surgeon and anaesthetist.

Complications of the combination of general and regional anaesthesia have been reported [15].

Intra-operative Care

Patient Position

It is axiomatic that positioning of the patient on the operating table is important in any surgical discipline and particularly so in orthopaedic surgery. The variety of positions necessary for orthopaedic procedures and the physical status of the patients mean that close attention must be paid to the positioning of the patient if complications such as nerve damage and ischaemic necrosis are to be avoided.

The majority of shoulder arthroplasty procedures are performed with the patient in the beach-chair position. This position brings with it advantages for the surgeon and both advantages and disadvantages for the patient and anaesthetist.

Advantages of the Beach-Chair Position

For the surgeon the beach-chair position gives ready access to both the front and back of the shoulder and positioning of the shoulder above the heart reduces local venous pressure, thereby reducing blood loss.

As mentioned above, the FRC affects the gas exchanging function of the lungs as a result of its relationship to the closing capacity. Functional residual capacity is affected by a number of factors including general anaesthesia (via its effect on diaphragmatic muscle tone), age, sex, lung disease and posture. Movement from the supine position to a 60° reverse Trendelenburg position can make as much as a 50 % difference in FRC, with FRC being higher, and therefore lung function better, in the reverse Trendelenburg position [32]. Overall lung function is therefore improved in the sitting position when compared with the supine position. Although this positional effect is unlikely to have as great an impact on the awake patient, it can have a significant effect on the anaesthetised patient. There is therefore a physiological advantage to the beach-chair position.

Disadvantages of the Beach-Chair Position

As mentioned above, adverse cardiovascular effects can derive from the beach-chair position. The anaesthetist should closely supervise the move into the position and should monitor the patient assiduously at this time. Treatment with intravenous fluids and vasoconstricting agents may become necessary if hypotension occurs.

As the operative site is above the heart, albeit by only a small distance, there is a possibility of venous air embolism (VAE). In this process, air can enter open veins when intravenous pressure is subatmospheric and can cause right ventricular outflow obstruction and a reduction in blood flow through pulmonary vessels, both of which cause an decrease in cardiac output. Clinically this occurrence is suggested by hypotension, arrhythmia and an acutely reduced end tidal concentration of carbon dioxide (which in itself is a result of an acute decrease in cardiac output). More sensitive detection can be provided by precordial Doppler ultrasound probes. If the anaesthetist suspects VAE, the surgeon should be informed immediately, and wet packs should be applied to the wound. The patient should be tipped towards the head-down position, and if nitrous oxide is being administered, it should be withdrawn and replaced with 100 % oxygen. The incidence of VAE can be reduced by ensuring adequate patient hydration with intravenous fluids, thus increasing central venous pressure, although care should be exercised in those patient as risk from left ventricular failure.

The patient's head can be relatively unstable in the beach-chair position. This may provide discomfort for some patients and dangers for others if they have a history of cervical spine instability or vertebro-basilar insufficiency. Care must be taken in securing the patient's head. Access to the head and neck may be difficult during surgery in the beach-chair position. The surgeon must be prepared to halt surgery to allow the anaesthetist to return the patient to the supine position if an airway problem occurs.

Use of Bone Cement

The volatile monomers derived from quick-setting bone cement are thought capable of provoking hypotension during prosthesis insertion, although some authors blame fat and bone marrow embolism [53]. A small study (9 patients) failed to identify any adverse haemodynamic or pulmonary events associated with methylmethacrylate cement in total shoulder arthroplasty [24].

Positioning the Patient

Care should be taken to ensure that the patient's head is in a neutral position or a position that is known to be comfortable for the patient. If the patient is under general anaesthesia, the anaesthetist should ensure that the head is well protected, and that it is unlikely to move during surgery. Sandbags and rubber or visco-elastic polymer head rings combined with padding and adhesive tape are often used. Evacuatable bean-bags are also used, although care should be taken that folds in the bag which, when evacuated, becomes very hard, do not press into the patients skin and create the risk of pressure necrosis.

The non-operated arm should be padded and protected. A pillow may be placed under the patient's knees to prevent uncomfortable over-extension of the knee and traction on the sciatic nerve and padding should, of course, be placed below the patient's heels or ankles.

Blood pressure cuffs placed on the non-operated arm interfere with the function of the intravenous infusion if, as is likely, it is placed in this arm. Although it is perfectly reasonable to use the leg as the site for automated non-invasive blood pressure monitoring, care must be taken to ensure that the cuff is an appropriate size for the size of the portion of the leg that is being used. Pulse oximeter probes can be conveniently placed on the patients' toes.

Postoperative Analgesia

The options for analgesia after shoulder arthroplasty include: (a) systemic opiate analgesia, (b) local opiate analgesia, (c) NSAIDs, and (d) regional analgesia, via: epidural catheter, suprascapular catheter, or brachial plexus catheter.

Systemic opiate analgesia remains the mainstay of postoperative analgesia for the majority of patients undergoing major surgery. Administration by subcutaneous, sublingual, intramuscular and intravenous routes can provide excellent analgesia with an acceptably low incidence of side effects. Patient-controlled intravenous opiate analgesia has become very popular in recent years and is undoubtedly effective in providing analgesia after shoulder arthroplasty. A full discussion of its use is not included as the vast majority of anaesthetists are familiar with the concepts and practice of patient-controlled analgesia (PCA).

Intra-articular administration of opiate drugs to provide postoperative analgesia is popular in arthroscopic knee surgery, although there is currently some doubt as to its efficacy. Little interest has been shown in the application of this technique to the upper limb, although there is one report of its use in the shoulder using buprenorphine [12]. To date, its use has been restricted to arthroscopic surgery, and the indications are that it is unlikely to be sufficiently effective to provide the sole source of analgesia for shoulder arthroplasty.

Epidural analgesia can be used for both anaesthesia during and analgesia after major shoulder procedures [3, 4, 74]. Although effective, it is unlikely that this technique will achieve widespread use because of the unfamiliarity of most anaesthetists with the technique and concerns about safety in terms of the danger of spinal cord damage and cardiovascular and respiratory complications.

It is possible to place a catheter near the suprascapular nerve [6, 30] and thereby provide analgesia of the shoulder, although its use for analgesia after shoulder arthroplasty has not been reported. Its routine use must therefore await published studies of its efficacy in this respect.

Regional analgesia after shoulder arthroplasty provides excellent pain relief and avoids many of the side effects common with systemic opiates such as nausea, pruritus, sedation, respiratory depression and urinary retention. A single-shot interscalene brachial plexus block with bupivacaine can provide up to and beyond 24 h of effective analgesia [5]. However, after shoulder arthroplasty it is often desirable to continue analgesia after this period as many patients are in significant pain on the second and third postoperative days. The provision of a pain-free early postoperative period facilitates the institution of passive physiotherapy.

Catheterisation of the Brachial Plexus

If a catheter can be passed into the brachial plexus, it is possible to extend the analgesia produced by a single shot block from hours to a period of days. Continuous brachial plexus blockade was first described in 1946. A needle was placed in the supraclavicular brachial plexus, and it was secured with a cork and a number of lengths of adhesive strapping. However, the advent of plastic intravenous cannulae led to the introduction of the concept of plexus sheath cannulation.

The placement of a catheter, rather than a cannula, into the interscalene brachial plexus is now becoming commonplace in the postoperative management of shoulder arthroplasty. There are currently a number of catheterisation kits designed for use with a nerve stimulator which aid the placement of a soft plastic catheter into the brachial plexus sheath. The Braun Contiplex and Polymedic Polyplex kits include a short-bevel or pencil-point needle over which can be passed a short cannula once the plexus has been located. A catheter, similar in size and design to an epidural catheter, is then passed through the cannula. Local anaesthetic can then be administered through the catheter by bolus injection, by infusion or, as recently described [26], by a PCA analgesia device.

Placement of Interscalene Brachial Plexus Catheters

Identification of the brachial plexus and confirmation of correct positioning are conducted exactly as for a single-shot block. Passage of the cannula over the needle into the brachial plexus at the axillary or subclavian perivascular level is relatively easy as at these locations the needle lies almost parallel with the plexus sheath at the point of insertion. However, when attempting to cannulate the brachial plexus at the interscalene level by the classical approach, the needle makes very nearly a right angle with the sheath. This can make it difficult to pass the cannula into the sheath. Kiking of the cannula can occur during insertion and impede the passage of the catheter. To avoid these problems many anaesthetists adjust their point of entry, the angle of the needle, or both, so that the needle and cannula make a more oblique angle with the sheath and the needle is thus more nearly parallel with the plexus. This can be done by entering the sheath at a slightly higher level than that of the sixth cervical vertebra and by angling the needle in a more caudal direction. Care should be exercised not to puncture the pleura if the needle is angled in a steeply caudad direction.

Another useful technique to aid the passage of the cannula is to inject the local anaesthetic solution down the needle having placed it within the plexus sheath. This "blows up" the plexus, separates the nerve trunks within it and aids the passage of the cannula. The Polymedic Polyplex kit has a side injection arm which facilitates this manoeuvre, but attempting this technique with the Braun Contiplex kit involves removing the stimulator lead from the needle. The movement involved in disconnecting the lead and connecting a manometer line for local anaesthetic injection can lead to dislodgement of the needle from the plexus sheath. Having blown up the sheath, the cannula should be passed a small distance into the sheath. Failing to resist the temptation to insert the full length of cannula can lead to kinking of the cannula and therefore difficult passage of the catheter. Even after blowing the sheath up with local anaesthetic, the passage of the catheter into the plexus is often associated with paraesthesiae, presumably as a result of the catheter coming into contact with nerves within the plexus. Once the catheter is in place, aspiration should be performed to exclude intravascular placement and the catheter should then be fixed in place.

Catheter Fixation

As Winnie [73] has pointed out, it is difficult to secure an interscalene catheter: "With the interscalene technique, the catheter is at right angles to the sheath and skin, so that movement of the head or shoulders tends to advance or withdraw the catheter". For this reason Winnie favours the subclavian perivascular approach for catheterisation of the brachial plexus. Insertion of subclavian perivascular catheters is more likely to lead to satisfactory fixation, but most shoulder anaesthetists who insert brachial plexus catheters favour the interscalene route as they are most familiar with this approach. Sutures, adhesive tape and adhesive bio-occlusive dressings (or a combination of these) have been used, but problems with catheter movement have been recorded in up to 25% of cases [63].

The authors currently favour the tunnelling of the interscalene catheter to a position above the middle portion of the clavicle, i.e. in a similar position to the insertion point of a subclavian perivascular brachial plexus block. Care should be taken not to tunnel the catheter too deeply within the tissues of the neck. We have had a successful experience of the technique although two complication have arisen. If the initial interscalene catheter insertion is just posterior to the external jugular vein, it is possible to tunnel the catheter through the vein. This leads, not surprisingly, to haemorrhage. Therefore the initial entry point of the block needle and cannula should be anterior to the external jugular vein. The other complication encountered is transection of the catheter with the tunnelling needle. Surgical neck exploration after this occurrence failed to retrieve the transected catheter.

Complications of Interscalene Brachial Plexus Catheterisation

The technique carries with it all the complications associated with single-shot block plus additional dangers of its own. The following adverse events have been reported:

- Failure of technique: the procedure takes some time to learn and early failures are common. With practice success rates should approach those of single shot interscalene block.
- Catheter failure (including dislodgement): reported as happening into up to 25% of cases [63].
- Accidental vertebral artery catheterisation [64].
- Accidental epidural catheterisation [8, 27].
- Plexus irritation causing severe pain on injection [41]: no neurological complications resulted in the reported case.
- Signs suggestive of local anaesthetic toxicity during local anaesthetic infusion such as tinnitus and dizziness [16], a metallic taste [63] and confusion [62].
- Breathing difficulty [16].
- Incorrect injection: an antibiotic solution was injected down the catheter causing pain but no long-term problems [35].

The following adverse effects appear not to have been reported yet:

- Catheter site infection. It is our practice to perform the technique under full aseptic conditions and to leave the catheter in place for up to four days. The record for a brachial plexus catheter (axillary) appears to be 41 days [61]. The catheter was removed because the patient became pyrexial but no local signs of infection were seen and no long-term problems were suffered by the patient.
- Catheter migration. Although it seems unlikely that a soft plastic catheter placed within the fascial sheath of the brachial plexus is unlikely to migrate in any direction other than outwards, epidural catheter migration is a recognised phenomenon, and this possibility must therefore be considered.

It should be mentioned that a patient should have a patent intravenous cannula in situ throughout the period of interscalene infusion and that nursing supervision and monitoring should be at appropriate levels to ensure the safety of the patient if migration of the cannula to another location such as intravascular occurs.

Bolus Injection or Infusion?

Local anaesthetic can be administered through an interscalene catheter by bolus injection or continuous infusion. The decision as to which mode of administration is chosen is largely determined by local staffing and supervision constraints. One advantage of bolus injection by a trained anaesthetist is that if the catheter has been placed in, or has migrated to, a potentially dangerous location, an anaesthetist is present at the time of greatest risk. However, if an infusion is used, there are three possibilities:

- That too much is being given, giving rise to the risk of toxicity.
- That too little is being given, which leads to inadequate analgesia
- That exactly the right amount is being given.

Infusion rates can of course be adjusted in an attempt to ensure that the third possibility pertains for as large a proportion of the time as possible. The use of interscalene PCA has been described [26]. Using a PCA pump that can infuse through catheters of small diameter, i.e. one that is not likely to alarm if the infusion is pumped at a relatively high pressure, it is possible to choose doses of local anaesthetic that can be safely given by the patient himself. The authors use a low level background infusion in addition to PCA bolus doses.

Choice of Infusion Drugs

Bupivacaine appears to be the currently favoured drug for use in this context. Bupivacaine infusion, in doses of up to 0.25 mg kg^{-1} h^{-1} has been shown to provide good analgesia without producing plasma bupivacaine levels that are thought to be associated with toxicity [16, 37, 62]. The addition of adrenaline to the local anaesthetic solution, in single-shot blocks at least, appears likely to be able to reduce the maximum plasma local anaesthetic concentration with bupivacaine, lignocaine, prilocaine and etidocaine [40, 71].

It is often said that the ideal drug for infusion in any situation is one that has a short duration of action and a low propensity to cause toxic reactions in overdose. It is therefore surprising that anaesthetists seem to have selected bupivacaine for interscalene brachial plexus infusion in view of the fact that lignocaine more closely resembles the ideal drug. The efficacy and safety of the use of lignocaine for brachial plexus awaits confirmation. Ropivacaine, which is reported to have a lower capacity for motor block and cardiac toxicity than bupivacaine, may prove to be a suitable drug for this application. Its presentation in a 0.1 % solution by the manufacturers also facilitates the preparation of infusion solutions.

As mentioned previously, the efficacy of opiate drugs when added to local anaesthetic drugs for peripheral nerve blockade is currently a subject of debate. There is anecdotal evidence of the beneficial effects on analgesia quality of the addition of fentanyl to bupivacaine for brachial plexus infusion [26, 33].

Future Prospects

It is likely that regional anaesthesia and analgesia will be used increasingly for shoulder arthroplasty. The placement of brachial plexus catheters will probably grow in popularity, but there are some potentially serious complications which have yet to be reported. When they are reported, there may be temporary reductions in the use of this technique. In particular, the use of opiate drugs via the interscalene route may produce complications as spread to the cervical epidural space is feasible. Ropivacaine will very likely find favour in postoperative analgesia via interscalene catheters. The continuing development of catheter placement kits will proceed, with new materials being used to produce kink-resistant cannulae that will aid the passage of catheters into the interscalene brachial plexus sheath.

References

1. Barutell C, Vidal F, Raich M, Montero A (1980) A neurological complication following interscalene brachial plexus block. Anaesth 35:365–367
2. Bashein G, Robertson HT, Kennedy WF Jr (1985) Persistent phrenic nerve paresis following interscalene brachial plexus block. Anesthesiology 63:102–104
3. Baylot D, Mahul P, Navez ML, Hajjar J, Prades JM, Auboyer C (1993) Cervical epidural anesthesia. Ann Fr Anesth Reanim 12:483–492
4. Boogaerts J, Guillaume C, Lafont N (1993) Loco-regional anesthesia for surgery of the shoulder. Cah Anesthesiol 41:173–15
5. Brandl F, Taeger K (1991) The combination of general anesthesia and interscalene block in shoulder surgery. Anaesthesist 40:537–542
6. Breen TW, Haigh JD (1990) Continuous suprascapular nerve block for analgesia of scapular fracture. Can J Anaesthesia 37:786–788
7. Chambers W (1992) Peripheral nerve damage and regional anaesthesia. Br J Anaesth 69:429–436
8. Cook LB (1991) Unsuspected extradural catheterization in an interscalene block. Br J Anaesth 67:473–475
9. D'Alessio JG, Weller RS, Rosenblum M (1995) Activation of the Bezold-Jarisch reflex in the sitting position for shoulder arthroscopy using interscalene block. Anesth Analg 80:1158–1162
10. Davidas JL, Blond JL, Rochette A, Manchom M, Degoute CS, Banssillon V (1992) Local analgesic action by direct effect of pethidine on nerve trunks. Therapie 47:485–487
11. Dutton RP, Eckhardt WF III, Sunder N (1994) Total spinal anesthesia after interscalene blockade of the brachial plexus. Anesthesiology 80:939–941
12. Fellahi JL, Magues JP, Marquer B, Guerot A, Mansat M, Cathala B (1995) Analgesia with intra-articular injection of buprenorphine after surgery of the shoulder. Cah Anesthesiol 43:313–318
13. Flory N, Van-Gessel E, Donald F, Hoffmeyer P, Gamulin Z (1995) Does the addition of morphine to brachial plexus block improve analgesia after shoulder surgery? Br J Anaesth 75:23–26
14. Fujimara N, Namba H, Tsunoda K, Kawamata T, Taki K, Igarasi M, Namiki A (1995) Effect of hemidiaphragmatic paresis caused by interscalene brachial plexus block on breathing pattern, chest wall mechanics and arterial blood gases. Anesth Analg 81:962–966
15. Gentili ME, Lefoulon-Gourves M, Mamelle JC, Bonnet F (1994) Acute respiratory failure following interscalene block: complications of combined general and regional anesthesia. Reg Anesth 19:292–293
16. Haasio J, Tuominen M, Rosenberg PH (1990) Continuous interscalene brachial plexus block during and after shoulder surgery. Ann Chir Gynaecol 79:103–107
17. Hendolin H, Mattila MA (1988) Comparison of bupivacaine hydrochloride 0.5 % and bupivacaine carbonate 0.5 % in interscalene plexus anesthesia. Reg Anaesth 11:12–15
18. Hickey R, Blanchard J, Hoffman J, Sjovall J, Ramamurthy S (1990) Plasma concentrations of ropivacaine given with or without epinephrine for brachial plexus block. Can J Anaesth 37:878–882
19. Hickey R, Candido KD, Ramamurthy S, Winnie AP, Blanchard J, Raza SM, Hoffman J, Durrani Z, Masters RW (1990) Brachial plexus block with a new local anaesthetic: 0.5 per cent ropivacaine. Can J Anaesthesia 37:732–738
20. Hickey R, Knape KG, Blanchard J, Hoffman J, Ramamurthy S (1990) Lidocaine hydrocarbonate is not superior to lidocaine hydrochloride in interscalene brachial plexus block. Reg Anesth 15:194–198
21. Hickey R, Hoffman J, Ramamurthy S (1991) A comparison of ropivacaine 0.5 % and bupivacaine 0.5 % for brachial plexus block. Anesthesiology 74:639–642
22. Hickey R, Rowley CL, Candido KD, Hoffman J, Ramamurthy S, Winnie AP (1992) A comparative study of 0.25 % ropivacaine and 0.25 % bupivacaine for brachial plexus block. Anesth Analg 75:602–606

23. Hirasawa Y, Katsumi Y, Kusswetter W, Sprotte G (1990) Experimental studies on peripheral nerve injuries caused by injection needles. Reg Anaesth 13:11-5
24. Huffnagle S, Seltzer JL, Torjman M, Marr A, Fenlin J (1993) Does the use of methylmethacrylate cement in total shoulder replacement induce haemodynamic or pulmonary instability? J Clin Anesth 5:404-407
25. Kumar A, Battit GE, Froese AB, Long MC (1971) Bilateral cervical and thoracic epidural blockade complicating interscalene brachial plexus block: report of two cases. Anesthesiology 35:650-652
26. Lucas MA, Harrop-Griffiths AW (1997) Interscalene patient-controlled analgesia. Anaesthesia 52:263-426
27. Mahoudeau G, Gaertner E, Launoy A, Ocquidant P, Loewenthal A (1995) Interscalene block: accidental catheterisation of the epidural space. Ann Fr Anesth Reanim 14:438-441
28. Markham A, Faulds D, Ropivacaine (1996) A review of its pharmacology and therapeutic use in regional anaesthesia. Drugs 52:429-449
29. McCaughey W (1992) Adverse effects of local anaesthetics. Drug Safety 7:178-189
30. Mercadente S, Sapio M, Villari P (1995) Suprascapular nerve block by catheter for breakthrough shoulder cancer pain. Reg Anesth 20:343-346
31. Moore D, Mulroy M, Thompson G (1994) Peripheral nerve damage and regional anaesthesia. Br J Anaesthesia 73:435-436
32. Nunn JF (1987) Applied respiratory physiology, 3rd edn. Butterworths, London
33. Parikh RK, Rymaszewski LR, Scott NB (1995) Prolonged postoperative analgesia for arthrolysis of the elbow joint. Br J Anaesth 74:469-471
34. Passannante AN (1996) Spinal anesthesia and permanent neurologic deficit after interscalene block. Anesth Analg 82:873-874
35. Patterson KW, Scanlon P (1990) An unusual complication of brachial plexus sheath cannulation. Br J Anaesth 65:542-543
36. Pere P (1993) The effect of continuous interscalene brachial plexus block with 0.125% bupivacaine plus fentanyl on diaphragmatic motility and ventilatory function. Reg Anesth 18:93-97
37. Pere P, Tuominen M, Rosenberg PH (1991) Cumulation of bupivacaine, desbutylbupivacaine and 4-hydroxybupivacaine during and after continuous interscalene brachial plexus block. Acta Anaesthesiol Scand 35:647-650
38. Pere P, Pitkanen M, Rosenberg PH, Bjorkenheim JM, Linden H, Salorinne Y, Tuominen M (1992) Effect of continuous interscalene brachial plexus block on diaphragm motion and on ventilatory function. Acta Anaesthesiol Scandi 36:53-57
39. Pihlajamaki KK (1991) Inverse correlation between the peak venous serum concentration of bupivacaine and the weight of the patient during interscalene brachial plexus block. Br J Anaesth 67:621-622
40. Pihlajamaki KK, Lindberg RL (1987) Bupivacaine with and without adrenaline in interscalene brachial plexus blockade. Studies in patients with rheumatoid arthritis. Br J Anaesth 59:1420-1424
41. Ribeiro FC, Georgousis H, Bertram R, Scheiber G (1996) Plexus irritation caused by interscalene brachial plexus catheter for shoulder surgery. Anesth Analg 82:870-872
42. Rice ASC (1996) Type of needle point and nerve damage. Anaesthesia 51:98-99
43. Rice ASC, McMahon SB (1992) Peripheral nerve injury caused by injection needles used in regional anaesthesia: the influence of bevel configuration, studied in a rat model. Br J Anaesth 69:433-438
44. Rice ASC, Andreev N, McMahon SB (1994) The consequences of microneurography electrode-induced injury of peripheral nerves observed in the rat and man. Pain 59:385-393
45. Roch JJ, Sharrock NE, Neudachin L (1992) Interscalene brachial plexus block for shoulder surgery: a proximal paresthesia is effective. Anesth Analg 75:386-388
46. Rosenberg PH, Pere P, Hekau R, Tuominen M (1991) Plasma concentrations of bupivacaine and two of its metabolites during continuous interscalene brachial plexus block. Br J Anaesth 66:25-30
47. Rosenberg PH, Lamberg TS, Tarkkila P, Marttila T, Bjorkenheim JM, Tuominen M (1995) Auditory disturbance associated with interscalene brachial plexus block. Br J Anaesth 74:89-91
48. Ross AF, Tinker JH (1994) Anesthesia risk. In: Miller RD (eds) Anesthesia. Churchill Livingstone, New York
49. Scammell SJ (1979) Case report: inadvertent epidural anaesthesia as a complication of interscalene brachial plexus block. Anaesth Intens Care 7:56-57
50. Selander D (1993) Peripheral nerve injury caused by injection needles. Br J Anaesth 7 1:323-324
51. Selander D, Dhuner K-G, Lundborg G (1977) Peripheral nerve injury due to injection needles used for regional anaesthesia. Acta Anaesthesiol Scand 21:182-188
52. Sharrock N (1991) Reg Anesth 15 [Suppl]:64
53. Sharrock NE, Savarese JJ (1994) Anesthesia for orthopaedic surgery. In: Miller RD (ed) Anesthesia. Churchill Livingstone, New York
54. Sukhani R, Winnie AP (1987) Clinical pharmacokinetics of carbonated local anesthetics. II. interscalene brachial block model. Anesth Analg 66:1245-1250
55. Sukhani R, Winnie AP (1989) Clinical pharmacokinetics of carbonated local anesthetics. III interscalene brachial block model. Anesth Analg 68:90-93
56. Sukhani R, Barclay J, Aasen M (1994) Prolonged Horner's syndrome after interscalene block: a management dilemma. Anesth Analg 79:601-603
57. Tetzlaff JE, Yoon HJ, Brems J (1994) Interscalene brachial plexus block for shoulder surgery. Reg Anesth 19:339-343
58. Tetzlaff JE, Yoon HJ, Dilger J, Brems J (1994) Subdural anesthesia as a complication of an interscalene brachial plexus block. Case report. Reg Anesth 19:357-359
59. Tetzlaff JE, Yoon HJ, Brems J, Javorsky T (1995) Alkalinization of mepivacaine improves the quality of motor block associated with interscalene brachial plexus anesthesia for shoulder surgery. Reg Anesth 20:128-132
60. Thiagarajah S, Lear E, Azar I, Salzer J, Zeiligsohn E (1984) Bronchospasm following interscalene brachial plexus block. Anesthesiology 61:759-761
61. Thomson S (1990) Long-term indwelling catheter for intermittent axillary plexus blocks with bupivacaine. Anaesth Intens Care 18:276-277
62. Tuominen M, Pitkanen M, Rosenberg PH (1987) Postoperative pain relief and bupivacaine plasma levels during continuous interscalene brachial plexus block. Acta Anaesthesiol Scand 31:276-278

63. Tuominen M, Haasio J, Hekali R, Rosenberg PH (1989) Continuous interscalene brachial plexus block: clinical efficacy, technical problems and bupivacaine plasma concentrations. Acta Anaesthesiol Scand 33:84–88
64. Tuominen MK, Pere P, Rosenberg PH (1991) Unintentional arterial catheterization and bupivacaine toxicity associated with continuous interscalene brachial plexus block. Anesthesiology 75:356–358
65. Urmey WF, Gloeggler PJ (1993) Pulmonary function changes during interscalene brachial plexus block: effects of decreasing local anesthetic injection volume. Reg Anesth 18:244–2449
66. Urmey WF, McDonald M (1992) Hemidiaphragmatic paresis during interscalene brachial plexus block: effects on pulmonary function and chest wall mechanics. Anesth Analg 74:352–357
67. Urmey WF, Talts KH, Sharrock NE (1991) One hundred per cent incidence of hemidiaphragmatic paresis associated with interscalene brachial plexus anesthesia as diagnosed by ultrasonography. Anesth Analg 72:498–503
68. Vainionpaa VA, Haavisto ET, Huha TM, Korpi KJ, Nuutinen LS, Hollmen AI, Jozwiak HM, Magnusson AA (1995) A clinical and pharmacokinetic comparison of ropivacaine and bupivacaine in axillary plexus block. Anesth Analg 81:534–538
69. Wajima Z, Nakajima Y, Kim C, Kobayashi N, Kadotani H, Adachi H, Inoue T, Ogawa R (1995) IV compared with brachial plexus infusion of butorphanol for postoperative analgesia. Br J Anaesth 74:392–395
70. Wajima Z, Shitara T, Nakajima Y, Kim C, Kobayashi N, Kadotani H, Adachi H, Ishikawa G, Kaneko K, Inoue T (1995) Comparison of continuous brachial plexus infusion of butorphanol, mepivacaine and mepivacaine-butorphanol mixtures for postoperative analgesia. Br J Anaesth 75:548–551
71. Wildsmith JA, Tucker GT, Cooper S, Scott DB, Covino BG (1977) Plasma concentrations of local anaesthetics after interscalene brachial plexus block. Br J Anaesth 49:461–466
72. Winnie AP (1970) Interscalene brachial plexus block. Anesth Analg 49:455–66
73. Winnie AP (1983) Plexus anesthesia. Saunders, Philadelphia
74. Zablocki AD, Baysinger CL, Epps JL, Bucknell AL (1987) Cervical epidural anesthesia for surgery of the shoulder. Orthop Rev 16:98–10

Section IV:

Advances in Humeral Design and Surgical Technique

Anatomical Study of the Proximal Humerus: Surgical Technique Considerations and Prosthetic Design Rationale

P. Boileau and G. Walch

Summary

In an effort to better understand the three-dimensional geometry of the proximal humerus, an anthropometric study was undertaken analyzing human cadaveric specimens using a digitized measuring device linked to a computer. The present study emphasizes the variable shape *of the proximal humerus over its variable dimensions because of the* variable orientation *(variable inclination and retroversion) and the* variable location *of the articular surface (variable medial and posterior offset). The shape of the proximal humerus is variable, much more variable in fact than the designs of most contemporary humeral components would suggest or can accommodate. Although good clinical results with shoulder replacement can be achieved using either the modular or the nonmodular components that are currently available, their relatively fixed geometry means that they are not truly anatomical when compared with our findings. We have developed a new type of humeral component based on these findings which is not only modular but also adaptable to the individual bony anatomy.* Prosthetic adaptability *is a new concept in the design of shoulder prosthesis which concentrates on correctly positioning the prosthetic head in relation to the individual anatomical neck.*

Introduction

Restoring normal anatomy of the humeral proximal epiphysis is important in reconstructive shoulder arthroplasty because it affects both deltoid and rotator cuff lever arms in the vertical plane and/or the soft tissue balance in the horizontal plane [2, 13, 24, 25]. Any change in this normal anatomy may lead to abnormal kinematics of the shoulder, by malpositioning of the joint line and/or deviation of the instant centers of rotation [12, 14, 15].

We designed the present anthropometric study of the proximal humerus because our experience with shoulder arthroplasty had encountered difficulties in consistently recreating the normal anatomy of the humeral proximal epiphysis, and because a previous cineradiographic study of active elevation of the prosthetic shoulder has shown abnormal kinematics [5]. Surface measurements were made on fresh human cadaveric specimens using a digitized measuring system connected to a computer, allowing three-dimensional computerized modeling of the bones [7].

The purpose of this anatomical study was to determine both the *shape* and the *dimensions* of the proximal humerus. There were three steps in planing this study: first, verifying the possible sphericity of the cartilaginous head surface; second, characterizing the distribution of sizes of this articular surface (diameter and thickness); and third, defining the orientation (inclination and retroversion) and location (possible anteroposterior and/or mediolateral offsets) of the articular surface.

Material and Methods

Sixty-five humeri (32 left, 33 right) of fresh cadavers were carefully dissected of all soft tissue, avoiding damage to the articular cartilage. The cadavers were from caucasiens (19 men, 20 women) aged 67–95 years (average 86±13 years). Of the 65 humeri, 52 were paired (26 pairs). Specimens that showed evidence of osseous pathology, previous fractures, or the presence of metallic hardware were excluded from the study.

The Metrologic MT1 (Metrologic Instruments, Meylan, France), a highly accuracy three-dimensional digitized measuring machine, precalibrated, was equipped with a special frame to receive the humeri. Each bone was fixed on this support at the humeral head and at the elbow so that it could rotate around its own axis (diaphyseal axis). Surface measurements were made with a probe that was moved manually, while the bones were rotated in 10° increments. This allowed parallel slices to be digitized: every 5 mm at the level of the proximal and distal epiphysis and every 10 mm at the level of the diaphysis. The probe digitized about 36 points for each slice. The bones were then fixed in rotation, and we digitized points on the humeral head articular surface. About 20 points were arbitrarily digi-

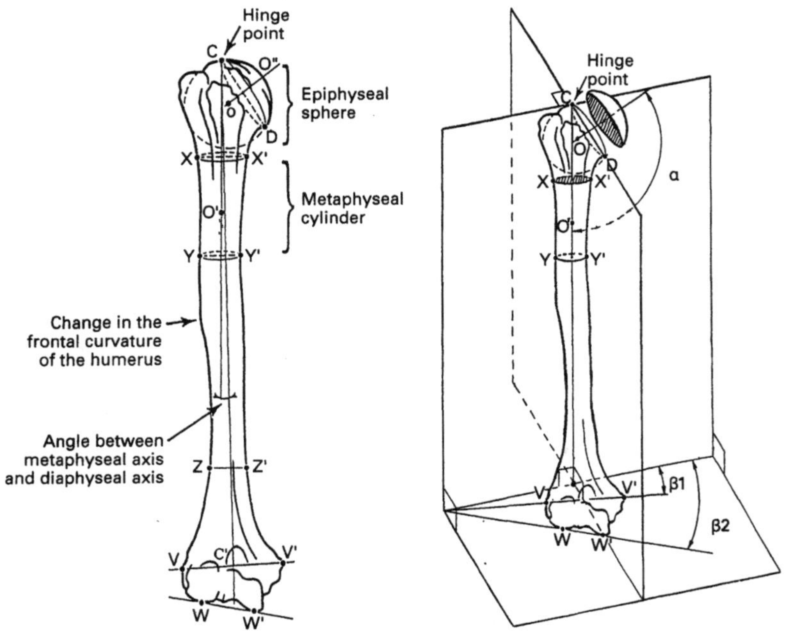

Fig. 1. a Axes used to characterize the morphological factors: 1, humeral head axis; 2, diaphyseal axis; 3, metaphyseal axis; 4, transepicondylar axis; 5, tangent elbow axis. **b** Three-dimensional coordinate system (see text)

tized on the hyaline cartilage of the humeral head and about 40 at the periphery of the articular surface. At least 1200 points were digitized for each humerus.

A computer connected with the digitizing machine and equipped with the Metrologic 3-D manual software (Metrologic Instruments, Meylan, France) collected the data and yielded three-dimensional images of the humeri. These were subsequently manipulated on a three-dimensional computer-assisted design workstation to produce surface reconstruction and multiplanar reformatted images. The computer software first calculated precisely the various morphological parameters (diameter, thickness, inclination, retroversion) and then modeled the proximal humeri with simple geometric figures (Fig. 1a): the plane which best fitted the periphery of the articular surface was called the *anatomical neck plane* (C–D), the sphere which best fitted the articular surface of the humeral head was called the *epiphyseal sphere*, and its center was calculated (O), and the cylinder which best fitted the shape of the upper humeral shaft was called the *metaphyseal cylinder*, and its center was calculated (O'). This metaphyseal cylinder was arbitrarily limited to the proximal half of the bone because of the altered curvature in the coronal plane one-half of the way down the humeral shaft after 13 cm (10.3–15.8).

The five following axes were defined (Fig. 1a):

- The humeral head axis defined perpendicular to the anatomical neck plane (O–O") fitted to a set of points taken on the periphery of the articular cartilage
- The diaphyseal axis, already mentioned, which represents the arbitrary axis of rotation of the bones (C–C')
- The proximal metaphyseal (intramedullary) axis, the axis of the metaphyseal cylinder which is of interest when implanting a humeral prosthesis because it represents the theoretical stem axis (C–O')
- The transepicondylar axis, defined by a line joining the most medial and the most lateral extremities of the distal humerus (V–V')
- The tangent elbow axis, defined by a line tangent to the trochlea and the condyle (W–W'). All morphological factors related to the orientation and location of the articular surface were calculated in relation to the proximal metaphyseal axis, i.e., the stem axis (inclination, anteroposterior translation, and mediolateral translation) and to the transepicondylar and tangent axis (retroversion).

The axes of reference in the three dimensions of the space were then defined (Fig. 1b). The images of each proximal humerus was inclined until the proximal metaphyseal (intramedullary) axis was positioned in a vertical position: *inferosuperior* or *X axis*. The images of the bones were rotated around the proximal metaphyseal axis until the anatomical neck plane appeared as a line. The projection of this line onto the plane perpendicular to the already defined X axis resulted in a vector which defined the *anteroposterior* or *Y axis*. The plane perpendicular to the X–Y plane allowed the *mediolateral* or *Z axis* to be defined. A three-dimensional coordinate axis system was established with the origin selected arbitrarily to lie within the metaphyseal cylinder. All the measurements were conducted according to these projections.

The surface measurements of the hyaline cartilage of the humeral head (Figs. 2a, 4) allowed the diameter of a potential humeral sphere to be determined (distance A–B) and thus the humeral head

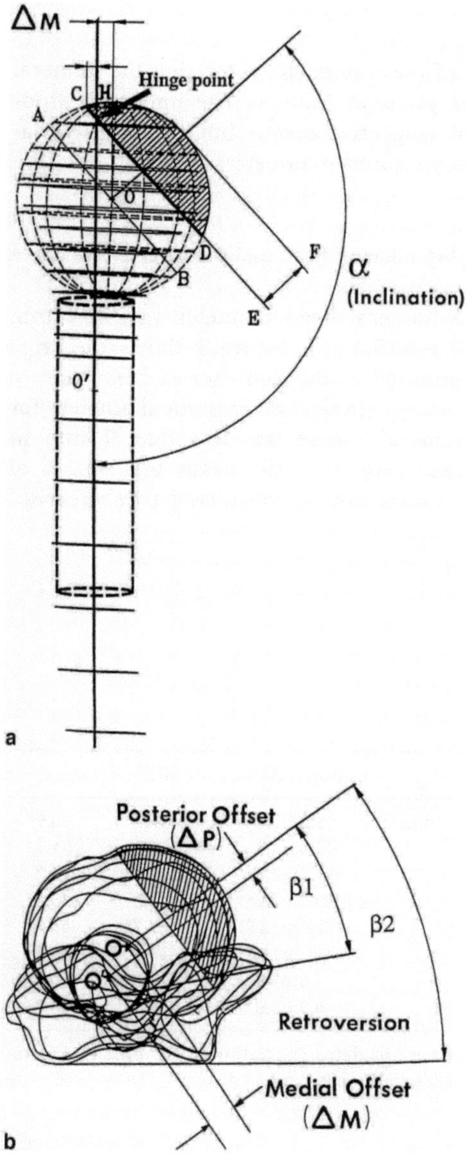

Fig. 2. a The anatomical measurements made in the frontal view: *A–B*, diameter of curvature; *C–D*, articular surface diameter; *E–F*, articular thickness; *ΔM*, medial offset; *C–H*, "hinge point" distance; α, *inclination angle*. **b** The anatomical measurements made in the axial view: retrotorsion angle related to the transepicondylar axis (*β1*) and to the tangent axis (*β2*). *ΔM*, Medial offset; *ΔP*, posterior offset

diameters to be evaluated. To verify the possible sphericity of the humeral head we used the classical method of least-squares optimization [32], defined as the thickness of a theoretical spherical shell of outer theoretical diameter (D1) and inner diameter (D2). All digitized points of the articular surface were located within the thickness of this shell. The standard deviation of all data points is a measure of the "sphercity" of humeral heads. We postulated in this study that a three-dimensional figure in which the difference between two extreme diameters measured is less than 1 mm (or 2 % of the average diameter), can be considered to be a true sphere (D1–D2<1 mm). The coronal views (Fig. 2a) allowed measurement of the diameter (distance C–D) and the thickness (distance E–F) of the articular surface for each specimen. The articular surface of the humeral head is known to face the shaft superiorly (inclination): this parameter was investigated (angle α).

Finally, we observed on the coronal views that the metaphyseal axis (theoretical stem axis) typically crossed near the top of the articular surface in most of the specimens (Fig. 2a); this point was called the "hinge point." On the axial views (Fig. 2b) we were able to measure the retroversion angle related to the transepicondylar axis (angle β1) or to the tangent elbow axis (angle β2). From the three-dimensional images obtained from the computer we observed that the head segment was not only variably oriented but was also variably located with a tendency to be translated medially (medial offset) and posteriorly (posterior offset) or both medially and posteriorly (combined offset). To quantify this variable translation of the articular head surface in both planes, the relationship between the center of the *epiphyseal sphere* (O) and the center of the *metaphyseal cylinder* (O') was investigated.

The anatomical humeral parameters measured from this procedure for each specimen included (Fig. 2):

- The diameter of curvature of the humeral head articular surface, measured in both coronal and axial planes (distance A–B)
- The articular surface diameter, measured in both coronal and axial planes defined by the diameter of the articular surface at the level of the margin of the cartilage (distance C–D)
- The articular surface thickness, defined by the perpendicular distance from the articular margin to the apex of the diameter of curvature (distance E–F)
- The inclination angle, the angle between the proximal metaphyseal (intramedullary axis), i.e., the stem axis and the perpendicular to the articular margin plane (angle α)
- The retroversion angle, the angle between the perpendicular to the articular margin plane and the transepicondylar axis (angle β1) or the tangent elbow axis (angle β2)
- The medial offset, the perpendicular distance between the axial planes containing the center of the epiphyseal sphere and the center of the metaphyseal cylinder (ΔM=distance O–O' in the frontal plane)

- The posterior offset, the perpendicular distance between the coronal plane containing the center of the epiphyseal sphere and that containing the axis of the metaphyseal cylinder (ΔP=distance O–O' in the axial plane)
- The hinge point distance, the distance between the axial plane containing the axis of the cylinder and the upper border of the articular surface (distance C–H).

The accuracy of the digitizing machine was in the order of l0 μm and was such that the margin of error may be considered insignificant for this application. To determine interobserver and intraobserver variability, ten specimens were chosen randomly and were digitized independently by two different observers. The measurements were repeated 3 weeks later and were made separately by the two observers without knowing previous measurements or the number of the specimens. Analysis of variance showed that the standard deviation for repeat readings by an observer and between two observers was negligible [26].

Results

A summary of the results characterizing the humeral specimens is given in Table 1. The important findings are not respective means but the large variations of the measured parameters.

Sphericity of the Humeral Head and Diameter of Curvature

The average humeral head diameter was 46.2 mm (range of 37.1–56.9 mm). Figure 3 shows the large variations observed in the diameter of curvature.

The difference between two extreme diameters for the same humeral sphere was less than 1 mm in 88.2 % of cases (Fig. 4). This means that 88.2 % of the humeral heads can be considered true spheres.

Table 1. Summary of the variables characterizing the humeral specimens

Dimensions	Mean±SD	Min.	Max.
Diameter of curvature (humeral head diameter; mm)	46.2±5.4	37.1	56.9
Articular surface diameter (mm)	43.3±4.3	36.5	51.7
Articular surface thickness (mm)	15.2±1.6	12.1	18.2
Inclination[a]	129.6°±2.9°	123.2°	135.8°
Retroversion (transepicondylar axis)	17.9°±13.7°	- 6.7°	47.5°
Retroversion (tangent elbow axis)	21.5°±15.1°	-10.3°	56.5°
Posterior offset (mm)[a]	2.6±1.8	- 0.8	6.1
Medial offset (mm)[a]	6.9±2.0	2.9	10.8

[a] Inclination, posterior offset, and medial offset are calculated in relation to the proximal intramedullary axis or theoretical stem axis of a humeral component.

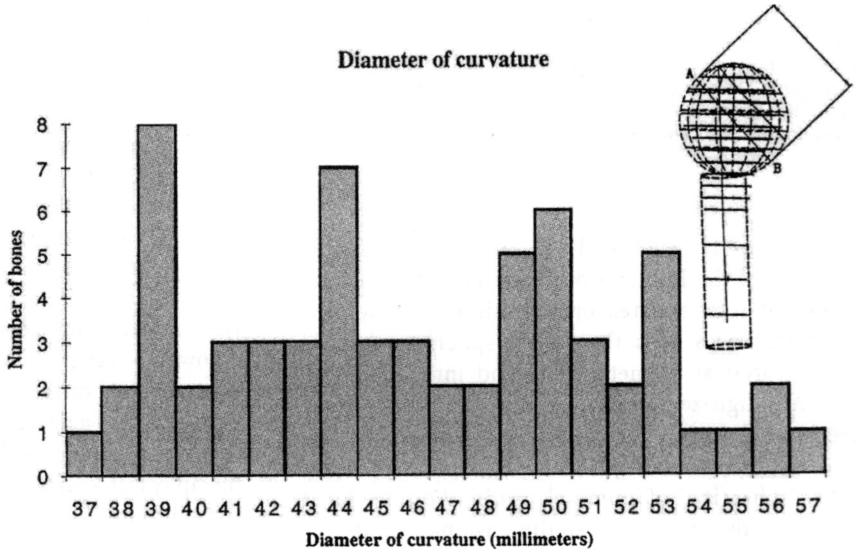

Fig. 3. Distribution of humeral head diameters

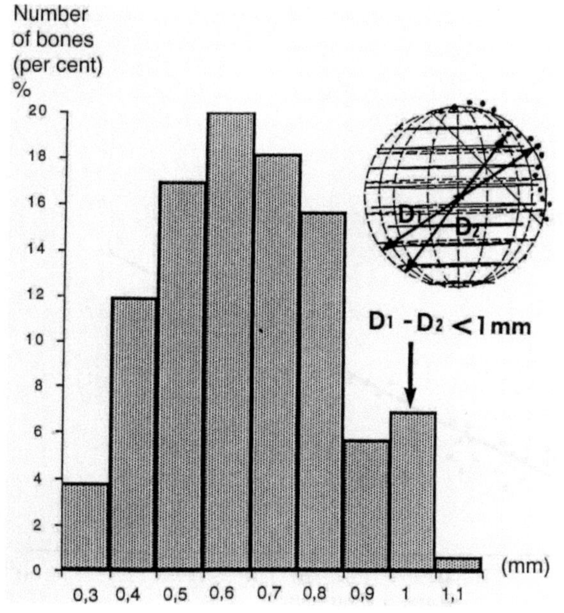

Fig. 4. Distribution of the difference between the extreme diameters (*D1*, inner diameter; *D2*, outer diameter) for the same humeral sphere. This difference was less than 1 mm in 88.2% of cases, meaning that the humeral head can be considered as part of a true sphere

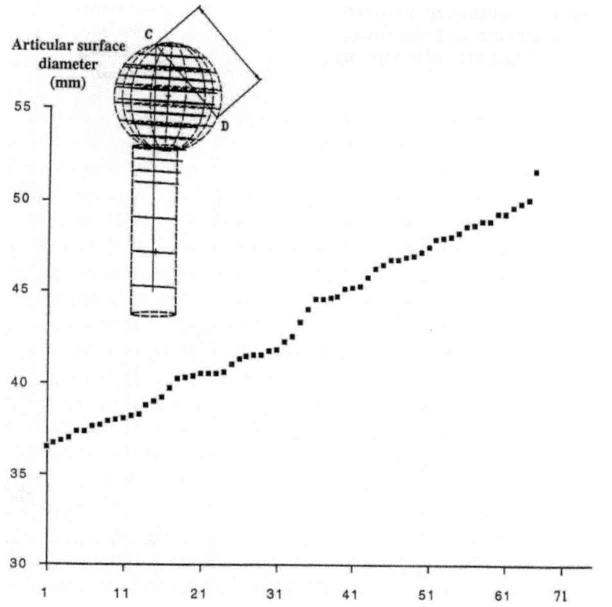

Fig. 5. Distribution of the articular surface diameters

Dimensions of the Articular Head Surface

Because of the large variations in the diameters of curvature observed, there were significant variations observed in the diameters and the thicknesses of the articular surface.

Figure 5 shows the distribution of the articular surface diameters (distance C–D): the mean articular surface diameter was 43.3 mm (range 36.5–51.7 mm).

Figure 6 shows the distribution of the height of the humeral head (distance E–F): the mean head segment thickness was 15.2 mm (range 12.1–18.2 mm).

There was a strong linear correlation between articular surface diameter and humeral head diameter (Fig. 7). Regression analysis determined the equation of the regression line as $y=0.78x+7.32$, where y was the articular surface diameter and x was the diameter of curvature ($r=0.96$).

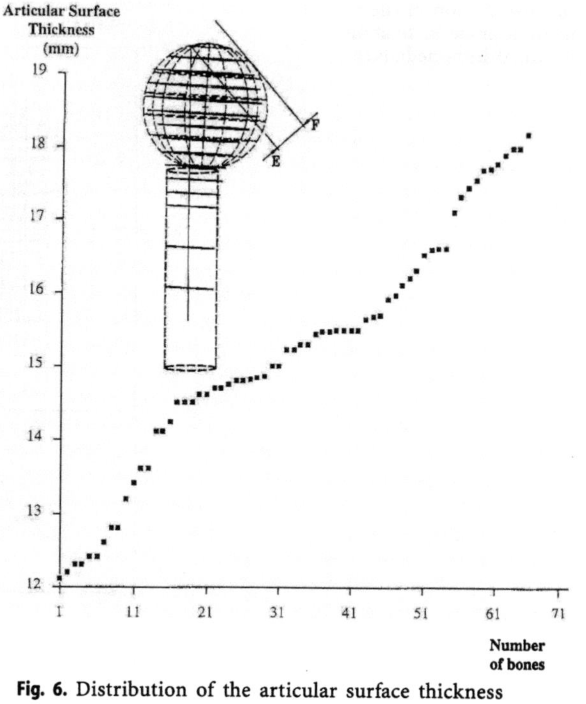

Fig. 6. Distribution of the articular surface thickness

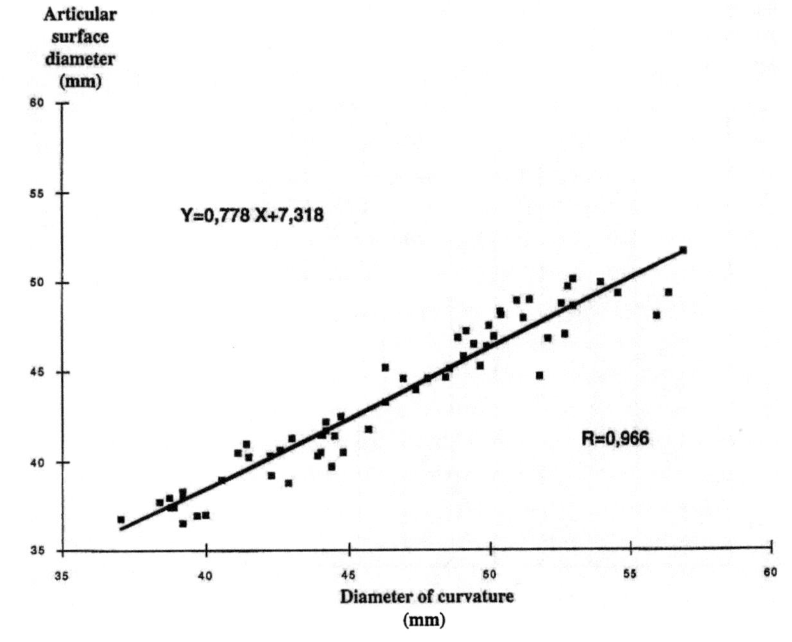

Fig. 7. Relationship between the diameter and the thickness of the articular surface

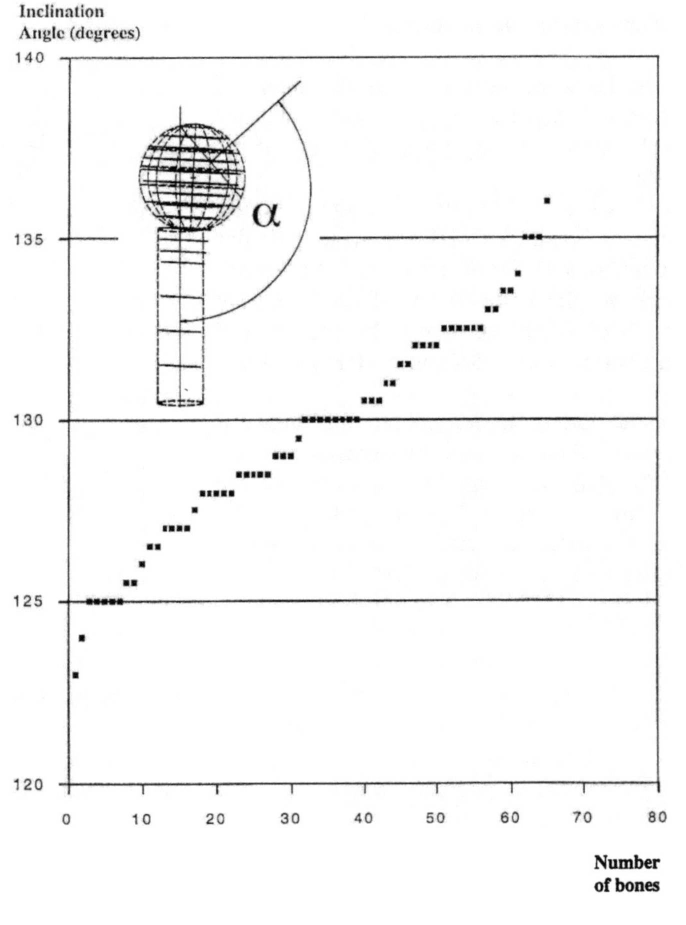

Fig. 8. Distribution of the inclination angle in relation to proximal intramedullary axis

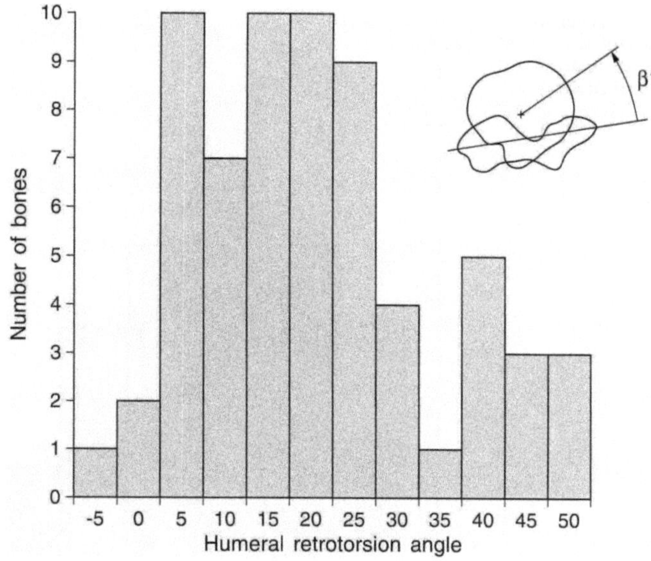

Fig. 9. Distribution of the retroversion angle in relation to the transepicondylar axis

Orientation of the Articular Head Surface

Significant variations of the inclination and retroversion angles were found.

Figure 8 shows the distribution of the inclination angles of the articular surface of the humeral heads with respect to the proximal metaphyseal (intramedullary axis) (angle α, neckshaft angle). The mean inclination was 129.6° (range 123.2°–135.8°).

Figure 9 shows the distribution of the retroversion angles of the articular surface of the humeral heads with respect to the transepicondylar axis: the mean retroversion (angle β1, Fig. 2b) was 17.9° (range -6.7° to 47.5°). This retroversion angle was 21.5° (range −10.3° to 56.5°) when measured in relation to a line tangent to the trochlea and the condyle (angle β2, Fig. 2b).

Translation of the Articular Head Surface

Our study showed that the epiphyseal sphere did not lie centrally on the base of the metaphyseal cylinder but was offset in both planes, leading to a combined offset (Fig. 10).

In the axial plane the center of the epiphyseal sphere (O) was usually translated posteriorly in relation to the center of the metaphyseal cylinder (O'; distance ΔP, Fig. 2b). Figure 11 shows the distribution of the posterior offset of the articular head surface in relation to the humeral shaft (average, 2.6 mm, with a 95° confidence limit of 0.8–6.1 mm).

In the coronal plane the center of the epiphyseal sphere (O) was translated medially in relation to the center of the metaphyseal cylinder (O'; distance ΔM, Fig. 2). The center of the epiphyseal sphere

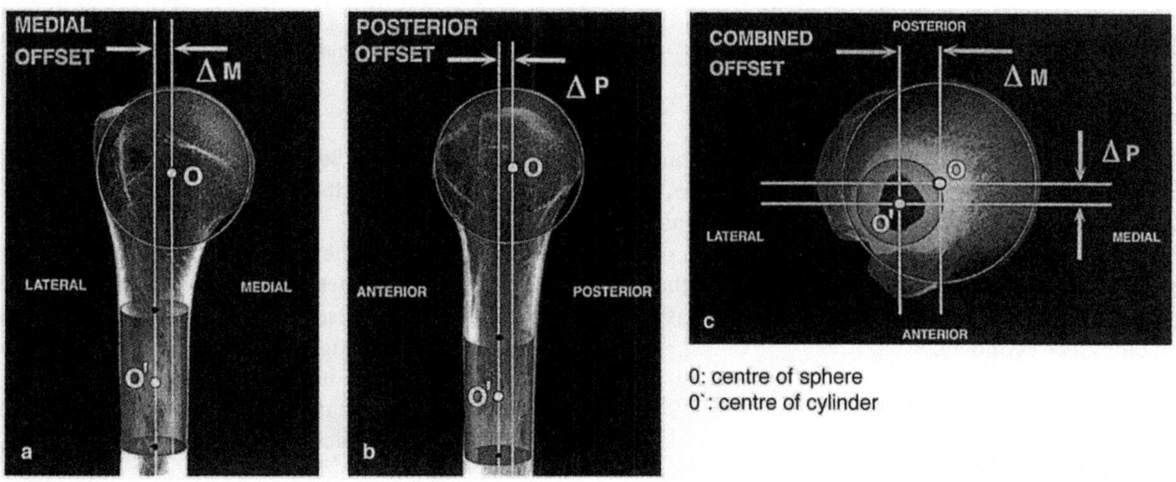

Fig. 10 a–c. Translation of the articular head surface related to a theoretical intramedullary stem axis in both coronal and axial plane illustrated on radiographs. **a** Medial offset. **b** Posterior offset. **c** Combined offset

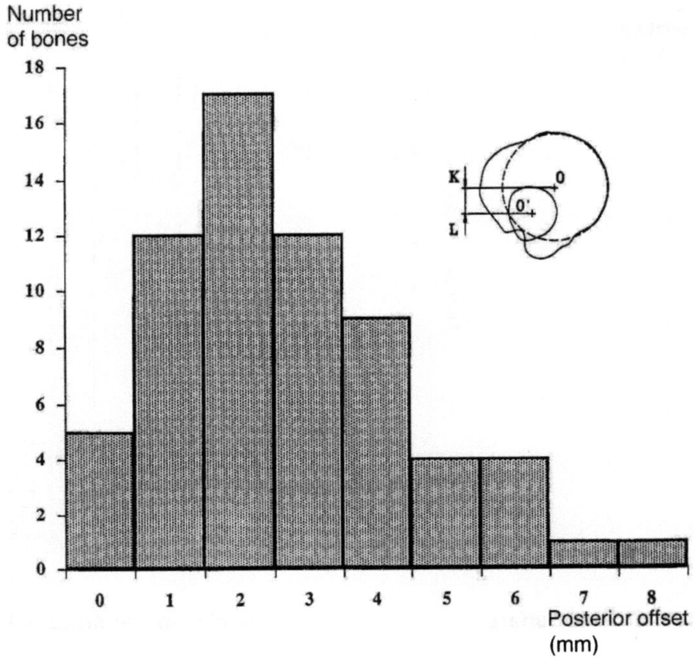

Fig. 11. Distribution of the posterior offset of the center of humeral head relative to the shaft (intramedullary stem axis)

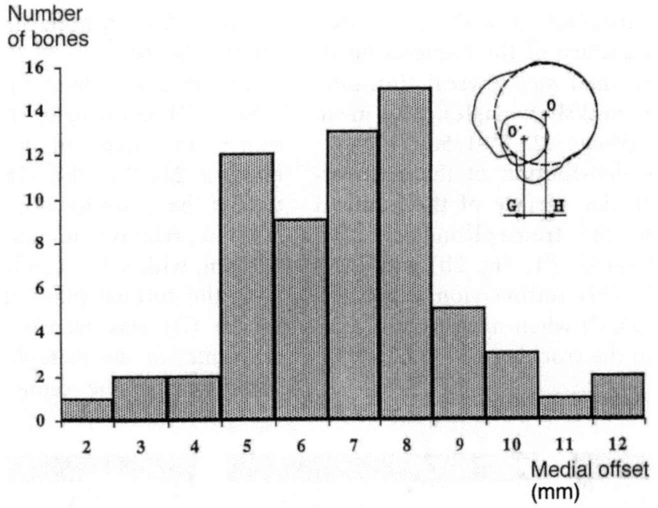

Fig. 12. Distribution of the medial offset of the center of the humeral head relative to the shaft (intramedullary stem axis)

and the center of the metaphyseal cylinder could be separated by up to 10 mm (average 6.9 mm, with 95% confidence limits of 2.9–10.8 mm). Figure 12 shows the distribution of the medial offset of the articular head surface (which is a portion of the epiphyseal shear) in relation to the humeral shaft (the metaphyseal cylinder).

Geometric Relationship Between Retroversion and Posterior Offset in the Axial Plane

Figures 1b and 2b show the geometric relationship in the axial plane between the retroversion angle and the posterior offset of the articular surface in one specimen. Although it has not been calculated in the present series, it is obvious from these drawings that part of what we call retroversion of the humeral head is in fact posterior offset.

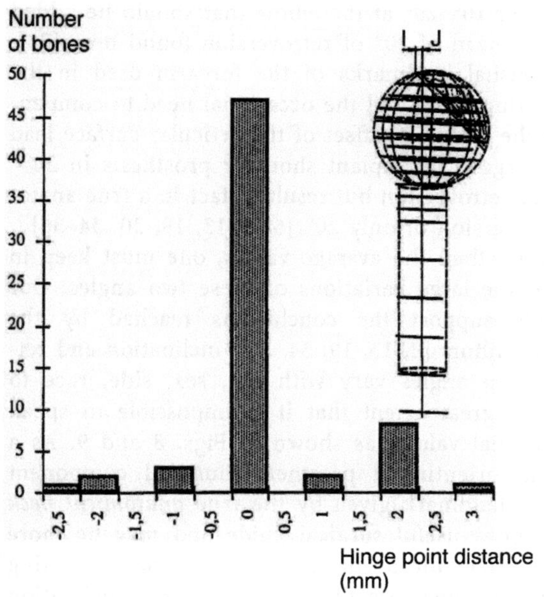

Fig. 13. Distribution of the "hinge point" distance (*C–H*): the proximal intramedullary axis intersects the plane of the anatomical neck (*C–D*) almost constantly at point C (top of the articular surface). The distance C–H was less than 1 mm in 72.3 % of the bones

Geometric Relationship Between Articular Surface and Metaphyseal (Stem) Axis in the Coronal Plane

In most of the specimens the metaphyseal axis, theoretical stem axis, intersected the plane of the humeral neck at the superior part of the anatomical neck, i.e., the superior margin of the articular head surface (Fig. 2a). The distance C–H, between the "hinge point" and the metaphyseal axis (hinge point distance), was less than 1 mm in 72.3 % of cases, meaning that the geometric relationship between the articular surface and the intramedullary axis of the proximal part of the humerus is almost constant in the coronal plane (Fig. 13).

Discussion

Our goal was to define the exact *dimensions* and *shape* of the proximal humerus. The results show that the geometry of the proximal humerus is variable: although the articular surface is spherical in about 90 % of cases, there are significant variations both in dimensions and in shape of the proximal humeri.

Surface measurements were made on *the outside* on the entire humeri. The proximal portion of the bones were modeled with simple geometric shapes: an epiphyseal sphere for the humeral head and a metaphyseal cylinder for the humeral shaft (Fig. 1). It may be argued that extramedullary measurements are less accurate than intramedullary measurements, and that fitting a cylinder to the data collected along the bone shafts is a poor geometric model. To obtain an indication of the adequacy of the geometric modeling of the shaft and the accuracy of the extramedullary measurements, we osteotomized ten humeri frontally and ten humeri sagittally and made manual measurements with a caliper inside and outside the proximal part of the bones. We observed that the cortical bone was parallel all along with less than 1 mm of difference, and that the maximum deviation of the cylinder diameter was less than 5 mm from the top to the bottom of the cylinder. This means that the errors made with extramedullary measurements are comparable to those made with intramedullary measurements, and that a cylinder is an acceptable representation of the geometry of the humeral shaft. Moreover, the fact that the humeral shaft is not a true cylinder does not prevent the axis of this shaft from being located and thus a theoretical stem axis. It may also be argued that it is arbitrary to use only the proximal half of the humerus to define the axis of the shaft (i.e., the proximal intramedullary axis). Our choice is based on two facts: first, a prosthetic stem usually locates in this proximal half of the bone, and, second, we observed both from the three-dimensional pictures of the bones obtained with the computer and from the coronal section of the humeri that there is a change in the curvature of the humeri in the frontal plane after the proximal 13 cm (Fig. 1a).

The diameters of curvature measured in this study are similar to those of others studies [9, 17, 18, 31]. However, some previous anthropometric studies of Saha [31], Maki and Gruen [21], Ishibashi et al. [18], and Ianotti et al. [17] analyzing the humeral head surface with gauge calipers, roentgenograms, or computed tomography have assumed that the central portion of the articular surface of the humeral head is spherical, but that the peripheral dimension of the articular surface is slightly elliptical. Iannoti [17], for instance, found that the axial plane is an average of 2 mm smaller than the coronal plane. Our results, as those of Roberts et al. [30] and Soslowsky et al. [32] do not support these conclusions. Using a 3D measuring machine, we found that the fit of the three-dimensional cartilage surface data to a theoretical sphere produced deviations from sphericity of less than 2 % of the diameters, indicating that the articular surface may indeed be represented by a portion of a sphere (Figs. 2, 4). Roberts et al. [30], using a similar, highly accurate and reproducible computer analysis technique, made the same observation and found that a sphere is a good representation of the geometry of the articular surface with an average accuracy of 1%. Soslowsky et al. [32], using a precise stereophotogrametry technique, also found that the humeral joint surface may be approximated by a portion of a sphere with small deviations from sphericity of less than 1% of the radius.

These various geometric models of the humeral head articular surface (spherical or slightly elliptical) are probably related to the fact that the margin of the cartilage, i.e., the anatomical neck, is not confined to one plane in space, as emphasized by Kronberg et al. [20]. Although the anterior margin of the cartilage is well demarcated and slightly elevated by a straight bony wall, the posterior margin of the articular surface is V-shaped. However, to date most of the nonconstrained shoulder prosthesis feature humeral components with a spherical head prosthesis [1, 7, 9, 22–24]. The large variations in diameter and thickness of the articular surface of the humeral head (Figs. 5, 6) are not in accordance with the conclusions reached by Neer [25], who found little variation in the normal humeral heads, regardless of the size of the patient. In contrast, our anatomical data are similar to those of others [9, 17, 18, 21, 30, 32] and support the need of a wider variety of sizes of humeral heads, which may explain the recent proliferation of modular prosthesis.

The mean inclination angle measured in our study (129.5°) corresponds to the values reported by Fick [13], Steindler [34], and Strasser [35] but is a little smaller than the value of 135° reported by Ianotti et al. [17]. The low average retroversion angle measured in the present study (17.9° in relation to the transepicondylar axis and 21.5° in relation to the tangent axis to the trochlea and condyle) agree with the values expressed by the other anatomical study of Broca [8], Khral [19], and Roberts et al. [30] who reported, respectively, 16°, 15.6°, and 21.4°. Using X-ray or computed tomography, other authors [20, 24, 27, 28] have found greater retroversion, ranging from 25° to 30°. The higher value of 30°–40° degrees of retroversion, currently recommended in the surgical literature for humeral head replacement, has been successful for many years because it probably represents a favorable compromise between true retroversion, posterior offset and carrying angle of the forearm [7, 30, 33].

As we have mentioned in a previous study [6], two important geometric considerations of the humerus should be taken into account when considering "surgical retroversion": (a) previous interpretation of retroversion did not take into account the posterior displacement of the articular surface, as shown in Fig. 2b; (b) there is a mean carrying angle of 10°–20° at the elbow that should be added to the mean of 20° of retroversion found here [33]. The visual landmarks of the forearm used in the operating room and the occasional need to compensate the posterior offset of the articular surface lead the surgeon to implant shoulder prosthesis in 30°–40° of retroversion but result in fact in a true anatomical version of only 20° [6, 8, 13, 19, 30, 34–36].

More than the average values, one must keep in mind the large variations of these two angles. Our results support the conclusions reached by the early authors [8, 13, 19, 34, 35]: inclination and retroversion angles vary with age, sex, side, race to such a great extent that it is impossible to speak of normal values, as shown in Figs. 8 and 9. As a result, orienting a prosthetic humeral component to the landmark given by the true *anatomical neck* may be a useful surgical guide and may be more appropriate for a specific shoulder than orienting every patient's prosthesis to the same inclination and the same retroversion [2].

This study shows that the shape of the proximal humerus varies according to the variable orientation of the articular surface (inclination, retroversion) and variable location of this articular surface (medial offset, posterior offset). Although a few recent studies have emphasized this variable shape of the proximal humerus [2, 17, 30, 36], it is interesting to note that some early investigators such as Broca [8], Fick [13], Khral [19], Steindler [34], and Strasser [32] were already aware of the significant variations in inclination and retroversion and even knew of the existence of possible medial and posterior offsets of the humeral head articular surface. The significant and variable posterior and medial offset of the articular surface found in the present study also contributes to a large extent to the variable shape of the proximal humerus. The average posterior offset measured in our study was 2.6 mm (range, 0.8–6.1 mm; Fig. 11). Roberts et al. [30], using an extramedullary method similar to ours, found a posterior offset of 4.7 mm (0–12 mm) while Ballmer et al. [2], using a intramedullary method, found an offset ranging from 3 mm anterior to 4 mm posterior, with an average of 2 mm posterior. This study reveals that part of what we call retroversion of the humeral head is in fact posterior offset (Fig. 2b) and should be considered by shoulder surgeons. The medial offset of the articular surface (average 6.9 mm) found in this study as well as the close geometric relationships between the theoretical stem axis and the articular surface in the coronal plane have never been reported in the previous literature. The constant intersection point between the metaphyseal axis and the superior margin of the articular head surface or "hinge point", observed in 72.3% of the humeri, represents a useful surgical guide: when performing a hemiarthroplasty, the medullary canal of the humerus should be reamed starting at a point lateral on the cut surface (Fig. 2a).

Surgical Relevance

Reproduction of the anatomical model may be difficult at arthroplasty. Lack of respect of the variable shape of the proximal humerus may have biomechanical consequences by malpositioning the joint line or deviating the instant centers of rotation [5, 12, 14, 15, 29]. Although it is difficult to know how precise the reconstruction of the proximal humerus should be, information in the literature shows that the possibilities are reduced. Fischer [12] has shown, for instance, that displacing the center of curvature by 20% of its radius (5 mm for an average radius of curvature of 25 mm) alters the lever arm of the rotator cuff by 20%.

Failure to respect the geometric features of the proximal humerus, related to the prosthesis design or a poor surgical technique, can lead to pathological situations, well described in the literature (Table 2). For instance, excessive superior "bulging" of the prosthetic head related to a prosthesis design that does not respect the medial offset of the articular surface or a humeral component scaled too high results in a *subacromial (superior) impingement* with excessive tension on the rotator cuff superiorly [25]. If the reverse mistake is made with a low placement of the humeral head prosthesis, the greater tuberosity is prominent and impinges against the posterosuperior margin of the glenoid: *glenoid (posterior) impingement* [25, 37]. Finally, eccentric placement, related to abnormal rotation and/or abnormal anteroposterior translation of the articular head surface, can lead to either coracoid *(anterior) impingement* [11, 16, 30] or *anteroposterior instability* with asymmetric tension on the external/internal rotators [10, 22, 24].

The concept defended by Neer [23–25], a pioneer in shoulder arthoplasty, was that "design of total shoulder arthroplasty should mimic the normal anatomy to provide the best function and durability." The design developed by Neer [23–25] for the humeral component was based on one radius of curvature for the humeral head (44 mm) with a choice of two different thickness (15, 22 mm). This first generation of shoulder prosthesis met the need of many patients even though it proposed only a midrange of sizes and did not respect exactly the coronal and axial geometry of the proximal humerus. This prosthesis remains the "gold standard" because it has been associated with excellent and good results with a long follow-up [7, 14, 24]. The present study helps to understand how the surgical technique may compensate the variable geometric features sometimes encountered in proximal humeri by meticulous attention to detail in placement of the component.

The surgeon's experience and judgement are required for appropriate placement (orientation and location) of the prosthesis and closer anatomical reconstruction (Table 2). For instance, the variable medial offset and variable inclination of the articular surface may be compensated by choosing a smaller diameter stem while increasing varus or medially translating the humeral component (Fig. 14). However, varus or medial positioning of humeral component may tighten soft tissues by increasing separation between their glenoid and humeral attachments, and may be questionable [10]. When the humeral head prosthesis sits eccentrically (anteriorly) in the axial plane, the surgeon has also two technical possibilities: one is to choose a smaller diameter stem to allow posterior translation and

Table 2. Variable orientation (inclination and retrotorsion) and variable location (medial offset and posterior offset) of the articular surface of the humeral head: pathological consequences if not matched and surgical possibilities of control while positioning and orientating a standard, loose-fit humeral component

Articular head surface orientation and location		Potential pathological consequences if not respected wiht a humeral component	Surgeon-controllable variables[a]
coronal plane	Inclination	Subacromial (superior) impingement (if superior "bulging" of the prosthetic head)	Varus/valgus tilt
	Medial offset	Glenoid (posterior) impingement (if inferior "sliding" of the prosthetic head)	Mediolateral translation
axial plane	Retroversion	Coracoid (anterior) impingement (if anterior "bulging" of the prosthetic head)	Anteversion/retroversion
	Posterior offset	Anteroposterior instability (if abnormal rotation and/or anteroposterior translation of humeral component)	Anteroposterior translation

[a] These possibilities are partially or totally reduced with cementless, close-fitting humeral components and/or a humeral components with too long stems.

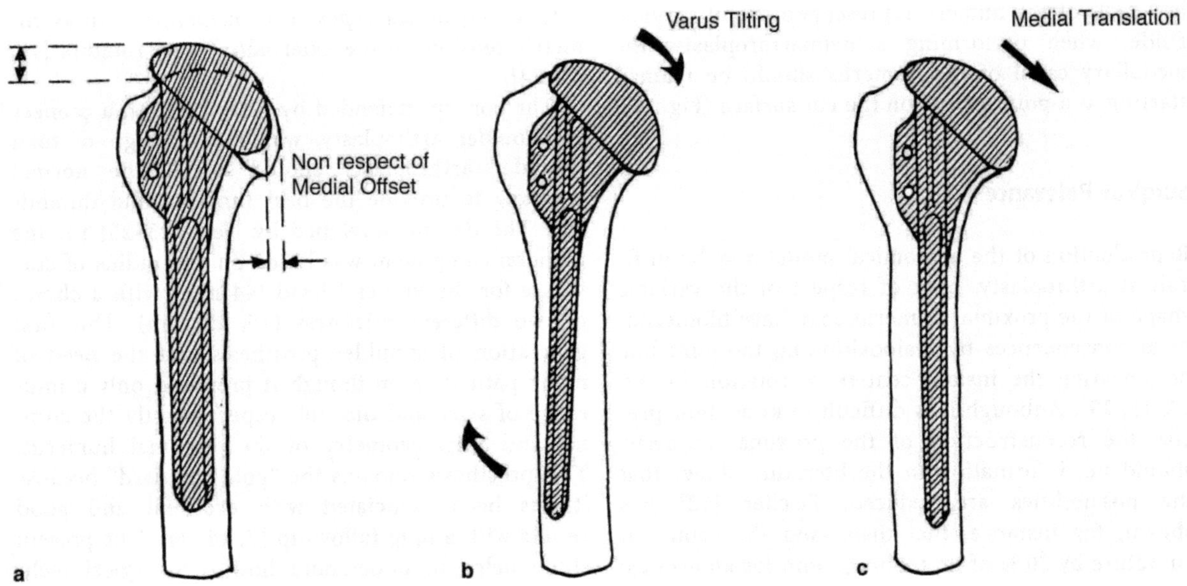

Fig. 14. Two ways of dealing with medial offset of the articular head surface at surgery, when using a prosthesis than does not respect the "hinge point": implanting the prosthesis with some varus (with a loose fit stem; *A*), implanting the prosthesis with some medial translation (also with a loose fit stem; *B*)

centralization of the prosthesis at the time of cement fixation; the other is to resect more bone posteriorly, taking care to the rotator cuff insertion, to allow increasing of prosthetic retroversion (Fig. 15). However, altering the version of the prosthesis to face more posteriorly may not restore the balance between the anterior and posterior structures and may be questionable [10, 11].

The second generation of shoulder prosthesis, currently being developed, is represented by modular prostheses which offer a greater selection of sizes for both the prosthetic head and stem. The greater number of prosthetic heads may help the surgeon to respect the variation in sizes of the articular surface and to improve the soft tissue balancing [2, 10, 14, 22]. The greater number of prosthetic stems is aimed, in theory, at improving primary stabilization and fixation of the humeral component. Our study suggests that filling of the medullary canal with the prosthetic stem may become a possible handicap to reproducing the anatomical model by seating the head prosthesis eccentrically. The close fitting of cementless stem prostheses may dictate the position of the prosthetic head and make it more difficult (if not possible) to respect the medial and posterior offset of the articular surface and thus achieve the covering of the bone cut. As emphasized by Ballmer et al. [2], prosthesis fit eliminates all but two of the six degrees of freedom, leaving only the depth of insertion and the rotation of the prosthesis stem to be adjusted. However, if a loose-fit prosthesis offers more surgical possibilities, fixation may become questionable. In addition to stem diameter, stem *length* may be limiting factor: a stem that is too long may prevent the surgeon from inserting a hum-

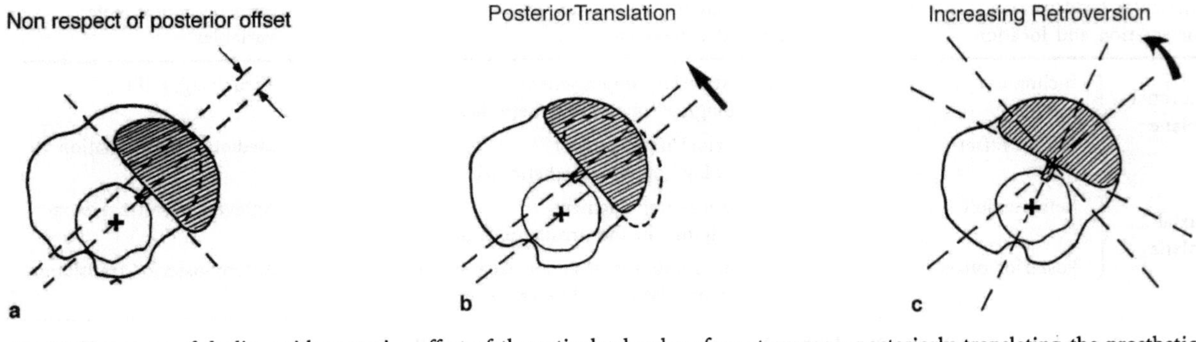

Fig. 15. Two ways of dealing with posterior offset of the articular head surface at surgery: posteriorly translating the prosthetic head with a loose fit stem (*A*), increasing prosthetic retroversion with a bone cut in excessive version (*B*)

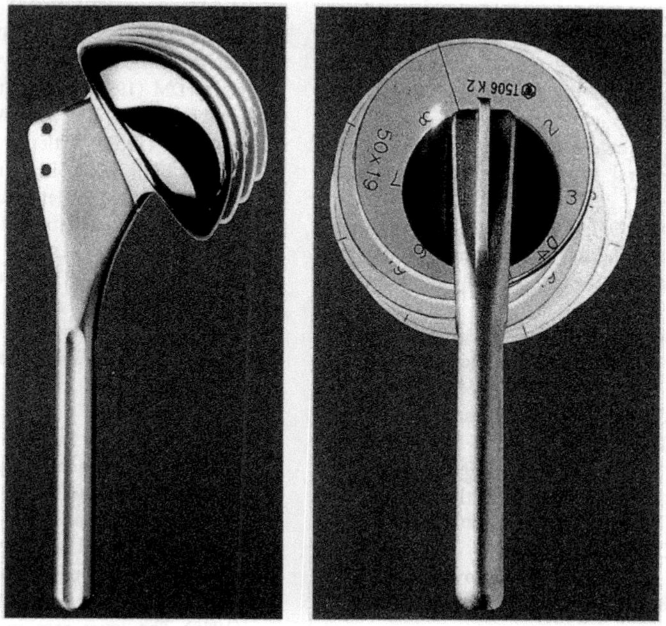

Fig. 16 a,b. The Aequalis prosthesis, an adaptable prosthesis. **a** Adaptation of inclination by a system of variable necks between the stem and the head; **b** Adaptation of mediolateral and anteroposterior offset through an eccentric indexing system

eral prosthesis with enough varus (trying to compensate for a large medial offset, for instance) because of the change in the coronal curvature of the diaphysis past the first 15 cm.

The geometric considerations in the present study are helpful for identifying the limits of humeral prosthetic design currently available and for understanding the importance and the limits of the surgical technique in shoulder arthroplasty. Hence, it is not unreasonable to suggest that if a third generation of shoulder prosthesis is needed, it should emphasize both the correct placement of the prosthetic head, to restore the normal glenohumeral anatomy and kinematics, and the filling of the medullary canal with the stem, to optimize component fixation. Although good clinical results with shoulder replacement can be achieved using both the modular and nonmodular components that are currently available, their relatively fixed geometry means that they are not truly anatomical when compared with the findings of our study. The shape of the proximal humerus is variable, much more variable in fact than most contemporary humeral component designs would suggest or can accommodate [3, 4, 34].

In order to restore the variable three-dimensional geometry of the proximal humerus, we have developed a new type of humeral component which is not only modular but also adaptable to the individual bony anatomy. *Prosthetic* adaptability is a new concept in shoulder arthroplasty that concentrates on the correct placement of the prosthetic head, allowing restoration of the normal glenohumeral anatomy and kinematics as well as filling the medullary canal with the stem to optimize component fixation. The design of this new type of prosthesis incorporates the variable inclination by using variably angled neck components between the stem and the prosthetic head and the variable, combined (posterior and medial) offset of the articular surface through an eccentric indexing system (Fig. 16). Individual head retroversion is provided by individual osteotomy of the articular surface after removal of the crown of osteophytes. Restoring soft tissue tension *(soft tissue balancing)* by performing an anterior and/or posterior release, in combination with the correct restoration of the spatial positioning of the humeral head relative to the humerus *(bony balancing)* by using this new type of adaptable prosthesis should result in *anatomical balancing.*

This new type of adaptable shoulder prosthesis, by placing the center of rotation back to its original position, should present at least three advantages: (a) restoring normal kinematics with better movements; (b) protecting the rotator cuff by avoiding its overtensioning; (c) decreasing abnormal eccentric loads on the glenoid component.

References

1. Amstutz HC, Sew Hoy AL, Clarke IC (1981) UCLA anatomic total shoulder arthroplasty. Clin Orthop 155:7–20
2. Ballmer FT, Sidles JA, Lippitt SB, Matsen FA (1993) Humeral head prosthetic arthroplasty: surgically relevant geometric considerations. J Shoulder Elbow Surg 2:296–304
3. Boileau P, Walch G (1994) The combined offset (medial and posterior) of the humeral sphere. J Shoulder Elbow Surg 3:6

4. Boileau P, Walch, G (1996) Varus shoulder prosthesis: error or necessity? J Shoulder Elbow Surg 62:186
5. Boileau P, Walch G, Liotard JP (1992) Cineradiographic study of active elevation of the prosthetic shoulder. Rev Chir Orthop 6:351–359
6. Boileau P, Walch G, Mazzoleni N, Urien JP (1993) In vitro measurement of humeral head retroversion. J Shoulder Elbow Surg 2:12
7. Boileau P, Walch G (1997) The three-dimensional Geometry of the proximal humerus: Implications for Surgical Technique and Prosthetic Design. J Bone and Joint Surg 75B 5:857–865
8. Broca P (1881) La torsion de l'humérus et le tropomètre, instrument destiné à mesurer la torsion des os. Rev Anthrop 4:193–210, 385–423, 1577–1592
9. Clarke IC, Gruen TAW, Sew Hoy A, Hirschowitz D, Maki S, Amstutz HC (1979) Problems in gleno-humeral surface replacements - real or imagined? Eng Med 8:161–175
10. Collins DN, Harryman DTII, Lippitt SB, Jackins SE, Matsen FA III (1991) The technique of glenohumeral arthroplasty. Techniques Orthop 6:43–59
11. Dines DM, Warren RF, Inglis AE, Pavlov H (1990) The coracoid impingement syndrome. J Bone Joint Surg Br 72:314–316
12. Fischer LP, Carret JP, Gonon GP, Dimnet J (1977) Etude cinématique des mouvements de l'articulation scapulo-humérale. Rev Chir Orthop 63 [Suppl II]:108–112
13. Fick R (1904) Anatomie und Mechanik der Gelenke. Fischer, Jena, pp 171–174
14. Figgie HE III, Inglis AE, Golberg VM, Ranawat CS, Figgie MP, Wile JM (1988) An analysis of factors affecting the long term results of total shoulder arthroplasty in inflammatory arthritis. J Arthroplasty 3:123–130
15. Friedman RJ (1990) Biomechanics of the shoulder following total shoulder replacement. In: Post M, Morrey BF, Hawkins RJ (eds) Surgery of the shoulder. Mosby–Year Book, St. Louis, pp 263–266
16. Gerber C, Terrier F, Zehnder R, Ganz R (1987) The subcoracoid space: an anatomic study. Clin Orthop 215:132–138
17. Ianotti JP, Gabriel JP, Schneck SL, Evans BG, Misra S (1992) The normal glenohumeral relationships. An anatomical study of the hundred and fourty shoulders J Bone Joint Surg Am 74:491–500
18. Ishibashi T, Mikasa M, Fukuda H (1990) A new humeral prosthesis for the Japanese. In: Post M, Morrey BF, Hawkins RJ (eds) Surgery of the shoulder. Mosby–Year Book, St. Louis, pp 273–281
19. Khral VE, Evans FG (1945) Humeral torsion in man. Am J Phys Anthrop 3:229–253
20. Kronberg M, Brostrom MD, Soderlund V (1990) Retroversion of the humeral head in the normal shoulder and its relationship to the normal range of motion. Clin Orthop 253:113–117
21. Maki S, Gruen T (1976) Anthropometric study of the glenohumeral relationships. Trans Orthop Res Soc 1:173
22. Moeckel BH, Altcheck DW, Warren RF, Wickiewicz TL, Dines DM (1993) Instability of the shoulder after arthroplasty. J Bone Joint Surg Am 75:492–497
23. Neer CS (1955) Articular replacement for the humeral head. J Bone Joint Surg Am 37:215–228
24. Neer CS (1990) Glenohumeral arthroplasty design In: Shoulder reconstruction, 1st edn. Saunders, Philadelphia, pp 146–160
25. Neer CS, Watson KC, Stanton FJ (1982) Recent experience in total shoulder replacement. J Bone Joint Surg Am 64:319
26. Neter J, Wasserman W (1974) Applied Linear statistical models. In: Irwin RD (ed) Regression analysis of variance and experimental designs. Homewood
27. Ovesen J, Nielsen S (1985) Prosthesis position in shoulder arthroplasty: a cadaver study of the humeral component. Acta Orthop Scand 56:330
28. Randelli M, Gambrioli PL (1986) Glenohumeral osteometry by computed tomography in normal and unstable shoulders. Clin Orthop 208:151
29. Rietveld ABM, Daanen HAM, Rezing PM, Obermann WR (1988) The lever arm in gleno-humeral abduction after hemi-arthroplasty. J Bone Joint Surg Br 70:561–565
30. Roberts SNJ, Foley APJ, Swallow HM, Wallace WA, Coughlan DP (1991) The geometry of the humeral head and the design of protheses. J Bone Joint Surg Br 73:647–650
31. Saha AK (1961) *. In: Theory of the shoulder mechanism: descriptive and applied. Thomas, Springfield, pp 1–55
32. Soslowsky LJ, Flatow EL, Bigliani LU, Mow VC (1992) Articular geometry of the glenohumeral joint. Clin Orthop 285:181–190
33. Steel FLD, Tomlinson JDW (1989) The carrying angle in man. J Anat. 92:315–317
34. Steindler A (1936) Mechanics of shoulder arm complex. In: Thomas CC (ed) Kinesiology of the human body under normal and pathological conditions. Thomas, Springfield, p 453
35. Strasser H (1936) Das Shultergelenk. Die obere Extremität. In: Lerbuch der Muskel- und Gelenkmechanik. Springer, Berlin, pp 17–21
36. Walch G, Boileau P (1992) Morphological study of the humeral proximal epiphysis. Orthop. Proc. J Bone Joint Surg Br 74 [Suppl I]:14
37. Walch G, Boileau P, Noel E, Donnell ST (1992) Impingement of the deep surface of the supraspinatus tendon on the postero superior glenoid rim: an arthroscopic study. J Shoulder Elbow Surg 1:238–245

Prosthetic Adaptability: A New Concept in Shoulder Arthroplasty

P. Boileau and G. Walch

Summary

The large variation in articular surface dimensions makes modularity a prerequisite for the design of a shoulder prosthesis. However, the variable shape of the proximal humerus, as observed in our anatomical study, has led us to develop a new generation of shoulder prosthesis which is not only modular but also adaptable to the individual anatomy. Prosthetic adaptability is a new concept which allows four geometrical parameters to be taken into account intraoperatively: inclination, retroversion, posterior offset and medial offset can be individualised for each shoulder, thanks to technological innovations.

Introduction

The goal of a surgeon inserting a shoulder prosthesis is, as with all prosthetic surgery, to come as close as possible to the anatomical model. This raises two questions: (a) Are we sure we are perfectly familiar with the anatomical model? (b) Do the standard prostheses at our disposal, including modular systems, allow us to reproduce this anatomical model? It was with the aim of answering these two questions that we have been working since 1988 on a morphological study of the gleno-humeral joint and the possibilities of reproducing the morphology using a shoulder prosthesis.

We discuss here the development of the humeral side of these studies and their consequences on the design of the shoulder prosthesis; the glenoidal side will be dealt with in a separate article.

Morphological Study of the Proximal Humerus

The aim of the anatomical study [3, 4, 5, 7, 21] was to establish precisely both the dimensions and shape of the proximal humerus. The study was carried out using dry bones taken from cadavers and using modern investigative techniques: precision measurement machines and computer-aided design programmes. The precalibrated precision measurement machine was fitted with a support designed to hold the humerus so that a number of points on the bone surface could be digitised (Fig. 1a).

Each humerus was fixed in the support by the top of the humeral head and at the level of the epicondyle and epitrochlea. With the bone turning 10° at a time, the digitisation of its surface points was made from parallel sections located every 5 mm on the proximal and distal epiphyses and every 10 mm on the diaphysis. A 1-µm precision probe was used to note the coordinates of 36 regularly spaced points for each bony section, amounting to 1200 points per humerus. Particular attention was paid to the digiti-

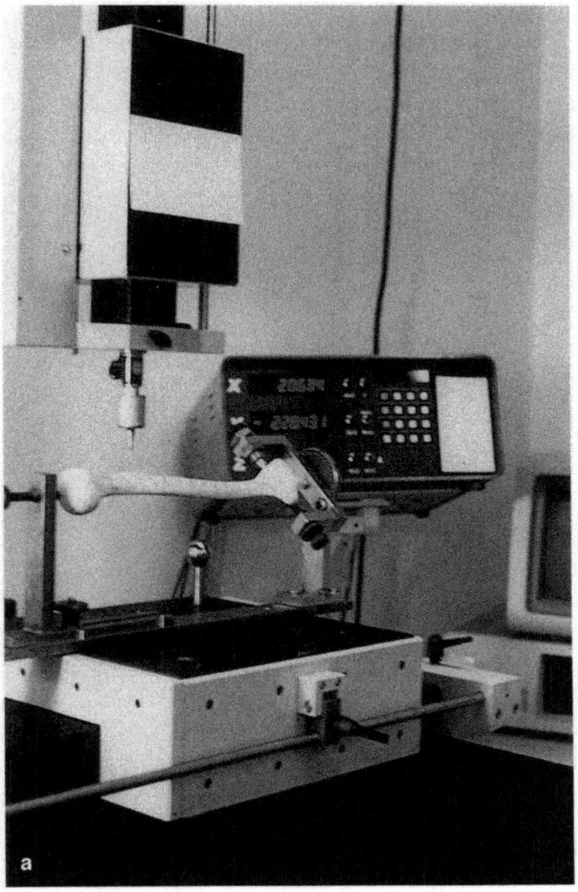

Fig. 1. a Digitalization of humeri using a precision measurement machine linked to a computer for analysis of the bone's shape and dimensions

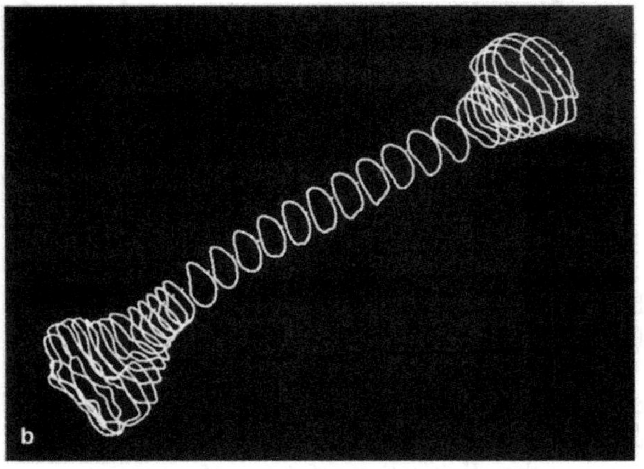

Fig. 1. (continued) **b** Resulting three-dimensional image of a humerus

sation of the articular surface of the humeral head in that a number of points at the periphery and over the entire stretch of the articular cartilage were noted. All of these coordinates were then transmitted to a computer fitted with a software programme giving a three-dimensional image of the humerus (Fig. 1b).

The computer was able to give a precise calculation of the different morphological parameters (diameter, thickness, inclination, retroversion) on the one hand and produce a model of the proximal end of the humerus using simple geometrical figures on the other: epiphyseal sphere and metaphyseal cylinder (Fig. 2a). Two axes were defined (Fig. 2a): the diaphyseal axis, rotational axis of the humeri, and the proximal metaphyseal axis, along which a prosthetic stem can be inserted.

Sphericity of the Humeral Head

We first wanted to verify the sphericity of the humeral head. Using the recorded articular surface points, we were able to determine the diameters of the potential humeral sphere. In order to verify this sphericity we used the classical method of least-squares optimization [21], defined as the difference between two extreme diameters: (E)=(D1)–(D2). Thus, a geometrical figure where the difference between the two most extreme diameters is less than 1 mm, may be considered as being a sphere. Of the 160 humeri studied, the difference between extreme diameters was less than 1 mm in 88.2% of cases.

We can therefore confirm that in almost 90% of cases, the humeral head is comparable to a sphere. The articular surface constitutes about a third of this sphere. This is an important concept that had not been previously fully acknowledged by other authors [14].

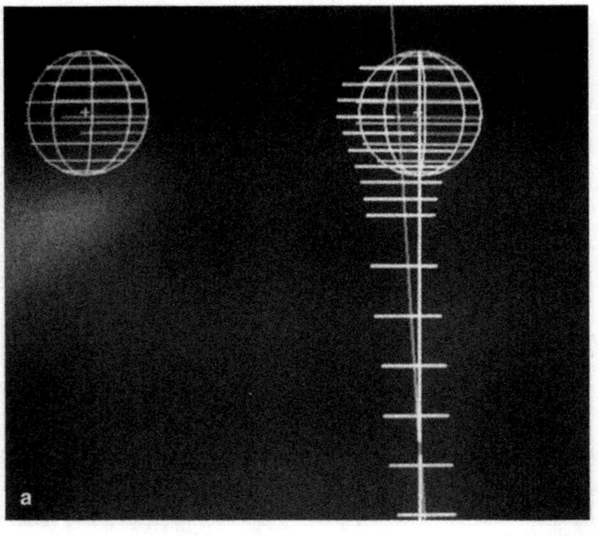

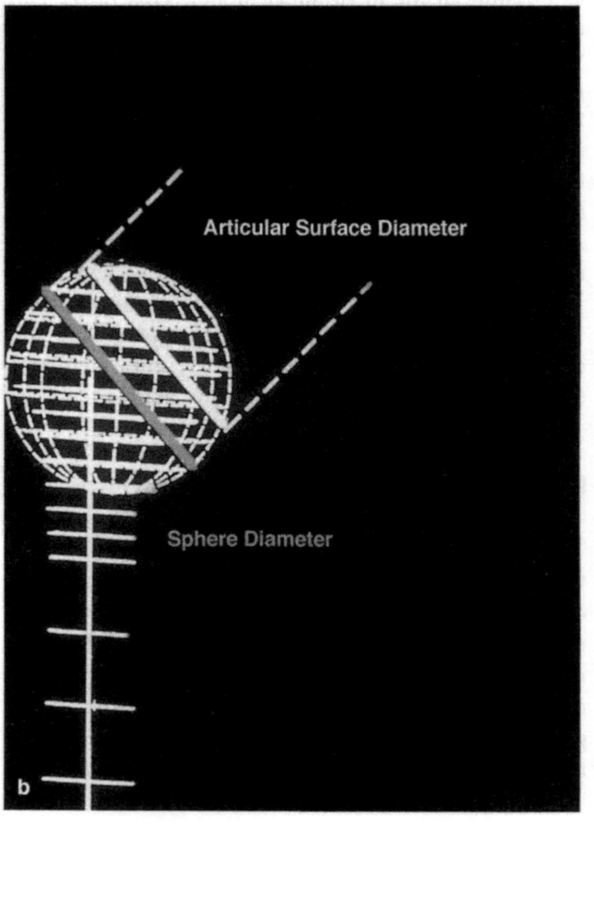

Fig. 2. **a** Model of the humerus produced using simple geometrical figures: epiphyseal sphere and metaphyseal cylinder. The metaphyseal axis is that of the metaphyseal cylinder along which a prosthetic stem can be inserted. **b** Humeral head sphericity and mathematical relationship linking the three parameters: diameter of the sphere, diameter of the head and thickness of the humeral head

Dimensional Variations of the Humeral Articular Surface

Since the humeral head is a sphere and the articular surface constitutes only part of this sphere, there is a mathematical relationship between the diameter of the humeral sphere, the diameter of the humeral head and the thickness of the humeral head (Fig. 2b). As two of these parameters are known, the third one can be calculated. The mean *diameter of curvature* (humeral head diameter) measured was 46.2 mm with a minimum of 37.1 and a maximum of 56.9 mm. Our anatomical studies showed that there were wide variations in the dimensions of the articular surface: (a) the diameter of the articular head surface was highly variable, averaging 43.3 mm, range 36.5–51.7 mm; (b) similarly, the thickness of the articular head surface was highly variable, averaging 15.2 mm, range 12.1–18.2 mm.

Prosthetic Modularity: The Consequences of Dimensional Variation

The large variation in the dimensions of the articular surface in both diameter and thickness makes the idea of modularity a prerequisite in the design of shoulder prostheses [5, 7, 9]. Standard humeral prostheses (first generation,"monoblock" prosthesis) cannot pretend to cope with the anatomical variations encountered. The Neer prosthesis, for example, with a single diameter of 44 mm and two head thicknesses (15 and 22 mm), can only rarely reproduce the anatomical model.

This undoubtedly explains certain poor functional results and certain abnormal biomechanical situations with reduction of gleno-humeral prosthetic mobility, such as we and others have observed during a radiocinematographic study of Neer prostheses [2, 11]. Thus a second-generation of modular prostheses have appeared in recent years. Three generations of unconstrained shoulder prosthesis are now available:

- First-generation prosthesis: "monoblock, non-modular"
  - Neer (3 M)
  - Cofield (Richards)
  - Fenlin (Zimmer)
- Second generation prosthesis: "modular"
  - Modular (3 M)
  - Bio-modular (Biomet)
  - Select shoulder (Intermedics)
  - Global (Depuy)
- Third generation prosthesis: "modular and adaptable"
  - Aequalis (Tornier).

The theoretical advantages of a modular prosthesis are: (a) the ability to select an exact diameter and thickness of articular head which is important in the muscular-ligamentous balance of the shoulder; (b) the ability to match the differing radii of curvature between the glenoid and the corresponding prosthetic humeral head. These two abilities to better match the anatomy led us to believe that the biomechanical behaviour achieved will be closer to normal behaviour.

However, the modularity only allows adaptation to dimensional variations of the articular surface and not to variations in orientation and position in space of this articular surface, in other words, to variations in the shape of the proximal end of the humerus.

Variations in the Orientation of the Humeral Articular Surface

Our anatomical studies have shown that the angular variations are very important, especially the inclination and retroversion of the articular surface. The idea of an average value here is completely relative, and it is the idea of variation which must be kept in mind (Fig. 3). The humeral inclination averages 129.6° varying between 123.2° and 135.8°. Similarly the humeral retroversion is highly variable depending on the individual and even between right and left sides of the same individual. This retroversion, averaged 17.9° varying from –6.5 to 47.5°.

Variation of Position in Space of the Humeral Articular Surface

The intra-medullary axis along which the humeral prosthesis is inserted is that of the proximal metaphysis since a change in curvature occurs at the humeral diaphysis. It is therefore possible to identify a proximal humeral metaphyseal cylinder which contain the stem. We have seen that the articular surface was spherical, and that the computer was able to determine the epiphyseal sphere which was best adapted to this articular surface. *The question therefore is to know what is the position in space of the sphere in relation to the cylinder?*

Our anatomical work showed that the spherical humeral head does not sit on the base of the cylinder but lies eccentrically in two planes (Fig. 4).

In the frontal plane the medial displacement of the spherical head defines a offset. This *medial offset* is characterised in practice by the proximal meta-

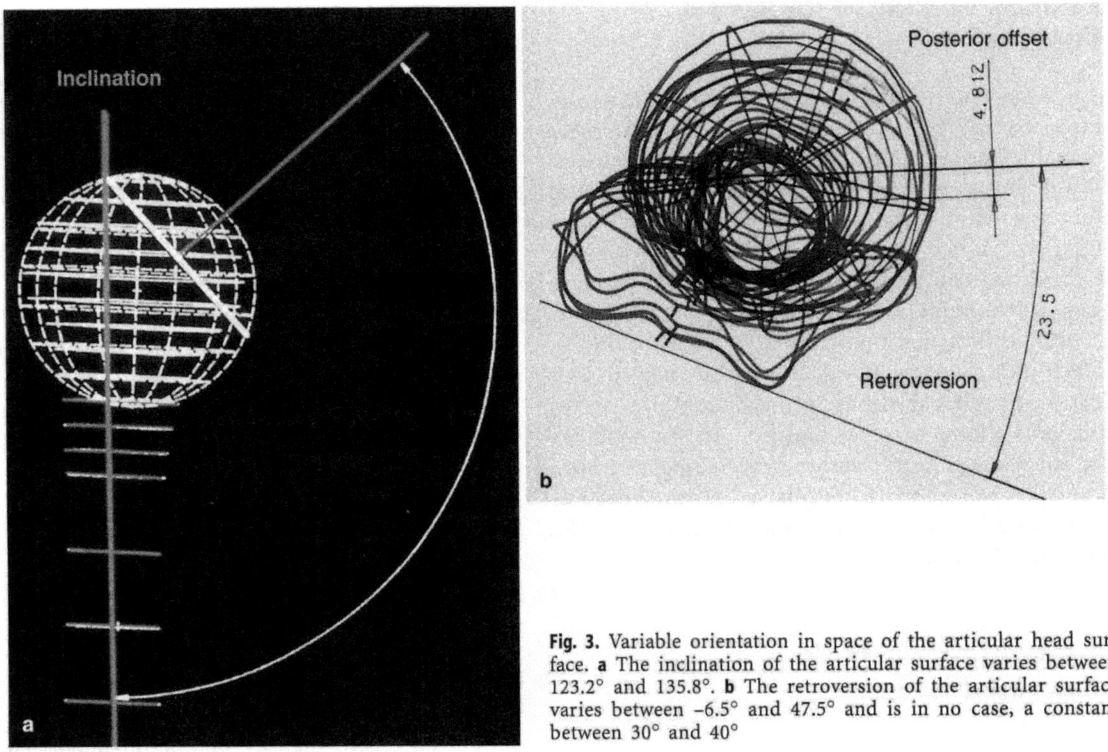

Fig. 3. Variable orientation in space of the articular head surface. **a** The inclination of the articular surface varies between 123.2° and 135.8°. **b** The retroversion of the articular surface varies between -6.5° and 47.5° and is in no case, a constant between 30° and 40°

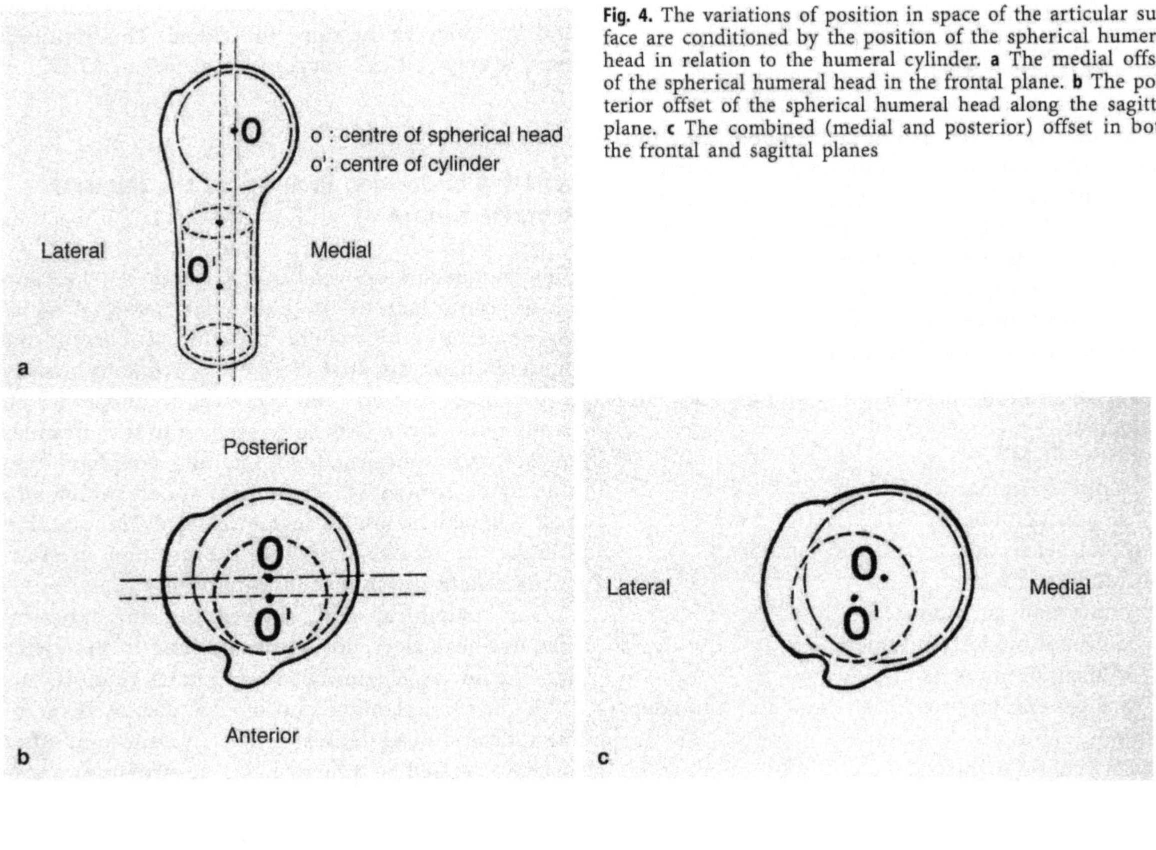

Fig. 4. The variations of position in space of the articular surface are conditioned by the position of the spherical humeral head in relation to the humeral cylinder. **a** The medial offset of the spherical humeral head in the frontal plane. **b** The posterior offset of the spherical humeral head along the sagittal plane. **c** The combined (medial and posterior) offset in both the frontal and sagittal planes

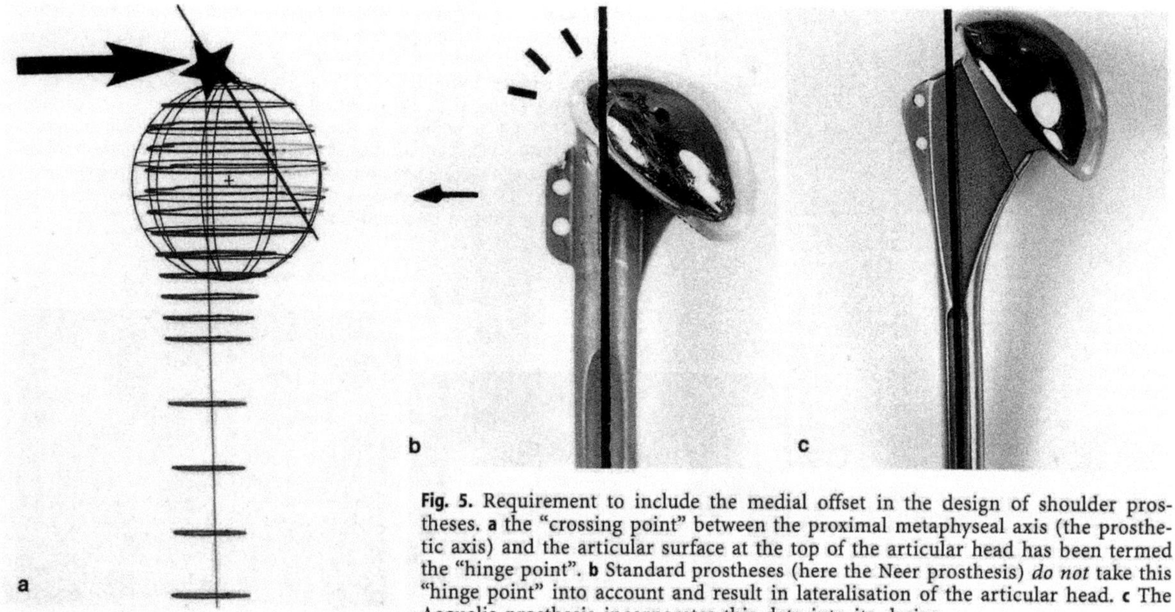

Fig. 5. Requirement to include the medial offset in the design of shoulder prostheses. **a** the "crossing point" between the proximal metaphyseal axis (the prosthetic axis) and the articular surface at the top of the articular head has been termed the "hinge point". **b** Standard prostheses (here the Neer prosthesis) *do not* take this "hinge point" into account and result in lateralisation of the articular head. **c** The Aequalis prosthesis incorporates this data into its design

physeal axis crossing the periphery of the articular head at a level we have called the "crossing point" or "hinge point" (Fig. 5a). Thus the centre of the sphere and the centre of the cylinder may be separated in the frontal plane by 6.9 mm on average with a range of 2.9–10.6 mm. This medial displacement of the articular surface had never before been described and must be an imperative integral part of the design of a humeral prosthesis (Fig. 5).

In the sagittal plane the posterior eccentricity of the spherical humeral head defines the *posterior offset* which is variable, averaging 2.6 mm with a range from -0.8 to 6.1 mm in our series. This posterior offset of the humeral articular surface, which has also been shown by Roberts et al. [19] must also be included in the design of a humeral prosthesis (Fig. 4b).

Finally the offset of the spherical humeral head usually occurs in both the frontal and sagittal planes resulting in a *true combined (medial and posterior) offset* (Fig. 4c).

Prosthetic Adaptability: The Result of Variations in the Orientation and Position in Space of the Articular Surface

"Prosthetic adaptability" is a new concept which allows morphological parameters to be taken into account intra-operatively. This new concept allows a practical "made to measure, on the spot" answer without the inconvenience of stocking multiple prostheses or having them made preoperatively [5, 7]. With regards to shoulder prostheses, the adaptability of the humeral implant allows integration of the *four parameters* whose wide variation we have seen above: (a) the inclination, (b) the retroversion, (c) the medial offset, and (d) the posterior offset. We consider these four parameters one by one.

The inclination of the articular head surface is a factor which is much too variable to be imposed in an arbitrary manner; cutting the humeral head along a fixed inclination corresponding to that of the prosthesis, or a cutting jig gives a very approximate result [6, 12, 18]. Conversely, cutting the humeral head along its anatomical angulation by following the limits of the anatomical neck does not always allow for the correct positioning of a standard prosthesis (Fig. 6a). This variation in inclination must be included in the design of the humeral implant. The Aequalis prosthesis allows variable inclination due to a system of variable necks between the stem and the prosthetic head (Fig. 6b). The inclination is chosen perioperatively using a template (Fig. 7).

The retroversion of the articular head surface is another very variable parameter which should be taken into account when implanting a shoulder prosthesis [1, 3, 17]. Indeed, imposing a fixed and arbitrary humeral retroversion ranging between 30° and 40°, as recommended in surgical articles [8, 15, 16] gives a very approximate result.

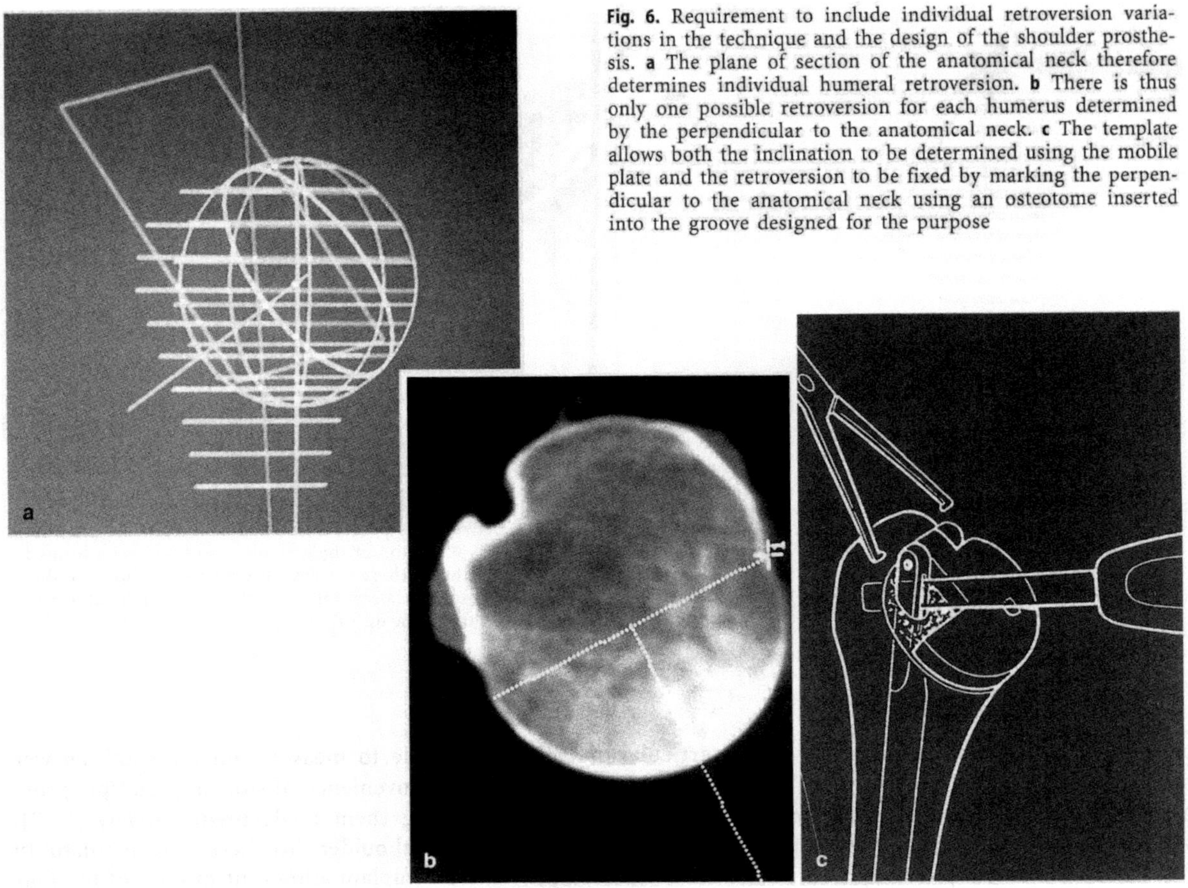

Fig. 6. Requirement to include individual retroversion variations in the technique and the design of the shoulder prosthesis. **a** The plane of section of the anatomical neck therefore determines individual humeral retroversion. **b** There is thus only one possible retroversion for each humerus determined by the perpendicular to the anatomical neck. **c** The template allows both the inclination to be determined using the mobile plate and the retroversion to be fixed by marking the perpendicular to the anatomical neck using an osteotome inserted into the groove designed for the purpose

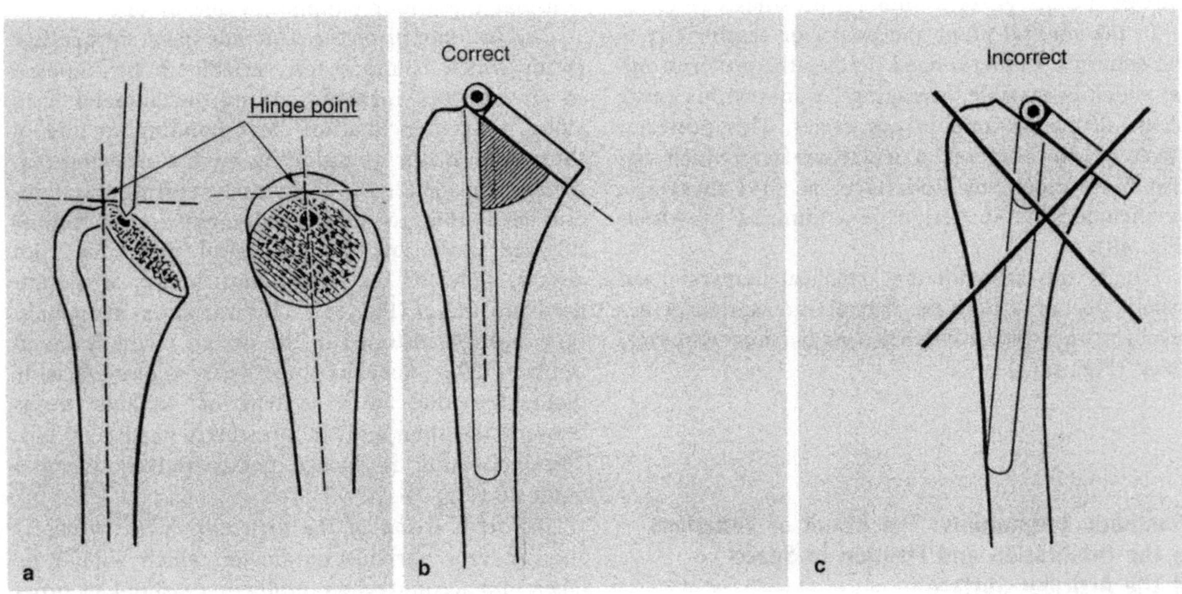

Fig. 7. Practical determination of the "hinge point"; articular surface medial offset control allowing the inclination to be measured. **a** The "hinge point" is located at the top of the humeral cut plane, posterior to the bicipital groove, marking the crossing between the proximal metaphyseal axis and the top of the articular surface. **b** The variations in inclination are determined intraoperatively using a template articulated from the "hinge point". **c** This template must be centered in the proximal medullary canal and not tilted so that the inclination can be measured correctly

At first sight, it appears very difficult (if not possible) to match the individual retroversion of the articular surface. In fact the problem is considerably simplified when we remember that the humeral retroversion is determined by the plane of section which goes through the anatomical neck (Fig. 6). There is therefore only one possible humeral retroversion for each humerus which is easy to determine by marking the perpendicular to the anatomical neck (Fig. 6b,c).

The template of the Aequalis prosthesis allows both determination of the inclination using the mobile plate and the angle of retroversion by marking the perpendicular to the anatomical neck using an osteotome inserted into the groove designed for this purpose. Thus marked, the slot in the cancellous tuberosity represents the future site of the prosthetic fin (Fig. 7).

Thus, looking for the original anatomical neck is a fundamental stage during shoulder arthroplasty, allowing both the individual humeral inclination and the retroversion to be determined and therefore *the orientation in space of the articular surface can be fixed.* This marking of the anatomical neck, which is a delicate part of the operation, can only be done after complete trimming of the crown of osteophytes (Fig. 8). Fat tissue, similar to that found at the bottom of osteoarthritic sockets, usually marks the limit between the healthy cortical bone and the pathological exuberant osteophytes.

The design of a humeral prosthesis should also take into account the *medial offset of the articular head surface* by respecting the "hinge point" between the proximal metaphyseal axis and the top of the articular head (Fig. 9a). The Neer prosthesis, for example, does not respect the medial offset of the articular surface which results in the reduction of the deltoid lever arm and rotator cuff (Fig. 9b).

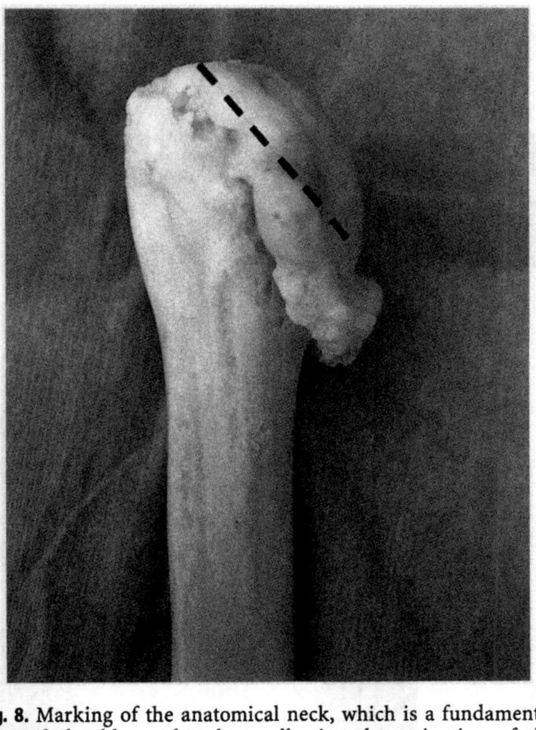

Fig. 8. Marking of the anatomical neck, which is a fundamental part of shoulder arthroplasty allowing determination of the humeral inclination and retroversion, can only be done after complete triming of the crown of osteophytes

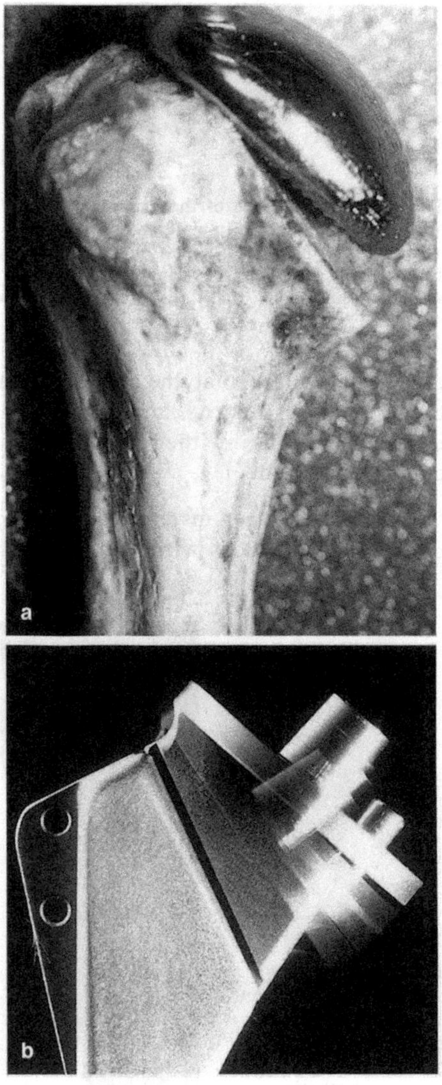

Fig. 9. Requirement to include individual angulation variations in the design of a shoulder prosthesis. **a** Anatomical osteotomy of the humeral head does not always allow one to correctly position a standard prosthesis. Conversely, cutting the humeral head according to a fixed inclination may change the rotational centres. **b** The Aequalis prosthesis allows adaptation to individual inclination through a system of variable necks between the stem and the prosthetic head

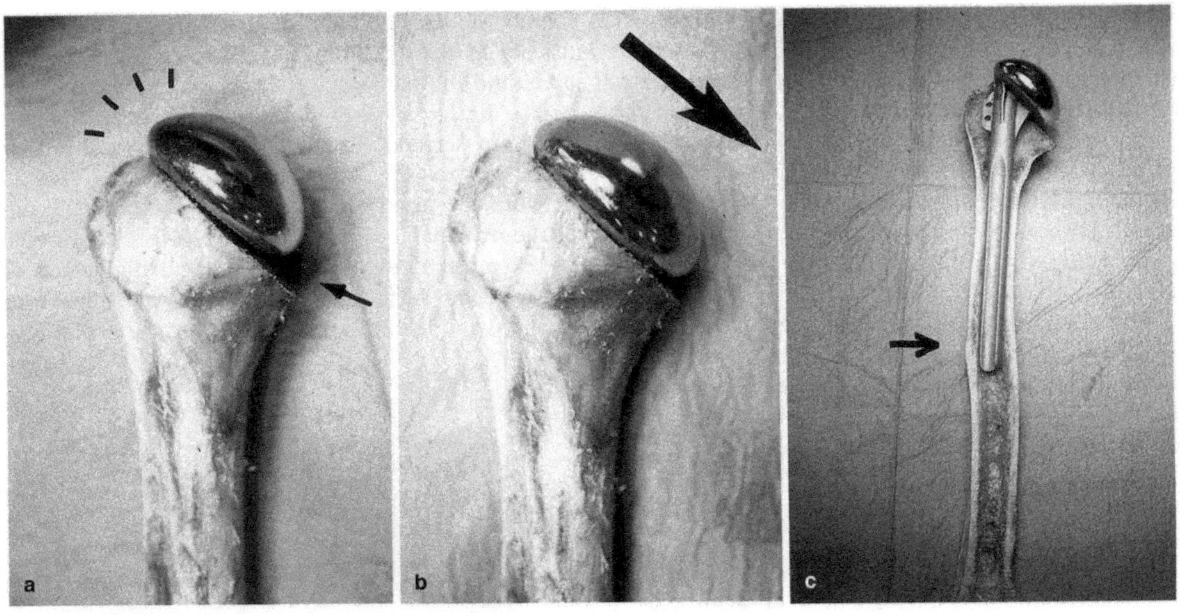

Fig. 10. Results of the absence of the articular surface medial offset and variable inclination in standard prostheses. **a** Superior protrusion of the prosthetic head, potentially damaging to the rotator cuff and absence of covering of the inferior part of the bone cut. Requirement to tilt the prosthesis in varus so that it better matches the anatomical model (**b**), which is not always possible because of the length of the stem which is "in conflict" with the change of diaphyseal curvature of the humerus in the frontal plane (necessity to use a smaller diameter stem) (**c**)

This lead us to believe that the implantation of a Neer type prosthesis in the humerus always lies between two situations, neither of which is really satisfactory (Fig. 10 and 11):

- The prosthesis is either inserted along the proximal intra medullary axis with the drawback of it being badly orientated to the humeral plane of section and protruding above the top of the prosthetic head which is potentially damaging to the rotator cuff (Fig. 10a).
- Or the prosthesis is tilted in varus or medially translated so that is better aligned and recon-

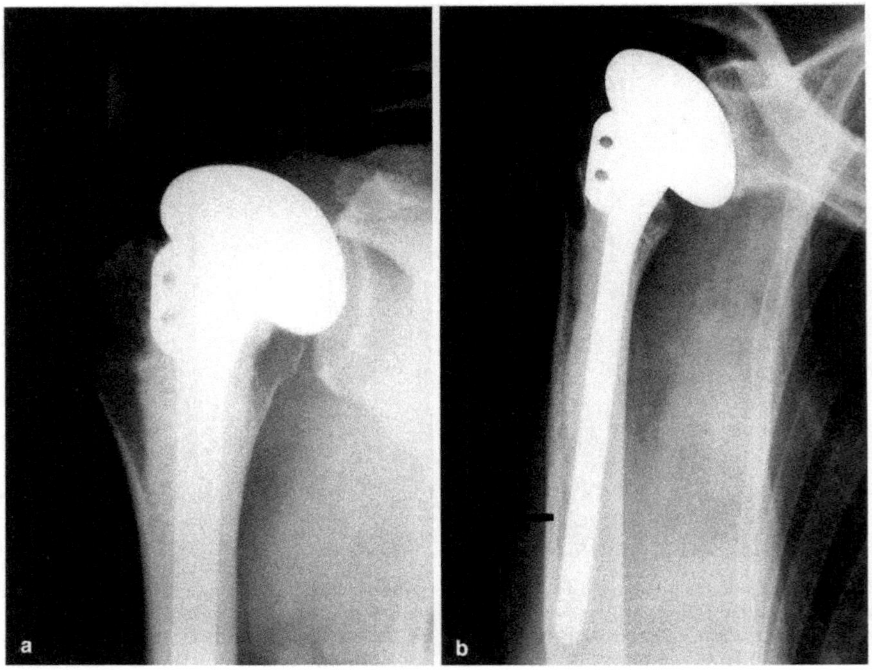

Fig. 11. Postoperative X-rays often observed after insertion of a standard humeral prosthesis. **a** Humeral centering of the prosthesis causing protrusion of the prosthetic articular surface due to the medial offset not having been taken into account in the design of the prosthesis. **b** Varus prosthesis allowing "cheating" in reproducing the articular surface medial offset and inclination

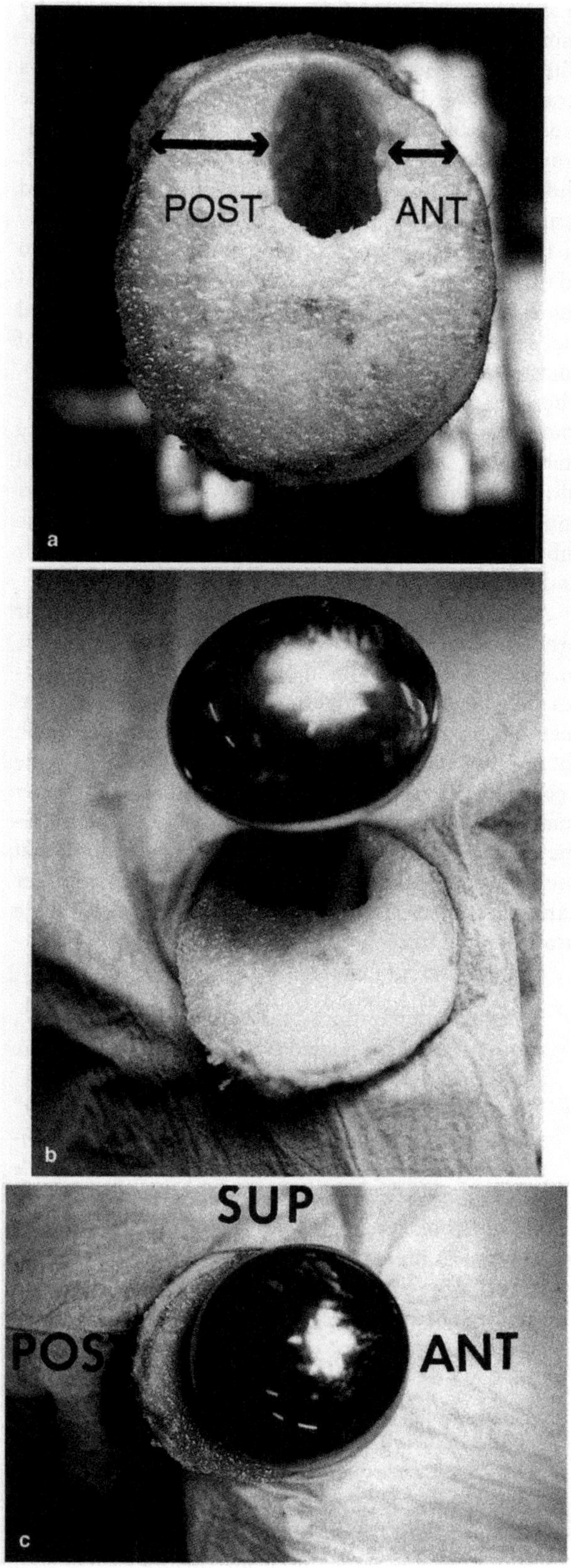

structs the anatomical model. This is not always possible due to the diameter or the length of the prosthetic stem: too long in the standard prosthesis are not taking into account the change in curvature of the humeral diaphysis in the frontal plane (Fig. 10 b,c). This enables us to understand the postoperative X-rays obtained with standard prostheses (Fig. 11 a,b).

With the Aequalis prosthesis the inclination can be measured from the hinge point with the help of a template (Fig. 7).

Finally, the design of a humeral prosthesis should take into account *the posterior offset of the articular head surface*. No currently available standard shoulder prosthesis, not even a modular one, allows this posterior articular surface offset to be respected. In certain cases, during implantation of a standard humeral prosthesis, the prosthetic head is found to be pushed forward so that it does not cover the bone cut (Fig. 12). The solution then consist in posterior translation and centralization of the prosthesis artificially on increasing retroversion after having modified the bony section to accommodate this new adaptation. Therefore, when this posterior offset is not taken into account in the design of shoulder prostheses, the biomechanical consequences are serious: the displacement of the rotation centres of the joint means that the action of the lever arm causing kinematic disturbance is modified [5].

There are, in fact, two solutions to incorporating the posterior offset of the articular surface:

- A different prostheses for the left and right sides, as proposed by Roberts et al. [19], with the drawbacks of having a fixed posterior offset and of stocking multiple implants.
- A prosthesis which would be adaptable to both sides, incorporating a variable anterio-posterior offset (as shown in our anatomical studies). We have concentrated on this solution, in designing an original prosthetic head eccentric displacement system which incorporates this adaptation (Fig. 13).

Fig. 12. Results of not respecting the articular surface medial offset in standard prostheses: After humeral head resection, reaming of the humeral shaft reveals the articular surface posterior offset. (**a**) Insertion of a standard humeral implant along the proximal metaphyseal axis (**b**) does not allow the posterior aspect of the cut surface to be covered, requiring resection of the neck with an artificial increase of the humeral retroversion or posterior translation of the prosthesis, using a smaller diameter stem (**c**)

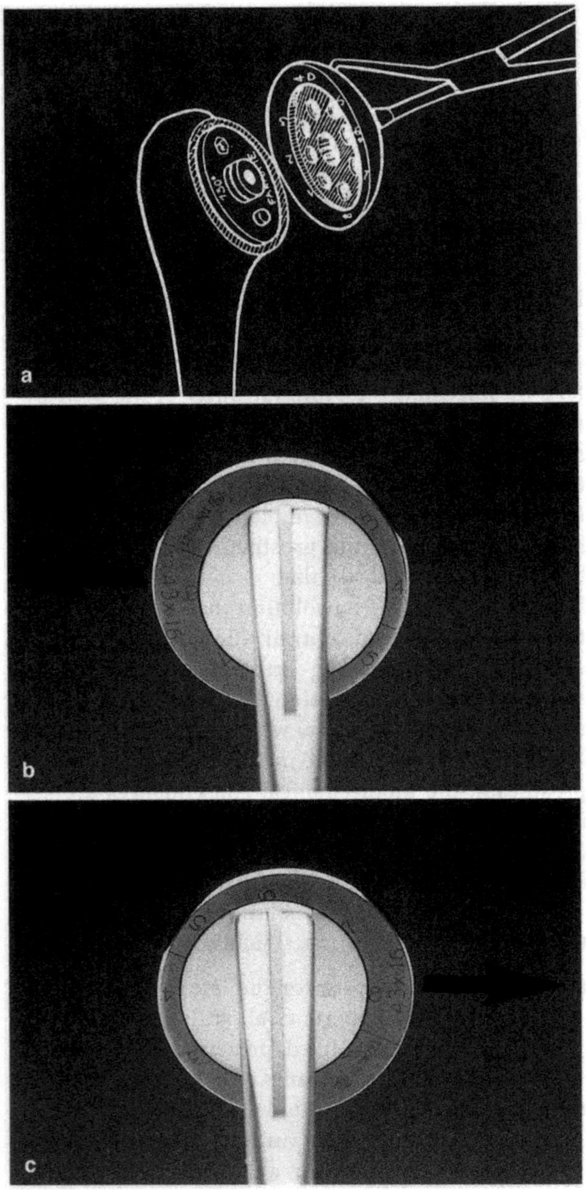

Fig. 13. Integration of the articular surface postero medial offset in the design of the Aequalis prosthesis. **a** An original and patented system with eccentric indexing allows the articular surface to be offset posteriorly. **b** From the right side. **c** From the left side, avoiding the need for different implants for each side

The Aequalis Prosthesis: A Modular and Adaptable Prosthesis

The Aequalis shoulder prosthesis is a non-constrained gleno-humeral prosthesis which is the result of fundamental studies performed in collaboration with engineers from the Tornier company over 10 years. Its development is based on two essential features which appear to us to be necessary to produce consistent clinical results: (a) Development of a prosthesis which precisely matches the anatomy by using an adaptable and modular humeral component. (b) The access to instrumentation which allows straightforward and reproducible implantation of the prosthesis by different surgeons. The humeral component consists of three parts (humeral stem, neck and head) which, through its technical design and range of components adapts perfectly to the anatomy of the joint rather than forcing the joint anatomy to adapt to the prosthesis. The length of the humeral stems has been shortened to adapt to the proximal metaphyseal humeral cylinder before the change of curvature at the humeral diaphysis (Fig. 10c). There is only one prosthetic stem length for the four diameters: 6, 9, 12 and 15 mm. The rotatory stability of the humeral stem is ensured by optimal filling of the metaphysis, a fin in the upper part containing two holes to allow reinsertion of the tuberosities in fracture cases and, finally, anterior and posterior grooves.

Modularity is provided by a range of ten articular heads of increasing size, the diameter and thickness of which were determined from our anatomical studies. A single head thickness is used for each diameter (up to the largest 50 mm diameter for which there are two available thicknesses) so that the anatomical variations encountered can be better matched. It is important that the thickness and diameter of the articular surface are respected so that the musculo-ligamentary balance of the shoulder can be recovered and that the differing radii of the head-glenoid complex are maintained.

Adaptability is ensured by:

- A variable inclination due to the 125°, 130°, 135°, and 140° necks, selected by the surgeon using the template (Figs. 7, 9).
- A variable retroversion selected "automatically" using the template (Fig. 6). *The use of the template and the possibility to dispose of variable necks allow to respect the variable orientation of the artivular head surface.*
- A variable medial and a posterior offset (Fig. 5), both incorporated in the prosthesis design and selected by the surgeon intraoperatively, using an *original eccentric indexing system,* located on the inferior aspect of each head. *Eight positions* are available allowing the articular head to be offset posteriorly or anteriorly and medially or laterally, until the cut bony surface is perfectly covered (Fig. 13). *The original prosthetic head eccentric displacement system allows to respect the variable location of the articular head surface.*

This movement of the prosthetic articular surface in all spatial planes helps the implant to adapt to all pathological situations encountered and thus the proximal humerus can be reconstructed according to the anatomical model.

Conclusion

The geometrical configuration of the proximal end of the humerus is much more complex than previously described. A standard humeral prosthesis can reproduce neither its shape nor dimensions. A modular prosthesis can respect the variable dimensions but cannot respect the variable orientation (variable inclination and retroversion) and the variable location (variable medial and posterior offset) of the articular surface. This led us to review the design and development of humeral prostheses. While the dimensional variations can be accounted for through the implant's modularity, the variation in shape must be matched by the implant's adaptability.

Until now the ideas of "prosthetic adaptability" has not been included in the design and development of the humeral implant. This undoubtedly partly explains the inconsistent clinical results achieved with shoulder prostheses. The Aequalis shoulder prosthesis has adopted all these characteristics and is the only third-generation prosthesis actually available. It allows for the individual inclination, individual retroversion, and individual combined (medial and posterior) offset of the articular surface (revealed in our studies) to be respected.

Thus it has been possible to solve a relatively complex geometrical problem through simple but original mechanical solutions, and the preliminary clinical results seem to confirm the merits of this new concept of adaptability.

References

1. Ballmer FT, Sidles JA, Lippitt SB, Matsen FA (1993) Humeral head prosthetic arthroplasty: surgically relevant geometric considerations. J Shoulder Elbow Surg 2:296–304
2. Boileau P, Walch G, Liotard JP (1992) Cineradiographic study of active elevation of the prosthetic shoulder. J Orthop Surg 6:351–359
3. Boileau P, Walch G, Mazzoleni N, Urien JP (1993) In vitro study of humeral retrotorsion. J Shoulder Elbow Surg 2:S12
4. Boileau P, Walch G (1994) The combined offset (medial and posterior) of the humeral sphere. J Shoulder Elbow Surg 3:21–6
5. Boileau P, Walch G (1995) Adaptability and modularity in shoulder arthroplasty. Acta Orthop Belgica 61 [Suppl I:49–61
6. Boileau P, Walch G (1996) Varus shoulder prosthesis: error or necessity? J Shoulder Elbow Surg 62:186
7. Boileau P, Walch G (1997) Product design and development: humeral considerations in a shoulder prosthesis. Orthop Special Edition 3:63–66
8. Cofield RH (1984) Total shoulder replaçement with the Neer prosthesis. J Bone Joint Surg Am 66:899–906
9. Fenlin JM, Vacaro A, Andreichik D, Lin S (1990) Modular total shoulder: early experience and impressions. Sem Arthroplasty 2:102–111
10. Fisher LP, Carret JP, Gonon GP et al (1977) Etude cinématique des mouvements de l'articulation scapulo-huméral. Rev Chir Orthop 63 [Suppl II]:108–112
11. Friedman RJ (1990) Biomechanics of the shoulder following total shoulder replacement. In: Post M, Morrey BF, Hawkins RJ (eds) Surgery of the shoulder. Mosby-Year Book, St. Louis, pp 263–266
12. Jobe CM, Ianotti JP (1995) Limits imposed on glenohumeral motion by joint geometry. J Shoulder and Elbow Surg 4:281–285
13. Hawkins RJ, Bell RH, Jallay B (1989) Total shoulder arthroplasty. Clin Orthop 242:188–194
14. Iannotti JP, Gabriel JG, Shnecks L, Evans BG, Misra S (1992) The normal gleno-humeral relationships. J Bone Joint Surg Am 74:491–500
15. Neer CS, Watson KC, Stanton FJ (1982) Recent experience in total shoulder replacement. J Bone Joint Surg Am 64:319–337
16. Neer CS (1990) Glenohumeral arthroplasty design In: Shoulder reconstruction. Saunders, Philadelphia, pp 146–160
17. Pearl ML Volk AG (1995) Retroversion of the proximal humerus relevant to prosthetic replacement arthroplasty. J Shoulder Elbow Surg 8:151–162
18. Pearl ML Volk AG (1996) Coronal plane geometry of the proximal humerus relevant to prosthetic arthroplasty. J Shoulder Elbow Surg 5:320–326
19. Roberts SNJ, Foley APJ, Swallow HM, Wallace WA, Coughlan DP (1991) The geometry of humeral head and the design of prosthesis. J Bone Joint Surg Br 73:647–650
20. Soslowsky LJ, Flatow EL, Bigliani LU, Mow VC (1992) Articular geometry of the glenohumeral joint. Clin Orthop 285:181–190
21. Walch G, Boileau P (1992) Morphological study of the humeral proximal epiphysis. J Bone Joint Surg Br 74:14

The Surgical Approaches for Shoulder Arthroplasty

J.C. Scheffer

Summary

Although the delto-pectoral approach is the most common approach used to insert a shoulder prosthesis, some surgeons still prefer to use superior approaches. Details of the different techniques are given to provide the best exposure possible.

Introduction

Although many possible surgical approaches to the shoulder are available, our experience has shown that surgeons tend to select the one with which they are most familiar (according to their 'school') rather than the one best suited to the lesion being treated [1–3, 5, 7, 10–13]. However, in our series the delto-pectoral approach was used in 95% of the cases with the superior approaches (transacromioclavicular Patte and transacromial Debeyre) used in only 5% (Fig. 1). There was one posterior approach.

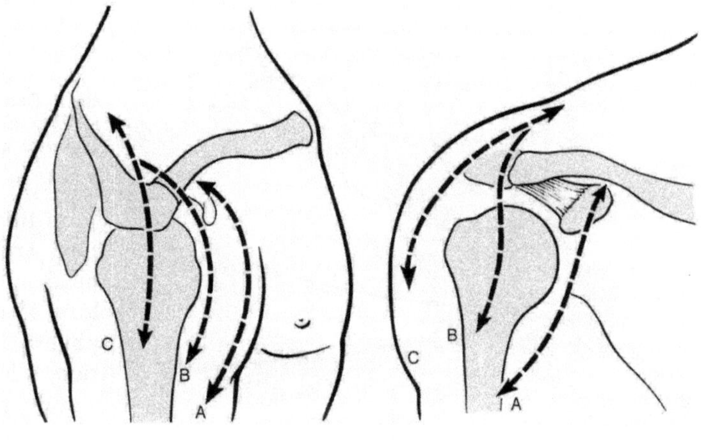

Fig. 1. The delto-pectoral approach (**A**) and the superior approaches: trans-acromio-clavicular (**B**) and trans-acromial (**C**)

The Delto-pectoral Approach

This was by far the most commonly used approach and was employed in virtually all the fracture cases (the technique in fracture surgery is detailed elsewhere.) Having been intubated under general anaesthesia the patient is installed in the semi-sitting or beach-chair position with the shoulder outside the table (Fig. 2).

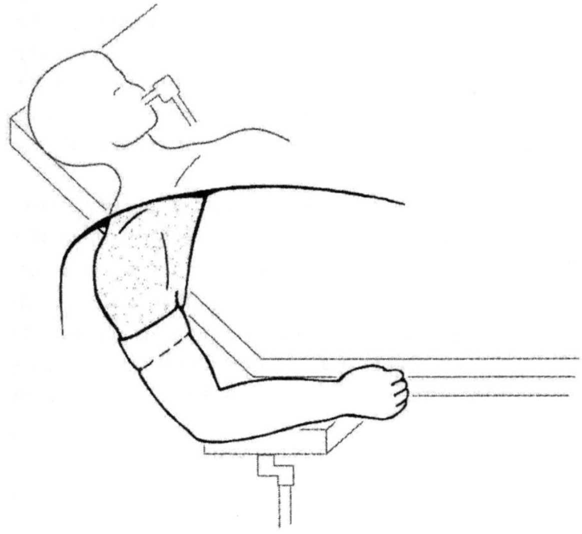

Fig. 2. Beach-chair position with the shoulder outside the table

Superficial Layers

An elongated straight or 'S' incision is made starting from the coracoid and running lateral to the delto-pectoral groove and this is then extended out from the axillary fold to avoid any scar retraction. The delto-pectoral groove can then be opened and the deltoid muscle and cephalic vein retracted laterally (Fig. 3). The conjoint tendon is retracted medially taking care to the musculo-cutaneous nerve [8]. The deltoid should never be detached from the clavicle [6, 9, 17, 18] The clavipectoral fascia is then incised along the lateral border of the conjoint tendon and the acromioclavicular ligament can be partially divided. This step can be made easier by placing a Homan retractor over the coracoid or over the acromio-clavicular ligament.

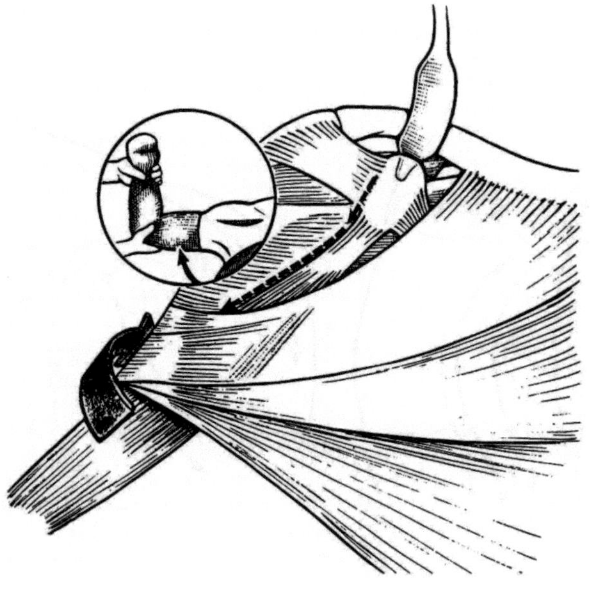

Fig. 3. Incision of the clavi-pectoral fascia after retracting the deltoid and the cephalic vein laterally

Subscapularis identification and release

Defining and releasing the borders of the subscapularis is an important step (Fig. 4):

- Onto the medial wall of the bicipital groove whose tendon can be located at the lower part of the incision by dividing the pectoralis major tendon for 1–2 cm.
- The *upper border* is easily defined beneath the fold of the subcoracoid bursa and can be followed under the coracoid.
- The *lower border* is marked by the anterior circumflex vessels. The axillary nerve is routinely located [4, 18].

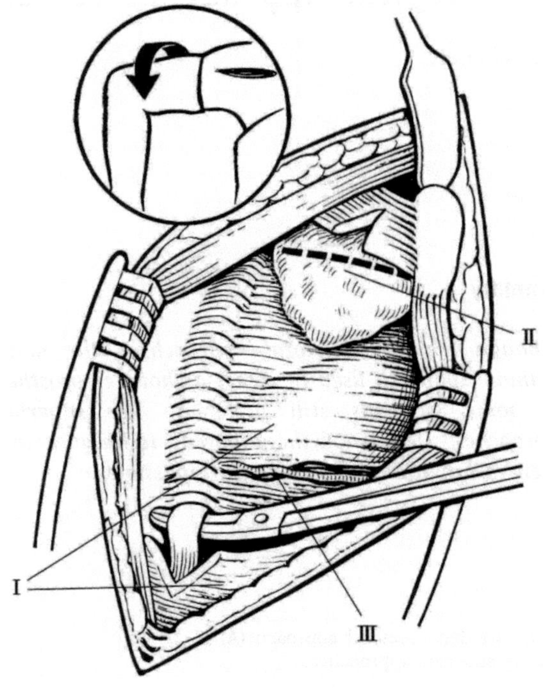

Fig. 4. Defining the three borders of the sub-scapularis: superior (tip of the coracoid), lateral (bicipital groove) and inferior (anterior axillary vessels)

At this stage it is important to test external rotation, and where this is limited, try to assess how much of it is due to adhesions of subscapularis or loss of elasticity, capsular contraction and osteophytes. If there is clearly a subscapularis contraction, a lengthening should be performed by making a complete release of the subscapularis.

Division of subscapularis is carried out at the same time as the capsule (except in the previous case) following a vertical line 1.5 cm medial to the bicipital groove and descending for three-fourths of its height. The division should stop just before the circumflex vessels where the cut turns horizontally and medially following the direction of the fibres.

The upper border and deep and superficial surfaces of the tendon must be fully released (especially beneath the coracoid) and then external rotation retested. The remaining fibres of subscapularis can then be progressively divided keeping in close contact to the humerus to avoid damage to the circumflex nerve. This results in a gradual increase in external rotation.

Dislocation and exposure of the Humerus

Having dislocated the humeral head anteriorly, exposure can be improved by extending and adducting the arm which is then pushed upwards. It is often necessary to perform a posterior vertical capsulotomy particularly when there is any retraction, and this facilitates the later steps especially in the preparation of the glenoid. The bone cuts made at the humeral level is detailed later.

Exposure of the Glenoid

Exposure of the glenoid is an essential step but can be rather difficult via the delto-pectoral approach. The humeral bone cut must be protected while the humerus is firmly retracted posteriorly. The arm is positioned in abduction and three retractors placed around the glenoid: above, in front and behind. Again, a posterior capsulotomy should be carried out if required. The actual preparation of the glenoid should be carried out as determined preoperatively from the computed tomographic findings, and this is detailed elsewhere.

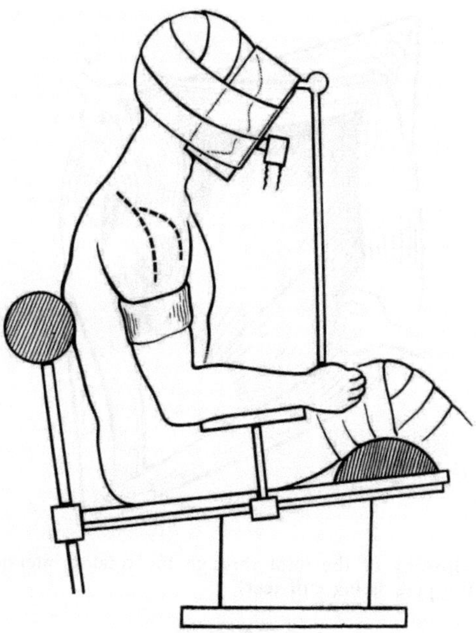

Fig. 5. Sitting position needed for the superior approaches

Superior Approaches

These have been suggested for use either as a routine approach (the transacromial Debeyre approach) or for specific indications related to the state of the rotator cuff or the glenoid (transacromioclavicular approach of Patte). These approaches do give a better exposure of the glenoid than the delto-pectoral approach [15].

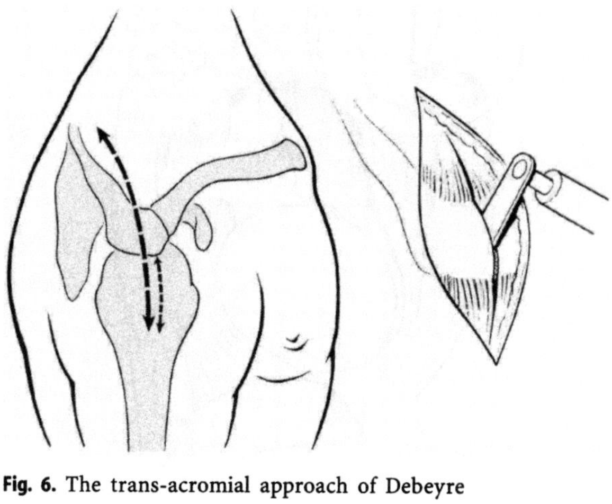

Fig. 6. The trans-acromial approach of Debeyre

The Trans-acromial Approach of Debeyre

This is one classical approach possible for repairing the rotator cuff and has also been described by Kessel [14, 15, 19].

The patient is positioned in the sitting position (Fig. 5) with the face being putting in a special support. Surgeons should take great care that no eye compresson is present. The incision centred on the posterior third of the acromion and extends medially upwards into the supraspinatus fossa to 1 cm in front of the scapular spine opening the trapezius and laterally downwards following the fibres of deltoid vertically for about 4 cm from the acromion (Fig. 6). This incision may be extended into the supraspinatus fossa for a cuff repair if so required. The acromion is divided using an oscillating saw and the anterior part elevated around the acromio-clavicular joint. This gives a complete view of the cuff from above.

The joint is approached via the rotator interval raising a flap of the coraco-humeral ligament based on the coracoid (Fig. 7) or via any preexisting cuff tear. The subscapularis is divided (Fig. 8) as required from above downwards medial to the bicipital groove having been released in the same manner as described above. The margins of the humeral head are certainly less well seen than when using the delto-pectoral approach, and therefore the humeral cut can be more difficult to perform. It should still, however, be made from above downwards with the cut coming out close to the insertion of the cuff into the anatomical neck (Fig. 9).

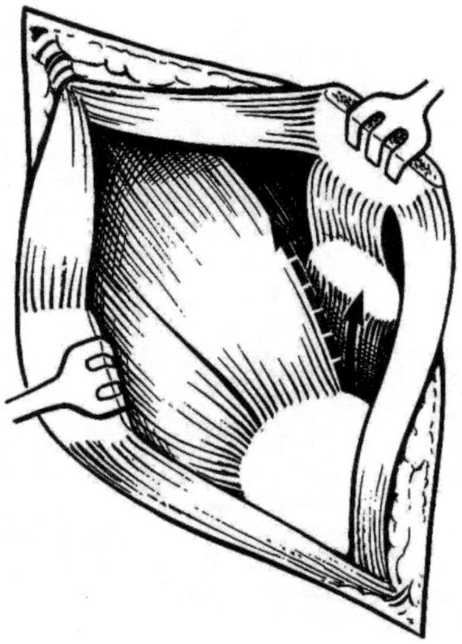

Fig. 7. Opening of the joint through the rotator interval (or through a preexisting cuff tear)

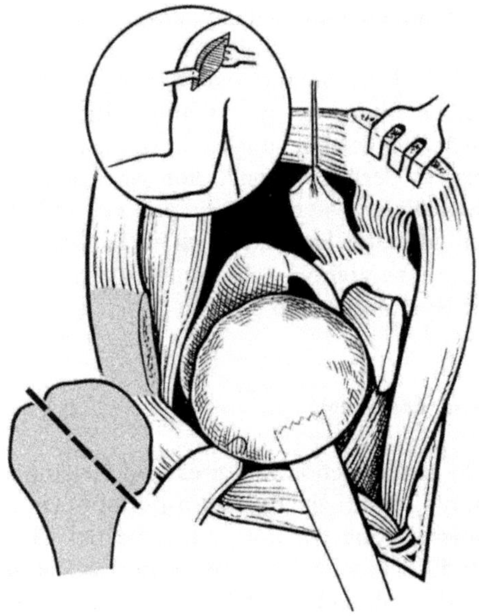

Fig. 9. Osteotomy of the humeral head from above downwards

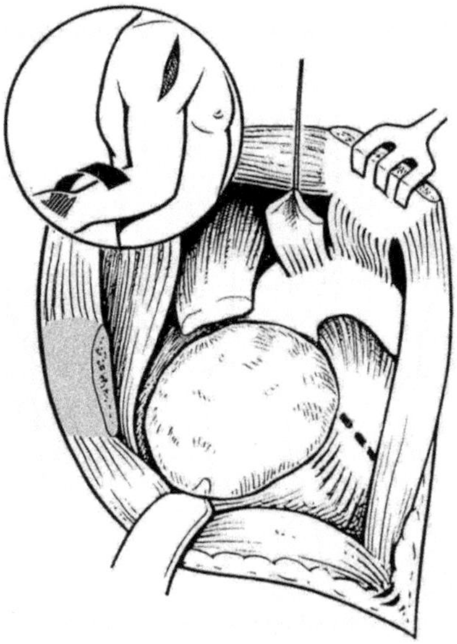

Fig. 8. Division of the subscapularis from above downwards

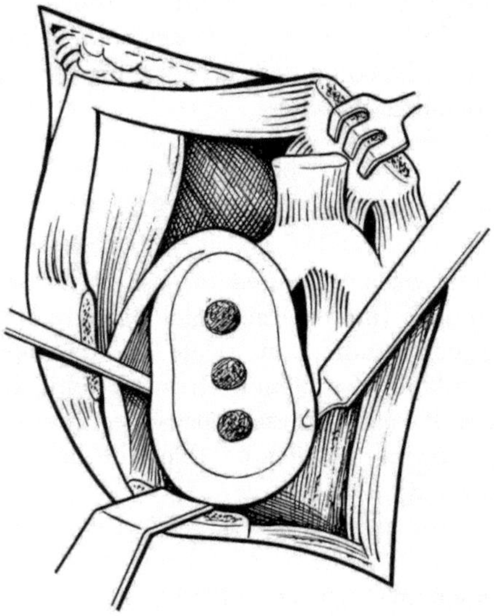

Fig. 10. Direct view on the glenoid with the superior approach

The glenoid on the other hand is seen face on from above and is more easily prepared (Fig. 10). Inserting the glenoid component does not usually present a problem, but it can prove more difficult with the humeral component, especially when a large head is used because the acromion cannot be retracted out of the way sufficiently. In this case it is possible to help by performing an osteotomy of the lateral quarter of the clavicle which does not seem to cause any problems in consolidating though care should always be taken with fragile acromions.

The layers are closed by repairing the coraco-humeral ligament or the cuff and using trans-osseous sutures or screws to fix the acromion.

The Trans-acromio-clavicular Approach of Patte

This combines the advantages of the delto-pectoral and transacromial approaches and also allows the problem of concomitant acromioclavicular joint arthritis to be dealt with.

The patient is operated on in the beach-chair or sitting position. The line of the incision is centred on the acromioclavicular joint (Fig. 1) and is extended upwards as required into the supraspinatus fossa and downwards vertically in the direction of the deltoid fibres for a maximum of 4 cm. The lateral 1 cm of the acromion is resected plus the acromial spur (Fig. 11).

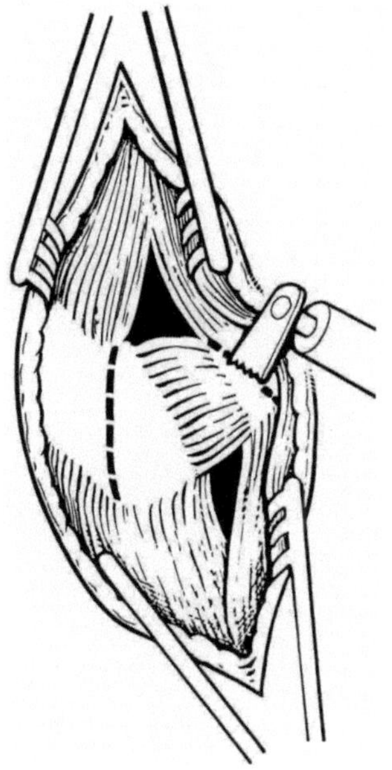

Fig. 11. Resection of the acromio-clavicular joint through the trans acromio-clavicular approach of Patte

The joint is approached, depending on the case, either via a preexisting cuff tear (Fig. 12a), by the rotator interval or, as in the delto-pectoral approach (Fig. 12b), by freeing and dividing the subscapularis in the same way as previously described but without having to extend the skin incision so low (it is not always necessary to cut the subscapularis when using the superior approaches).

This approach allows the head to be disengaged equally as well as it can be in the delto-pectoral approach and to have a view of the glenoid and to repair any cuff tear equally as well as with the trans-acromial approach. In specific cases the incision can be combined with a delto-pectoral approach if required.

If the cuff is of poor quality or unrepairable, particular care must be taken with the transacromioclavicular approach because it increases the risk of the humeral head migrating further upwards: wherein lies the importance of a good preoperative clinical examination and computed tomographic arthrogram. However, these conditions are also the ones that limit the indications for the insertion of a shoulder arthroplasty.

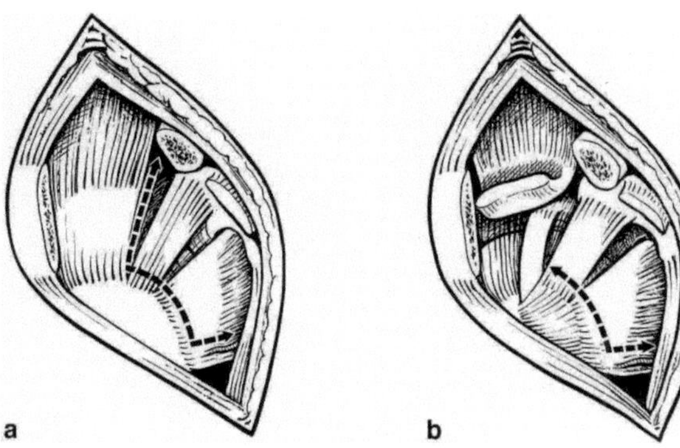

a b

Fig. 12. Opening of the joint through the rotator interval (*a*) or through a preexisting cuff tear (*b*)

References

1. Abbott LC, Saunders JBM, Hogey H et al (1949) Surgical approaches to the shoulder joint. J Bone Joint Surg Am 31:235–244
2. Banks SW, Laufman H (1953) Surgical exposures of the extremities. Saunders, Philadelphia
3. Bateman JE (1980) Surgical approaches to the shoulder. Orthop Clin North Am 11:349–366
4. Burkhead WZ, Schheinberg RR, Box G (1992) Surgical anatomy of the axillary nerve. J Shoulder Elbow Surg 1:31–36
5. Cadenat FM (1948) Les voies de pénétration des membres. 2nd edn, Doin, Paris
6. Cofield RH (1984) Total shoulder arthroplasty with the Neer's prosthesis. J Bone Joint Surg Am 66:899–906
7. DePalma AF (1983) Surgery of the shoulder, 3rd edn. Lippincott, Philadelphia
8. Flatow EL, Bigliani LU, April EW (1989) An anatomical study of the musculocutaneous nerve and its relationship to the coracoid process. Clin Orthop 244:166–171
9. Groh GI, Rockwood CA (1992) Loss of deltoid following shoulder operations: an operative disaster. Presented at the meeting of the Western Orthopaedic Association. October, Monterey Calif, USA
10. Henry AK (1945) Extensile exposure applied to limb surgery. Livingstone, Edinburgh, p 15
11. Hollinshead WH (1969) Anatomy for surgeons, 2nd edn. Harper & Row, New York
12. Hoppenfeld D, de Boer P (1990) Surgical exposures in orthopaedics. Saunders, Philadelphia
13. Johnston TB (1988) Gray's anatomy, 27th edn. Longmans Geen, New York, pp 769–776
14. Kessel J, Watson M (1977) The trans-acromial approach to the shoulder for ruptures of the cuff. Int Orthop 2:153
15. Patte D (1985) Voies d'abord de l'épaule et de l'extremité supérieure de l'humérus. Encycl. Méd. Chir., (Paris, France). Techniques chirurgicales, Orthopédie-Traumatologie, 44250-4.10.06, 12 pages
16. Neer CS, Watson KC, Stanton FJ (1982) Recent experience in total shoulder replacement. J Bone Joint Surg Am 64:319–337
17. Neer CS (1990) Shoulder reconstruction. Saunders, Philadelphia
18. Rockwood CA (1990) The technique of total shoulder arthroplasty. Inst Course Lect 39:437–447
19. Scheffer JC, Patte D (1987) Prothèses totales d'épaule. Encycl Méd Chir, Orthopédie-Traumatologie, 44294, 10, p 10, Techniques Chirurgicales, Paris

Technical Problems Encountered with Subscapularis and the Superior Cuff in Shoulder Arthroplasty

G. Walch, P. Boileau, N. Riand, and I. Pozzi

Summary

Using the delto-pectoral approach to insert a shoulder arthroplasty allows any of the inherent problems of the rotator cuff to be dealt with: retraction or rupture. Subscapularis lengthening, using whichever technique (release through glenoid capsulotomy, coronal 'Z-plasty' of the tendon, medial reattachment of the tendon), is an essential step in the operation, but the axillary nerve must be identified before it is carried out.

Introduction

The subscapularis is the 'keystone' when performing a total shoulder arthroplasty for two reasons: firstly, the vast majority of surgeons use the delto-pectoral approach which requires division of its muscle, and secondly because external rotation is often limited in whatever the aetiology and can be improved by lengthening or liberation of this musculo-tendinous structure. Moreover, the upper part of the rotator cuff, consisting of the supraspinatus and infraspinatus, may be torn, and it is important when doing a shoulder arthroplasty that this is repaired.

Subscapularis Division and Repair

Subscapularis is very rarely torn in degenerative conditions but is practically always contracted [2, 8]. Releasing and lengthening the tendon must be considered as an essential step in the intervention in order to regain external rotation [3, 4]. Theoretically an elongation of 1 cm should allow an increase in external rotation of 20° [5].

The first step is to define the insertion of the tendon into the lesser tuberosity. The upper border is well known to arthroscopists being pearly white, rounded and measuring about 6–8 mm in diameter and is clearly identified via the anterior approach. It is most easily located with the arm in maximum external rotation-extension with the elbow at the side when the tendon can be seen running horizontally and passing directly behind the tip of the coracoid (Fig. 1). It is covered by the subscapular bursa which is often thickened in arthritic conditions and hangs above and in front of the tendon. The bursa is easily opened using dissecting scissors and this usually releases a few drops of articular fluid.

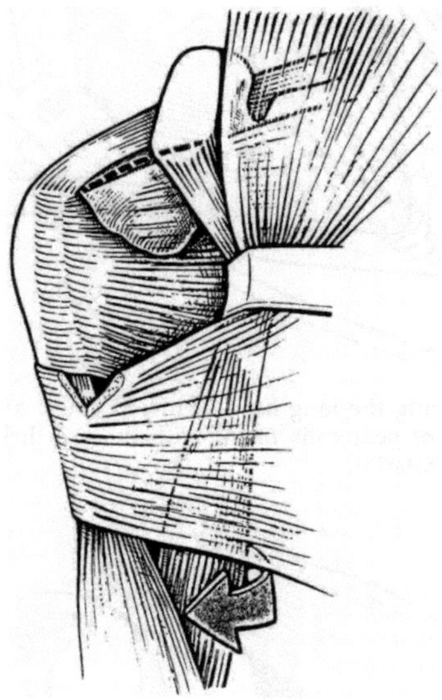

Fig. 1. The superior tendon of the subscapularis is located directly behind the tip of the coracoid. It is covered by the subscapular bursa

The lateral border of subscapularis is marked by the long head of biceps which can be found just above and medial to the insertion of pectoralis major when the arm is abducted and internally rotated (Fig. 2). The inferior border is identified by the presence of the anterior axillary vessels which must be ligated. Identifying the axillary nerve is a simple and indispensable step to take so that the subscapularis can be released completely and safely. For this the arm should be flexed anteriorly by 10°–20° and held in neutral rotation and 10° of adduction. Having retracted the lower part of the conjoined tendon, two or three gentle sweeps with fine dissecting scissors will demonstrate the nerve as it circles from above downwards and from medial to lateral in contact with the subscapularis muscle (Fig. 3).

The second step, after having placed the muscle on traction using sutures and performed a vertical arthrotomy is to open the sub-scapularis. There are three methods of opening the subscapularis:

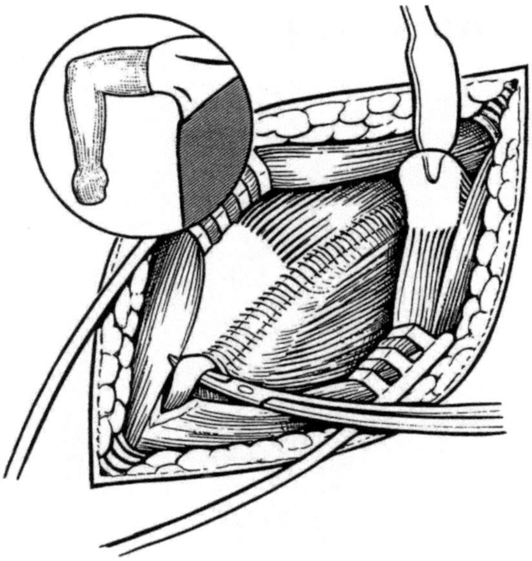

Fig. 2. Identifying the long head of biceps above and medial to the insertion of pectoralis major with the arm held in abduction-internal rotation

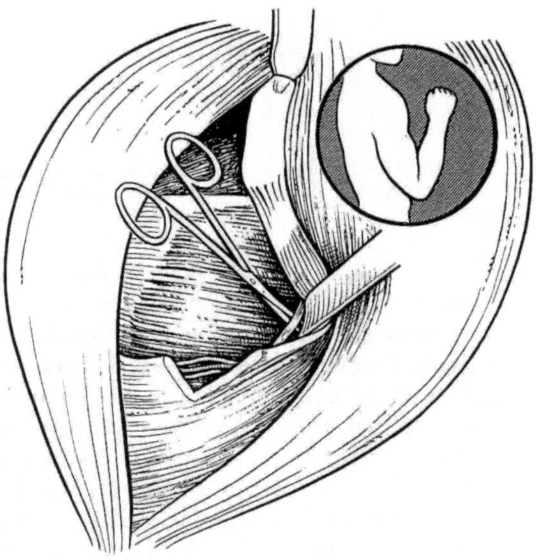

Fig. 3. Identifying the axillary nerve with the arm flexed anteriorly by 10°–20° and held in neutral rotation and 10° of adduction. The nerve runs from above downwards and from medial to lateral in contact with the subscapularis muscle

- Starting at the bicipital groove the entire tendon can be divided close to the lesser tuberosity using sharp dissection. At the end of the procedure the tendon can be 'elongated' by reinserting it at the level of the anatomical neck close to the prosthesis rather than back onto the lesser tuberosity [3, 6, 10] (Fig. 4).
- The subscapularis and the capsule can be divided together using a vertical incision about 15–20 mm medial to the bicipital groove. This leaves a stump of tendon still attached to the tuberosity which allows for an end-to-end reattachment (Fig. 5).
- The subscapularis can be opened in a Z fashion by splitting the tendon in the frontal plane, and the two sections can be sutured together end-to-end at the end of the procedure [7, 8]. This technique is not always easy because in the arthritic patient the layers created are paper thin (Fig. 6).

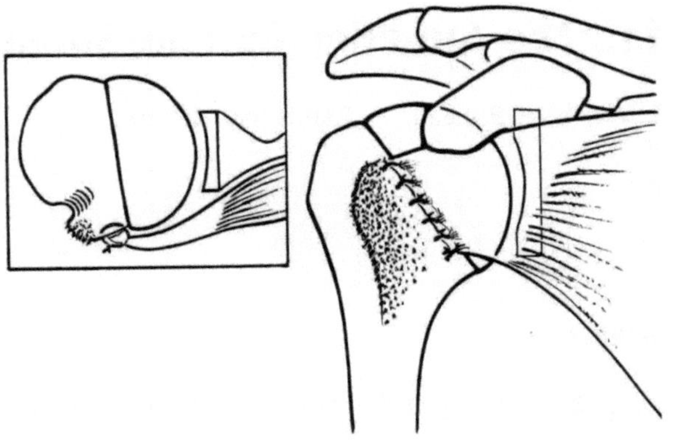

Fig. 4. Starting at the bicipital groove the tendon can be divided close to the lesser tuberosity. At the end of the procedure the tendon can be elongated by reinserting it at the level of the anatomical neck with non absorbable sutures

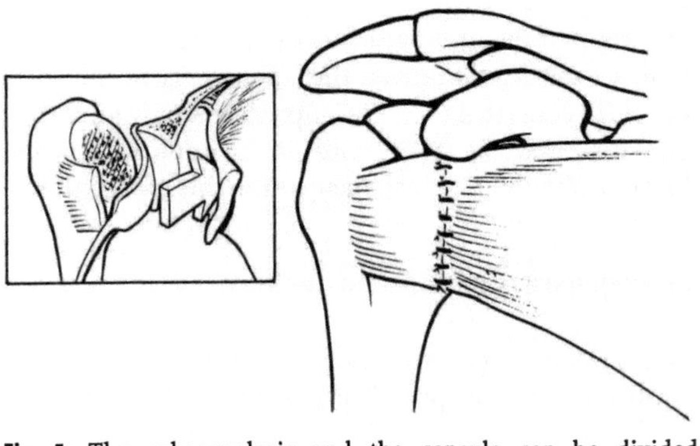

Fig. 5. The subscapularis and the capsule can be divided together. This leaves a stump of tendon which allows for an end to end reattachment

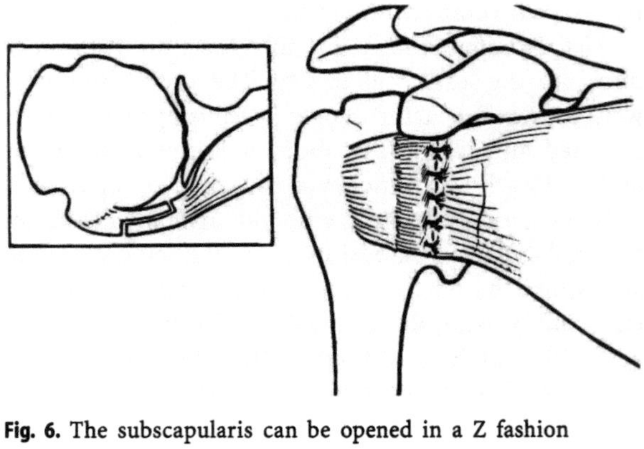

Fig. 6. The subscapularis can be opened in a Z fashion

Having divided or released the insertion of subscapularis it then needs to be freed [6]. Firstly, the upper border is released using open dissecting scissors (the tendon is adherent to the foot of the coracoid and the sub-acromial bursa). Then a juxta-glenoid capsulotomy is performed to free the muscle from the scapular neck (Fig. 7). When the anterior capsule is very pathological (synovial proliferation or significant retraction), it is preferable to resect it but otherwise it can be left. The release of the deep face of the subscapularis is then continued by dissecting the muscle from the subscapular fossa using a periosteal elevator. Finally, the lower part of the muscle and the capsule are freed using dissecting scissors under direct vision whilst gently retracting the axillary nerve. This release should give 1–2 cm of subscapularis lengthening (Fig. 8). There is not usually anything to be gained by freeing the anterior face of the muscle where the brachial plexus and axillary vein and subscapularis nerves are situated [1].

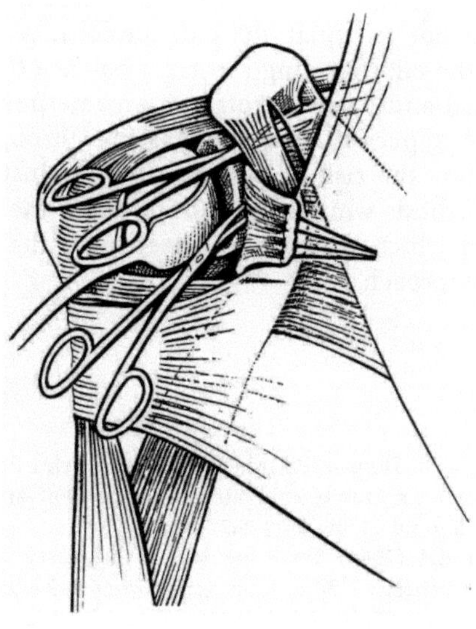

Fig. 7. The upper border and the deep part of the subscapularis are released using dissecting scissors

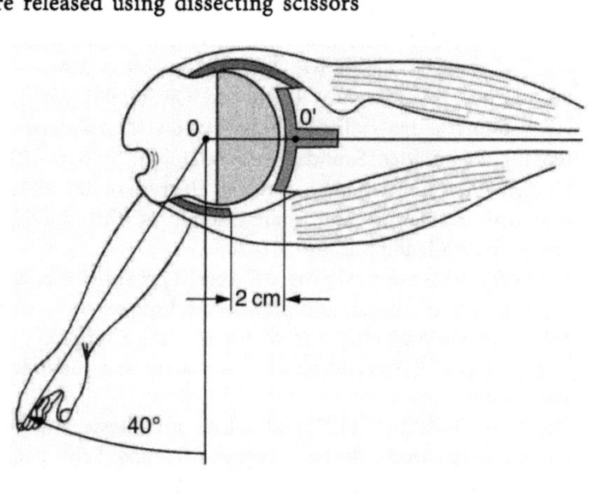

Fig. 8. Subscapularis lengthening of 2 cm allows for an increase in external rotation of 40° [5]

At the end of the procedure an end-to-end repair is carried out using simple or doubled non-absorbable sutures. The superior, horizontal part of the tendon should also be sutured to the coraco-humeral ligament which has been left intact.

The Superior Cuff: managing cuff tears

In order to explore the cuff via the delto-pectoral approach the arm should be placed in abduction and internal rotation. A Homann type retractor can be positioned under the anterior deltoid and levered against the anterior acromial spur (Fig. 9). The acromial insertion of the coraco-acromial ligament is clearly seen and an acromioplasty or resection of the inferior acromio-clavicular osteophytes can be carried out. However, if a resection of the distal centimeter of the clavicle is envisaged it is better to opt for a short counter incision in the skin over the acromio-clavicular joint.

A rupture of the supraspinatus can be repaired via the delto-pectoral approach. It is advisable to insert all the sutures that will be used to reattach the cuff to the greater tuberosity before implanting the prosthesis and to tie them after the component has been cemented (Fig. 10). It seems preferable to simply roughen up the greater tuberosity surface rather than making a trough in the bone. When the rupture extends beyond the supraspinatus reinserting it places a significant strain on the cuff, which increases the forces acting on the glenoid (Fig. 11). An other option in cases where there is a massive cuff tear with an eccentric head is to ignore the cuff tear and implant a hemi-arthroplasty. In fact, even if the head is still centered at the time of the arthroplasty, the natural history of the cuff

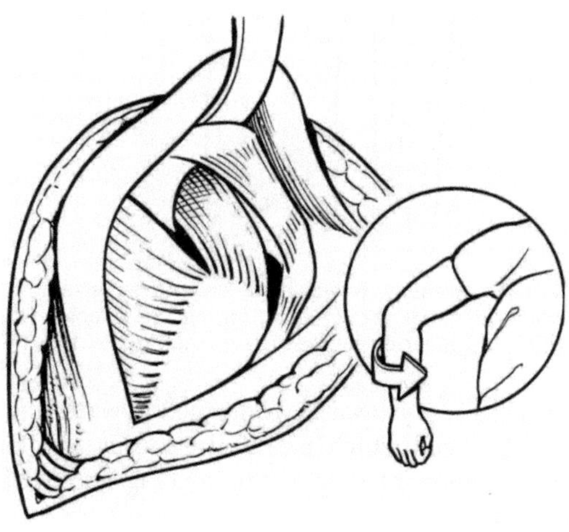

Fig. 9. In order to explore the cuff via the delto-pectoral approach the arm should be placed in abduction and internal rotation

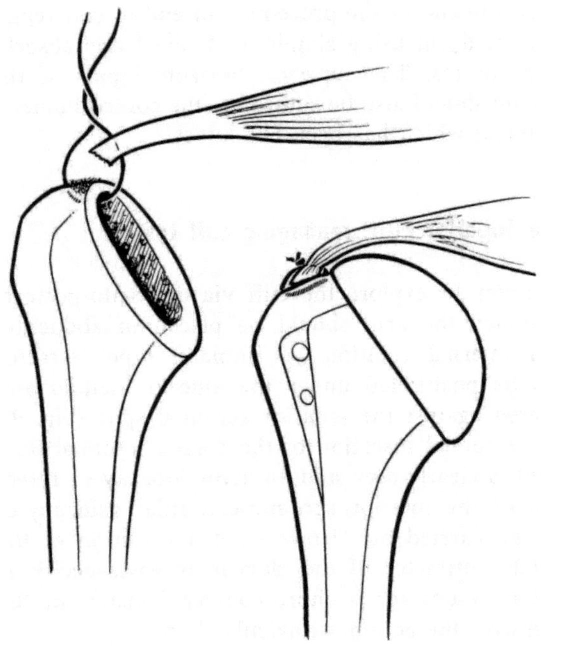

Fig. 10. To repair a supra-spinatus tear it is advisable to insert all the sutures before implanting the prosthesis and to tie them after the component has been cemented

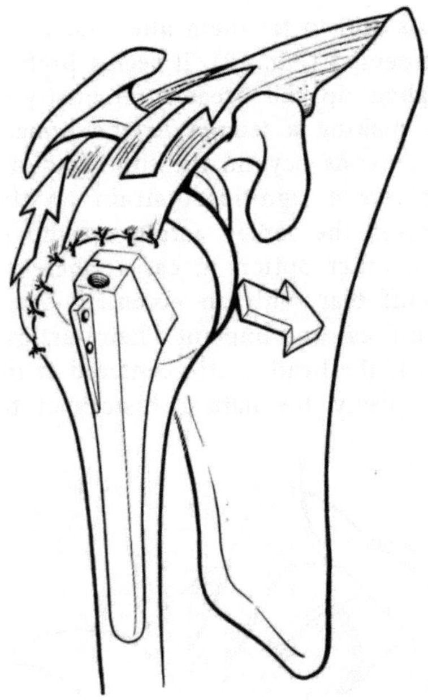

Fig. 11. Repair of a massive tear place a significant strain on the cuff, which increases the forces acting on the glenoid. This is responsible for anterior subluxation of the prosthesis

tear is a tendency towards continued upward migration of the head which may cause loosening of the glenoid component due to the rocking-horse effect [6] (Fig. 12).

When the superior cuff has a massive tear and a large headed hemi-arthroplasty is being considered, it seems preferable to use the anterior delto-pectoral approach releasing subscapularis, to avoid doing an acromioplasty, to leave the coracoacromial ligament intact and not to repair the cuff tendons. A partial repair of the cuff allowing a correct balance between the internal and external rotators is sometimes possible. The superior approach passing through the rupture runs the risk of causing superior instability of the prosthesis which may end up under the skin – a problem which we have not seen with the delto-pectoral approach.

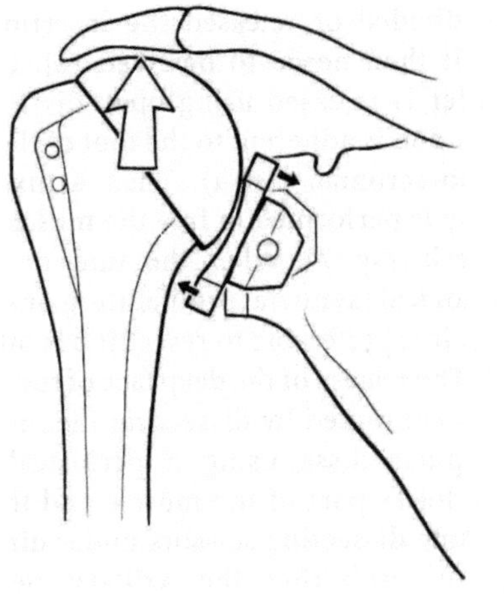

Fig. 12. Upward migration of the humeral head due to rotator cuff tear may cause loosening of the glenoid component due to the rocking-horse effect [6]

References

1. Checchia SJ, Doneux PS, Martins MG, Meireles FS (1996) Subscapularis muscle enervation: the effect of arm position. J Should Elbow Surg 5:214–218
2. Cofield RH (1984) Total shoulder arthroplasty with the Neer prosthesis. J Bone Joint Surg Am 66:899–906
3. Connor PM, Bigliani LU (1996) Total shoulder replacement. In: Copeland S (ed) Shoulder surgery. Saunders, London, pp 251–289
4. Fenlin JM (1994) Soft tissue management in gleno-humeral arthroplasty. Operative Tech Orthop 4:203–209
5. Matsen FA, Thomas SC, Rockwood CA (1990) Anterior gleno-humeral instability. In: Rockwood CA, Matsen FA (eds) The shoulder. Saunders, Philadelphia, pp 526–622
6. Matsen FA, Lippitt S B, Sidles JA, Harryman DT (1994) Practical evaluation and management of the shoulder. Saunders, Philadelphia, pp 202–205
7. Neer CS (1982) Surgical protocol Neer II proximal humerus arthroplasty of the shoulder: Neer technique. Saint Paul MN: Minessota Mining and Manufactoring Company
8. Neer CS (ed) (1990) Shoulder reconstruction. Saunders, Philadelphia
9. Walch G, Boileau P (1991) Shoulder prosthesis. Surgical technique in chronic disease. Aequalis. Tornier, Saint Ismier
10. Wirth MA, Basamania C, Rockwood CA (1994) Fixation of glenoid component: keel versus pegs. Operative Tech Orthop 4:218–225

The Surgical Anatomy and Osteotomy Technique for the Humeral Head

P. Boileau and G. Walch

Summary

The technique of resection of the humeral head has had to be completely changed since the introduction of the concept of ***prosthetic adaptability*** *which allows a more precise replication of the bone anatomy of the proximal humerus. Prosthetic adaptability is a new concept which allows individual inclination and retroversion to be matched and also any possible mediolateral or anteroposterior offset to be covered. Orienting and positioning a humeral prosthesis using as landmarks the boundaries of the* ***anatomical neck*** *is more accurate than positioning the prosthesis following the same, fixed inclination and retroversion. The landmarks of the anatomical neck can be found, even in a humeral head deformed by degenerative or inflammatory disease, as long as the osteophytes are removed* ***before*** *doing the osteotomy. This means adopting a new surgical technique aided by a preoperative radiographic assessment, by the optimal surgical exposure, and above all by abandoning the old concepts of making a bone cut with a fixed inclination and retroversion.*

Introduction

Repositioning the articular surface in its original location and recreating normal anatomic relationships are critically important when using a nonconstrained shoulder prosthesis [1, 8, 9, 18, 22, 24]. Because our previous anthropometric studies have shown that the humeral head is variably inclined to the shaft, variably retroverted to the transepicondylar axis of the elbow, and its center is offset medially and posteriorly from the axis of the shaft, we have changed both the design of the prosthesis and the technique for its implantation [2–6, 27].

Resection of the humeral head is a critical stage in shoulder arthroplasty, and the technique has had to be completely changed since adaptability of the prosthesis to the individual bone anatomy of the proximal humerus has been made possible through technological innovations [4, 6]. *Prosthetic adaptability* is a new concept which allows a more precise replication of the bone anatomy of the proximal humerus because individual inclination and retroversion can be matched and also any possible mediolateral or anteroposterior offset can be covered.

This paper describes the new osteotomy technique of the humeral head with the Aequalis shoulder prosthesis, a third-generation (adaptable) prosthesis.

Geometric and Biomechanical Considerations

With first-generation (monoblock Neer type) and second-generation (modular) prostheses, resection of the head was carried out based on two arbitrarily fixed angles: inclination and retroversion [8, 9, 12, 18, 19]. *Inclination* was selected depending on the prosthesis used and varied from make to make (Fig. 1). The humeral cut was made using a template or the prosthesis itself as a guide. The humeral head was positioned slightly above the level of the greater tuberosity, and the stem was aligned parallel to the proximal diaphysis which then allowed the level of the cut to be marked. *Retroversion* was fixed at an angle of 30°–40°, corresponding to the average angle recommended in the surgical literature. This was achieved by flexing the elbow to 90° and turning the arm into 30°–40° of external rotation before carrying out the osteotomy.

Our previous anatomical studies [2–6, 27], as with others both older and more recent [1, 7, 10, 15–17, 20, 21, 23, 25, 26], have shown these two angles to be very variable both between and within individuals. Inclination and retroversion vary with age, sex, race, and side to such an extent that one cannot talk of an average value. In our study inclination varied from 125°–140° and retroversion from 0°–50°. These results confirm that the geometry of the proximal humerus is extremely variable, and that these two angles (inclination and retroversion) should be individualized if one wishes to reproduce the anatomical model. Moreover, our anthropometric studies have shown that the articular surface is medially and posteriorly offset in relation to the medullary canal: these variable geometric parameters should also be taken into account both in

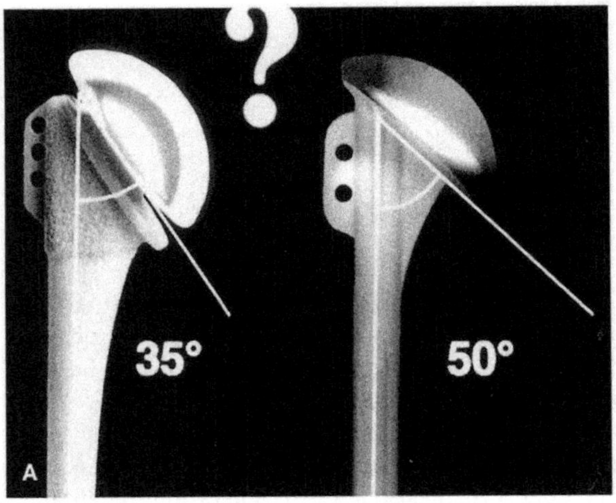

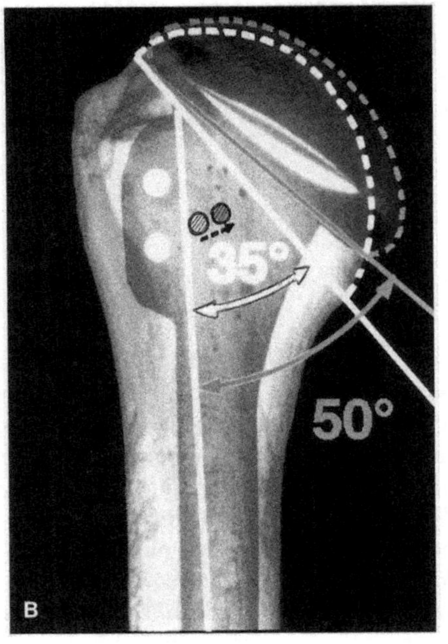

Fig. 1 A–B. Variable inclination angle. **A** Most shoulder prosthetic designs have only one shaft angle. **B** This fixed inclination limits the surgeon's ability to replicate the original anatomy and displaces the center of rotation and the medio-lateral offset

the design of the humeral component and in the technique of implantation.

However, most prosthetic designs for the replacement of the proximal humerus have only one shaft angle [8, 9, 12]. This fixed inclination limits the potential for the surgeon to reproduce the original anatomy (Fig. 1). Making a humeral cut of 140° of inclination in a patient who has only 125° displaces the center of rotation proximally and alters the kinematics of the glenohumeral joint [4, 5, 21]. In the same way, resecting the head at a fixed retroversion of 30°–40° (in relation to the forearm) in an individual who has only 5°–10° of retroversion can lead to posterior cuff tear damage and also alters the kinematics (Fig. 2). Moreover, using the forearm as a goniometer is inaccurate, particularly in patients with rheumatoid arthritis where there is often a significant valgus deformity at the elbow and an increased carrying angle [1, 2, 20].

Thus the determination of individual inclination, individual retroversion, and individual posterior and medial offset requires defining the edges of the proximal humeral articular surface. Orienting and positioning a humeral prosthesis using as landmarks the boundaries of the *anatomical neck* is a more interesting surgical answer and is certainly more accurate than positioning the prosthesis fol-

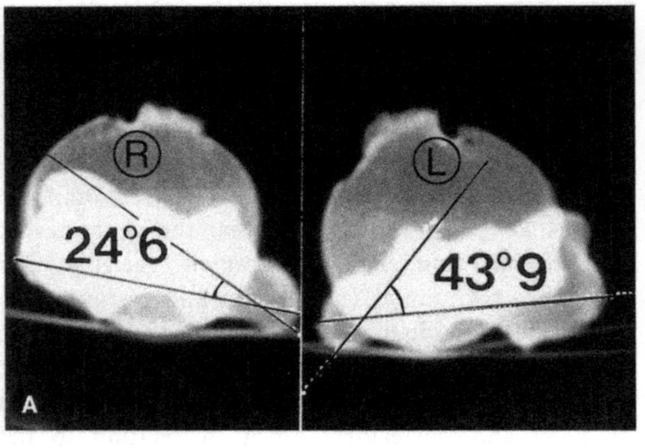

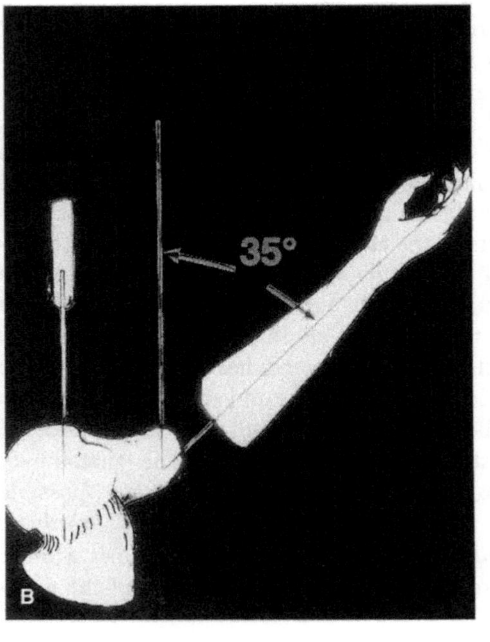

Fig. 2 A–B. Variable retroversion angle. **A** Example of different retroversion angles on both sides in the same individual. **B** Cutting the humeral head with a fixed retroversion angle can place the posterior cuff at risk. (Reproduced from [20])

lowing the same, fixed inclination and retroversion and fixed posteromedial offset. However, to do this requires two conditions to be met: (a) to be able to find the limits of the anatomical neck even in arthritic conditions of the shoulder where the bone anatomy of the proximal humerus may be markedly distorted, and (b) to have a prosthesis available which can be adapted to each individual shoulder which is now possible with the Aequalis shoulder prosthesis (Tornier) because of technological innovations.

Surgical Exposure

The landmarks of the anatomical neck can be found, even in a humeral head deformed by degenerative or inflammatory disease, as long as the osteophytes are removed *before* doing the osteotomy in order that the normal anatomy can be demonstrated. This means adopting a new surgical technique aided by preoperative radiographic assessment, by optimizing the surgical exposure and above all by abandoning the old concepts and especially the idea of using a humeral cutting guide.

The preoperative radiographic investigations allow the degree of cartilage wear to be assessed and, importantly, localizes the osteophytes to help guide their removal (Fig. 3). The anteroposterior, double-obliquity, radiograph shows the extent of the infero-medial "droplet" osteophytes and also the superolateral osteophytes "dribbling" onto the greater tuberosity (Fig. 3A). Computed tomography allows the size of the posterior and anterior osteophytes to be judged (Fig. 3B).

The surgical exposure is of over-riding importance and must allow the head to be dislocated anteriorly out of the wound (Fig. 4). The patient is positioned on a standard operating table in the beach-chair position. The patients head should be secured to avoid lateral flexion or hyperextension of the neck which may cause stretching of the cervical roots. The whole shoulder, including the scapula, should be outside the table to allow complete extension (vertical humerus) and external rotation of the arm greater than 90°. A cheap and "home-made" arm support (classical Trillat knee support) is used to keep the arm in abduction during the deltopectoral approach, the soft tissue release, and the glenoid preparation. This arm support should be retracted alongside the table during preparation of the humerus. The axilla is separated from the sterile surgical field using adherent plastic drapes. Before making any incision the surgeon must evaluate the degree of retraction of the anterior soft tissue by measuring the amount of passive external rotation under anesthesia. This determines the technique of soft tissue release (see next paragraph). The skin incision is made in a straight line from the coracoid process to the distal insertion of the deltoid on the humerus, avoiding the axillary fold because of possible scars retraction.

The *deltopectoral approach*, passing medial to the cephalic vein, maximizes the exposure once the clavipectoral fascia has been divided (Fig. 4D). *Superiorly* the incision reaches the clavicle and a Hohmann-type retractor is placed above the coracoid process and the acromio caracoid ligament is preserved. *Inferiorly* the upper insertion of the pectoralis major into the humerus should be released (2 cm) to allow better visualization of the inferior

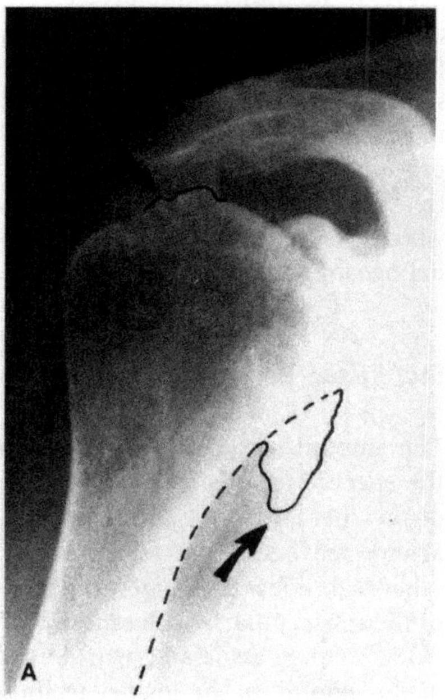

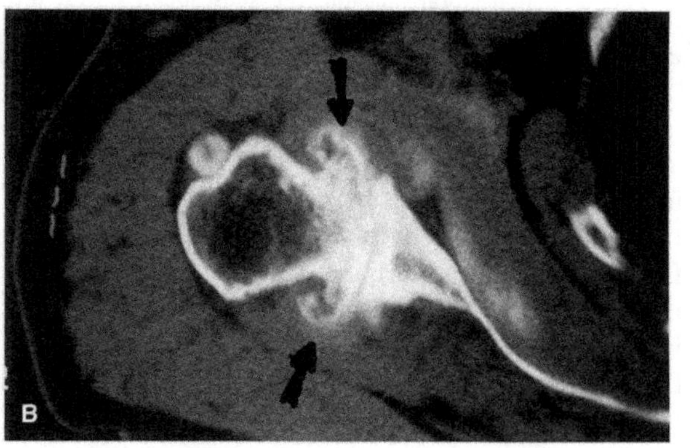

Fig. 3 A–B. Preoperative planing. **A** AP view of the shoulder helps to localize inferior and possible superior osteophytes. **B** Computed tomogram helps to localize anterior and posterior osteophytes

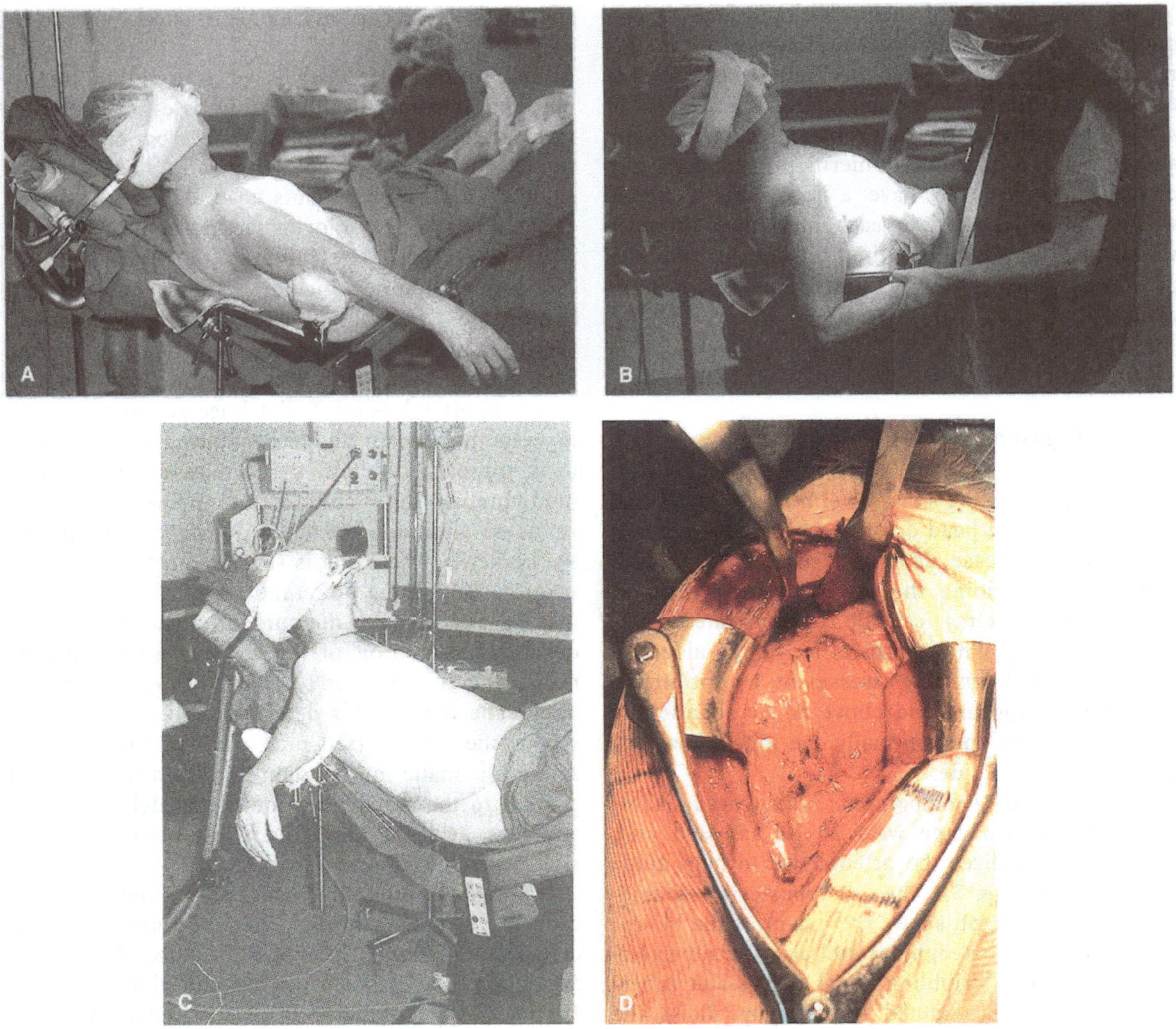

Fig. 4 A–D. Installation and surgical exposure. **A** Patient in the beach-chair position with the whole shoulder outside the table with the arm is positioned on a "U" support. **B** The arm support can be retracted medially to allow extension and preparation of the humerus (*vertical*). **C** The arm can be placed in abduction to allow exposure and preparation of the glenoid. **D** Deltopectoral incision: the subscapularis with the capsule is usually divided 2 cm medial to the biceps groove with an oblique incision. The coracoacromial ligament is preserved

aspect of the glenohumeral joint. The tendon is usually not repaired at the completion of the operation. *Laterally* the deep surface of the deltoid is freed from the underlying tissues and from the humerus while putting the arm in abduction and internal rotation. *Medially* the conjoint tendon is freed from the underlying subscapularis and retracted using a Richardson- or Farabeuf-type retractor. This step is facilitated by putting the arm in flexion and neutral rotation with the elbow flexed to slacken the conjoint tendon. After following the anterior humeral circumflex vessels, the axilary nerve is identified and protected. A self-retaining, asymmetric retractor is put in place. By placing the arm in extension again the three borders of the subscapularis are identified: the lateral border of the subscapularis insertion lies medial to the bicipital groove; the upper border lies immediately below the tip of the coracoid process and the lower border, which is only muscular (without any tendon), is defined by the anterior circumflex vessels.

Soft Tissue Release

The amount of passive external rotation determines the specific *technique for release and/or lengthening of the subscapularis*. The coronal Z-plasty has been abandoned because it weakens the tendon and two other techniques are currently used: (a) a 360° release of the subscapularis with anterior capsulotomy or (b) a 360° release associated with a medial advancement of the tendon. In the former technique the tendon is incised medially while in the latter the tendon is incised laterally, closed to the bicipital groove.

In the majority of cases there is a contracture in internal rotation with an external rotation limited to -10° or -20°. In these common cases the subscapularis should be divided in the middle of the tendon 2 cm medial to its insertion, after tagging it with stay sutures. The incision should be oblique to preserve enough tendon laterally to allow an easy repair [8, 24]. The upper three-quarters of the tendinous part of the subscapularis and the capsule should be divided together in an "L" fashion, temporarily preserving the inferior muscular part with the anterior circumflex vessels (Fig. 5A). A simple release of the superior three-quarters of the subscapularis is done by performing a capsulotomy along the anterior and inferior border of the glenoid (Fig. 5B–D). During this step the axillary nerve is protected by the lower muscular part of the subscapularis. Lengthening of the subscapularis is about 1.5 to 2 cm and gives usually an increased external rotation of about 40° (1 cm $\simeq$ 20°). At the time of closure, a tendon to tendon is performed.

When the internal contracture of the subscapularis is severe, with less than -20° (usually previous operated shoulders), the tendon is released from its insertion into the lesser tuberosity, just medial to the bicipital groove. The juxtaglenoid capsulotomy is performed in the same manner as previously. At the time of closure, the tendon of the subscapularis is reattached to the anatomical neck with a bone to tendon repair using transosseous sutures. This gives another one to two cm of lengthening, providing another 20°–40° of external rotation. Once the subscapularis has been lengthened, it is placed in the glenoid fossa and kept in place with a "fourk" retractor until the end of the procedure.

On the humeral side, the capsule is released anteriorly and inferiorly from the neck beyond the 6 o'clock position, even where there is a large inferior osteophyte (Fig. 5E). The division of the lower (muscular) part of the subscapularis is completed after

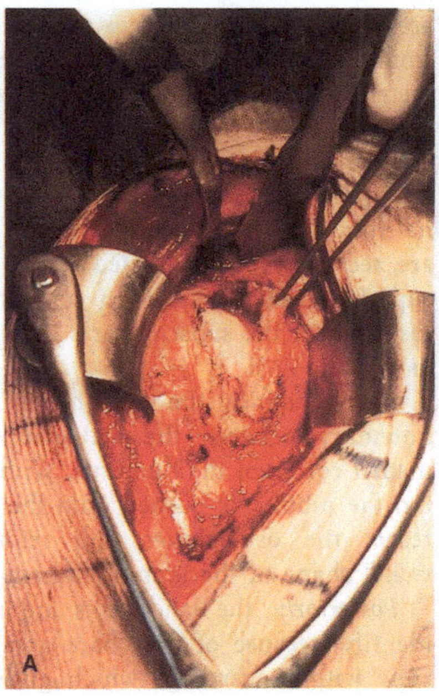

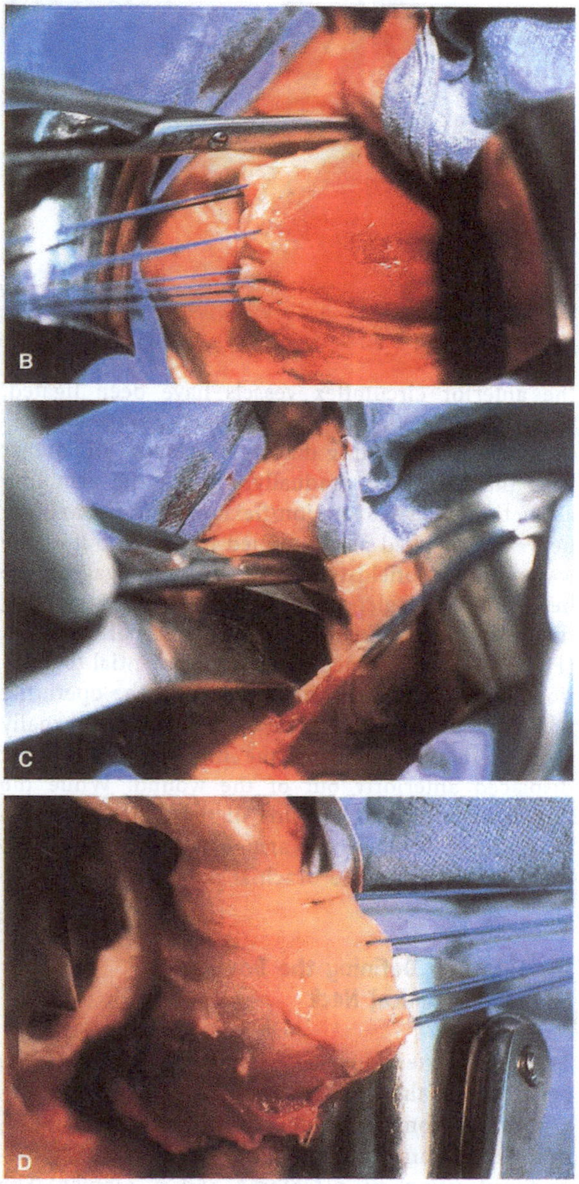

Fig. 5 A–F. Soft tissue release and humeral dislocation. **A** The lower part of the subscapularis with the anterior circumflex vessels is preserved in this first step. **B** The superior part of subscapularis is separated from its coracoid attachments ("the mooring pile"). **C** An anterior capsulotomy close to the glenoid enables the deep surface of the muscle to be freed from the subscapularis fossa. **D** After performing an inferior capsulotomy while protecting the axillary nerve the subscapularis is lengthened about 2 cm

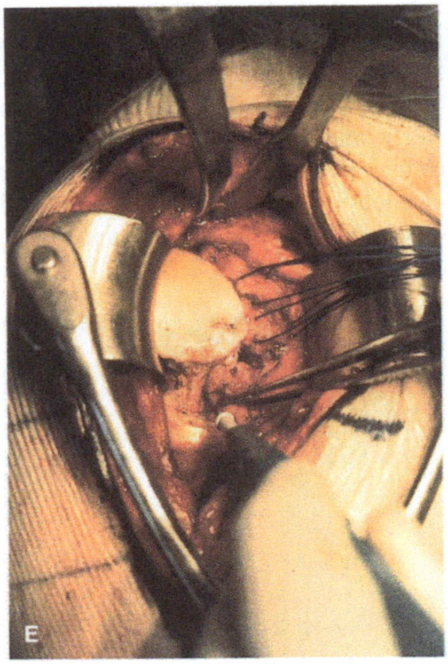

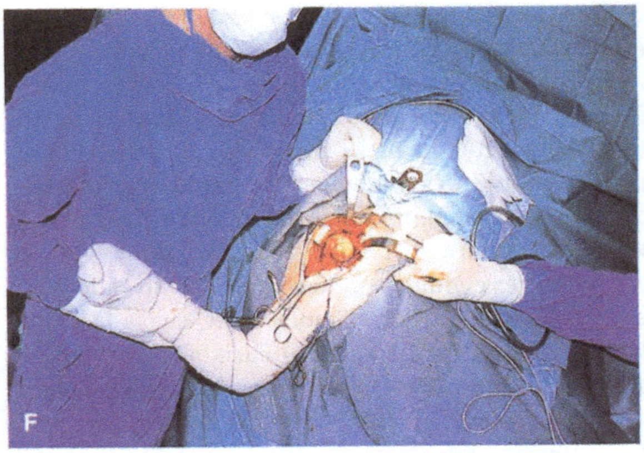

Fig. 5 A–F. (continued) E With the arm in adduction, flexion, and external rotation the capsule is released from its attachment on the humerus beyond the 6 o'clock position. The lower part of the subscapularis is now divided after ligature of the anterior circumflex vessels. **F** The humeral head is then dislocated anteriorly by extension with the arm abducted and externally rotated

the anterior circumflex vessels have been ligated. The risk of damage to the axillary nerve is minimized by using cutting diathermy, staying in contact with the bone and gradually moving the arm into adduction/external rotation/flexion while the axillary nerve is protected and retracted inferiorly out of the way with a Scofield-type retractor. Disengaging the head from the glenoid is made easier by moving the arm into extension and external rotation (Fig. 5F). As mentioned above, it is essential to position the patient's torso on the edge of the operating table so that the arm can be extended and externally rotated, thereby allowing the humeral head to be displaced anteriorly out of the wound. While the arm is extended off the side of the table, the assistant should support the arm and push upward to prevent stretch on the brachial plexus.

Locating and Defining the Boundaries of the Anatomical Neck

The osteophytes must be trimmed from around the periphery of the humeral head as guided by radiography and computed tomography so that the anatomical neck can be identified. The trimming is carried out using an osteotome and a nibbler. The osteotome is used to start the trimming, working from superior to inferior with the arm in adduction-extension-external rotation (Fig. 6A–C). Then the nibbler is used to finish the trimming, working from inferior to superior and keeping pressure on the humeral cortex. As in the acetabulum a layer of fatty tissue is found which marks the division between cortical bone and osteophytes. The boundaries of the anatomical neck are gradually revealed. The key point is to use a "dynamic technique" moving the arm into flexion-extension and/or internal-external rotation according to the need of the exposure.

Superolaterally, the anatomical neck marks the limit between the surface and the top of the greater tuberosity. A small "ice pick" is inserted into the greater tuberosity, protecting the tendon of the long head of biceps and the insertion of supraspinatus, nicely exposing the superior aspect of the articular surface and the top of the greater tuberosity. The trimming is often limited here because there are usually few osteophytes at this level. Because the frontal diameter is a little longer than the axial diameter, a small peace of cartilage is usually kept in place superiorly at the time of the osteotomy.

Anteriorly, the boundaries of the anatomical neck are usually easy to find by placing the arm in internal rotation. Here the edges of the articular surface are rectilinear and situated about 5 mm from the superior insertion and 15 mm from the inferior insertion of the subscapularis onto the lesser tuberosity (Fig. 7A).

Inferomedially, the anatomical neck marks the boundary between the articular surface and the medial cortex of the humerus. With the arm in flexion the nibbler is pushed onto the medial cortex to resect the osteophytes and reform the "Gothic vault" shape of the scapulohumeral curve.

Posteriorly, the landmarks are more difficult to identify because of the "bare area," an anatomical zone without cartilage which gives the anatomical

Fig. 6 A–C. Locating and defining the anatomical neck. **A** The key point is to remove all the osteophytes which obscure the anatomical neck: the osteophytes are trimmed away using an osteotome and a nibbler. **B** Some fat tissue usually lies between cortical bone and osteophytes. **C** The crown of osteophytes before and after trimming

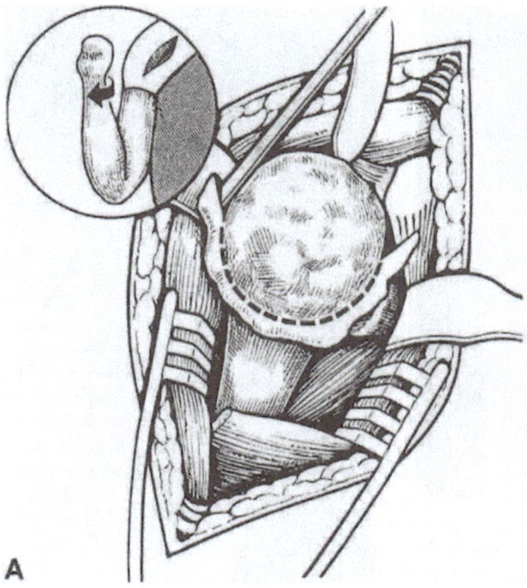

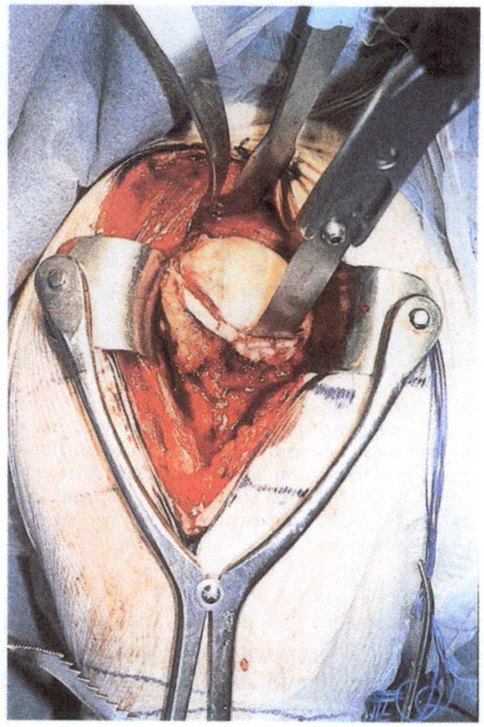

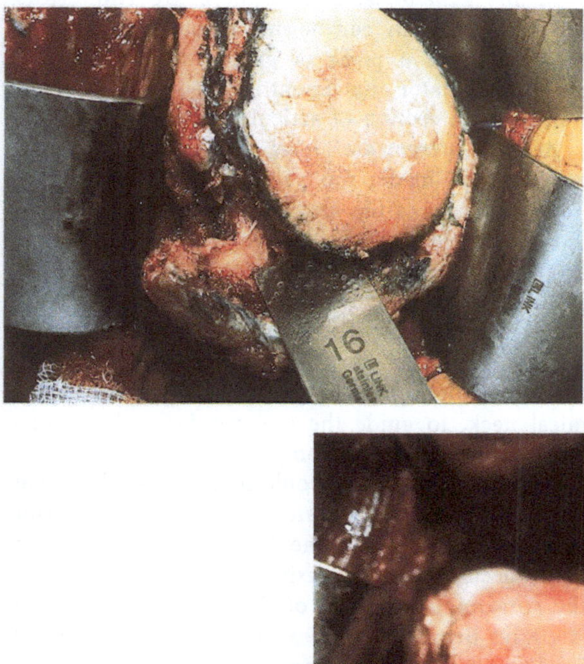

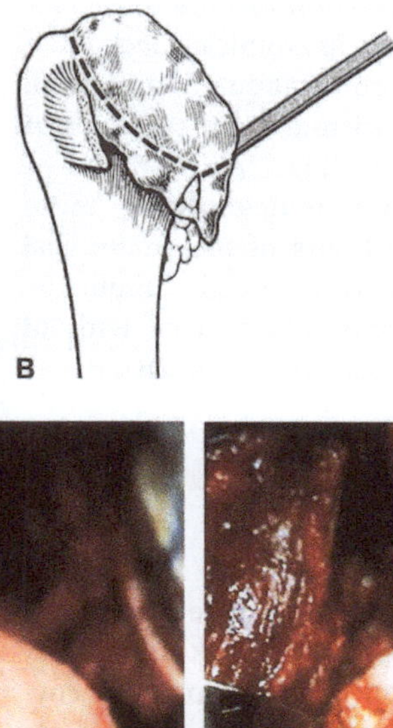

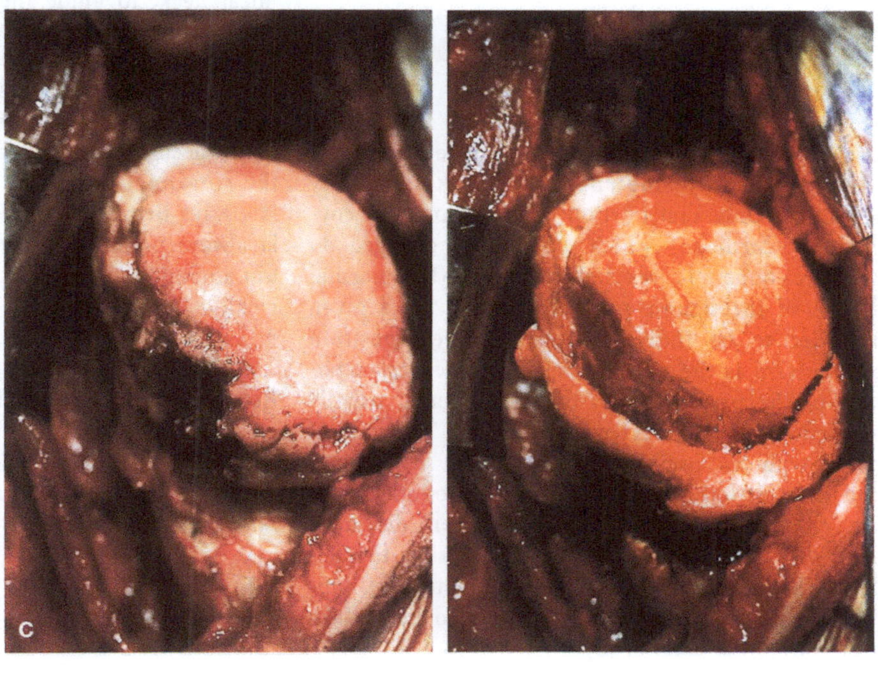

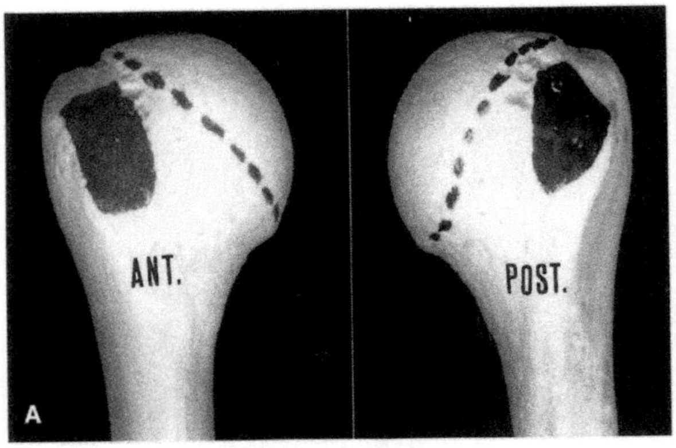

Fig. 7. **A** Dry bone demonstrates the location of the anatomical neck in relation to the tendinous insertions: insertions of the subscapularis (anterior) and the infraspinatus (posterior). **B** Computed tomogram of dry bone demonstrates that the anatomical neck is located about 5–10 mm from the lesser (LT) and greater (GT) tuberosities above the equator (depth of the osteotomy)

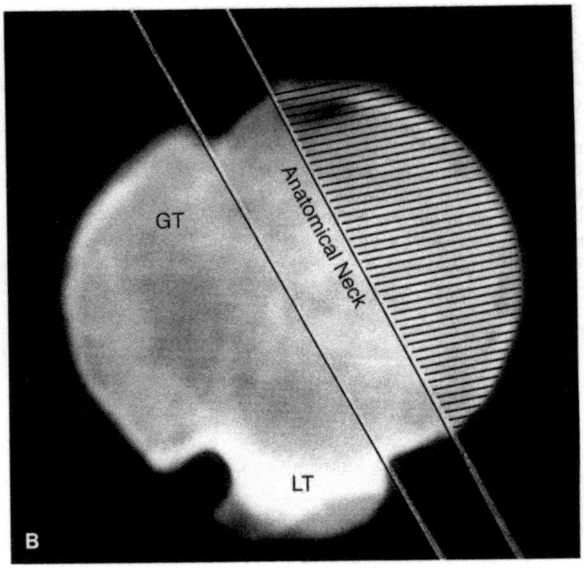

neck an italic "S" shape, and which should be respected. These landmarks are located with the arm in flexion and maximal external rotation and the posteroinferior osteophytes are resected using the nibbler. Again, the insertion of the posterior cuff marks the limit of the anatomical neck, and this boundary is usually found about 5 mm from the superior insertion and 15 mm from the inferior insertion of the infraspinatus (Fig. 7A).

The depth of the osteotomy is determined "automatically" by following the limits of the anatomical neck. The osteotomy should be made about 5–10 mm from the rotator cuff attachment without compromising the tendon insertion (Fig. 7B).

Humeral Head Osteotomy

Osteotomy of the humeral head can be performed when the limits of the anatomical neck are clearly identified. Only that portion of head normally covered by cartilage (which may have changed to sclerotic bone) is resected to allow the normal degree of inclination and retroversion for a given shoulder to be individualized. The best position for the arm is the one which allows the best exposure of the proximal part of the humerus, usually adduction-extension-external rotation. The cut is made with an oscillating saw (or an osteotome) and must strictly follow the normal boundaries of the anatomical neck which have been displayed (Fig. 4B). When using an oscillating saw, the left hand (for a right-handed person) should be supported by resting it on the humerus to help make an accurate cut (Fig. 8A,B).

At the superolateral level there are two errors which theoretically can be made: too large an excision may take a piece of greater tuberosity with the lateral rotator attachment and too small an excision leaves a section of articular surface (Fig. 9A).

At the inferomedial level two further mistakes may also be made: too valgus an osteotomy may leave a section of the articular surface in place and too varus a cut may damage the inferior cortex (Fig. 9B). This is by far the most common mistake because the articular surface of the head of the humerus is almost always distorted into a varus position. Therefore the surgeon should remove all the medial osteophytes necessary to find the anatomical neck, to guide the saw cut *before* beginning the humeral head osteotomy.

Posteriorly a mistake would be to make a bone cut with too much retroversion placing the posterior cuff at risk. However, the bone cut can be made quite accurately and easily free-hand. Whenever the surgeon is not sure of the normal anatomy, it is always better to cut less than too much! A recut is always possible, and one should remember that the amount of bone removed is usually surprisingly small.

Reproducing the Bony Anatomy

Prosthetic adaptability allows individual inclination and retroversion to be matched and also any mediolateral or anteroposterior offset to be covered.

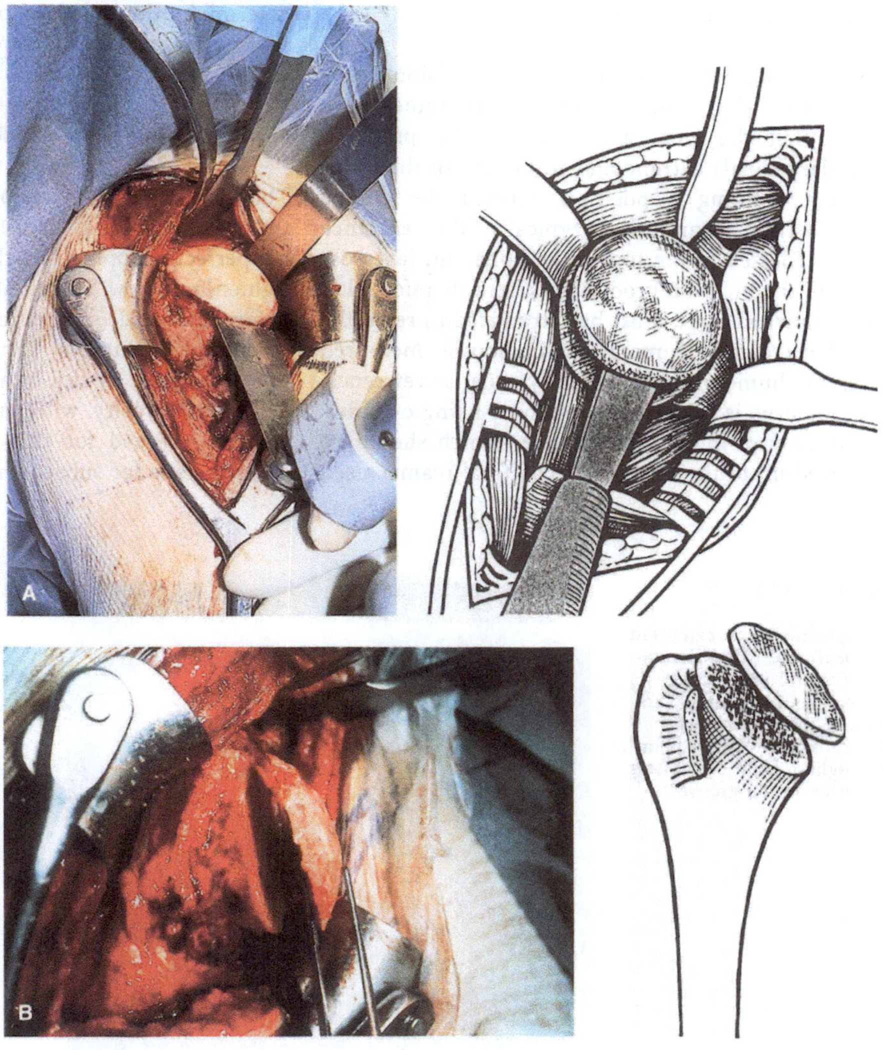

Fig. 8 A,B. Humeral head osteotomy. **A** Once the anatomical neck has been identified, the humeral head is cut using a saw. **B** The amount of the bone resected is usually surprisingly small

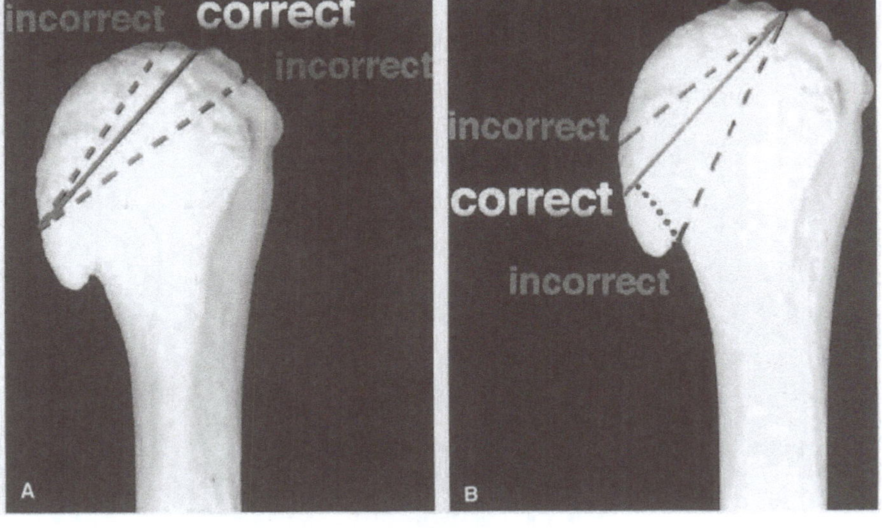

Fig. 9 A,B. Theoretical errors possible while performing head osteotomy: cutting too much or too less. **A** Superolaterally. **B** Inferomedially

Preparing the Medullary Canal

This is performed with the arm in extension-external rotation (Fig. 10). Our anatomical studies have shown that the stem axis (axis of the proximal medullary canal) extrapolates to the top of the humeral cut defining a position, termed the "hinge point." This means that typically the entrance point is located at the top of the bone cut, just posterior to the bicipital groove. It is here therefore that the cylindrical rasps must be introduced to ream the medullary canal. Humeral inclination is measured using the humeral intramedullary canal as reference. The humerus is reamed progressively using cylindrical reamers of increasing diameter which should be advanced up to the last ridge. The final reamer used determines the diameter of the *inclination-retroversion guide* and the diameter of the humeral stem.

Reproducing Inclination and Retroversion

The inclination-retroversion guide is introduced into the medullary canal (Fig. 11). The mobile plate must be perfectly applied to the humeral cut with the tightening screw in contact with the "hinge point" before the guide is secured at that angle using the screwdriver. Humeral retroversion is marked with the neck-guide in situ by marking a slot on the cancellous tuberosity with an osteotome, through the groove designed for this purpose. This slot represents the site for subsequent positioning of the hum-

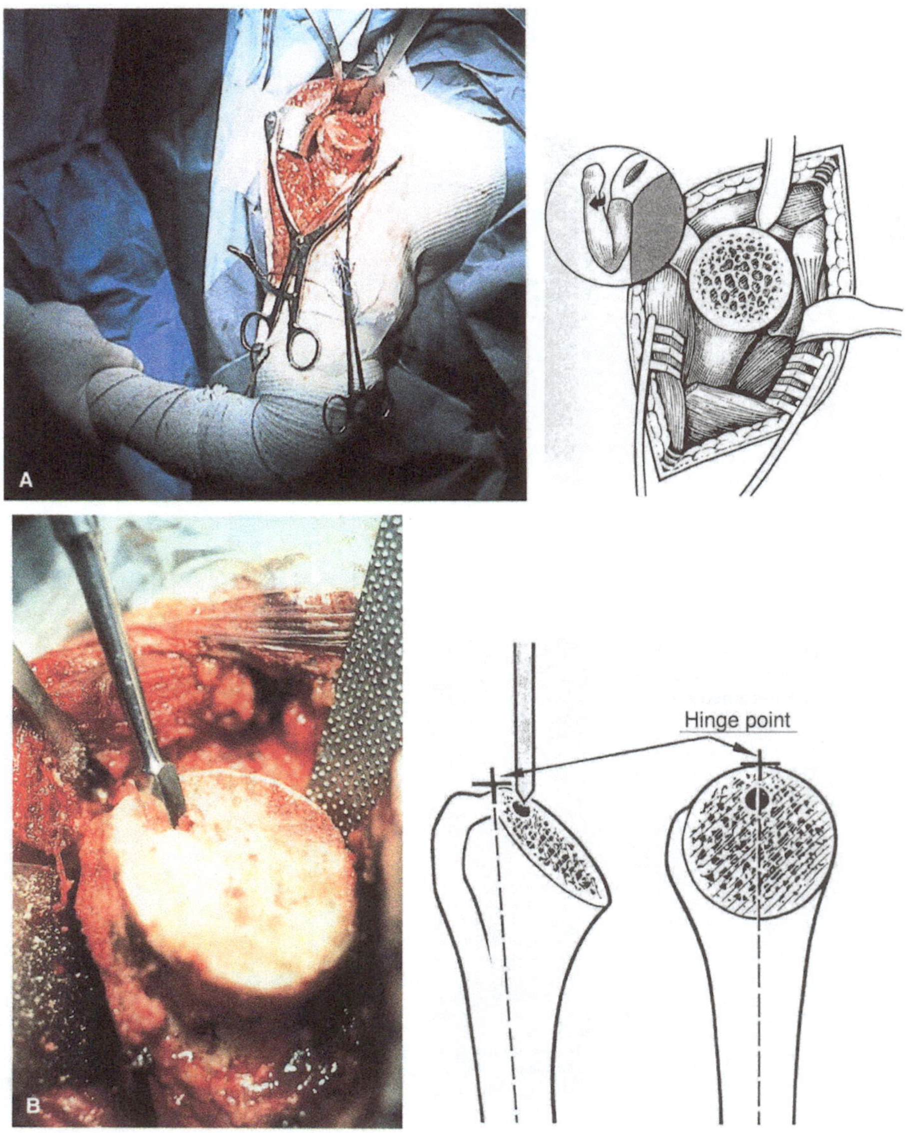

Fig. 10 A–C. Preparing the medullary canal. **A** The arm is kept positioned in extension (*vertical*) and external rotation (careful progressive movements in order not to cause a spiral fracture). **B** Locating the "hinge point": the highest point of the cut posterior to the groove

Fig. 10 A–C. (continued)
C Broaching the medullary canal with the cylindrical broaches of increasing diameter: the final broach determines the diameter of the neck guide and of the stem

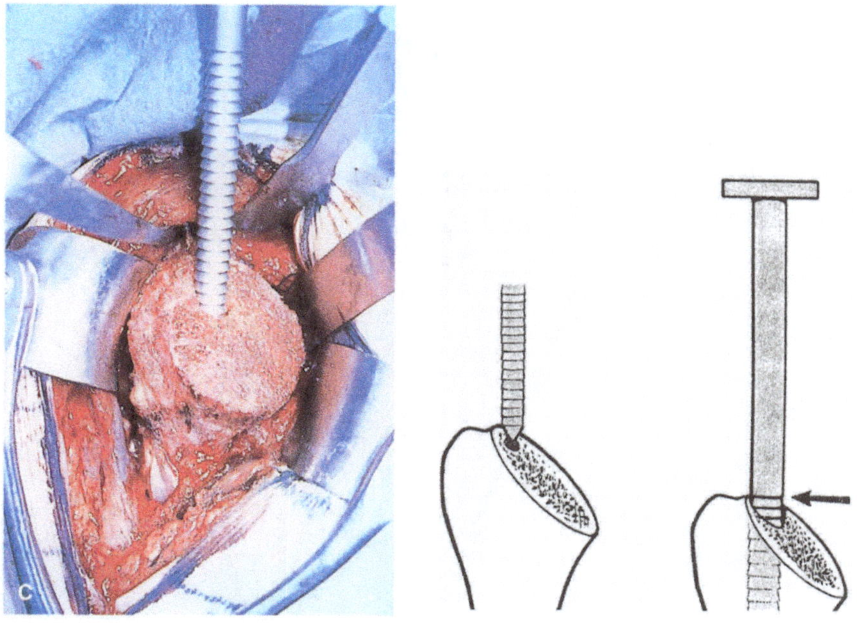

eral fin (Fig. 11C,D). The plane of section of the anatomical neck therefore determines inclination and retroversion of the humerus. After removing the guide, the angle of humeral inclination is read directly from a template (Fig. 11E). There are four possible angles of inclination from 125°–140°, each provided by one of four trial neck components. If an angle lies between two values, the lower should be chosen for the prosthesis. If, for example, the angle is between 135° and 140°, the 135° prosthesis should be chosen.

Definitive broaching of the humeral stem is performed using the corresponding broach. Retroversion is expected by aligning the fin of the broach with the slot created by the osteotome as described above. The broach should be advanced up to its last ridge for a 125° slope, or to one of three marks for slopes of 130°, 135° or 140° (Fig. 12A,B). The trial stem-neck unit is introduced into the humeral shaft, observing the correct position for the fin and impacted (Fig. 12C–E).

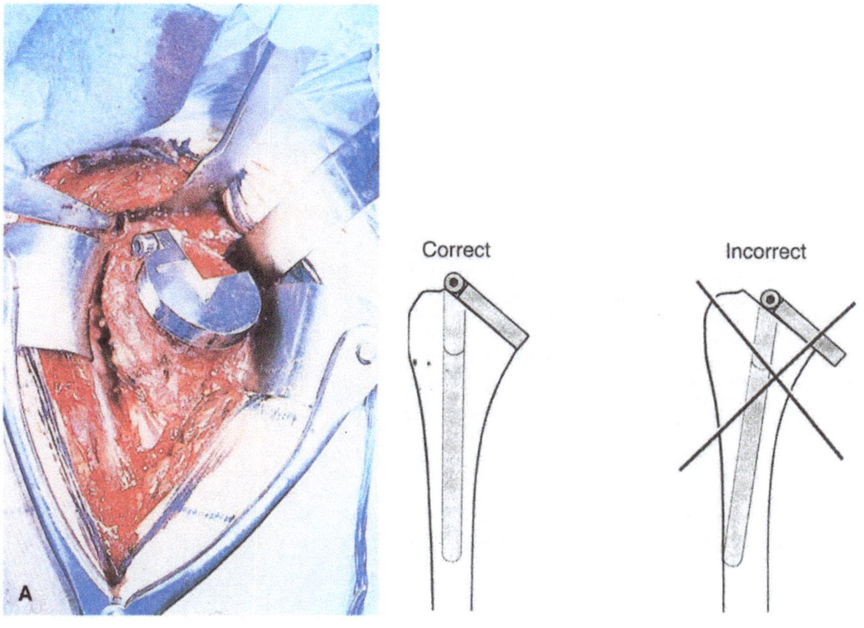

Fig. 11 A–E. Reproducing humeral inclination and retroversion. **A** The neck guide is introduced in the medullary canal

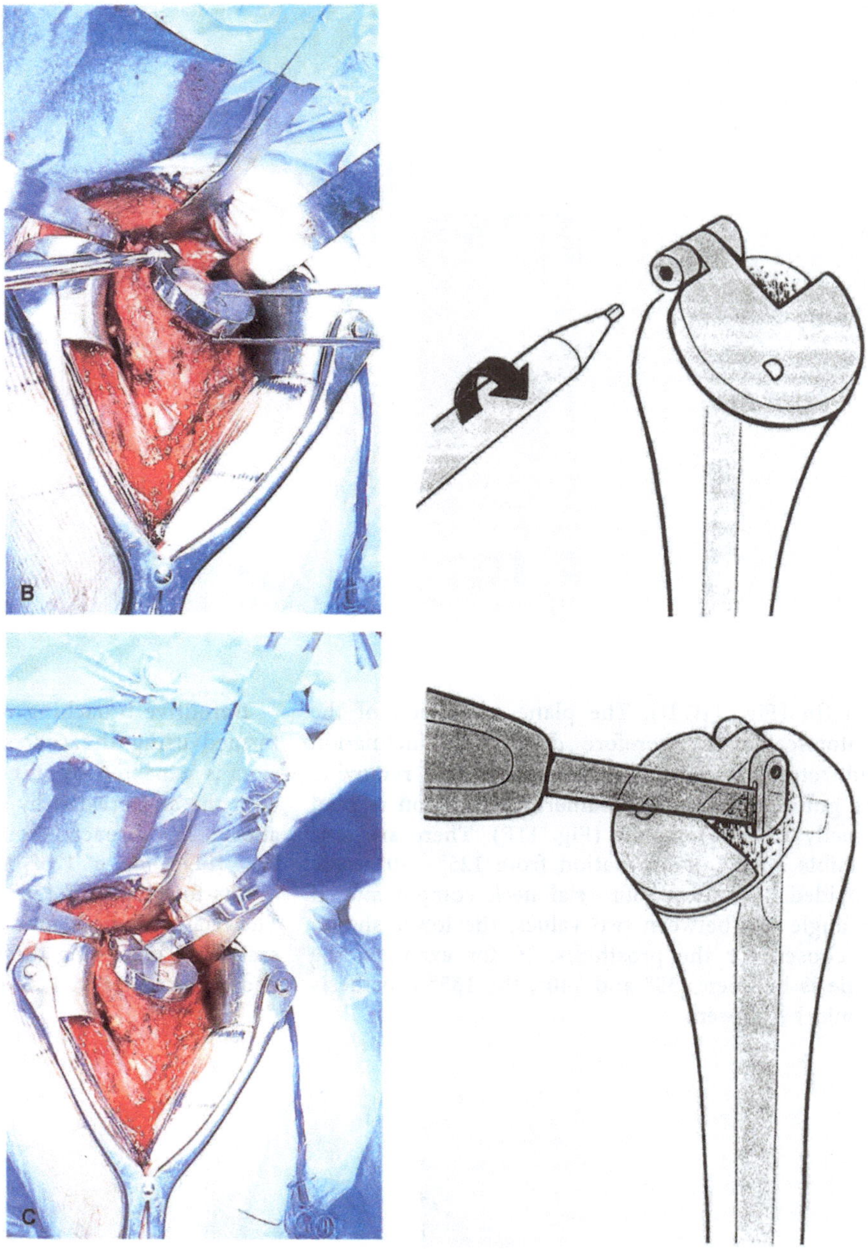

Fig. 11 A–E. (continued) B With the neck guide flat on the bone cut, the tightening screw fixes the inclination. **C** Humeral retroversion is marked with an osteotome (do not try to cover the bone cut with the tray of the neck guide)

Fig. 11 A–E. (continued)
D Marking the slot for the fin of the prosthesis (note that the tray of the neck guide does not cover the humeral cut). **E** Humeral inclination is measured using a template (if an angle lies between two values, the lower one should be chosen for the prosthesis)

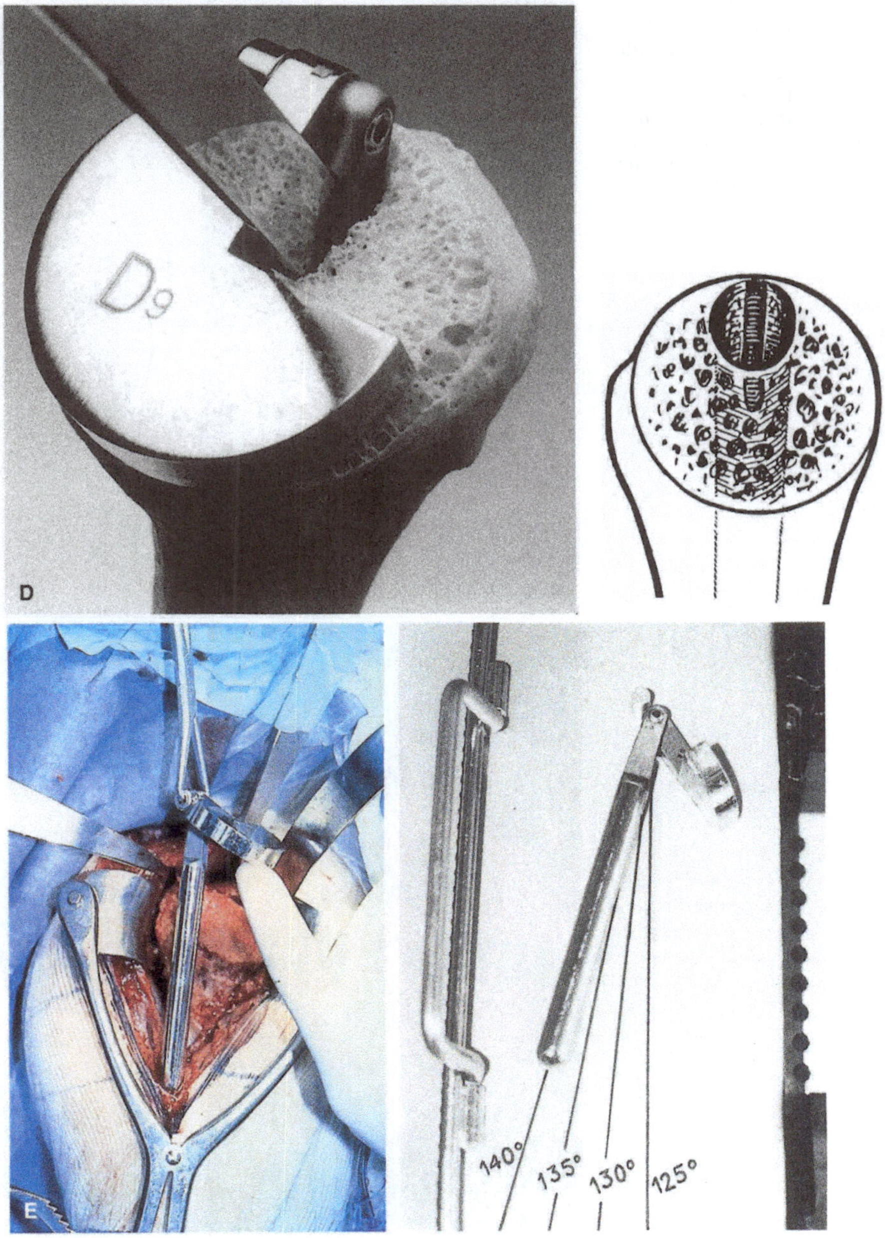

Fig. 12 A–E. Introducing the trial stem-neck. **A** The definitive broach is advanced with respect to the previously marked retroversion and measured inclination. **B** Posterior offset of the articular surface is often obvious after preparing the medullary canal

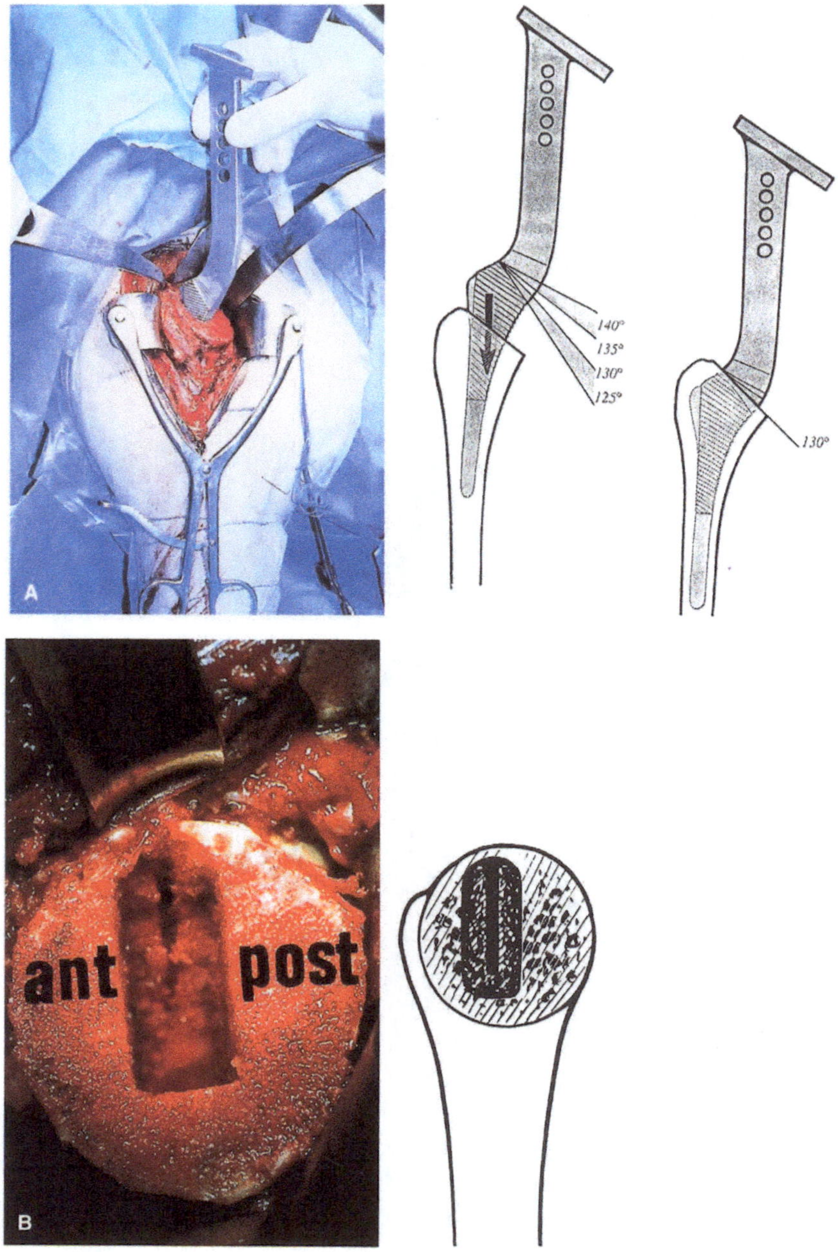

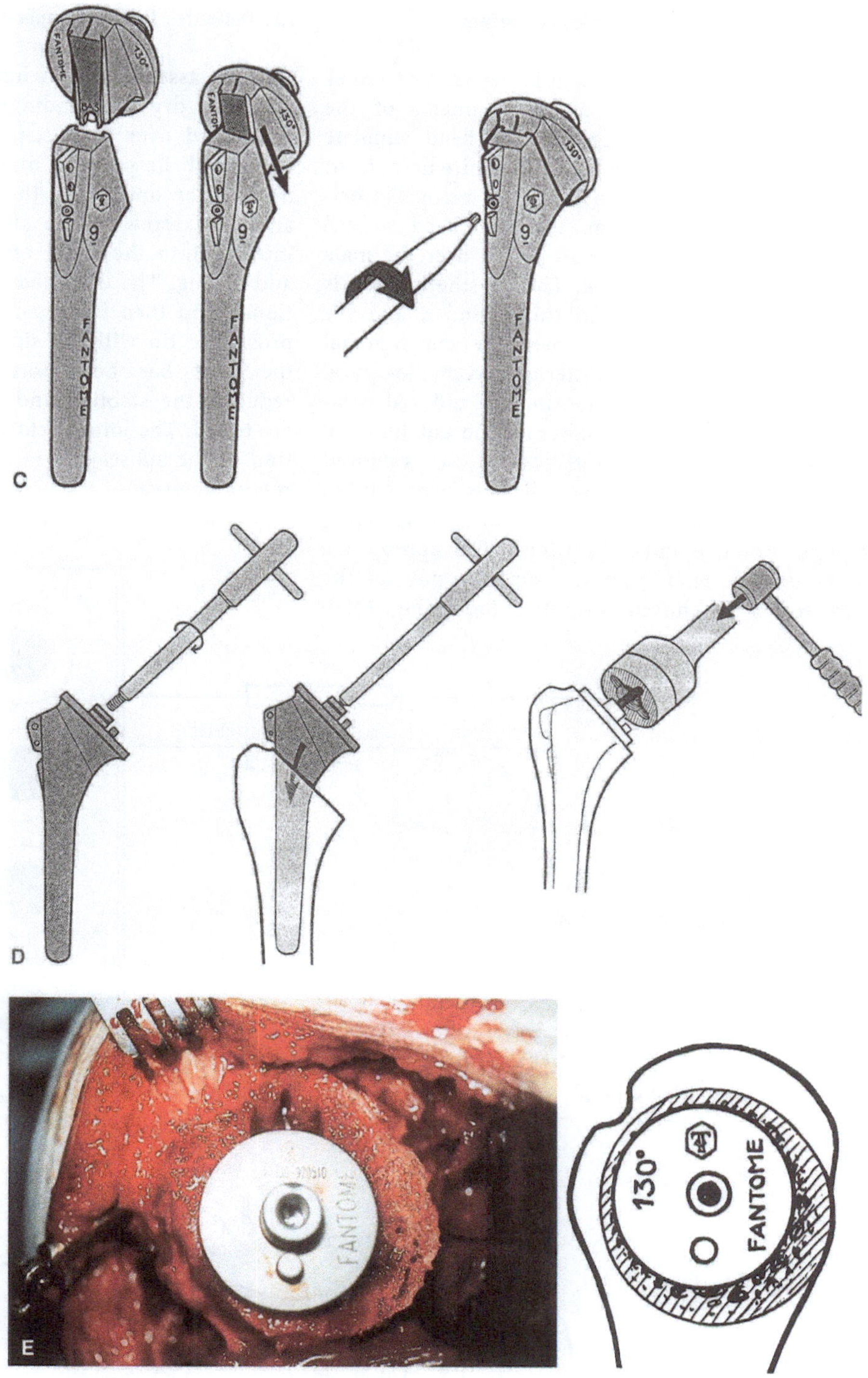

Fig. 12 A–E. (continued) C The trial stem and neck are assembled. **D** The trial stem-neck is introduced into the humeral shaft and impacted. **E** The bone cut with the trial stem-neck into the humeral shaft

Reproducing Offsets of the Articular Surface

The size of the trial head size is determined either by caliper measurement of the diameter of the resected head or by using the trial head template (Fig. 13A). The only remaining requirement is to reproduce the articular surface offset using the original eccentric dial system. The trial head is held with the trial head clamp and placed over the male cylindrical part of the neck. The prosthetic head is rotated eccentrically around this cylinder, and the ideal position selected to cover the cut humeral neck (Fig. 13B,C). Anteroposterior and medio-lateral offsets are preserved by choosing the indexed position which allows perfect cover of the cut humeral surface. The entire trial prosthesis is then removed using the extractor hammer. The posterior face of each trial head is marked from 1–8, corresponding to eight possible index positions. The appropriate figure is then read from the superior pole of the neck to give the chosen anatomical index (Fig. 13D).

The Definitive Humeral Implant

This is assembled proximal to distal with clean gloves in dry surroundings. The definitive head is positioned over the neck, aligning the anatomical index with its position marked on the upper of the neck. After impaction, the head can be fixed with an union screw to the stem-neck unit. Cement is injected into the canal after diaphyseal obturation and drying. The definitive humeral implant is positioned and then impacted, taking care to align the prosthetic fin with its slot in the tuberosity. After the joint has been washed and the prosthesis reduced, the stability and mobility of the shoulder are tested. The joint is closed by meticulous reinsertion of the subscapularis and partial closing of the rotator interval.

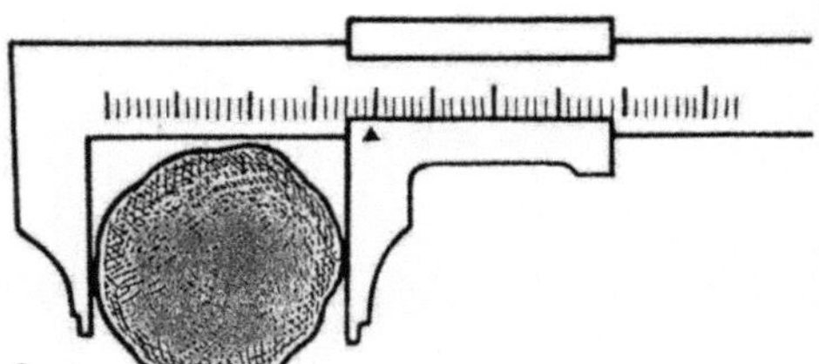

A

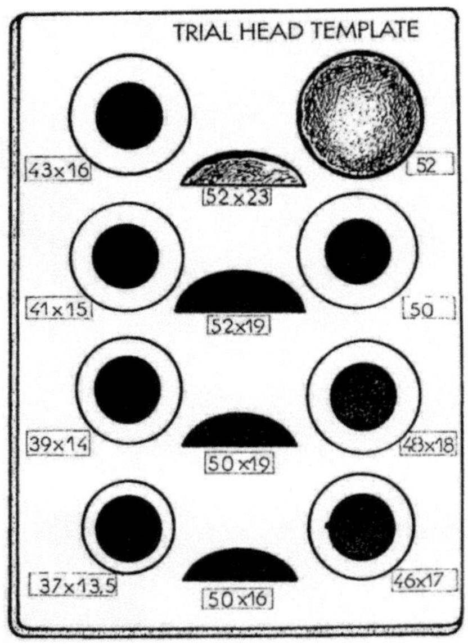

Fig. 13 A–E. Reproducing offsets of the articular surface. **A** The diameter of the resected head is measured with a calliper or a template. **B** Mediolateral and anteroposterior offsets are preserved by choosing the indexed position which allows perfect cover of the cut humeral surface

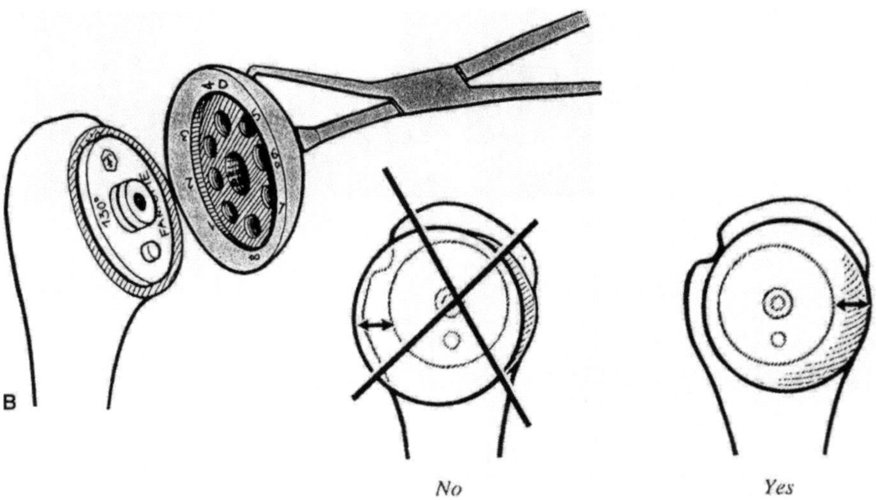

B

Fig. 13 A–E. (continued)
C Checking for restoration of the bony anatomy. **D** The trial prosthesis is removed using the extractor and the anatomical index (1–8) is then read from the superior pole of the neck. **E** Respect of the mediolateral and anteroposterior offsets with perfect match between the prosthetic head and the bone cut

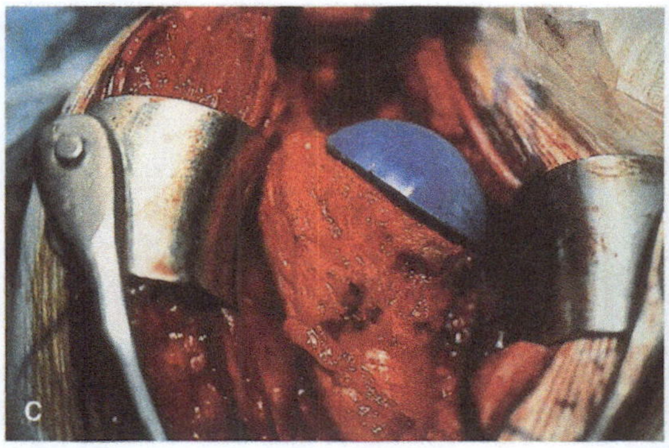

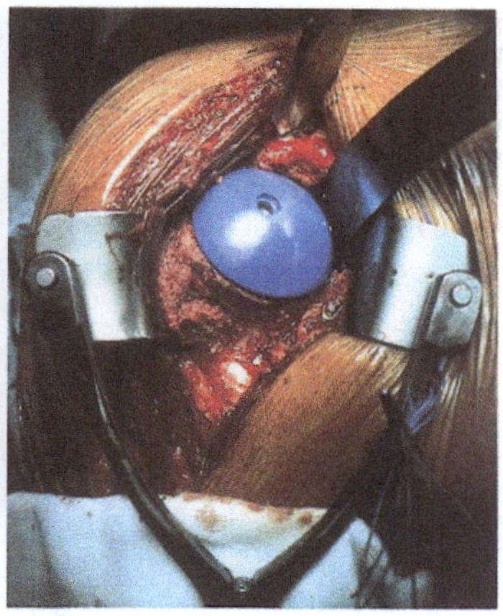

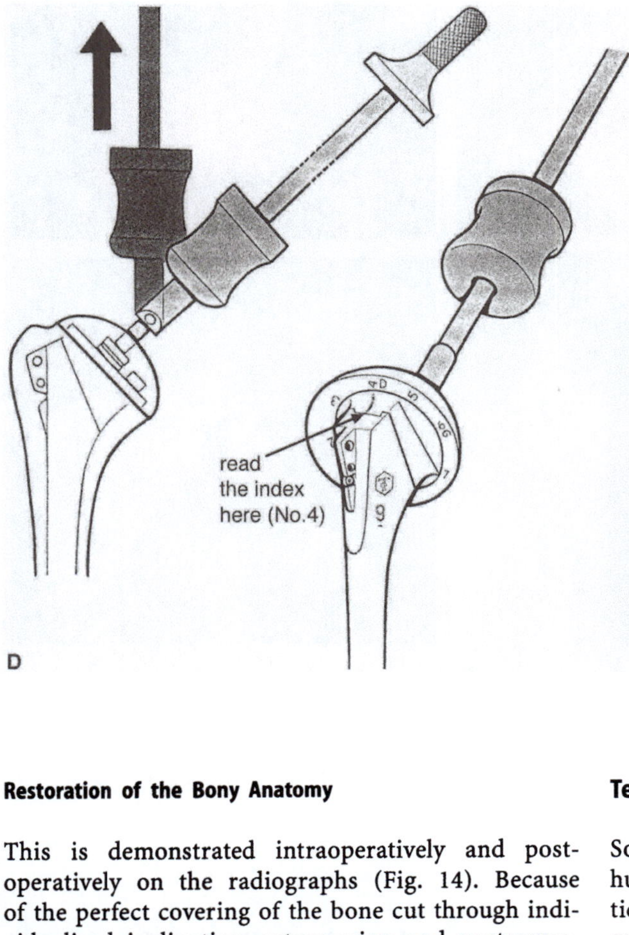

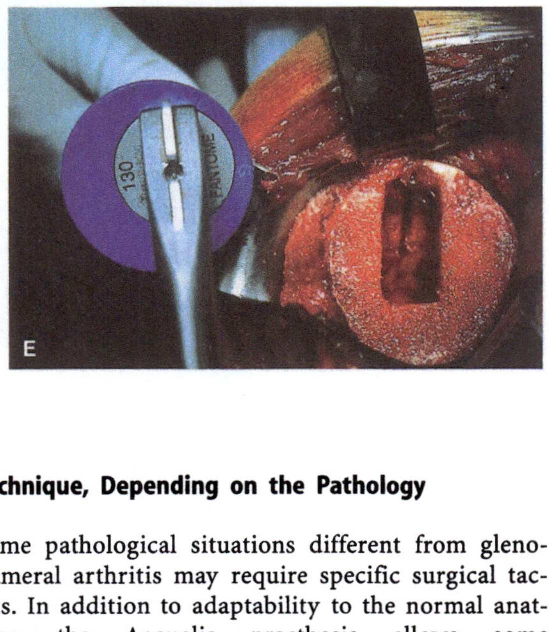

Restoration of the Bony Anatomy

This is demonstrated intraoperatively and postoperatively on the radiographs (Fig. 14). Because of the perfect covering of the bone cut through individualized inclination, retroversion and posteromedial offset and through the direct relationship between head height and diameter, incorrect placements of the head are avoided with the Aequalis shoulder prosthesis. Once the prosthesis is seated the head of the prosthesis is just superior to the greater tuberosity of the humerus allowing smooth passage of the supraspinatus. Restoration of the bony anatomy allows perfect tensioning of the cuff and avoids overtensioning the glenohumeral joint which is known to decrease range of motion and increase loads across the glenoid component.

Technique, Depending on the Pathology

Some pathological situations different from glenohumeral arthritis may require specific surgical tactics. In addition to adaptability to the normal anatomy, the Aequalis prosthesis allows some adaptability to the pathological anatomy.

Version of the humeral component and/or anteroposterior offset sometimes requires individualization based on the pathology present. For instance, in patients with arthritis of *recurrent anterior dislocation*, more retroversion may be required for stability. It is also possible to decrease the anterior offset or to put a posterior offset. By, contrast, in patients with *sequelae of chronic, unreduced posterior fracture dislocation*, less retroversion or an anterior offset may be appropriate.

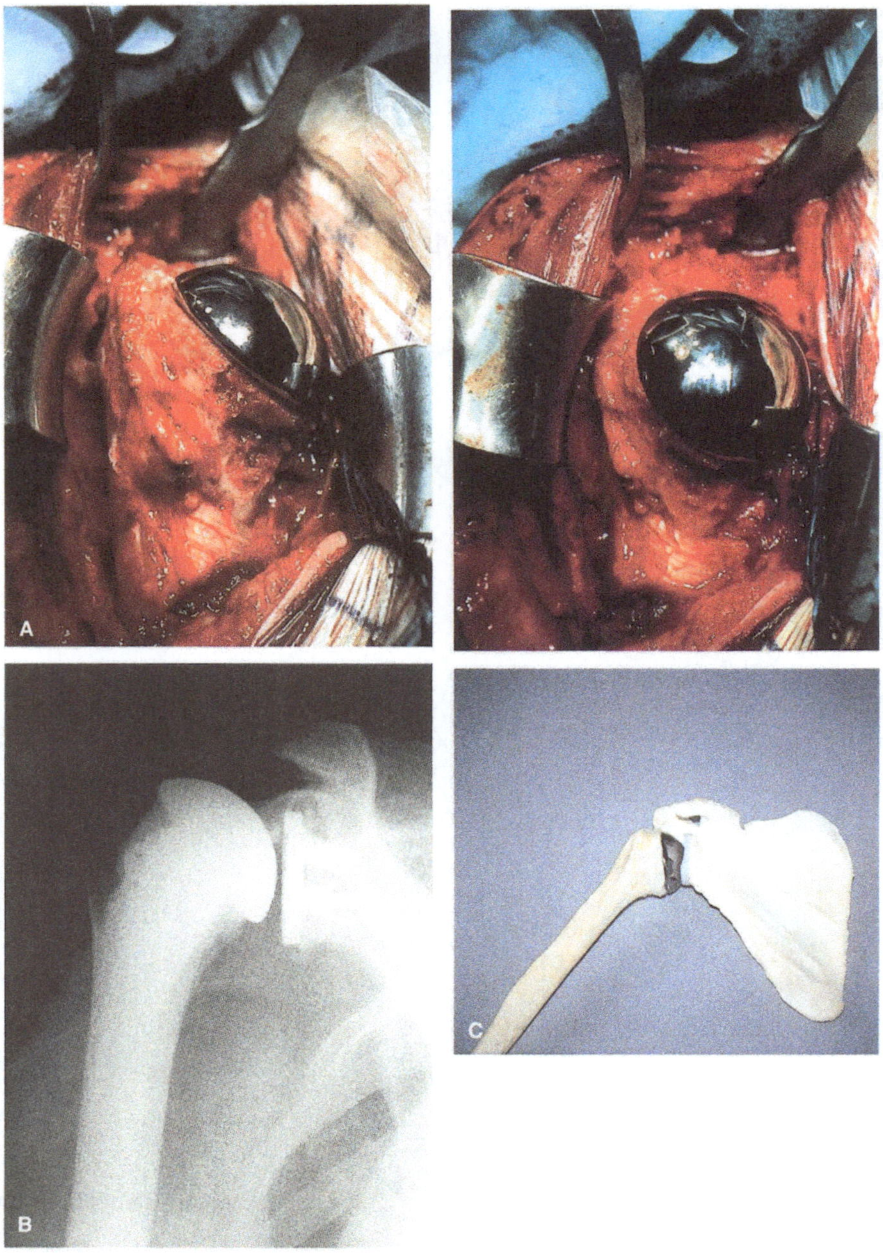

Fig. 14. Restoration of the bony anatomy of the humerus. **A** Demonstrated intraoperatively. **B** Demonstrated postoperatively on the radiographs. **C** Demonstrated on dry bones

Inclination of the humeral component may also be individualized, taking into account the pathology. For instance, in patients with *cuff tear arthritis* it may be appropriate to increase the inclination angle, to allow the prosthetic head to face more superiorly, and to articulate with both the glenoid medially, and the acromion, superiorly. In some advanced arthritic conditions, the bone in the proximal humerus may be deficient, especially medially. In these cases the medial humerus should be reconstructed using bone graft and cement while inclination should be individualized (usually decreased).

Finally, *complete individualization of the four geometric parameters* (the inclination and retroversion angles as well as the posteromedial offsets) may be appropriate in some *sequelae of four-part impacted fractures (either in valgus or in varus).* In some of these cases by using all the possibilities offered by prosthetic adaptability, the surgeon may avoid the need to perform an osteotomy of the greater tuberosity. Approximation of the anatomy of the proximal humerus without performing a greater tuberosity osteotomy allows immediate postoperative rehabilitation and in our experience gives better functional result.

Conclusion

Humeral osteotomy is perhaps the most critical step in total shoulder arthroplasty. The prosthetic modularity and adaptability creates the intraoperative flexibility needed to achieve optimal restoration of the normal bony anatomy as well as correct tensioning of the rotator cuff and deltoid. Both the "*bony balancing*" (precision with which prosthetic components replicate the bony anatomy) and the "*soft tissue balancing*" (release and lengthening of the contracted soft-tissue or shortening of the stretched soft tissue) increase the chance of achieving greater postoperative motion.

References

1. Ballmer FT, Sidles JA, Lippitt SB, Matsen FA (1993) Humeral head prosthetic arthroplasty: surgically relevant geometric considerations. J Shoulder Elbow Surg 2:296–304
2. Boileau P, Walch G, Mazzoleni N, Urien JP (1993) In vitro measurement of humeral head retroversion. J Shoulder Elbow Surg 2 (2):S12
3. Boileau P, Walch G (1994) The combined offset (medial and posterior) of the humeral sphere. J Shoulder Elbow Surg 3:6
4. Boileau P, Walch G (1995) Adaptabilité et modularité dans les prothèses d'épaule. Acta Orthop Belgica 61 [Suppl I]:49–61
5. Boileau P, Walch G (1995) Varus shoulder prosthesis: error or necessity? J Shoulder Elbow Surg S62:186
6. Boileau P, Walch G (1997) The three dimensional geometry of the proximal humerus: implications for surgical technique and prosthetic design. J Bone Joint Surg Br 79B:857–865
7. Broca P (1881) La torsion de l'humérus et le tropomètre, instrument destiné à mesurer la torsion des os (rédigée par L Mamouvier). Rev Anthrop 2(4):193–210, 385–423, 1577–1592
8. Collins DN, Harryman DT II, Lippitt SB, Jackins SE, Matsen FA III (1991) The technique of glenohumeral arthroplasty. Techn Orthop 6:43–59
9. Fenlin JM, Vacaro A, Andreichik D, Lin S (1990) Modular total shoulder: early experience and impressions. Semin Arthropl 1(2):102–111
10. Fick R (1904) Anatomie und Mechanik der Gelenke. Fischer, Jena, pp 171–174
11. Figgie HE III, Inglis AE, Golberg VM, Ranawat CS, Figgie MP, Wile JM (1988) An analysis of factors affecting the long term results of total shoulder arthroplasty in inflammatory arthritis. J Arthropl 3:123–130
12. Flatow EL (1995) Prosthetic design considerations in total shoulder arthroplasty. Semin Arthropl 6(4):233–244
13. Friedman RJ (1990) Biomechanics of the shoulder following total shoulder replacement. In: Post M, Morrey BF, Hawkins RJ (eds) Surgery of the shoulder. Mosby Year Book, St Louis, pp 263–266
14. Harryman DT, Sidles JA, Harris SI, Lippitt SB (1995) The effect of articular conformity and the size of the humeral head component on laxity and motion after glenohumeral arthroplasty: a study in cadavera. J Bone Joint Surg Am 77:555–563
15. Ianotti JP, Gabriel JP, Schneck SL, Evans BG, Misra S (1992) The normal glenohumeral relationships. An anatomical study of the hundred and forty shoulders. J Bone Joint Surg Am 74:491–500
16. Jobe CM, Ianotti JP (1995) Limits imposed on glenohumeral motion by joint geometry. J Bone Joint Surg 77:281–285
17. Khral VE, Evans FG (1945) Humeral torsion in man. Am J Phys Anthrop 3:229–253
18. Neer CS II (1990) Glenohumeral arthroplasty design. In: Shoulder reconstruction, 1st edn. Saunders, Philadelphia, pp 146–160
19. Ovesen J, Nielsen S (1985) Prosthesis position in shoulder arthroplasty: a cadaver study of the humeral component. Acta Orthop Scand 56:330
20. Pearl ML, Volk AG (1995) Retroversion of the proximal humerus relevant to prosthetic replacement arthroplasty. J Shoulder Elbow Surg 8:151–162
21. Pearl ML, Volk A G (1996) Coronal plane geometry of the proximal humerus relevant to prosthetic arthroplasty. J Shoulder Elbow Surg 5:320–326
22. Rietveld ABM, Daanen HAM, Rezing PM, Obermann WR (1988) The lever arm in gleno-humeral abduction after hemi-arthroplasty. J Bone Joint Surg Br 70:561–565
23. Roberts SNJ, Foley APJ, Swallow HM, Wallace WA, Coughlan DP (1991) The geometry of the humeral head and the design of protheses. J Bone Joint Surg Br 73:647–650
24. Romeo AA (1995) Total shoulder arthroplasty: pearls and pitfalls in surgical technique. Semin Arthropl 6(4):265–272
25. Steindler A (1936) Mechanics of shoulder arm complex. In: Thomas CC (ed) Kinesiology of the human body under normal and pathological conditions. Thomas, Springfield, Illinois, p 453
26. Strasser H (1917) Das Schultergelenk. Die obere Extremität. In: Lehrbuch der Muskel- und Gelenkmechanik. Springer, Berlin, pp 17–21
27. Walch G, Boileau P (1992) Morphological study of the humeral proximal epiphysis. Orthop Proc J Bone Joint Surg Br 74 [Supppl I]:14

Section V:

Advances in Glenoid Design and Surgical Technique

Normal and Pathological Anatomy of the Glenoid: Effects on the Design, Preparation, and Fixation of the Glenoid Component

P. Boileau and G. Walch

Summary

In an effort to better understand anatomical and pathological aspects of the glenoid that may be of surgical importance, we reviewed the literature and performed ourselves several studies analysing (a) the size and shape of the normal glenoid surface, (b) the radius of curvature of the glenoid surface and the corresponding humeral head, (c) the horizontal orientation of the glenoid (glenoid version), (d) the vertical orientation of the glenoid (glenoid inclination), (e) the possibilities of bony fixation of a glenoid component. All the results are discussed in terms of their surgical relevance for glenoid orientation, glenoid fixation and glenoid design.

Introduction

Knowledge of the normal anatomy of the glenoid is essential for surgical planning, preparation and positioning of the prosthesis. It also may be a basis for future glenoid component design. However, since total shoulder replacements are generally performed not in normal shoulders but in grossly arthritic shoulders with extensive anatomic distorsions, knowledge of the pathological anatomy is also necessary.

Using our own studies and those reported in the literature, this article reviews the normal and pathological anatomy of the glenoid that may have some surgical relevance regarding (a) the size and shape of the normal glenoid surface, (b) the radius of curvature of the glenoid surface and the corresponding humeral head, (c) the horizontal orientation of the glenoid, (d) the vertical orientation of the glenoid, (e) the possibilities of bony fixation of a glenoid component.

Size and Shape of the Glenoid Surface

Anatomy

We made surface measurements of 34 glenoids from human cadaveric specimens using a digitised measuring system linked to a computer, allowing three dimensional computerised modelling of the bones. The Metrologic MT1 (Metrologic, France), a highly accurate three-dimensional digitised measuring machine, pre-calibrated, was equipped with a special frame to hold the scapula. A computer linked to the digitizing machine and equipped with Metrologic 3D manual software, collected the data and produced three-dimensional pictures of the scapula. The accuracy of the digitising machine was in the order of 10 μm and was such that the margin of error may be considered insignificant for this application (Fig. 1). Our anatomical measurements are summarised in Fig. 2.

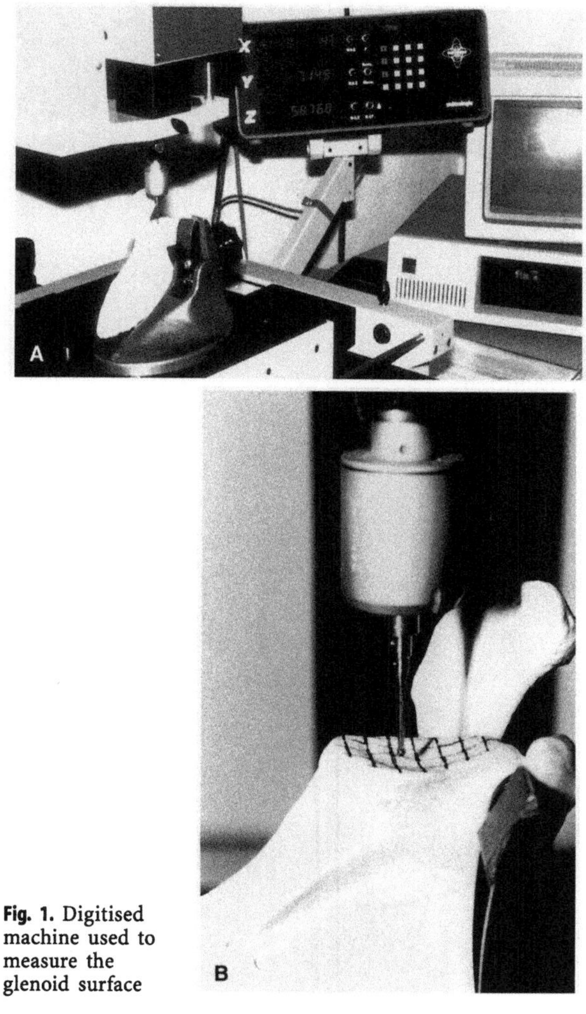

Fig. 1. Digitised machine used to measure the glenoid surface

Table 1. Dimensions of the glenoid articular surface according to the literature and to our own studies

	Glenoid dimensions		
	Vertical diameter (mm)	Small horizontal diameter (mm)	Large horizontal diameter (mm)
Fick 1904 [27]	35–40	–	25–30
Mallon 1992 [51] (n=28)	35±4.1 (28.5–43.5)	-	24±3.3 (16–29.5)
Iannotti 1992 [45] (n=140)	39±3.7 (30–48)	-	29±3.1 (21–34)
Boileau and Walch 1997 [8] (n=34)	34.9±3.4 (30.5–42)	18.9±2.4 (15–26)	25.5±2.8 (30.5–42)

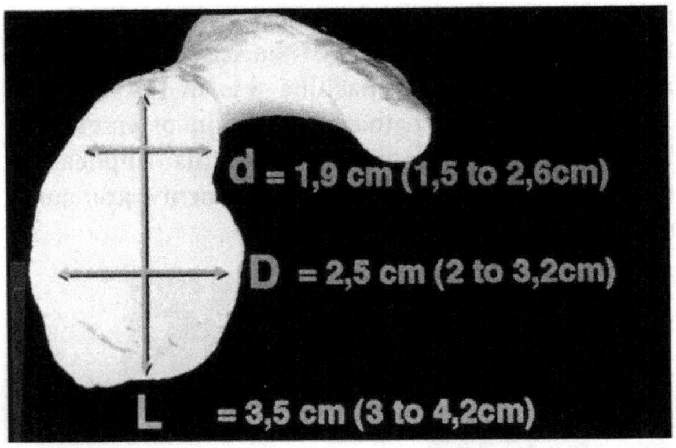

Fig. 2. Glenoid dimensions according to our measurements

Our study has confirmed the characteristic pear shape of the glenoid; the glenoid surface being larger in its lower half than in its upper half. Two horizontal diameters, perpendicular to the vertical diameter can be defined: a small horizontal diameter and a large horizontal diameter.

Table 1 summarizes the results of other authors [27, 45, 51]: the glenoid surface averages 35–40 mm in height (vertical diameter) and 25–30 mm in width (large horizontal diameter).

Pathology

The glenoid surface may be decreased because of the aggressiveness aspect of the disease as in rheumatoid arthritis [20, 28]. By contrast, the glenoid surface may also be enlarged because of the proliferation of peripheral osteophytes as in osteoarthritis [25, 49, 51, 72] (Fig. 3). Depending on the pathology, the peripheral osteophytes can be anterior, posterior, superior and/or inferior.

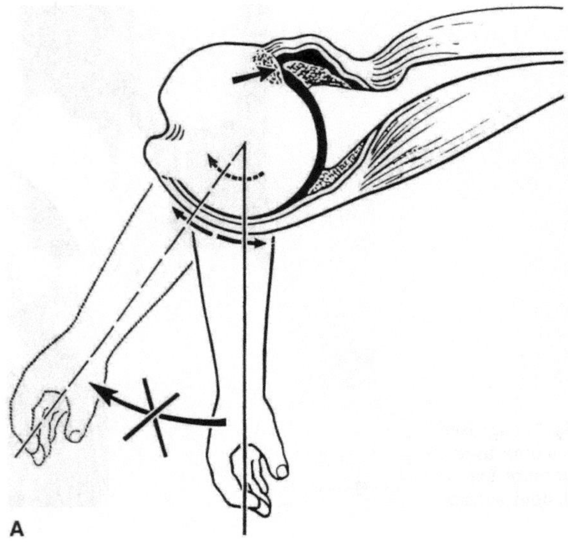

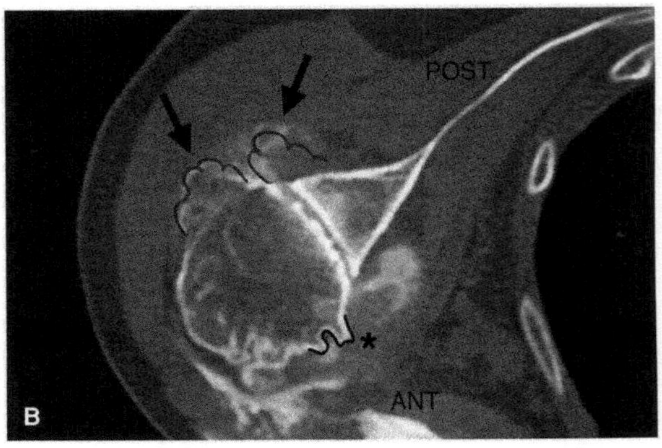

Fig. 3. Limited external rotation because of posterior osteophytes (arrows), responsible for posterior impingement with the greater tuberosity and because of anterior osteophytes (star), responsible for overtensioning of the anterior capsule and subscapularis

Surgical Relevance

Preserving the exact size and shape of the glenoid fossa is critical in total shoulder arthroplasty in order to restore the normal glenohumeral kinematics.

The surgical technique should try to restore the normal dimensions and shape of the glenoid surface.

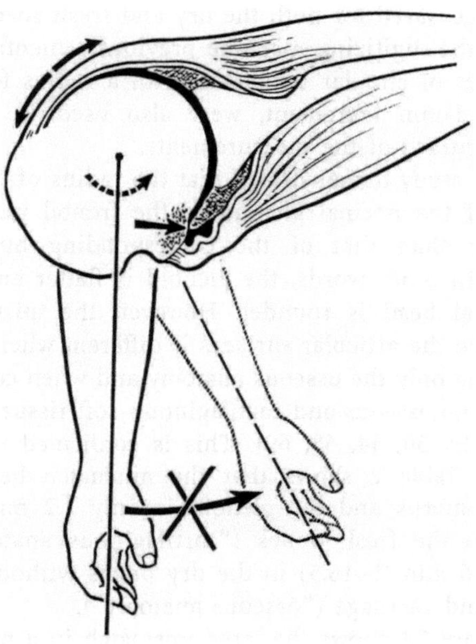

Fig. 4. Limited internal rotation because of anterior osteophytes (responsible for anterior impingement with the lesser tuberosity) and because of posterior osteophytes (responsible for overtensioning of the posterior capsule and subscapularis)

Removal of the peripheral osteophytes around the glenoid must be first carried out using an osteotome or a rongeur before reaming the glenoid or preparing the slo+ for the keel. The preoperative planning of glenoid preparation should include both AP view and a CT. Leaving osteophytes around the glenoid surface can lead to a significant malpositioning of the implant, either too anterior, too posterior or too low. The possible consequences include glenohumeral instability and/or limitation of the glenohumeral mobility due to an inadequate prosthetic component size and to the osteophytes themselves. Both external and internal rotation may be limited because of residual osteophytes (Figs. 3, 4).

Residual *posterior glenoid osteophytes* may limit external rotation because of posterior glenoid impingement with the greater tuberosity and simultaneously internal rotation because of overtensioning of the posterior soft tissue (infraspinatus and posterior capsule). Similarly, residual *anterior glenoid osteophytes* may limit external rotation by overtensioning the anterior soft tissues (subscapularis and anterior capsule) and simultaneously internal rotation because of anterior impingement with the lesser tuberosity. Finally, abduction may be limited because of *inferior osteophytes* which may overtension the inferior capsule and because of *superior glenoid osteophytes* which may lead to early impingement with the greater tuberosity (Fig. 5).

The design of a glenoid component should also try to match the pear shape and dimensions of the glenoid surface. First generation of glenoid compo-

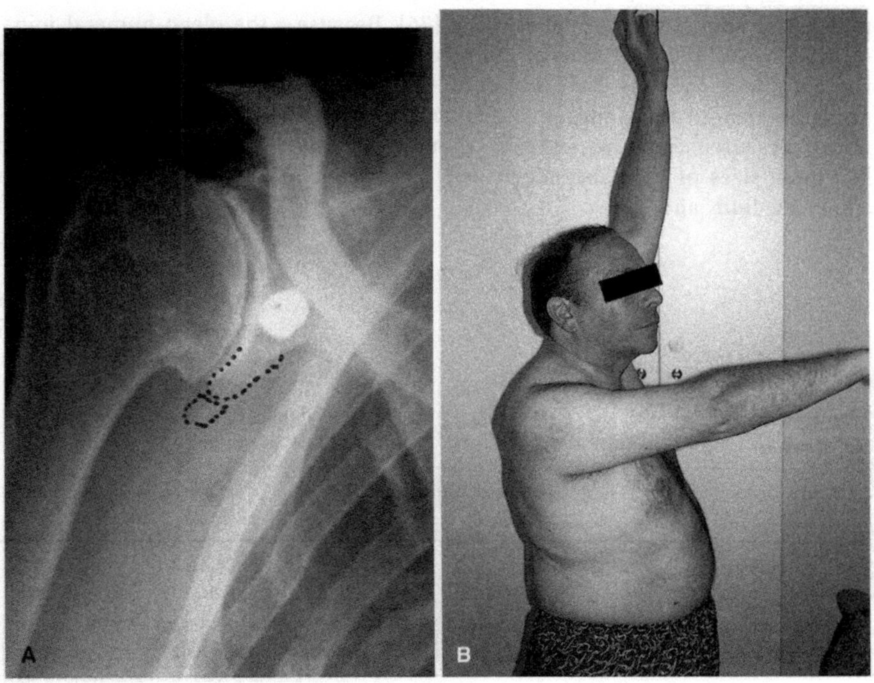

Fig. 5. A Inferior osteophytes may limit abduction because of overtensioning of the inferior capsule. **B,C** Clinical example

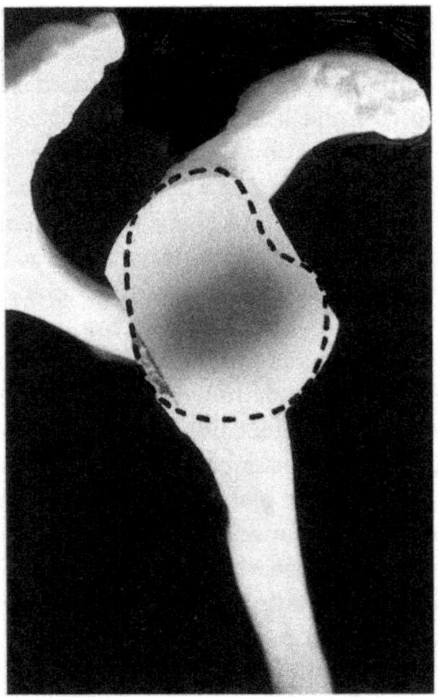

Fig. 6. First generation glenoid components were rectangular: they did not respect the pear shape of the glenoid leading to a potential internal impingement

nents, like the Neer glenoid component, were rectangular shaped and only available in one size [55, 58]. A non-pear shaped or over-large component (e.g. rectangular) may cause erosive lesions on the deep face of the rotator cuff because of overhanging of the prosthetic component (Fig. 6). An intrinsic mechanical impingement with the greater tuberosity *posteriorly* and the lesser tuberosity *anteriorly* is theoretically possible during abduction-external rotation or adduction-internal rotation [76]. Because of the variability in the size of the glenoid most of the prosthetic systems have enlarged the stock of available glenoid components. Based on our anatomical measurements, the Aequalis shoulder system has three sizes of pear shaped glenoid components: small, medium and large.

Glenohumeral Conformity and Constraint

Anatomy

We performed an anatomical study on twenty fresh frozen gleno-humeral joints in which the labrum was preserved and fourteen dry shoulders without any soft tissue attachment. The radius of curvature of the glenoid and corresponding humeral head were measured for both the dry and fresh specimen using the digitizing machine previously mentioned. A series of circular templates, with a radius featuring a 1-mm increment, were also used to verify the accuracy of the measurements.

Our study demonstrated that the radius of curvature of the normal glenoid in the frontal plane is greater than that of the corresponding humeral head. In other words, the glenoid is flatter and the humeral head is rounder. However, the mismatch between the articular surfaces is different when considering only the osseous anatomy and when considering the osseous and cartilaginous–soft tissue anatomy [29, 36, 44, 68, 69]. This is confirmed in our study: Table 2 shows that the mismatch between the humerus and the glenoid is only 2.2 mm (0–6.5) in the fresh bones ("cartilaginous anatomy") and 9.6 mm (5–16.5) in the dry bones without labrum and cartilage ("osseous anatomy").

Figure 7A shows the large mismatch in a normal osseous glenohumeral joint without soft tissue attachment. The vertical radius of curvature of the normal glenoid bone exceeds in a large amount that of the matching humeral head (0 to 13 mm for the diameters). This allows for some laxity in the gleno-humeral joint [16, 29, 33, 36, 41, 68, 71]. Figure 7B shows the small mismatch in a glenohumeral joint with the labrum and soft tissue attachments.

Finally, our measurements reveal that the depth of the glenoid is different in the vertical and horizontal planes, defining two different radii of curvature for each glenoid: the glenoid is more conforming in the coronal plane when compared with the sagittal plane (Table 3). It has been suggested that this unique geometrical configuration of the glenoid sur-

Table 2. Glenohumeral mismatch in the frontal plane in fresh shoulders (with labrum) and in dried shoulders (without labrum) in our studies

Anatomic specimens (n=34)	Glenoid radius of curvature (mm)	Humeral radius of curvature (mm)	Glenohumeral conformity (mismatch; mm)
Fresh shoulders, with labrum (n=14)	29.3±5.1 (23–44.3)	24.4±2.1 (21.5–29)	2.2±2.1 (0–6.5)
Dried shoulders, without labrum (n=20)	32.9±5.6 (26.5–36.5)	23.3±2.0 (19.5–27)	9.6±3.2 (5–16.5)

Table 3. Glenohumeral conformity according to our measurements

Glenohumeral conformity	Mean±SD (mm)	Range (mm)
Glenoid depth in the vertical plane	6.1±1.6	4.1–10
Glenoid depth in the horizontal plane	3±0.8	1.6–4.8
Vertical radius of curvature of the glenoid	29.3±5.1	23–44.3
Vertical radius of curvature of the corresponding humeral head	24.4±2.1	21.5–29

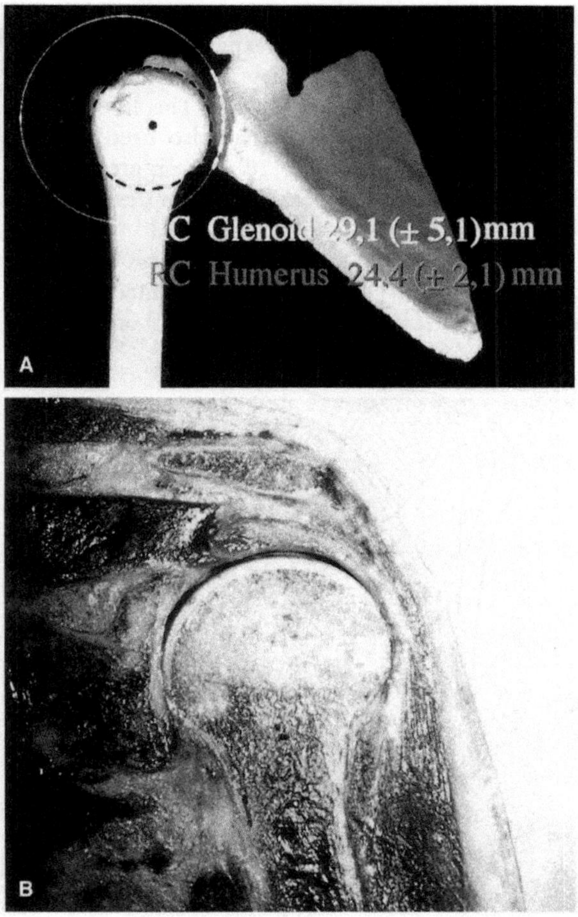

Fig. 7. A When considering only the osseous anatomy, the articular surfaces of the glenoid and humeral head have a large radius mismatch. **B** However, when taking into account the cartilage and the labrum, then the joint surfaces of the glenoid and the humerus have almost identical radii of curvature

face assists the musculotendinous force couple mechanism in keeping the humeral head from translating in a infero-superior direction while allowing some antero-posterior translation to occur [35, 50].

Pathology

Although the glenoid surface is usually flat in osteoarthritis, wear can lead to a conforming shape [13, 39, 54, 55]. Glasson et al. have observed that hemiarthroplasty can give good and acceptable functional results in these cases, suggesting that resurfacing the glenoid may not be necessary and that hemiarthroplasty may be an effective treatment for these specific patients with a concentric glenoid [39].

Surgical Relevance

The optimum degree of glenohumeral conformity desirable in total shoulder replacement is still controversial [5, 6, 11, 17, 34, 36, 41, 58, 70, 71].

Conforming Glenoid Component

Neer originally chose the same radii of curvature for the head and the glenoid to improve stability (he observed that the heads could sublux on the flat, arthritic glenoids) and to provide a fixed fulcrum for the muscles [54, 55, 58] (Fig. 8).

The advantage of a conforming glenoid component is that it provides a more stable joint with increased contact with the head so decreasing the stresses and keeping the head centered in the socket [29, 34, 36, 41, 75].

The disadvantages of a conforming design are twofold: firstly, if the prosthetic head remains centered, the glenohumeral mobility may be decreased, as demonstrated in radiographic studies by us [6] and others [36]; secondly, if any translation occurs in a conforming shoulder replacement, the head immediately tips up onto the rim of the glenoid, causing polyethylene wear and deformation and introducing a "rocking horse phenomena" [3, 9, 17, 30, 33, 70, 73]. This rocking horse effect can happen in the vertical plane (in case of cuff deficiency) and/or in the horizontal plane (in case of antero-posterior instability). A conforming glenoid design does not prevent some AP translation to occur as

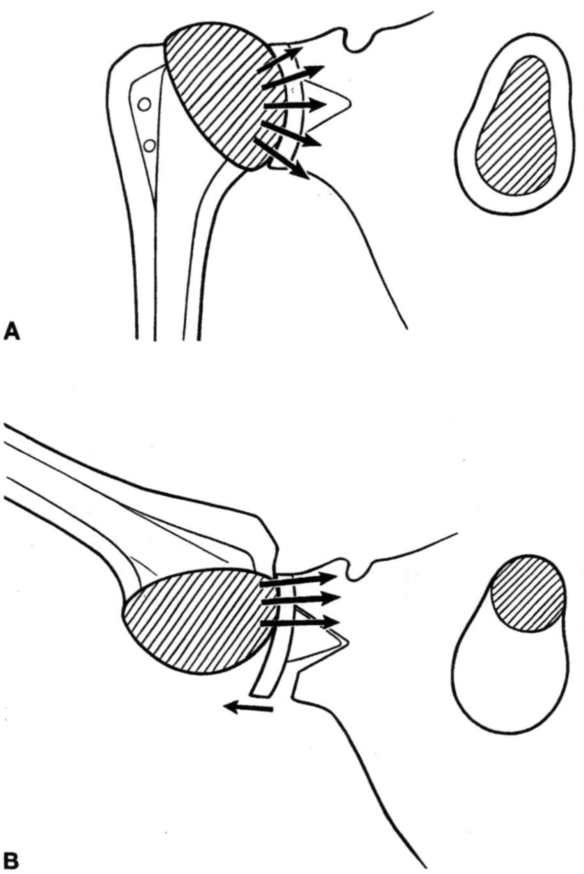

Fig. 8. Conforming design of glenoid component. **A** In a static position, when the articular surfaces of the humeral and glenoid components are matched, there is a large contact between the articular surface which provides maximal joint stability. **B** However, in a dynamic position any translation of the humeral component may cause eccentric rim loading and high contact pressures. This will result in asymmetric polyethylene wear, cold flow and "rocking horse" loosening of the glenoid component with predominant lucent lines at the inferior part of the tray and keel

demonstrated by radiological studies [33, 36], biomechanical studies [83] and retrieval studies of failed glenoid components [82] where the polyethylene has been found to be worn asymmetrically, either anteriorly or posteriorly.

In summary, the theoretical advantage of conforming glenoid designs (low pressures) has not been verified in surgical practice because of the existing translation which leads to eccentrics shear loads and loosening.

Non-conforming (Flat) Glenoid Components

Most of the newer design prostheses have a glenoid radius of curvature 2–6 mm larger than the humeral head to allow a certain degree of roll and slide (Fig. 9).

The advantage of a non-conforming (flat) glenoid component is to allow some glenohumeral translation without overbacking the rim thus decreasing the potential for polyethylene wear and deformation. A 6-mm mismatch between the humeral and glenoid components has been shown experimentally to allow translation and shock absorption without loading the glenoid rim [29, 36, 41, 42]. The limits seem to be fairly tight because it has also been demonstrated that a mismatch of 10 mm or greater produces pressures greater than the compressive yield strength [36].

On the other hand, the *disadvantages of a non-conforming (flatter) design* is that contact stresses are higher because they are focused on a small

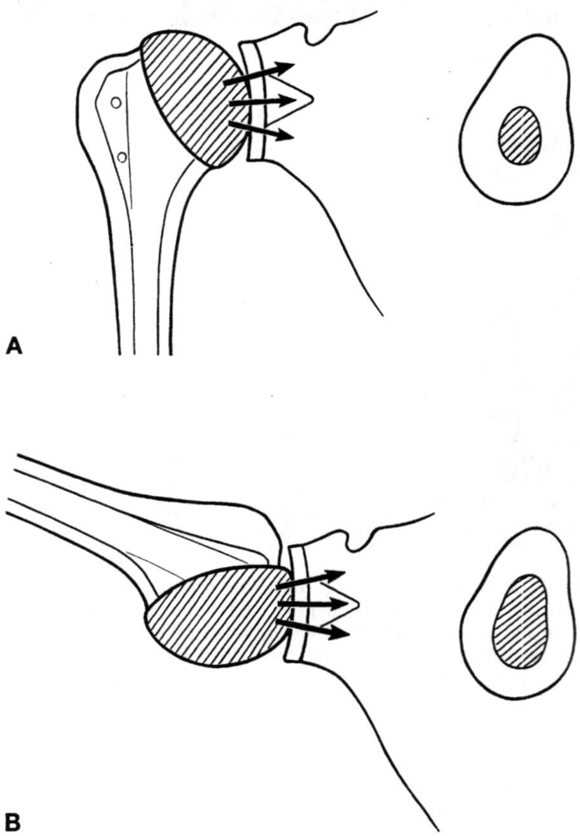

Fig. 9. Non-conforming design of glenoid component. **A** In a static position, when the radius of curvature of the glenoid component is larger than which of the humeral component, there is an increase in joint pressure (with higher contact stress). **B** However, in a dynamic position in case of translation, the load remains closer to the centre and thus has a smaller movement arm to rock the glenoid. Nevertheless, polyethylene wear can be increased

area and may increase wear if the contact pressures exceed the limits of the polyethylene and the joint is less stable [5, 29, 36, 41, 50].

As previously mentioned, the glenohumeral joint is *conforming* when the labrum is taken into account but truly *non-conforming* when only the flat osseous glenoid is taken into account (Fig. 7). In physiological conditions the labrum is present but is compliant and deformable, as shown by cine-MRI studies. Because polyethylene is rigid and also because no material as compliant and deformable as the labrum is currently available, the surface geometry of a glenoid component can only be a compromise. Neer himself recognised that it might be necessary to increase the size of the radius of curvature of the articular surface of the glenoid component if clinical follow-up showed a significant rate of loosening that could be attributed to this cause [58]. However, today, the optimum difference in the radius of curvature between the humeral head and the glenoid component to achieve clinical success has yet to be determined [29, 36, 41, 50]. Further studies of glenohumeral congruency in total shoulder arthroplasty and further prospective clinical trials will be necessary to determine the optimum range to minimize long-term polyethylene deformation and wear while allowing normal kinematics of the glenohumeral joint.

The posterior surface of the glenoid prosthetic component which is in contact with the bone, may be either flat or convex. No study in the literature allows us to conclude whether one shape is better than the other. The only important consideration, reported by Collins et al., is the need for congruent subchondral contact between the bony surface of the glenoid and the prosthesis to reduce the rocking-horse effect [16, 17]. Appropriate reamers must allow for a perfect match, whichever design is used (flat or convex).

Horizontal Orientation of the Glenoid (Glenoid Version)

Anatomy

The horizontal orientation of the glenoid with regard to the scapula plane is usually posterior with a retroversion angle averaging between -2° and -8°. However, these values are highly variable [10, 21, 35, 51, 53, 64]. Friedman, for instance, using CT scans, described an average anteversion of 2° in normal shoulders ranging from 14° of anteversion to 12° of retroversion [35]. Table 4 summarizes the measurements of the horizontal orientation of the glenoid. One could suggests that the horizontal glenoid slope is zero: the glenoid surface is grossly perpendicular to the axis of the scapula (+/- 10°). In fact, things are probably more complex and it would appear that the glenoid may be retroverted superiorly and anteversed inferiorly, as shown by Deutsch [22] and Mulladji [53].

Pathology

Both Friedman [35] and Mulladji [53] found that the amount of retroversion was significantly greater in the arthritic shoulders than in the normal shoulders. Friedman et al. found that the mean glenoid orientation was 2°±5° of anteversion (range +14° of anteversion to –12° of retroversion) in a control group of 63 patients while the mean retroversion was –14° in the patients with osteoarthritis and –7° in the patients with inflammatory arthritis [35]. Mulladji et al. found that the mean retroversion was –7.6° in rheumatoid arthritis (-15.1° to +8.2°) and –12.5° in osteoarthritis (–14.1° to +3°) while the mean retroversion in the normal shoulders was -3° [53].

In fact, the potential error when measuring glenoid version is high. Studying the shape of the worn glenoid and evaluating the degree of bone loss is probably more accurate. We performed CT arthrograms in 101 cases of glenohumeral osteoarthritis [1, 77]. We were then able to extrapolate

Table 4. Horizontal orientation of the glenoid in the normal shoulder according to the literature: (+) corresponds to an anteversed glenoid and (–) corresponds to a retroversed glenoid

		Horizontal orientation of the glenoid (glenoid version)	
	Method	Mean±SD	Range
Cyprien et al. 1983 [21] (*n*=50)	X-ray	–8°±5.01°	–
Randelli and Gambrioli 1986 [64] (*n*=40)	CT	–7°	-2° to -15°
Friedman et al. 1992 [34] (*n*=63)	CT	+2°±5°	-12° to +14°
Mulladji et al. 1994 [53] (*n*=19)	CT	–3°±4.2°	-5.1° to +2.2°
Mallon et al. 1992 [51] (*n*=32)	CT	–6°±4.2°	-13° to +2°
Mallon et al. 1992 [51] (*n*=28)	X-ray	–2°±4.2°	-12° to +7°

and analyse the glenoid morphology in the horizontal plane and also the glenoid version. Three types of glenoid were described: type A (53.5 %) with predominantly central wear, type B (39.5 %) with predominantly posterior wear with biconcavity and type C (5 %) with glenoid retroversion greater than 25° (see Walch et al. "Primary Gleno-humeral Osteoarthritis: Clinical and Radiographic Classification," this volume). In arthritis of dislocations, the glenoid wear can be either *anterior in patients who have not been operated* because of glenoid abrasion or fractures along the anteroinferior rim secondary to recurrent subluxations and dislocations or *posterior in patients who have been operated* because of too-tight anterior repairs which squeeze the head out of the back of the glenoid and produce the characteristic changes of osteoarthritis [54].

Surgical Relevance

Glenoid version should be adjusted during surgery to improve stability of the prosthesis and to try to avoid asymmetric wear of the polyethylene. Osteoarthritis often features a posterior glenoid wear which can be corrected by using a number of potential options. Cement should not be used as a structural support for the glenoid component since it will fracture and become displaced, causing toggling and loosening of the glenoid component [65, 66]. In glenoids with severe increased retroversion or wear, it may be necessary to reorientate the articular surface with the help of a posterior bone graft. However, in our experience glenoid bone grafts are extremely rare. In a series of 463 shoulder arthroplasties, Neer and Morisson [57] reported that bone-grafting for a deficient glenoid cavity was performed in only twenty patients (4.3 %). Although augmented polyethylene glenoids, initially proposed by Neer [58], have been abandoned, augmented metal-backed glenoids with elevated metal-trays to correct bony defect may have some place in the future. In surgical practice, purposeful eccentric or asymmetric reaming of the glenoid surface in the horizontal plane is usually the best option: posterior wear, which is the most common, can be addressed by decreasing the bone anteriorly, based on the glenoid centering pilot holes (Fig. 10).

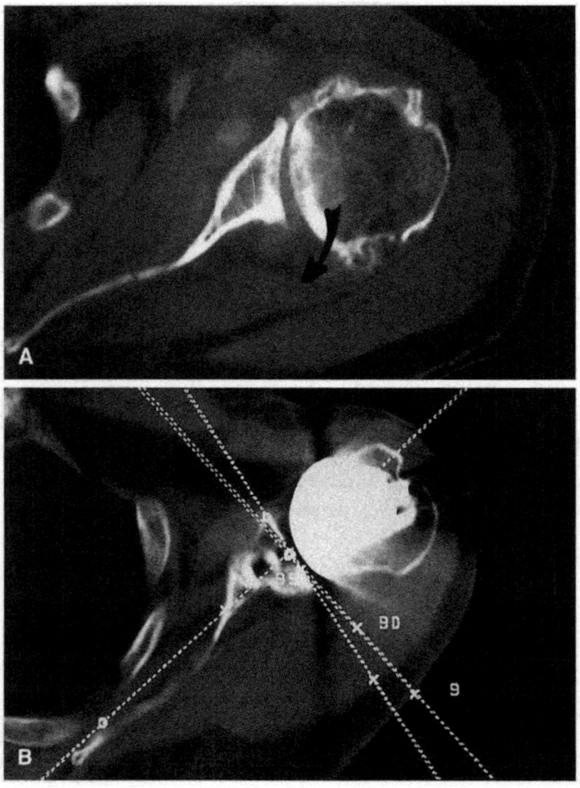

Fig. 10. Correcting posterior glenoid wear by decreasing the bone anteriorly with purposeful eccentric reaming of the glenoid articular surface. Postoperatively, the glenoid component is grossly perpendicular to the scapula

Vertical Orientation of the Glenoid (Glenoid Inclination)

Anatomy

The vertical orientation or inclination of the glenoid is variable as demonstrated by Gouaze et al. [40]. They showed that the slope of the glenoid may be ascendant in 45 % of cases with an average angle of 3° (between 1° and 10°), strictly vertical in 22 % and descendant in 33 % with an average angle of 4° (1°–12°; Fig. 11). The values found in the literature regarding the vertical orientation of the glenoid are variable [4, 11, 25, 26, 40, 62, 75, 80]. Basmajian

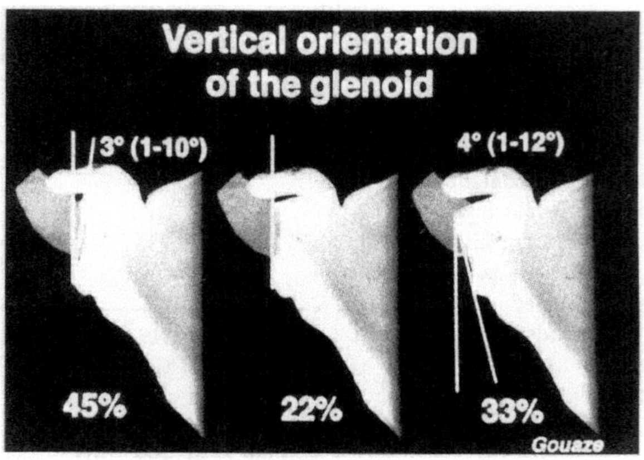

Fig. 11. Vertical orientation of the glenoid according to Gouaze et al. [40]

and Bazan found that the glenoid surface is superiorly oriented and stated that the upward slope of the glenoid fossa is of primary importance in preventing inferior subluxation of the glenohumeral joint [4].

By contrast, Mallon et al reported that the glenoid sloped downward, averaging 4° with a range from 13° of downward slope to 8° of upward slope [51]. Results found by Freedman and Munro are similar [31]. It can be stated that the normal vertical slope of the glenoid is between a downward slope of 10° and a upward slope of +10°. A localised hypoplasia of the posteroinferior glenoid has been found to be frequent (20%–30%) in an anthropometrical study on 1150 scapular bone specimens performed by Edelson [24, 25]. Finally, one should also realise that the vertical tilt of the scapula is dynamic and highly variable [23, 51, 75].

Pathology

We made radiographic measurements of the glenoid slope in the frontal plane preoperatively and at revision using true A-P view of the shoulders with the arm at side in 36 arthritic and 21 rheumatoid shoulders [8]. This study demonstrated that superior inclination of the glenoid surface is more specific to rheumatoid arthritis (Fig. 12) while inferior inclination of the glenoid surface is more specific to osteoarthritis (Fig. 13). This pattern of inclination was still present and even more obvious after total shoulder arthroplasty with a tendency to orientate the glenoid component superiorly in rheumatoid shoulders and inferiorly in osteoarthritic shoulders. Moreover, there was a linear relationship between the glenoid slope and the acromio-humeral distance: as the slope of the glenoid increased, so did the superior humeral translation with a narrowing of the acromio-humeral translation distance ($p<0.0001$).

Surgical Relevance

Our findings have important implications for the planning, preparation and positioning of the glenoid component in total shoulder replacements: one of the goals of total shoulder arthroplasty should be to vertically reorientate, or at least not to exacerbate, any abnormal glenoid slope [7]. This should be taken into account particularly in rheumatoid arthritis where there is a tendency to superiorly increase of the glenoid slope thus leading to a superior migration of humeral head. Correction of the abnormal glenoid slope (visible on the true A-P view) should aim at restoring the normal kinematics of the shoulder and protecting the rotator cuff as well as the glenoid component fixation. Superior wear of the glenoid can be addressed by

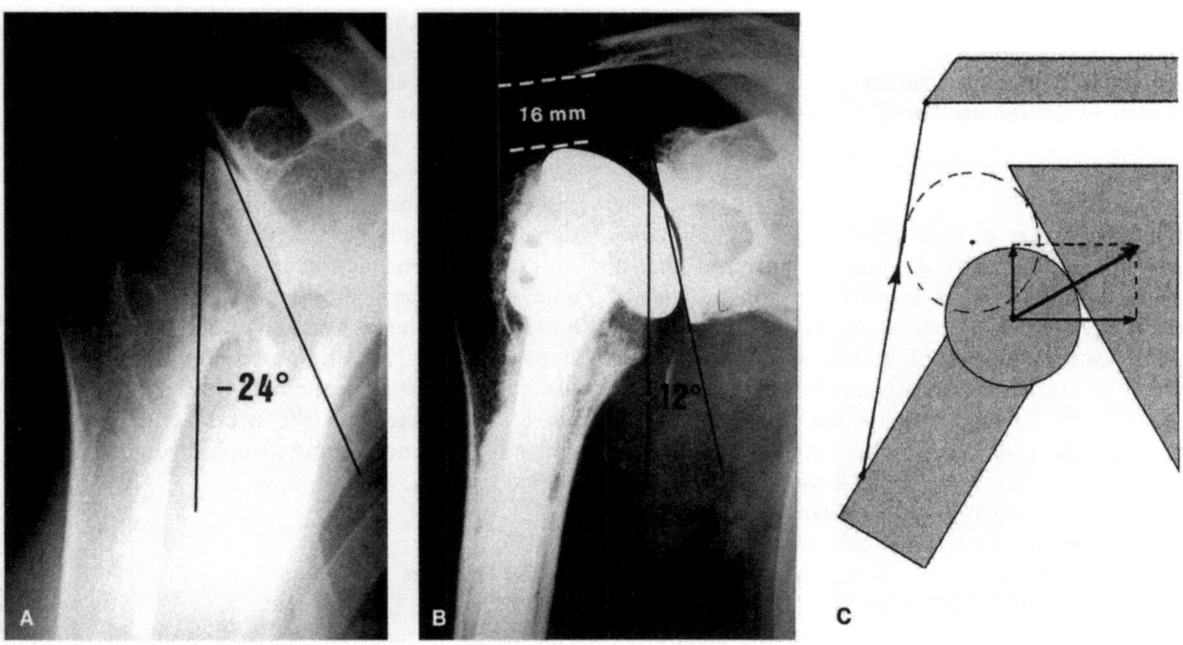

Fig. 12. Typical inferior inclination of the glenoid surface in primary osteoarthritis. **A** Preoperative AP view. **B** Consistent inferior inclination and increased acromio-humeral distance after shoulder replacement. **C** Possible biomechanical consequence of inferior inclination of the glenoid surface with distal humeral migration

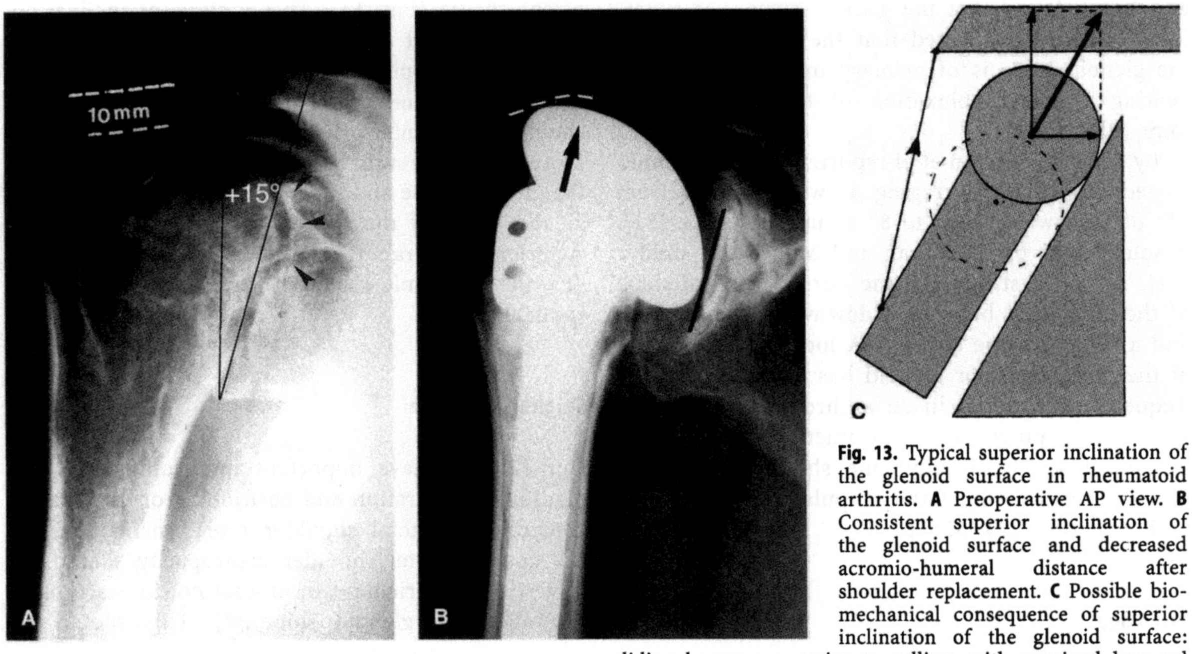

Fig. 13. Typical superior inclination of the glenoid surface in rheumatoid arthritis. **A** Preoperative AP view. **B** Consistent superior inclination of the glenoid surface and decreased acromio-humeral distance after shoulder replacement. **C** Possible biomechanical consequence of superior inclination of the glenoid surface: gliding becomes superior to rolling, with proximal humeral migration and compression of the cuff under the acromial arch

decreasing the bone inferiorly with purposeful eccentric reaming of the glenoid articular surface. If the bone loss is substantial, a superior bone graft may be used. However, from a practical point of view, a glenoid bone graft is rarely possible in long-standing rheumatoid arthritis because of the cirumferential contraction of the joint volume and the tight extracapsular muscles [18].

Possibilities of Bony Fixation (Depth of Cancellous Bone)

Anatomy

The possibilities of bony fixation of a glenoid component are limited by the poor volume and quality of the cancellous bone located beneath the glenoid surface [7, 11, 12, 32, 37, 38, 53, 77]. Using anatomical measurements and CT studies, we determined the depth of cancellous bone beneath the glenoid fossa available for fixation of a glenoid component in 34 dry scapula (Fig. 14A). The depth of cancellous bone beneath the glenoid fossa was a maximum of 26 mm in a normal scapula. Where there is significant erosion this cancellous anchorage may measure only 15 or 10 mm deep and may disappear altogether (Fig. 14B). Mallon et al. [51] measured the distance between the midpoint of a line connecting the inferior and superior edge of the glenoid fossa with the most medial edge of the visible cancellous bone: this averaged 31.5 mm (range 26–40 mm; SD 2.9)

Pathology

Prevalence of radiolucent lines of the bone-cement interface of glenoid components was reported to be between 30 % and 96 % [3, 5, 7, 9, 14, 43, 48, 52, 55, 59, 66, 74, 78]. In a recent report on total shoulder arthroplasty revision, the incidence of glenoid loosening was 28 % for failed unconstrained implants [82]. One should realize that glenoid lucent lines and loosening are likely to be underestimated because of the absence of standardised methods of measurement or fluoroscopically positioned radiographs [9, 47]. The clinical follow-up in the literature which was estimated to be 38 months for 700 cases, can also be considered insufficient [65]. Additionally, positioning of the glenoid in a nonanatomical position (tendency to low placement of the glenoid) as well as gleno-humeral loading caused by muscular imbalance because of rotator cuff insufficiency (vertical "rocking horse effect" or of soft tissue contracture or stretching (horizontal "rocking horse effect") increases the stress across the gleno-humeral joint and therefore jeopardize glenoid component fixation.

Surgical Relevance

The depth of cancellous bone beneath the glenoid fossa (and its range) gives the surgeon more knowledge of how much cancellous bone is available for fixation of the glenoid component of a total shoulder

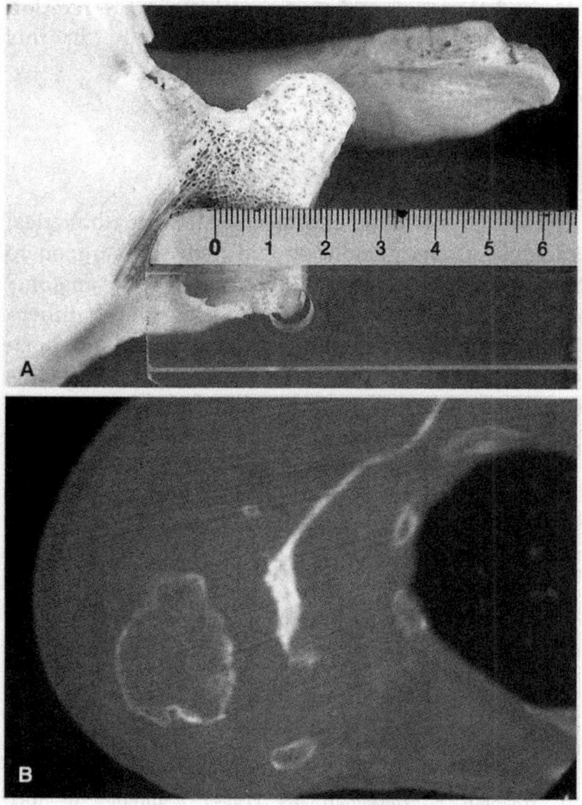

Fig. 14. The small area of cancellous bone available in the scapula limits the possibilities of glenoid fixation (A). In some agressive diseases, the cancellous bone may even totally disappear as shown on this CT scan of a rheumatoid shoulder (B)

arthroplasty. This fixation of a glenoid component is often difficult and may even be impossible in which case a hemi-arthroplasty must be carried out [9, 18, 63, 65, 79].

Cemented glenoid component are the most popular and remain the gold standard. However, it carries the usual disadvantages of high rate of lucent lines. Although the published rates of loosening (between zero and 28 %) and reoperation (2.9 %) are still low, lucent lines remains a concern for the future [9, 66, 82]. Brems [9] observed that 69 % of lucent lines could be seen on the immediate post-operative radiographs, while Collins et al. [17] have reported that appropriate bone preparation using mechanical reaming enhances glenoid fixation, suggesting that surgical technique could be critical in preventing lucent lines. A meticulous surgical technique is essential to improve glenoid fixation and the surgeon should focus on: (a) proper exposure, for adequate visualisation and placement of the glenoid component; (b) proper reaming to ensure improved conformity between the glenoid component and glenoid bone; (c) use of pulse-lavage and haemostatic agents to clean, dry and control bleeding from the cancellous bone; (e) pressurisation of the cement.

Uncemented metal-backed glenoid component fixation carries the theoretical advantage of achieving osteointegration with potentially longer term survival (Fig. 15). Friedman et al. [34] demonstrated with a finite element analysis, that all-polyethylene

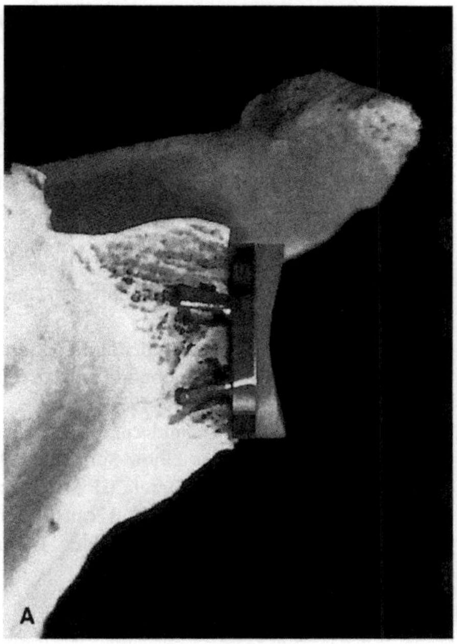

Fig. 15. Uncemented fixation of the Aequalis glenoid component through expanded screws and secondary bone ingrowth

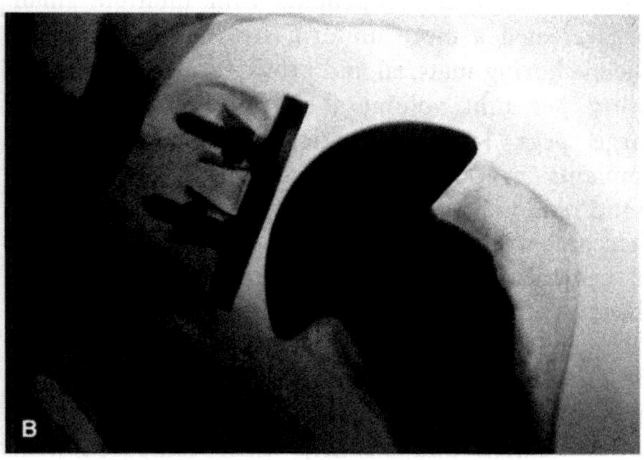

implants appear to provide a more physiologic distribution for non-axial loads. By contrast, Orr et al. [60] reported that all-polyethylene glenoid components transmit the loads centrally while metal-backed component distribute the forces more evenly to the underlying bone and prevent deformation of the polyethylene. Although the results of uncemented glenoid components with bony ingrowth are promising, some concerns about their use remain [5, 15, 29]: (a) *increased component thickness*, because of the metal tray, may lateralise the joint, thus over-tightening the cuff and diminishing mobility; (b) *thinness of the polyethylene* which may lead to increased wear because of the metal tray, as seen with the experience in patella resurfacing; (c) *glenoid component dissociation* is possible; (d) *stress shielding* of cancellous bone beneath the tray because of strong fixation of the metal keel or pegs to surrounding bone.

Fixation of Glenoid Component: Keel Versus Pegs

Keel design, as developed by Charles Neer, still remains the most popular design for glenoid components. Pegs glenoid components have been recently introduced but many controversies still exist. No scientific evidence can favor one design versus the other (keel versus pegs) for implant stability and fixation. For instance, in 1988 Orr et al. [60] used finite element analysis to examine several glenoid component design parameters and concluded that keel geometry could be altered to approximate the stress distribution found in the natural glenoid and to improve the glenoid component stability. By contrast, in 1992 Friedman et al. [34] studied the stress distribution of several glenoid component designs using two-dimensional finite element analysis and concluded that physiological stresses were approximated when the subchondral bone was preserved and when a tapered all-polyethylene keel component was used. Giori et al. in a parametric study found that components with multiple small pegs created a more uniform stress distribution in the anchoring material and provided more sheer stability per unit volume than implants with fewer large pegs [38]. Theoretical advantages of peg implants over the keel counterpart include less bone removal during bone preparation, greater surface area for cement contact and a smaller volume of cement required for fixation [80]. However, the disadvantages of multiple small pegs is the potential fragmentation of the glenoid, because of multiple drill holes in the bone which may lead to intra-operative fractures of the glenoid surface and a lower fixation and stability when compared with the keel design (see Lacaze et al., Primary fixation of glenoid implants: an in vitro study, in this volume).

Conclusion

Knowledge of both the normal and pathological anatomy of the glenoid should help the surgeon to anticipate the reconstruction of the bony anatomy of the glenoid surface (normal shape and dimensions, normal orientation in the vertical and horizontal planes) as well as to obtain the most stable implantation and safe fixation for the glenoid component. However, many technological aspects of glenoid components are not solved yet and remain under investigation: the optimum degree of glenohumeral conformity and constraint, the best biomaterial used (polyethylene or metal backed), the optimum design of the stem or anchorage (keel versus pegs) and finally, the best type of fixation (cemented versus uncemented).

References

1. Aliabadi P, Weissman BN (1994) Radiology of total shoulder arthroplasty. In: Friedman RJ (ed) Arthroplasty of the shoulder. Thieme Medical, New York, pp 53–69
2. Badet R, Boileau P, Noël E, Walch G (1995) Arthrography and computed arthrotomography study of seventy patients with primary glenohumeral osteoarthritis. Rev Rhum 62(9):555–562
3. Barret WP, Franklin JL, Jackins SE, Wyss CR, Matsen FA III (1987) Total shoulder arthroplasty. J Bone Joint Surg An 69:865–872
4. Basmajian JV, Bazant FJ (1959) factors preventing downward dislocation of the adducted shoulder joint: an electromyographic and morphological study. J Bone Joint Surg Am 41:1182
5. Boyd AD, Tornhill TS (1994) Glenoid resurfacing in shoulder arthroplasty. In: Friedman RJ (ed) Arthroplasty of the shoulder. Thieme, New York, pp 306–316
6. Boileau P, Walch G, Liotard JP (1992) Video-fluoroscopy of shoulder arthroplasties during active elevation. J Orthop Surg 6:4
7. Boileau P, Walch G, Liotard JP, Noel E (1994) Neer shoulder prosthesis: results related to the etiology. Rev Rhum 61:539–547
8. Boileau P, Walch G (1997) Glenoid slope in osteoarthritic and rheumatoid shoulders before and after arthroplasty. J Shoulder Elbow Surg 6:194–195
9. Brems J (1993) The glenoid component in total shoulder arthroplasty. J Shoulder Elbow Surg 2:47–54
10. Brewer BJ, Wubben RC, Carrera GF (1986) Excessive retroversion of the glenoid cavity. A cause of non traumatic posterior instability of the shoulder. J Bone Joint Surg Am 68:724–731

11. Buechel FF (1977) Glenohumeral joint in the chimpanzee: comparative anatomical analysis for use in endoprosthic replacement. J Med Primatol 6:108–113
12. Burkhead WZ, Hutton KS (1995) Biologic resurfacing of the glenoid with hemiarthroplasty of the shoulder. J Shoulder Elbow Surg 4:263
13. Cofield RH, Briggs BT (1979) Gleno-humeral arthritis. J Bone Joint Surg Am 61:668–677
14. Cofield RH (1984) Total shoulder arthroplasty with the Neer prosthesis. J Bone Joint Surg Am 64:319–337
15. Cofield RH, Daly PJ (1992) Total shoulder arthroplasty with a tissue-ingrowth glenoid component. J Shoulder Elbow Surg 1:77–85
16. Collins DN, Harryman DTII, Lippitt SB, Jackins SE, Matsen FA III (1991) The technique of glenohumeral arthroplasty. Techniques Orthop 6:43–59
17. Collins D, Tencer A, Sidles J, Matsen FA III (1992) Edge displacement and deformation of glenoid components in response to eccentric loading. The effect of preparation of the glenoid bone. J Bone Joint Surg Am 74:501–507
18. Connor PM, Flatow EL (1997) Surgical considerations of bony deficiency in total shoulder arthroplasty. In: Warner JJP, Iannotti JP, Gerber C (eds) Complex and revision problems in shoulder surgery. Lippincott-Raven, Philadelphia, pp 339–354
19. Copeland S (1989) Cementless total shoulder replacement. Presented at the 4th international conference on surgery of the soulder, New York, Oct 1989
20. Crossan JF, Vallace R (1980) Clinical and radiological features of the shoulder joint in rheumatoid arthritis. J Bone Joint Surg Br 62:116
21. Cyprien JM, Vasey HM, Burdet A, Bonvin JC, Kritsikis N, Vuagnat P (1983) Humeral retrotorsion and glenohumeral relationship in the normal shoulder and in recurrent anterior dislocation (scapulometry). Clin Orthop 175:8–17
22. Deutsch AL, Resnick D, Minck JH (1985) Cumputed tomography of the glenohumeral joint and sternoclavicular joints. Orthop Clin North Am 16:497–511
23. Dras SP, Roy GS, Saha RR (1966) Observations of the tilt of the glenoid cavity of the scapula. J Anat Soc Ind 15:114
24. Edelson JG (1995) Localized glenoid hypoplasia. An anatomic variation of possible clinical significance. Clin Orthop 321:189–195
25. Edelson JG (1995) Pattterns of degenerative change in the glenohumeral joint. J Bone Joint Surg Br 77(2):288–292
26. Engelbrecht E, Heinert (1987) More than ten Years' experience with unconstrained shoulder replacement. In: Kölbel R, Helbig B, Blauth W (eds) Shoulder replacement. Springer, Berlin Heidelberg New York, pp 85–91
27. Fick R (1904) Anatomie und Mechanik der Gelenke. Fischer, Jena, pp 171–174
28. Figgie HE, Inglis AE, Goldberg VM et al (1988) An analysis of factors affecting the long term results of total shoulder arthroplasty in inflammatory arthritis. J Arthroplasty 3:123–130
29. Flatow EL (1995) Prosthetic design considerations in total shoulder arthroplasty. Semin Arthroplasty 6:233–244
30. Franklin JL, Barrett WP, Jackins SE et al (1988) Glenoid loosening in total shoulder arthroplasty. Association with rotator cuff deficiency. J Arthroplasty 3:39–46
31. Freedman L, Munro RR (1966) Abduction of the arm in the scapular plane: scapular and gleno-humeral movements. J Bone Joint Surg Am 48:1503
32. Frich LA, Jensen NC, Odgaard A, Pedersen CM, Sjøbjerg JO, Dalstra M (1997) Bone strength and material properties of the glenoid. J Shoulder Elbow Surg 6:97–104
33. Friedman RJ (1992) Gleno-humeral translation after total shoulder arthroplasty. J Shoulder Elbow Surg 1(6):312–316
34. Friedman RJ, La Berge M, Dooley RL et al (1992) Finite element modeling of the glenoid component: effect of design parameters on stress distribution. J Shoulder Elbow Surg 1:261–270
35. Friedman RJ, Hawthorne KB, Genez BM (1992) The use of computerized tomography in the measurement of glenoid version. J Bone Joint Surg Am 74:1032–1037
36. Friedman RJ (1994) Biomechanics and design of shoulder arthroplasties. In: Friedman RJ (ed) Arthroplasty on the shoulder. Thieme, New York, pp 27–40
37. Fukuda K, Chen CM, Cofield RH et al (1988) Biomechanical analysis of stability and fixation stength of total shoulder prosthesis. Orthopedics 11:141–149
38. Giori NJ, Beaupre GS, Carter DR (1990) The influence of fixation peg design on the shear stability of prosthetic implants. J Orthop Res 8:892–898
39. Glasson JM, Djurasovic M, Levine WN, Pollock RG, Flatow EL, Bigliani LU (1996) Hemiarthroplasty for glenohumeral osteoarthritis in patients with an intact rotator cuff: results correlated to degree of glenoid wear. Presented at the American Academy of Orthopaedics Surgeons, annual meeting, Atlanta, Georgia, USA
40. Gouaze A, Castaing J, Soutoul JH, Chantepie G (1962) Sur l'orientation de l'omoplate et de sa cavité glenoïde. Arch Anat Pathol 10(3):175–181
41. Harryman DT, Sidles JA, Harris SL, Lippitt SB, Matsen FA (1995) The effect of articular conformity and the size of the humeral head component on laxity and motion after gleno-humeral arthroplasty. J Bone Joint Surg Am 77:555–564
42. Harryman DT, Sidles JA, Clark JM, Mc Quade KS, Gibb TD, Matsen FA (1990) Translation of the humeral head on the glenoid with passive gleno-humeral motion. J Bone Joint Surg Am 72(9):1334–1343
43. Hawkins RJ, Bell RH, Jallay B (1986) Experience with the Neer shoulder arthroplasty. A review of 70 cases. Orthop Trans 10:232
44. Howell SM, Galinat BJ (1989) The glenoid-labral socket. A constrained articular surface. Clin Orthop 243:122–125
45. Ianotti JP, Gabriel JP, Schneck SL, Evans BG, Misra S (1992) The normal glenohumeral relationships: an anatomical study of one hundred and forty shoulders. J Bone Joint Surg Am 74:491–500
46. Kelkar R, Newton PM, Armengol J et al (1993) Three dimensional kinematics of the glenohumeral joint during abduction in scapular plane. Trans ORS 18:136
47. Kelleher IM, Cofield RH, Becker DA et al (1992) Fluoroscopically positioned radiographs of total shoulder arthroplasty. J Shoulder Elbow Surg 1:306–311
48. Kelly IG, Foster RS, Fisher WD (1987) Neer total shoulder replacement in rheumatoid arthritis. J Bone Joint Surg Br 69:723–726
49. Kerr R, Resnick D, Pineda C, Haghighi P (1985) Osteoarthritis of the gleno-humeral joint: a radiological study. Am J Roentgenol 144:967–972
50. Mac Pherson EJ, Friedman RJ, An YH, Chokesis R, Dooley RL (1997) Antropometric study of normal glenohumeral relationships. J Shoulder Elbow Surg 6:105–112

51. Mallon WJ, Brown HR, Vogher JB III, Martinez S (1992) Radiographic and geometric anatomy of the scapula. Clin Orthop 277:142–154
52. Matsen FA, Lippit SB, Siddles JA, Harryman DT (1994) Smoothness. In: Pratical evaluation and management of the shoulder. Saunders, Philadelphia, pp 151–219
53. Muladji AB, Beddow FH, Lamb GHR (1994) CT- measurement of glenoid erosion in arthritis. J Bone Joint Surg Br 76:384–388
54. Morrison DS (1993) Glenoid deficiency in total shoulder arthroplasty. In: Bigliani LU (ed) Complications in shoulder surgery. William and Wilkins, Baltimore, pp 73–80
55. Neer CS II, Watson KC, Stanton FJ (1982) Recent experience in total shoulder replacement. J Bone Joint Surg Am 64:319–337
56. Neer CS II, Craig EV, Fukuda H (1983) Cuff tear arthropathy. J Bone Joint Surg Am 65:1232–1244
57. Neer CS II, Morison DS (1988) Glenoid bone-grafting in total shoulder arthroplasty. J Bone Joint Surg Am 64:319–337
58. Neer CS (1990) Glenohumeral arthroplasty. In: Neer CS (ed) Shoulder reconstruction. Saunders, Philadelphia, pp 146–271
59. O'Driscoll SW, Wright TM, Cofield RH (1993) Radiographic analysis of the glenoid component in total shoulder arthroplasty. J Shoulder Elbow Surg 2:S13
60. Orr TE, Carter DR, Schurman DJ (1988) Stress analyses of glenoid component designs. Clin Orthop 232:217–224
61. Peterson CJ (1983) Degeneration of the gleno-humeral joint: an anatomical study 54:277–283
62. Pizon P (1959) Osteométrie scapulo-humérale. Presse Med 67(40):1531–1533
63. Pollock RG, Deliz ED, McIlveen SJ et al (1992) Prosthetic replacement in rotator cuff deficient shoulders. J Shoulder Elbow Surg 1:173–186
64. Randelli M, Gambrioli PL (1986) Glenohumeral osteometry by computed tomography in normal and unstable shoulders. Clin Orthop 208:151–156
65. Rodosky MW, Bigliani LU (1994) Surgical treatment of nonconstrained glenoid component failure. Oper Tech Orthop 4:226–236
66. Rodosky MW, Bigliani LU (1996) Indication for glenoid resurfacing in shoulder arthroplasty. J Shoulder Elbow Surg 5(3):231–248
67. Roper BA, Paterson JMH, Day WH (1990) The Roper-Day total shoulder replacement. J Bone Joint Surg Br 72:694–697
68. Saha AK (1973) Dynamic stability of the glenohumeral joint. Acta Orthop Scand 44:668–678
69. Smith CM, Pichora D, Wyss UP et al (1992) Challenges in glenoid implant technology: a three dimensional finite element analysis. Orthop Trans 16:99
70. Severt R, Thomas BJ, Tsenter MJ et al (1993) The influence of conformity and constraint on translational forces and frictional torque in total shoulder arthroplasty. Clin Orthop 292:151–158
71. Soslowky LJ, Flatow EL, Bigliani LU, Mow VC (1992) Articular geometry of the glenohumeral joint. Clin Orthop 285:181–190
72. Sillar P, Meszaros T, Horvath F, Keri L, Lengyel E (1979) Gerontological aspects of degenerative changes of the shoulder-joint (radiological and clinical sudies). ZFA 34:411–421
73. Tomaszewski PR, Ondrla JM (1992) Incongruity and its relation to stress in prosthetic shoulder components. Trans ORS 17:425
74. Torchia ME, Cofield RH (1995) Long term results of Neer total shoulder arthroplasty. Orthop Trans 18:1994–1995
75. Toris T (1981) Roentgenographical examination of the tilted angle of the scapula in the resting position. Jpn Orthop Assoc 55:295
76. Walch G, Boileau P, Noel E, Donnell ST (1992) Impingement of the deep surface of the supraspinatus tendon on the postero-superior glenoid rim: an arthroscopic study. J Shoulder Elbow Surg 1:238–245
77. Walch G, Boileau P, Riand N (1997) Morphological study of the glenoid in primary glenohumeral osteoarthritis. J Shoulder Elbow Surg 6(2):226 (abstract 22)
78. Wilde AH, Borden LS, Brems JJ (1984) Experience with the Neer total shoulder replacement. In: Bateman JE, Welsh RP (eds) Surgery of the shoulder. Mosby, St Louis, pp 224–228
79. Wilde AH (1992) Shoulder arthroplasty: what it is good for and how good it is. In: Matsen FA III, Fu FH, Hawkins RJ (eds) The shoulder: a balance of mobility and stability, 1st edn. American Academy of Orthopaedic Surgeons, Rosemond, IL, pp 459–481
80. Wirth MA, Lyons FR, Rockwood CA Jr (1993) Hypoplasia of the glenoid. J Bone Joint Surg Am 75(8):1175–1184
81. Wirth MA, Basamania C, Rockwood CA Jr (1994) Fixation of glenoid component: Keel versus pegs. Oper Tech Orthop 4:218–225
82. Wirth MA, Seltzer DG, Senes HR et al (1994) An analysis of failed humeral head and total shoulders athroplasty. Presented at the Americal Shoulder and Elbow Surgeons, 10th open meeting, New Orleans, Febr 1994
83. Wuelker N, Schmotzer H, Thren K et al (1994) Translation of the glenohumeral joint with simulated active elevation. Clin Orthop 309:193–200

Primary Fixation of Glenoid Implants: An In Vitro Study

F. Lacaze, J.F. Kempf, F. Bonnomet, P. Boutemy, and F. Colin

Summary

We compared the different methods of primary fixation available within the glenoid components: cemented triangular keel, round backed and flat-backed, two cemented pegs, uncemented expansion screws. The implants were subjected to pull-out and eccentric load tests in a bone substitution material: a polyurethane foam loaded with aluminium. Experimental validation obtained from the measurements taken on the cadaveric specimens allowed us to make the following conclusions: (a) primary implant fixation was superior for the cemented implants during the tests, (b) the presence of cement beneath the tray added stability, (c) the cemented triangular keel had better fixation than the cemented pegs.

Introduction

The literature shows that loosening of the glenoid implant occurs in between 0% and 16% of unconstrained total shoulder arthroplasties. Glenoid loosening occurs for a number of reasons:

- *Anatomical* [13, 14]; small weight-bearing area (6 cm) and small volume anchoring zone (bone stock).
- *Mechanical:* gleno-humeral loads equal to 1–2 times body weight during normal activities [18].
- *Pathological* [3, 5]: mechanical and biological changes in the tissues alter the normal function of the joint.
- *Surgical* [16]: difficulties in glenoid exposure and cementing the implant [7].
- *Implant type*: the implant design (radius of curvature, gleno-humeral congruence, dimensions) determines movement at the bone/cement/implant interfaces and this can vary by a multiple of 2.5 [19]; polyethylene debris and wear particles; method of fixation [4, 6, 8].

This study was designed to look at the quality of primary implant fixation depending on the type of anchorage and the design of the glenoid tray. With this in mind, two series of tests were carried out: fixation tests [11] and implant displacement under eccentric loading [7, 11, 12, 15, 19]. Different implants configurations were used: cemented/uncemented, cement beneath the tray or not, triangular keel/ pegs and round backed/ flat backed implants.

Material and Methods

Implants Tested

The pull-out tests on the polyethylene implants were carried out on implants which had been left unmachined on their lateral part to facilitate their fixation in the hydraulic press (Fig. 1).

The different implants used were the middle sizes from the Aequalis range (Tornier, St. Ismier, France) with identical dimensions and radius of curvature of 30 mm. The pull-out test were carried out on the following implants:

- 4 implants, triangular keel, flat-backed, cemented
- 4 implants, triangular keel, round-backed, cemented
- 4 implants, pegs, flat backed, cemented
- 3 implants, expansion screws, metal-backed, flat, uncemented.

The displacement study was carried out on the following implants which had the same geometrical characteristics as before:

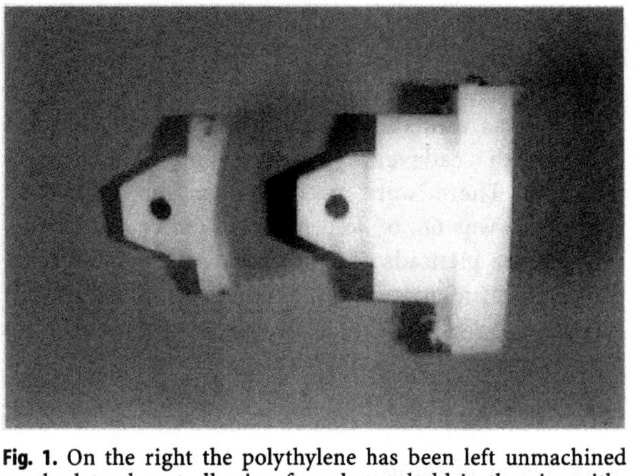

Fig. 1. On the right the polythylene has been left unmachined on the lateral part allowing for a better hold in the vice without affecting the fixation device (here, a cemented, triangular keel)

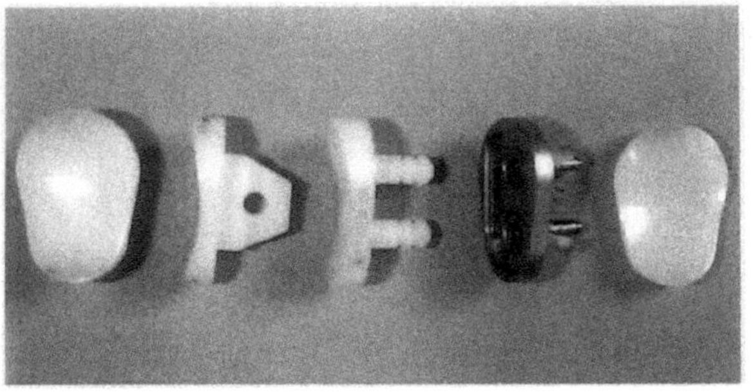

Fig. 2. The different implant tested for fixation and displacement under eccentric loading (see text)

- 3 implants, triangular keel, flat-backed, cemented
- 3 implants, triangular keel, flat-backed, cemented, no cement under the tray.
- 1 implant, triangular keel, round-backed, cemented
- 3 implants, pegs, flat-backed, cemented
- 3 implants, expansion screws, flat, metal-backed uncemented.

The cement used throughout the experiments was CMW1. Figure 2 shows the different implants tested.

Bone Substitution Material

Having tested several materials we selected a polyurethane foam loaded with aluminium at a density of 200 kg/m^3 whose mechanical characteristics where the closest to cancellous glenoid bone. The material is isotropic and was used in 50 mm cubes. The mechanical characteristics of the materials were determined following the test schedule NF T 51-034 (Dec. 1981). Young's modulus (E) was 80 Mpa and the Poisson coefficient (v) was 0.3.

Bone Sections

The test was validated against three paired shoulders from fresh cadavers preserved at -40 °C until required. There were two females and one male whose age was 68, 69 and 69 years. After defrosting, each of the glenoids was prepared using the appropriate instrumentation to achieve optimal fixation for the type of implant. The bone specimens were seated in blocks of PMMA resin.

Measurement of Forces

The hydraulic press used was an Instron 8500 with Digital Control linked to a Pentium (66) PC computer with a GPIB PCII card. The results were analysed using Max and Excel. The maximum force generated was 5000 N. The displacement measuring device used (LVDT) had a range of 2.5 mm with a 1% degree of precision over the distances measured. These results were analysed in the same way on Max and Excel.

Pull-Out Tests

The pull-out tests on the cemented implants was carried out by screwing the implant to the machine via the unmachined flange which did not effect the fixation characteristics of the implant. The foam block was held in a fixed vice. For the metal-backed implants, the tray was fixed into the vice and the foam block held with screws. The tests were carried out at a speed of 100 N/s and the results recorded at a frequency of 0.25 kHz. The mode of fixation failure was recorded for each test (cement fracture, pull-out from the foam, etc.).

Loading and Displacement of the Implants

The implants were subjected to a compressive force of 650 N, corresponding to the stresses on the glenoid when the arm is in abduction at 90° in the scapular plane in a 75-kg patient. The load was transmitted via a middle sized humeral prosthetic head. The radius of curvature of the head matched

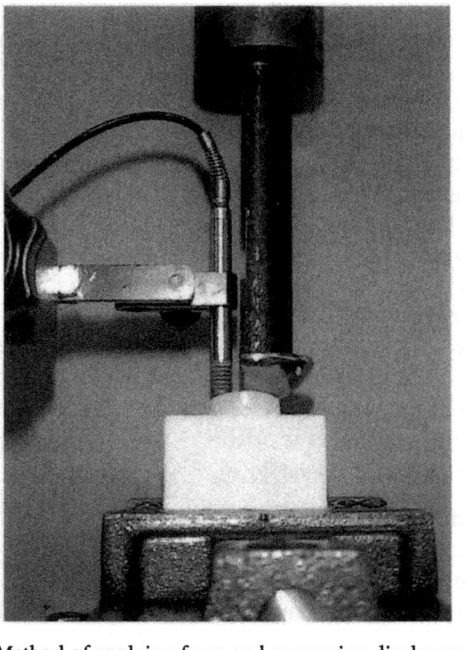

Fig. 3. Method of applying force and measuring displacement of the implants

that recommended for each glenoid tested and in these cases was 22.5 mm (Fig. 3)

The position of the loads was as follows: *central* (C), applied to the centre of the implant, *anterior*, force applied to the anterior part of the implant with an eccentricity of 10 mm (Le) and 7.5 mm (L) and *superior*, force applied to the upper part of the implant with an eccentricity of 10 mm (He) and 7.5 mm (H).

A grid was drawn on the glenoid to mark the load points. To ensure the correct loading positions had been set up an initial test was carried out using carbon paper between the head and the glenoid to mark the actual pressure point and any adjustment to the position could then be made (Fig. 4).

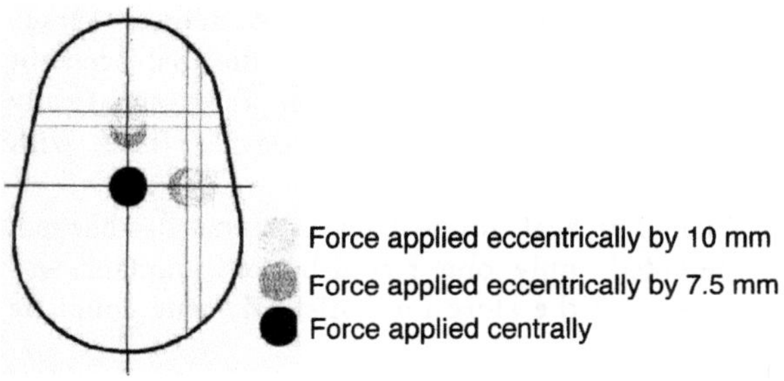

Fig. 4. Position of the forces applied to the glenoid

For each load two measurements of displacement were made. The first (M1) was made at the posterior edge of the implant and a second (M2) was made 10 mm directly beneath M1 (Fig. 5).

Complimentary measurements were made on the foam or resin block and on the vice to ensure there was no secondary movement. The first measurement (CM1) was repeated for each implant to insure that the results were comparable. For each type of loading (CM1, LM1), 3 load cycles were carried out. The loads were applied at a speed of 65 N/s and the results recorded at a frequency of 0.05 kHz.

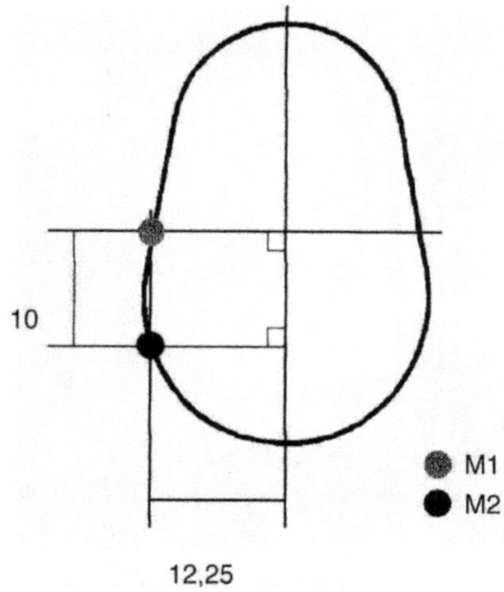

Fig. 5. Position of the points of measurement

The results were calculated using Excel, Statview on Pentium/PC and Macintosh 68LCO4O.

Results

Pull-Out Tests

Figure 6 summarises the pull out strength for the different glenoid components. Fixation failure for the *cemented, triangular keeled implants, both flat and round-backed*, occurred due to fracture of the cement mantle and pull-out of the foam. The cement mantle fracture occurred at the level of the transverse notch on the keel with the inferior part of the cement remaining encased in the foam block. Pull-out from the foam occurred at the superior part of the cement mantle surrounding the implant. There was no significant difference between the two implant types (Fig. 7).

The method of fixation failure for the two *implants with pegs* was identical, with the cement

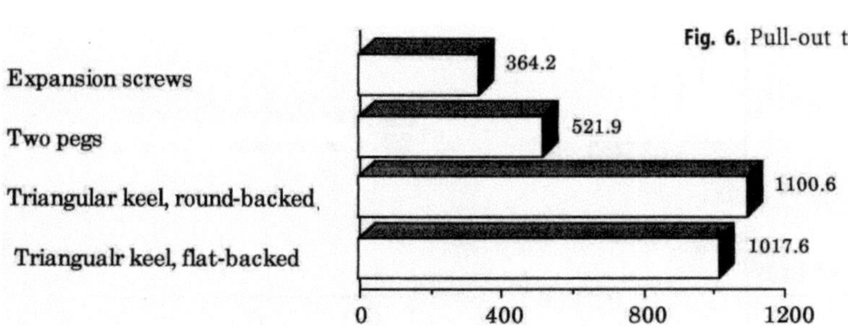

Fig. 6. Pull-out test results (N)

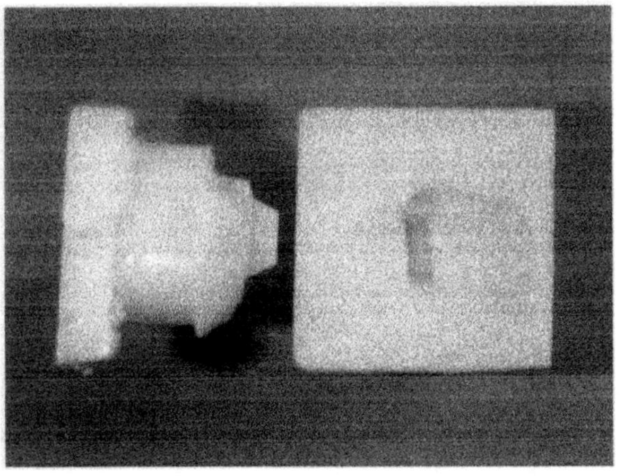

Fig. 7. Fracture of the cement mantle seen on the foam block with pull-out of the foam from around the cement situated immediately below the tray

mantle fracture occurring at the level of the transverse notch in the polyethylene. There was a statistical difference between the triangular keeled implants ($p<4\times10^{-4}$, Student's t test, bilateral, unmatched). For the *uncemented implants* we noted that pull-out from the foam occurred around the expansion screws. The difference in the force required to pull-out the uncemented glenoids with expansion screws and the cemented pegged implants was statistically significant ($p=0.01$, Student's t test, bilateral, non-apparided, ddl=6).

Fig. 8. Displacement (mm) measured at M2 for *eccentric loads on the upper part of the implant.* Two distances were used: 10 and 7.5 mm. Positive values indicate tilt and negative values indicate sinkage

Displacement with Load in the Polyurethane Foam

Figures 8 and 9 summarises the results for the loading tests:

- Triangular keel, flat-backed, cemented versus two pegs cemented: the displacements observed with the polyurethane foam were statistically larger for the cemented fixations. For LeM2, HM1, HM2 and Hem1 there was no significant difference.
- Triangular keel, flat-backed, cemented with and without cement beneath the tray: the displacements recorded using polyurethane foam were statistically greater in the absence of cement beneath the tray. For LeM2 and Hem1 there was no statistical difference.
- Triangular keel, flat-backed, cemented versus uncemented, expansion screws: the displacement recorded under all the forces were statistically greater in the uncemented device fixed with expansion screws.
- Triangular keel, round-backed versus flat-backed, cemented: only one round-backed implant was tested and therefore no statistical value could be calculated.

Displacement with Load in the Cadaveric Specimens

The measurements carried out on the cadaveric specimens could not be subject to statistical analysis due to the small numbers involved (1 shoulder per implant). However, we were able to observe similar behaviour patterns. The displacements occurred in the same directions though the degree was less by a factor of 1.5–3 depending on the specimen. The relationship between the results obtained in foam and in bone were conserved for two unmatched shoulders.

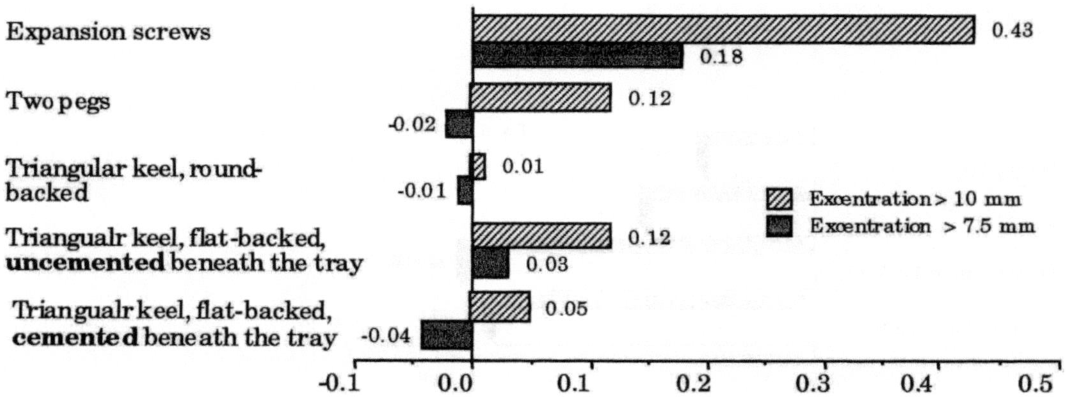

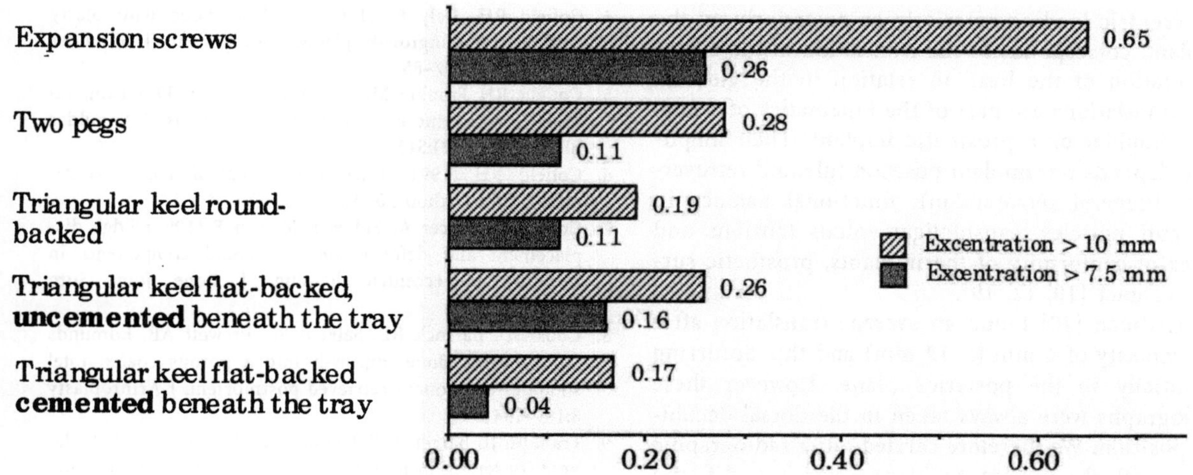

Fig. 9. Displacement (mm) measured at M1 for *lateral displacement* simulating translation of the humeral head. Two distances were used: 10 and 7.5 mm

Table 1 shows the results obtained during the tests carried out on the first pair of shoulders using a triangular keel with a round-back, cemented on the right and an uncemented, expansion screw glenoid on the left.

Table 1. Displacement values (mean±SD, mm) for triangular keeled, flat-backed, cemented glenoids versus uncemented metal-back components in cadaveric specimens: positive values indicate tilt and negative values indicate sinkage

	Triangular keel, round-backed, cemented (right)	Expansion screws, metal-backed, uncemented (left)
CM_1	−0.24±0.002	−0.25±0.006
LM_1	0.20±0.004	0.24±0.002
LeM_1	0.20±0.004	0.37±0.002
HM_2	0.01±0.001	0.08±0.008
HeM_2	0.08±0.001	0.18±0.006

Discussion

Pull-Out Tests (fixation of the glenoid components)

Before making any interpretation of the results, we accept that the pull-out tests do not correspond to physiological conditions. These tests do though, give an indication of the implant hold. The values for pull-out loads obtained for the different fixation modes can therefore only be compared within the body of a similar study.

Furthermore the experimental model has not been validated by an additional study on cadaveric specimens such that the results have no real scientific value.

The mode of fixation failure for the different cemented implants was identical and consisting of a cement mantle fracture at the level of the notch in the keel or the pegs with pull-out of the subjacent foam.

The implants with a triangular keel cemented in position presented the best results without any significant difference between the flat-back and round-back implants. However, it should be noted that the round-back prostheses always needed larger forces to achieve pull-out.

Only Fukuda et al. [11] have carried out pull-out tests – using the cemented, metal-backed Neer I and II, Cofield and Gristina implants. The authors observed fractures of the polyethylene keel, the metal tray or the fixation screws for traction values of 810–2780 N.

Displacement Under Load (fixation and stability of the glenoid components)

To evaluate the quality of the primary fixation of the different implants we used eccentric loading which is the most damaging to glenoid fixation [7, 9, 12, 17, 20] and the most likely to produce implant displacement especially where the conformity index is close to 1 [12].

Superior eccentricity of the humeral head corresponds clinically to the upward migration of the head which is due to a number of factors [1, 2]: rotator cuff tears, functional imbalance between the cuff muscles and the deltoid, excessive inclination of the glenoid implant upwards and medially suspended humeral implant and division of the coracoacromial ligament.

Under load, the triangular keeled implants with flat or round-backs, cemented gave the lowest tilt values (Fig. 8).

Eccentric loading anteriorly or posteriorly on the implant, corresponds to the translation of the centre of rotation of the head in relation to the glenoid. The translations are part of the kinematics of a normal shoulder or a prosthetic implant. Their amplitude depends on: implant position (glenoid retroversion, humeral retrotorsion), functional balance in the cuff muscles, capsuloligamentous tensions and index of conformity of the implants, prosthetic surface contact [10, 12, 19].

Friedman [10] found an average translation after arthroplasty of 4 mm (0–12 mm) and this occurring essentially in the posterior plane. However these radiographs were always taken in the dorsal decubitus position. We therefore carried out a radiographic study with the patient positioned sitting and found that the average translation distance (10 Aequalis arthroplasties) was 2.9±2.8 mm (0–10) and essentially occurred anteriorly.

During the tests we used forces applied laterally at 7.5 and 10 mm. In these load conditions the triangular keeled, flat-backed, cemented implants gave the lowest tilt values (Fig. 9).

Conclusion

Experimental validation obtained from the measurements taken on the cadaveric specimens allowed us to make the following conclusions: (a) primary implant fixation was superior for the cemented implants during the tests, (b) the presence of cement beneath the tray added stability, (c) the cemented triangular keel had better fixation than the cemented pegs.

References

1. Boileau P, Walch G, Liotard JP (1992) Etude radiocinématographique de l'élévation active de l'épaule prothésée. Rev Chir Orthop 78:355–364
2. Boyd AD Jr, Aliabadi P, Thornhill TS (1991) Postoperative proximal migration in total shoulder arthroplasty. Incidence and significance. J Arthroplasty 6:31–37
3. Brantschen R, Gerber C (1991) Possibilities of shoulder protheses in arthritis. Ther Umsch 48:645–57
4. Cofield RH, Daly PJ (1992) Total shoulder arthroplasty with a tissue-ingrowth glenoid component. J Shoulder Elbow Surg 1:77–85
5. Cofield RH Frankle MA, Zuckerman JD (1993) Humeral head replacement in glenohumeral arthritis. J Shoulder Elbow Surg 2(2):S13
6. Cofield RH (1994) Uncemented total shoulder arthroplasty. Clin Orthop 307:86–93
7. Collins D, Tencer A, Sidles J, Matsen F (1992) Edge displacement and deformation of glenoid components in response to eccentric loading. J Bone Joint Surg 74A:501–507
8. Cook SD, Barrack RL, Salkeld SL, Prewett AB, Edmunds JO Jr (1993) Bone ingrowth into a porous coated total shoulder component retrieved postmortem. J Arthroplasty 8:189–194
9. Franklin JL Barrett WP, Jackins SE, Matsen FA (1988) Glenoïd loosening in total shoulder arthroplasty (association with rotator cuff deficiency). J Arthroplasty 3:39–46
10. Friedman RJ (1992) Glenohumeral translation after total shoulder arthroplasty. J Shoulder Elbow Surg 1:312–316
11. Fukuda K, Chen CN, Cofield RH, Chao EY (1988) Biomechanical analysis of stability and fixation strength of total shoulder prostheses. Orthopaedics 11:141–149
12. Harryman DT, Sidles JA, Harris SL, Lippitt SB, Matsen FA (1995) The effect of articular conformity and the size of the humeral head component on laxity and motion after glenohumeral arthroplasty. J Bone Joint Surg 77A:555–563
13. Howell SM, Galinat BJ (1989) The glenoid-labral socket (A constrained articular surface). Clin Orthop 243:122–125
14. Iannotti JP, Gabriel JP, Schneck SL, Evans BG, Misra S (1992) The normal glenohumeral relationships (An anatomical study of 140 shoulders). J Bone Joint Surg 74A:491–500
15. Lippitt SB, Vanderhooft JE, Harris SL, Sidles JA, Harryman DT, Matsen FA (1993) Glenohumeral stability from concavity-compression: a quantitative analysis. J Shoulder Elbow Surg 2(1):27–35
16. Matsen FA, Tencer A (1991) Glenoid component stability is enhanced by accurate preparation of the bone surface. Presented at the 10th closed meeting of the American Shoulder and Elbow surgeons, Seattle
17. Neer CS II (1974) Replacement arthroplasty for glenohumeral osteoarthritis. J Bone Joint Surg 56A:1–13
18. Poppen NK, Walker PS (1978) Forces at the glenohumeral joint in abduction. Clin Orthop 16:165–170
19. Severt R, Thomas BJ, Tsenter MJ, Amstutz HC, Kabo JM (1993) The influence of conformity and constraint on translational forces and frictional torque in total shoulder arthroplasty. Clin Orthop 292:151–158
20. Thomas BJ, Amstutz HC, Cracchiolo A (1991) Shoulder arthroplasty for rheumatoid arthritis. Clin Orthop 265:125–128

Technique of Glenoid Resurfacing in Shoulder Arthroplasty

P. Boileau, D. Molé, and G. Walch

Summary

Glenoid resurfacing is technically challenging and this may explain why many surgeons still prefer to perform hemiarthroplasty. In our experience, total shoulder replacement has proven to give better functional results for many pathological conditions of the glenohumeral joint. Shoulder surgeons should be capable of performing glenoid resurfacing while anticipating technical errors responsible for most of glenoid component failures. Accurate preoperative planing using both standards radiographs and CT, as well as glenoid exposure are two key points. All the technical steps should be controlled including: (a) meticulous reaming with correct vertical and horizontal reorientation of the glenoid surface; (b) management of glenoid deficiencies; (c) correct positioning of the glenoid component; (d) secure fixation of the glenoid component; (e) finally, soft tissue reconstruction and balancing which should avoid any eccentric loads on the glenoid rim, responsible for glenoid lucent lines and loosening and for assymetric polyethylene wear.

Introduction

Resurfacing of the glenoid with a cemented polyethylene device was introduced by Neer in the 1970s for patients with significant glenoid erosion [42]. The reasons for resurfacing the glenoid were firstly, that severe erosion of the glenoid articular surface was thought to be a contributing factor towards the production of painful shoulder, and secondly, that glenoid resurfacing may facilitate reorientation and stabilisation of the prosthetic shoulder. Over the last twenty years several authors have reported the results of glenoid resurfacing and have documented the benefits in total shoulder arthroplasty [2, 6, 8, 15, 17, 18, 27, 28, 33, 36, 52, 54, 56]. However, the incidence of radiolucency at the glenoid bone-cement interface, reported in these series is high, ranging from 30 % to 96 %. Although clinical significance is not clear and long-term consequences are unknown there are still concerns about glenoid component fixation and longevity. The incidence of symptomatic glenoid loosening ranges from 0 % to 16 % in series with short or medium follow-up (35 months on average). For these reasons the authors and others have looked for fixations other than cement for the glenoid and bony ingrowth through a metal-back design has been proposed [10, 21, 22]. This article reviews considers in detail all the technical aspects of glenoid resurfacing with cemented and uncemented components as well as the potential complications.

Indications and Contraindications for Glenoid Resurfacing

Advantages and Disadvantages of Glenoid Resurfacing

Our experience as other surgeons have shown better results in respect to pain relief with total shoulder arthroplasty than with hemiarthroplasty alone [6, 8, 16, 19, 33, 42, 52]. However, the decision as to whether or not use a glenoid component should be left to the surgeon's discretion and should take into account the benefits and risks of this procedure. Glenoid resurfacing is a challenging procedure which involves increased operative time, blood loss, and anaesthesia because of the increased tissue dissection and exposure required for component implantation. Surgeons should control all steps of the procedure including correct exposure, meticulous reaming with accurate horizontal and vertical orientation of the glenoid surface, management of glenoid deficiency and soft tissue reconstruction in case of instability or rotator cuff tears. Surgeons should also be aware of all potential complications, including glenoid fracture, neurovascular injury, component failure, subluxation or dislocation, secondary cuff tears and component loosening.

Contraindications to the Use of a Glenoid Component

It is essential that patients selected for glenoid resurfacing have adequate glenoid bone, both in quantity and in quality, and no major soft tissue deficiencies.

Table 1. Contraindications to glenoid resurfacing are related to bone and/or soft tissue conditions

Glenoid bone deficiencies	• *Poor bone quality*: absence of cancellous bone, osteoporosis. • *Poor bone quantity*: severe glenoid wear.
Soft-tissue deficiencies	• *Loose glenohumeral joint*: massive cuff tears, with proximal humeral migration or antero-posterior instability. • *Tight glenohumeral joint*: medialisation because of soft tissue contracture.

A glenoid component should not be used in four circumstances (Table 1): (a) when the glenoid bone stock is not sufficient to allow intimate contact between the tray and the glenoid bone; (b) when the quality of the glenoid bone is inadequate with insufficient cancellous bone and severe osteoporosis; (c) when the glenohumeral joint is grossly unstable either in the vertical plane (because of proximal migration of the humerus secondary to long-standing massive cuff tears) or in the horizontal plane (because of anteroposterior instability with poor or impossible soft tissue balancing). It must be remembered that any eccentric loads can lead to glenoid component failure because of excessive polyethylene wear or dissociation from the metal tray; (d) when medialisation of the glenohumeral is excessive because of important glenoid erosion, as seen in some aggressive rheumatoid arthritis or because of severe soft tissue retraction and scars, as seen in some post-traumatic arthritis. In these case, the reduction in joint volume as well as the definitive shortening of the capsular and rotator cuff may preclude placement of a glenoid component and especially of a thick glenoid component. Forcing a glenoid component into a tight joint space can severely limit postoperative range of motion and function and lead to subscapularis rupture [25].

Preoperative Planning Before Glenoid Resurfacing

Preoperative planning is critical before deciding to resurface the glenoid and should include evaluation of the horizontal and vertical orientation and wear of the glenoid [1]. Standards radiographs (AP and axillary views) are not sufficient, in our experience, to accurately appreciate glenoid bone loss and we systematically perform narrow-cut (3 mm) CT or even CT arthrogram before total shoulder arthroplasty.

Vertical Orientation and Wear of the Glenoid

Vertical orientation and wear of the glenoid may be assessed using *true antero-posterior radiographs* and *CT scans*. One should remember that the normal articular surface of the glenoid is oriented approximately vertically and that the superior or inferior tilt of the articular surface is usually less than 10°. Superior erosion of the glenoid is known to occur more often in rheumatoid arthritis: it is therefore essential to determine if this erosion has reached, or even destroyed, the foot of the coracoid process. Depending on the importance of this superior glenoid wear, the surgeon will have the choice between (a) preferential inferior reaming, (b) superior glenoid bone grafting or (c) no glenoid resurfacing.

True antero-posterior radiographs also help to appreciate proximal migration of the humerus. It is usually accepted that narrowing of the acromiohumeral distance to less than five mm is synonymous with old and massive cuff tears. However, a false image of acromiohumeral narrowing is possible, due to excessive retroversion of the glenoid [3]. Because of the presence of eccentric shear loads associated with a massive cuff tear, termed the "rocking horse effect", glenoid resurfacing is usually contra-indicated in this condition [4, 28, 43, 44, 50, 57].

Horizontal Orientation and Wear of the Glenoid

Horizontal orientation and wear of the glenoid are best assessed by CT. As emphasized by Neer [46], *axillary views* may give false information depending on the rotation of the scapula. CT is helpful in the preoperative assessment of the glenoid and allows for assessment of the glenoid orientation and glenoid bone stock [3].

Evaluation of glenoid orientation in the horizontal plane is critical. One should remember that the glenoid surface is roughly perpendicular to the axis of the scapula or slightly retroverted (usually less that 10°). Posterior tilt of the glenoid surface, greater than 10°, or asymmetric posterior glenoid erosion should be considered as pathological and should be corrected surgically.

Evaluation of the glenoid bone stock is also essential to allow the location and orientation of the medullary canal to be determined. For instance, glenoid erosion in osteoarthritis is said to be predominantly posterior. In fact, we have described three types of glenoid in osteoarthritis: centralised glenoid wear, asymmetrical (predominantly posterior) glenoid wear, and dysplastic glenoid with retroversion greater than 25° [3, 55].

In addition CT allows for *evaluation of the degree of posterior humeral subluxation* and the amount of *fatty degeneration of the muscles of the rotator cuff.*

All these parameters should be taken into account in the decision-making process for glenoid resurfacing.

Glenoid Exposure and Preparation

Glenoid resurfacing is usually performed as the third step in total shoulder arthroplasty after soft tissue release and humeral preparation. However, in some inflammatory arthritis with very fragile bone, it may be appropriate to begin with the glenoid step before humeral osteotomy to avoid humeral fracture or bone impaction.

Exposure of the Glenoid Surface

Exposure of the glenoid surface is probably the most important step because it determines the rest of the procedure. An anterior glenoid retractor is placed in the subscapular fossa to retract the subscapularis muscle and tendon allowing the direction of the anterior wall or neck to be seen. The key step in glenoid exposure is the complete posterior dislocation of the proximal humerus (Fig. 1). Early detachment of the superior part of the pectoralis major is essential to achieve adequate exposure of the posterior scapula without forceful retraction on the deltoid. Complete detachment of the capsule on the humeral side reaching to at least the 6 o'clock position and possibly a posterior capsulotomy on the glenoid side, help to dislocate the proximal humerus posteriorly. The stem-neck trial component equipped with the humeral cut protector, should be inserted into the humerus to protect the cut surface and to avoid compression fracture or deformation during the glenoid preparation (Fig. 2A).

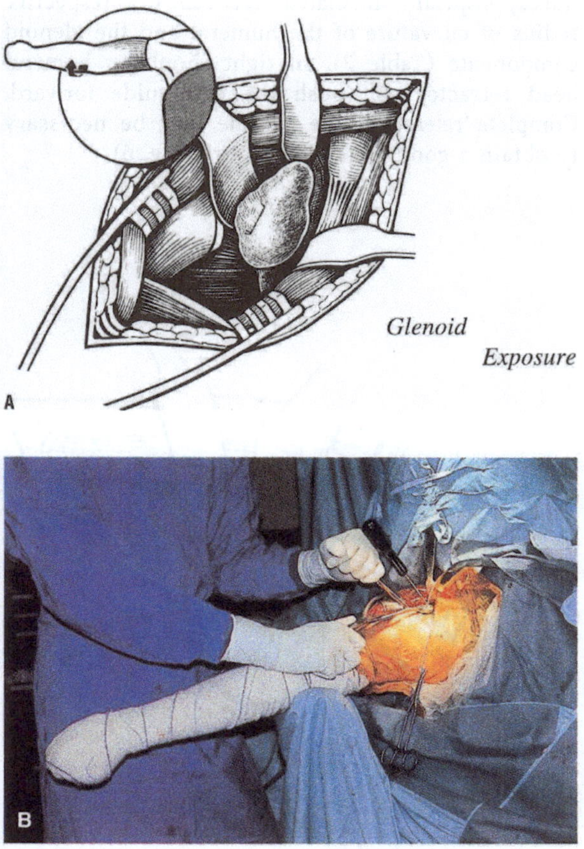

Fig. 1. Glenoid exposure: the arm abducted and optimally externally or internally rotated (**A**) and is held on a support to avoid stretchnig of the neurological structures (**B**)

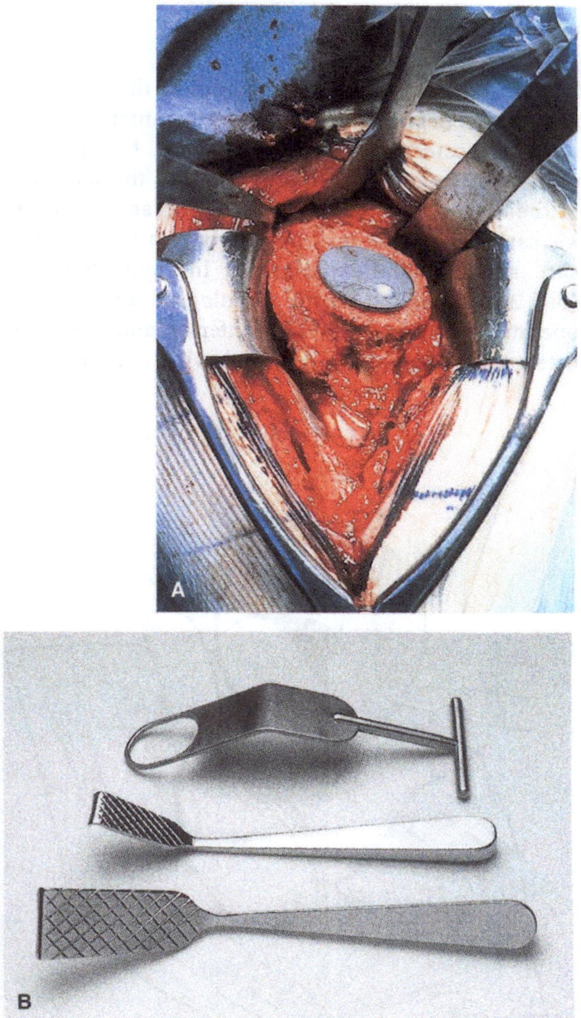

Fig. 2. A humeral cut proctrector is inserted into the humerus to avoid compression fractures or deformation during the glenoid preparation (**A**) Ring (Fukuda) or curved (Aequalis) humeral head retractors are prefered (**B**)

Then, with the arm held in abduction, a posterior glenoid retractor (i.e. Fukuda or Trillat or Aequalis type) is placed on the posterior glenoid border allowing the proximal humerus to be dislocated posteriorly (Fig. 2B). The arm can be held on a special support to avoid stretching of the neurologic structures and the degree of rotation (internal or external) of the arm depends on the degree of capsulomuscular retraction: it is different for each shoulder and should be individually checked. In our opinion, visualisation of and ease of working on the glenoid are optimised if the surgeon faces the glenoid instead of staying in the axillary fold. Finally, the self retainer should be removed from underneath the conjoint tendon in order to avoid stretching the axillary and musculocutaneous nerves and not deepen the surgical field.

Location of the Anatomical Glenoid

Location of the anatomical glenoid is the next step and should begin with excision of the anterior, inferior and posterior labrum. Care must be taken in removing the posterior labrum so that the insertion of the long head of the biceps is left intact. A posterior capsular release may help to have a better exposure and should be performed in tight shoulders (Fig. 3). Depending on the radiological and CT preoperative planning, anterior, inferior and posterior osteophytes should be removed with a rongeur or an osteotome to avoid eccentrical positioning of the glenoid component. One should be particularly aware of osteophytes on the inferior edge of the glenoid which may mislead the surgeon into placing the glenoid component too low. To avoid this error it is critical to determine the exact location of the vertical diameter of the normal glenoid. Two landmarks are particularly useful: superiorly, the base of the coracoid and inferiorly, the lateral margin of the scapula. Using diathermy or a sterile pen a vertical line is drawn based on these two landmarks and horizontal line marks the middle of the glenoid (Fig. 4).

Drilling of the Pilot Holes in the Medullary Canal

Drilling pilot holes into the medullary canal should be done using a drill guide (Fig. 4 and 5). Three drill guides are available (small, medium and large) corresponding to the sizes of the prosthetic glenoid components. The selection of the drill guide is made considering the vertical diameter of the glenoid and the humeral head size already selected, to select the appropriate mismatch between the respective radius of curvature of the humeral and the glenoid components (Table 2). In tight shoulders humeral head retractor can push the drill-guide forward. Complete release of the capsule may be necessary to obtain a good glenoid exposure (Fig. 6).

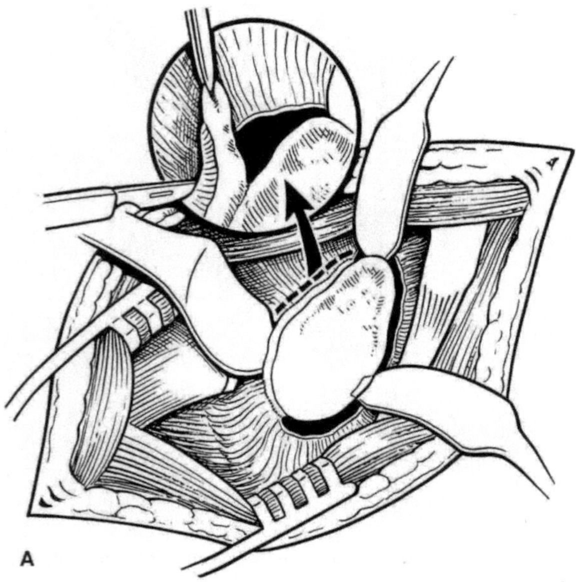
A

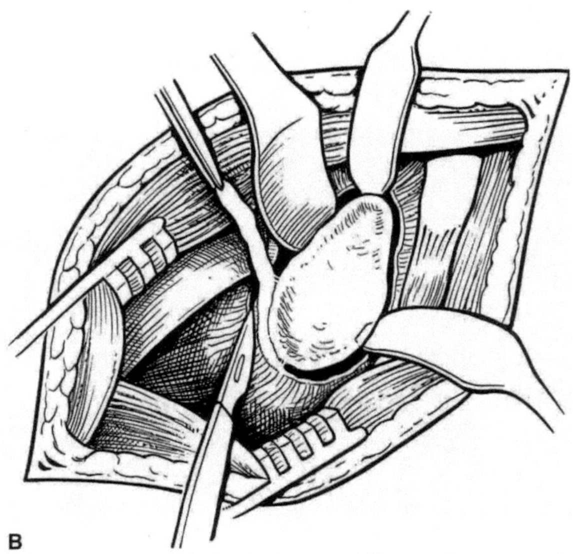
B

Fig. 3 A,B. Resection of the labrum and posterior release

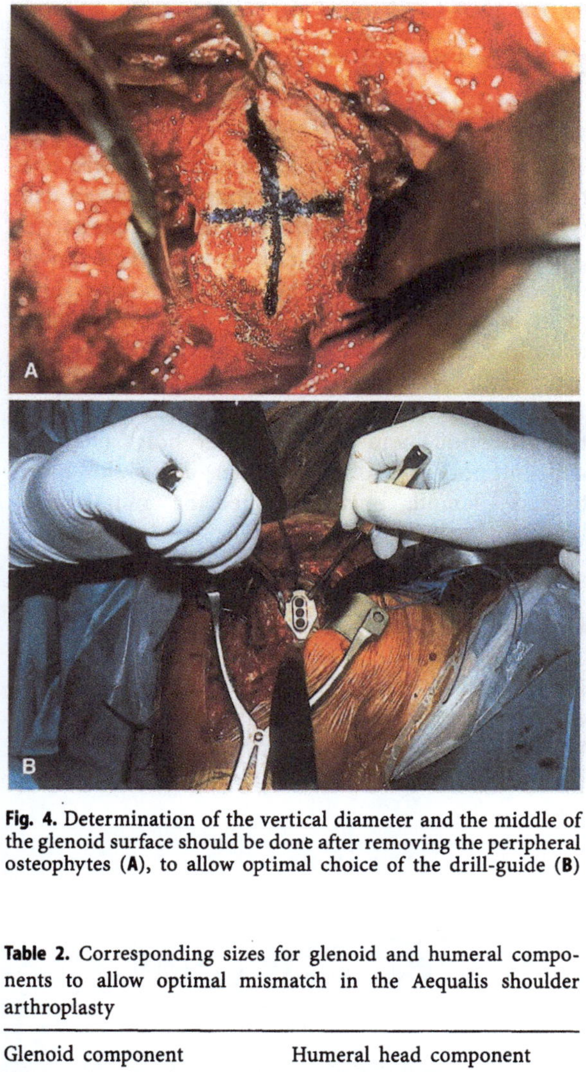

Fig. 4. Determination of the vertical diameter and the middle of the glenoid surface should be done after removing the peripheral osteophytes (**A**), to allow optimal choice of the drill-guide (**B**)

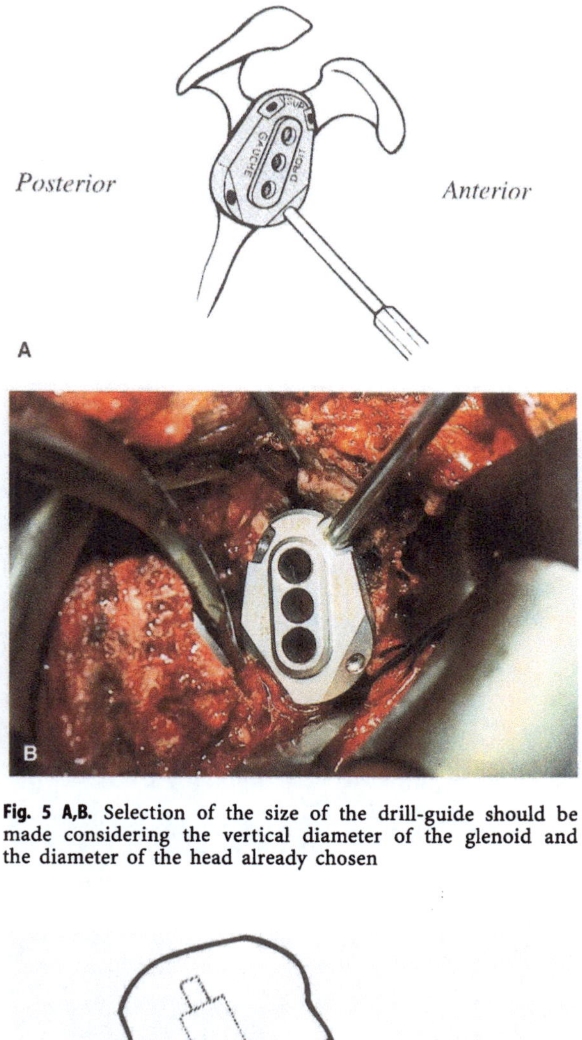

Fig. 5 A,B. Selection of the size of the drill-guide should be made considering the vertical diameter of the glenoid and the diameter of the head already chosen

Table 2. Corresponding sizes for glenoid and humeral components to allow optimal mismatch in the Aequalis shoulder arthroplasty

Glenoid component	Humeral head component
Small	37/13.5 39/14 41/15
Medium	43/16 46/17
Large	48/18 50/16 and 50/19 52/19 and 52/23

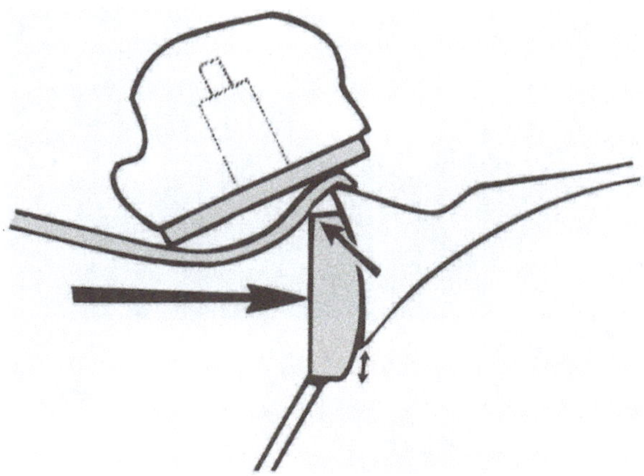

Fig. 6. In tight shoulders, the humeral head retractor can push the drill-guide forward. This can be corrected by changing the type of retractor, changing the rotation of the arm or completing the posterior capsular release

Although we recommend preserving the biceps insertion, the smallest size should not be systematically selected. The medullary canal is usually perpendicular to the glenoid surface. However, in osteoarthritis and rheumatoid arthritis, because of predominant posterior wear, there is a risk of perforating the anterior cortex if the drill guide is held parallel to the exposed surface. Horizontal anterior tilt of the drill guide may be necessary to allow the drill bit to be oriented perpendicular to the glenoid neck (Fig. 7). If a perforation is accidentally made through the cortex of the scapula, it should be closed with cortical bone graft taken from the humeral head.

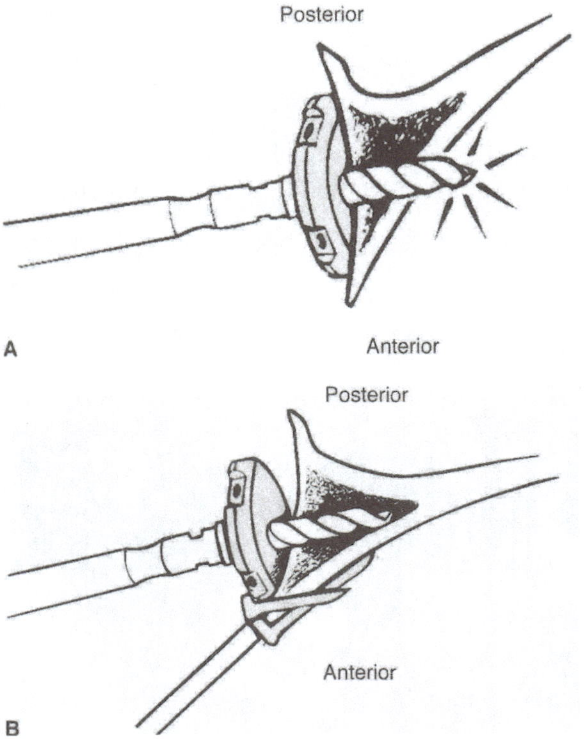

Fig. 7. A Posterior wear can lead to drill bit misplacement. **B** This can be corrected by using the gelnoid orientation guide or more simply by anteriorly tilting the drill guide

The humerus is usually sufficiently displaced posteriorly to allow the use of a straight powered drill (Fig. 8). When the proximal humerus cannot be greatly posteriorly displaced, a 45° angle power drill is available. The drill guide features three alignment holes: the middle hole is drilled first when using the polyethylene component. The diameter of the drill bit is 6 mm and the maximum depth is 17 mm (Fig. 9). A peg is then inserted to stabilize the drill guide and the two other holes (superior and inferior) are drilled. When using the metal backed glenoid, only the superior and inferior holes are drilled.

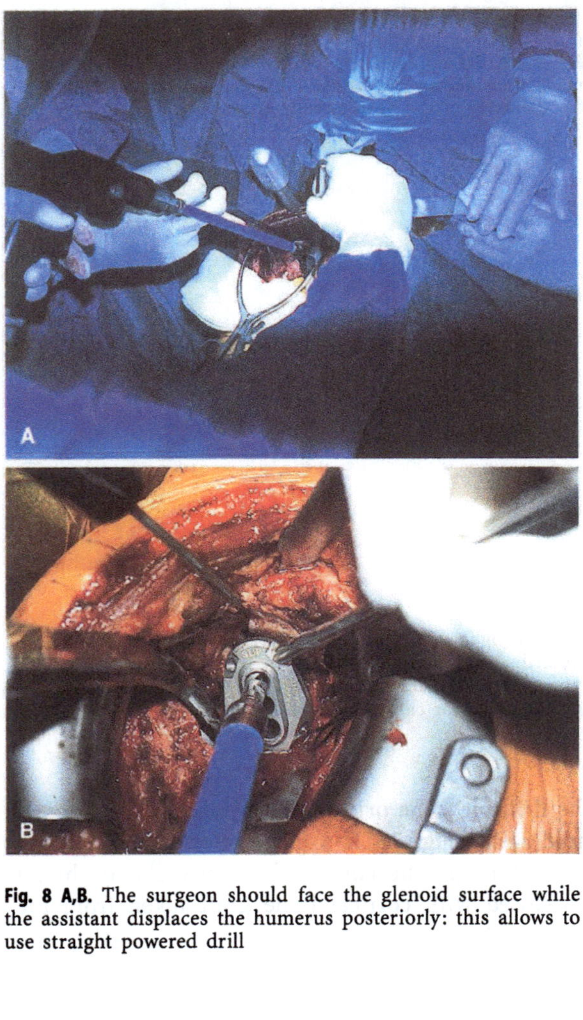

Fig. 8 A,B. The surgeon should face the glenoid surface while the assistant displaces the humerus posteriorly: this allows to use straight powered drill

Reaming of the Glenoid Surface

Resurfacing of the glenoid should allow for congruent reaming or mating of the subchondral plate to the back of the glenoid component. Collins et al. [23, 24] have shown that the glenoid bone should

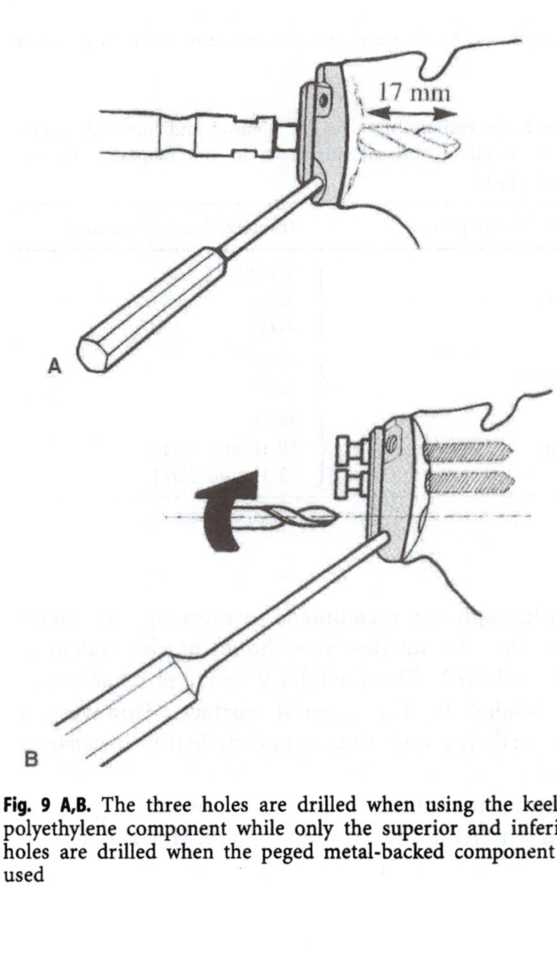

Fig. 9 A,B. The three holes are drilled when using the keeled polyethylene component while only the superior and inferior holes are drilled when the peged metal-backed component is used

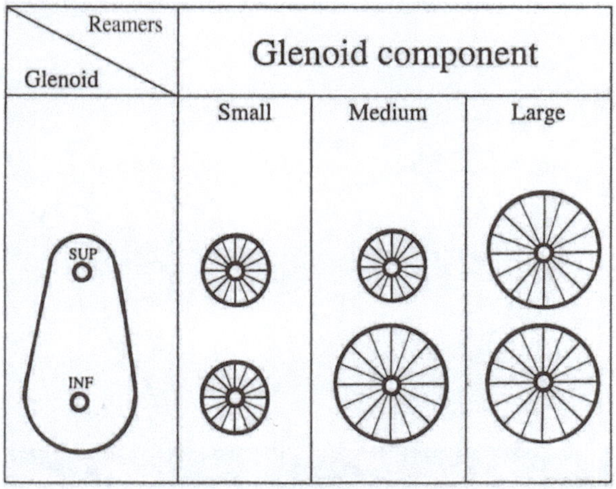

Fig. 10. Selection of the size of the glenoid reamers according to the glenoid size

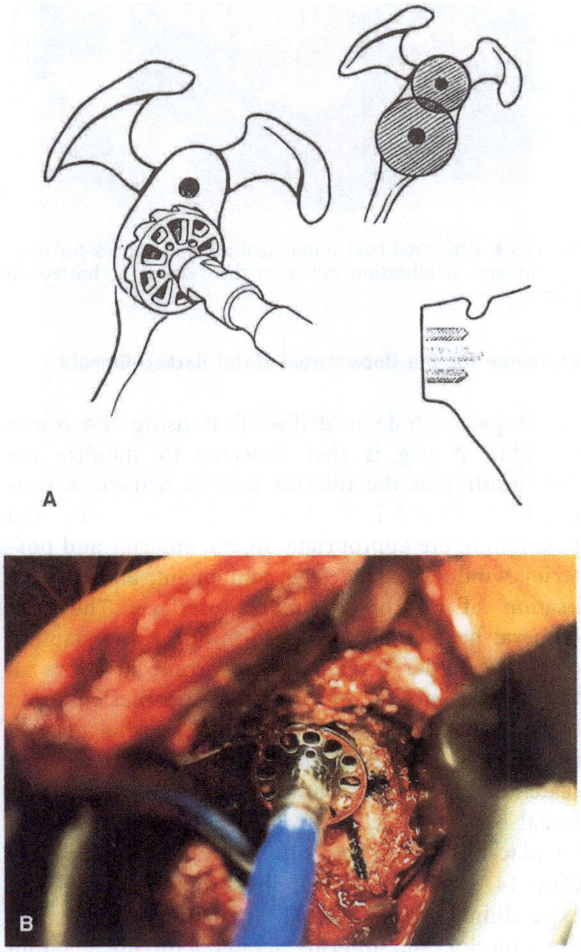

Fig. 11 A,B. Resurfacing the glenoid by reaming superior and inferior parts

be carefully prepared so that it matches the contour of the back of the glenoid component. This conforming reaming provides substantial stability for the glenoid component even without the use of any fixation system (cement, screws, metal-backing or keel). Glenoid reamers specifically designed are preferred to burr for resurfacing the glenoid surface. The pear-shape of the Aequalis glenoid component requires two reamer sizes, small and large (Fig. 10 and 11). These reamers are equipped with a pilot-guide (10 mm long) which is inserted into the previously drilled superior and inferior holes. The selection of the reamer sizes is made as follows: the small reamer is used for the small glenoid the large reamer is used for the large glenoid and both small and large reamers are used for the medium glenoid component (Fig. 10). The pilot-guide allows the reamer to remain perpendicular to the medullary canal. The goal is to obtain a perfectly planed surface. Preferential anterior reaming is usually required in osteoarthritis because of posterior wear. The glenoid component is 5 mm in depth and glenoid reaming should allow to restore the anatomical position of the joint line without medialisation or lateralisation.

Positioning and Fixation of the Glenoid Component

Positioning and fixation of the glenoid component depends upon the use of a cemented or uncemented glenoid component.

Technique for the Cemented Polyethylene Glenoid

The remaining bony bridges between the three holes are removed with a rongeur or a burr. Although, it has been recommanded to drill two small canals to enhance the cement anchorage (one superior towards the coracoid and one inferiorly along the external border of the scapula), we do not recommand this techniques. The space prepared for the keel is always the same size, whichever glenoid component size is selected. The glenoid punch must be inserted completely within the keel space and the cancellous bone is compacted (Fig. 12). A trial glenoid component is used to check that its size and positioning are appropriate. Anterior and posterior, windows on the trial component allow visualisation of the bone-implant interface. Impossibility to "rock" the trial component demonstrate its stable position (Fig. 13). The keel space and the glenoid surface are carefully cleaned and dried. Pulse lavage and haemostatic agents are used to control bleeding. Cementing is then performed. It has been claimed

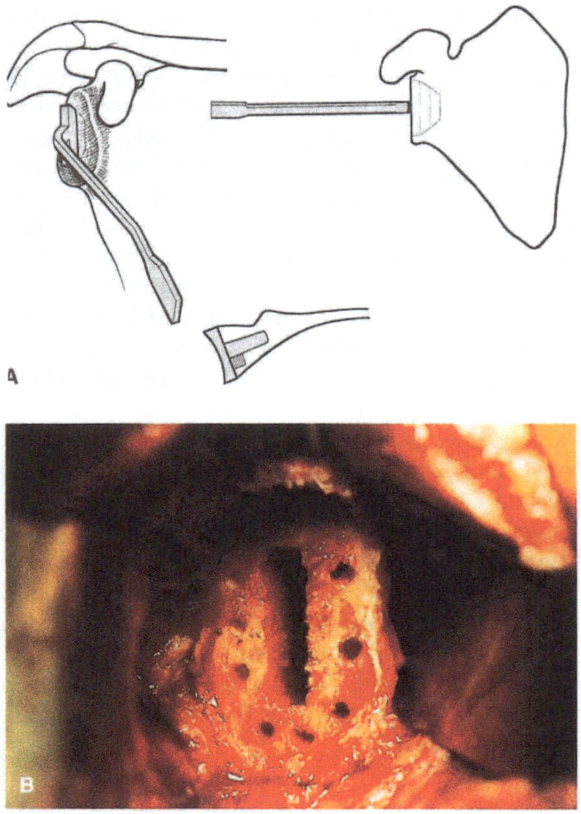

Fig. 12. A slot is created in the glenoid fossa when the keeled glenoid is used. **A** The straight glenoid punch is used to compact the cancellous bone inside the keel space. **B** The keel space and the glenoid surface are carelully cleaned and dried. Small peripheral holes can be drill to enhance cement fixation

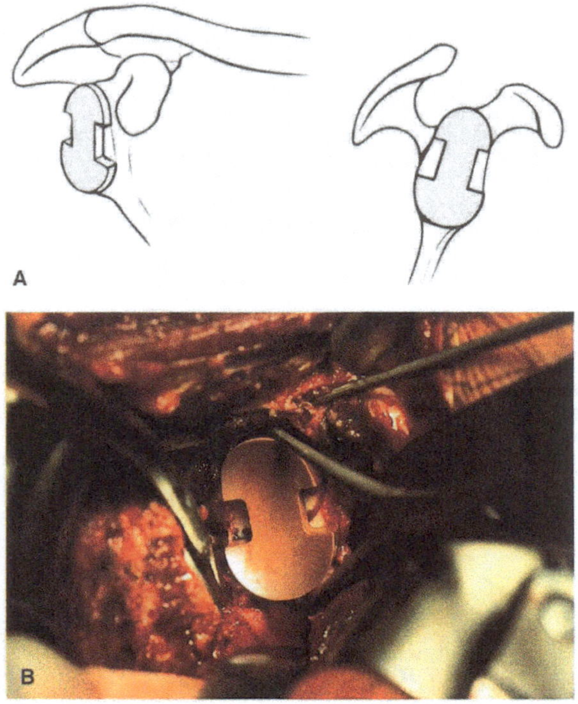

Fig. 13 A,B. Fenestred trial component allows to check for optimal fit and stabilization either in the vertical or horizontal plane

that the vast majority of lucent lines around the glenoid component are the result of poor technique and can be seen on the immediate postoperative radiographs [14, 15, 20, 42, 46].

Neer and Morrison have found that these lucent lines can be minimised through the use of a *double cementing technique* [39, 42]. Dry gauze or haemostatic tissue is packed in the medullary canal of the glenoid neck. The packing is then removed and the methylmethacrylate is injected into the canal with a syringe while still in a liquid state. The cement can be pressurised using a gauze or the metal glenoid punch covered with a wetted rubber glove [23]. The dry canal is then immediately refilled with the semisoft methylmethacrylate which is pressurised manually. After removing the excess cement on the articular surface, the glenoid component is inserted, impacted into place, and held manually or with the glenoid impactor until the cement has hardened. The final step is to check for stability of the glenoid component. In case of component instability, the cement and glenoid should be removed and the same procedure performed again.

Technique for the Uncemented Metal Backed Glenoid

The superior hole is drilled first using the 6-mm drill bit. A peg is then inserted to stabilise the drill guide and the inferior hole is drilled. A two-peg trial glenoid is used to check that its size and positioning are appropriate. Again, anterior and posterior windows in the trial component, allow visualisation of the bone-implant interface. The trial humeral head is then reduced to check the stability of the shoulder joint. Eighty percent or more of the bearing surface of the metal prosthesis should be in contact with glenoid bone. The trial glenoid is removed and the glenoid tray is positioned and seated with the impactor. Before impacting, additional bone graft taken from the humeral head can be placed between the bone and the glenoid tray (Fig. 14). Once impacted, the three petals of each expanding peg are opened, tightening alternatively the superior and inferior screws with the 4.5 mm screwdriver (Fig. 15). Tightening must be performed until strong, primary stability is obtained and usually corresponds to a minimum of 8 screwdriver turns, but should not exceed 8.5 turns. The polyethylene insert is then positioned posteriorly and

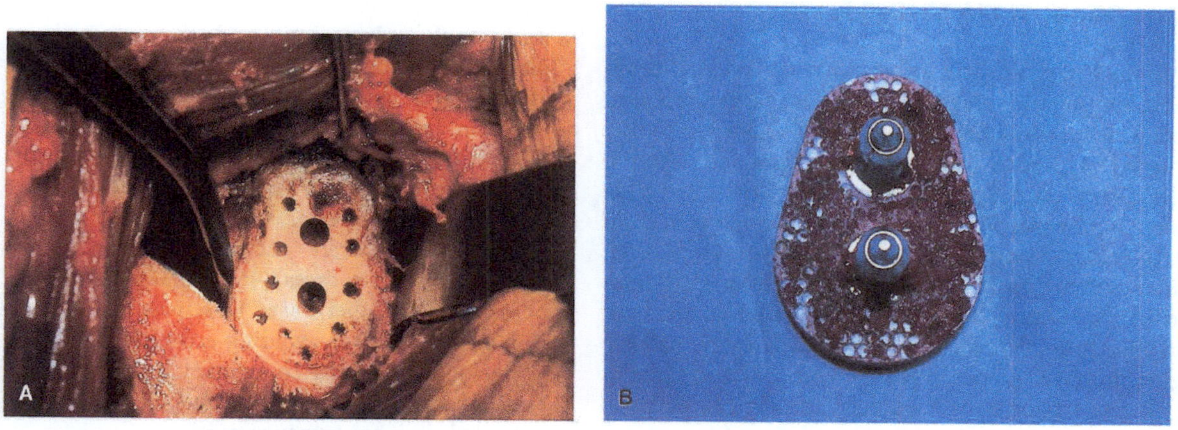

Fig. 14 A,B. Flat reamed glenoid surface will receive the metal tray filled with cancelous bone

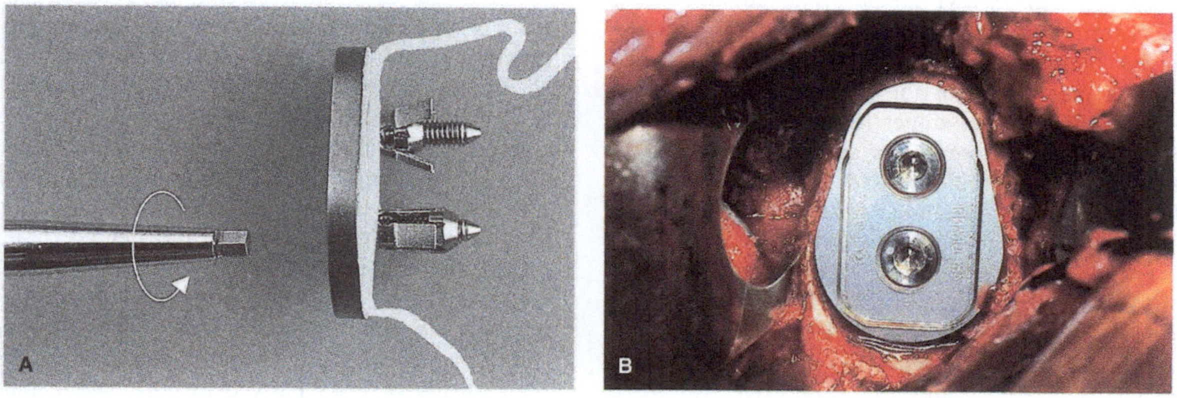

Fig. 15 A,B. Expanding screws are alternatively opened

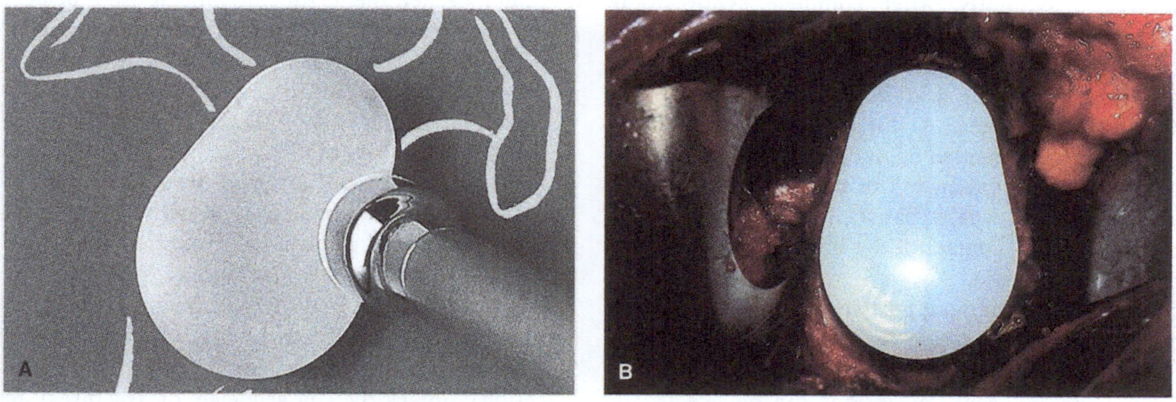

Fig. 16 A,B. The polyethylene insert is impacted in a direction perpendicular to the glenoid surface

click-locked in place by engaging the anterior edge with the polyethylene insert impactor. The direction of the impactor should be perpendicular to the glenoid surface (Fig. 16).

With properly sized prosthetic components and appropriate soft tissue balancing, testing of the shoulder should allow: (a) partial subluxation of the humeral head posteriorly out of the glenoid prosthesis (50 % posterior drawer), (b) 30°–40° of external rotation with reapproximation of the subscapularis, (c) 90° of internal rotation with the arm at the side (forearm across the chest) and 60° of internal rotation in abduction (forearm parallel to the chest) [23, 37].

Management of Glenoid Deficiencies

Although glenoid deficiency is not considered as an absolute contraindication to total shoulder replacement, it certainly brings a technical challenge to the surgical approach of the arthritic shoulder. Glenoid deficiency can be posterior (osteoarthritis, arthritis after tight repair), central and superior (rheumatoid arthritis), anteroinferior (glenoid fractures or erosion after arthritis from instability) or superior (cuff tear arthritis). Secure fixation of the glenoid component in the case of major glenoid deficiency is a very challenging problem. As described by Neer [46] and Cofield [19, 20], six methods have been explored to address this problem depending on the severity of bone loss, the location of available bone and the type of pathology: (a) methyl methacrylate augmentation, (b) custom built-up glenoid component, (c) coracoid (high) placement of the glenoid component, (d) altering the version of the glenoid component, (e) bone grafting, (f) asymmetric (anterior or inferior) bone reaming. However, in surgical practice only the last two are regularly used, the two first procedures have been abandoned and condamned while the others are used occasionally.

From a practical point of view, glenoid deficiencies can be classified into three forms: cavity, segmental and combined (total) defects.

In cavity glenoid defects, the cortical rim of the scapula is preserved and thus supportive. This type of cavity defect, often seen in rheumatoid arthritis and other inflammatory arthritis, is the result of aggressive synovitis. After complete synovectomy and cleaning of the cystic defects, the cavity defect can be filled with *morsellised bone grafts* or *monobloc cancellous* bone graft shaped to the size of the defect and impacted. A slot or hole pegs are then created and a cemented or uncemented glenoid component can be implanted. The stability of the glenoid components is usually satisfactory because of the close peripheral contact of the implant with well vascularised bone rim.

In segmental non-supportive deficiencies, the scapular rim is non-supportive and cannot transmit correctly the mechanical forces to the subchondral bone. Different technical options can be selected:

- *Cement augmentation* should be avoided because it may break out leaving the glenoid component unsupported and leading to toggle motion and possible breakage of the keel [39, 46, 51].
- *Customised glenoid components* (augmented, angulated or oversized components) have been proposed in the past. They are not desirable because of the higher constraint on the components with increased stress at fixation [39, 46]. However, this fist generation of customised glenoid components were made with polyethylene and there may be a place for customised glenoid components with asymmetrical metal-back tray in the future.
- *Coracoid (high) placement of the glenoid component* in the cancellous bone at the base of the coracoid may be helpful in certain situations with predominantly superior wear and bone loss, as seen in some severe rheumatoid arthritis and cuff tear arthritis cases [46]. This solution may be suitable in other cases with proximal migration of the humerus avoiding eccentric (superior) loads on the glenoid component. In our experience, lowering the humerus when it has already ascended, has been unsuccessful.
- *Positioning the glenoid component with more retroversion* in cases of excessive retroversion or wear of the glenoid, is rarely a solution in our experience and this should be compensated for by decreasing humeral retroversion. For instance if the glenoid component is positioned with 20° of retroversion (because of posterior wear) then the humeral component should be placed in neutral version. In order to avoid protrusion of the keel outside the anterior cortex, the glenoid component should be placed high (in the base of the coracoid) when using this technique [46]. This principle is applicable to specific pathological conditions, such as old posterior dislocation and the arthritis of Erb's palsy deformity, where the external rotators are weak, contractured and shortened. Any attempt to lengthen these muscles would weaken them. Any attempt to use a posterior bone graft for the glenoid component and to position the humerus in its normal retroversion would fail because of increased medio-lateral offset which may lead to pull-off or fracture of the soft greater tuberosity.
- *Bone grafts* can be obtained from the resected humeral head and then appropriately shaped to restore the normal glenoid bony architecture, where there are major defects [10, 14, 20, 25, 39, 45]. The graft is usually secured with screws under compression. The bone graft may be implanted posteriorly (in osteoarthritis), anteriorly (in arthritis of dislocation), inferiorly (in sequelae of fractures) or superiorly (in rheumatoid arthritis). However, in our experience, indications for glenoid grafting are limited because of the frequent associated muscular and capsular contracture seen in arthritic conditions. We have observed that positioning a glenoid bone graft in a medialised and tight shoulder with retracted capsular structures and short external rotators may overtighten the joint and limit mobility. Moreover, the rate of glenoid loosening is higher after bone grafting [20].

It is difficult to know what size of a glenoid osseous deficiency requires bone-grafting. Collins et al. [24] in an in vitro study, have demonstrated that a bony deficiency of 25 % or even 33 % of the glenoid did not increased displacement of the posterior edge of the component in response to a posteriorly directed load. When bone grafting is necessary, large cortical cancellous graft are obtained from a portion of the humeral head already removed. The worn area of the glenoid is debrided down to bleeding bone and the bone graft is shaped to fit the defect. Fixation of the bone graft is obtained with the use of screws. To make the procedure easier and to avoid doing a posterior counter incision we developed a technique with cannulated screws. Two pins are passed through the deltoid through the posterior bone graft and then perforating the anterior cortex of the scapula. A cannulated drill is then passed through the first pin. The screws should be long enough to obtain a solid cortical grip and lag the bone graft in place. Once the graft is perfectly stabilised, the reamer is used again to reshape the glenoid surface and to restore a stable support for the glenoid component. The graft is then further stabilised by the glenoid component. Although Neer has suggested that if it is impossible to use screw fixation, the bone graft may be wedged into the defect and held in place with heavy nonabsorbable sutures passed through the graft and the reamed glenoid bone, we have never used this technique [45, 46].

- *Asymmetric bone reaming* is the simplest and safest technique and may be used in many arthritic conditions. Preferential reaming may be done in the horizontal plane by *lowering the anterior high side in osteoarthritis* and/or in the vertical plane by *correcting the superior tilt in rheumatoid arthritis.* This can be performed with a glenoid reamer which allows bone contouring. It has the advantages to reorientate the articular surface and then to avoid overtensioning of the glenohumeral joint which always jeopardises the fragile soft tissues and increases the polyethylene wear.

In combined (total) glenoid defects, the technical options are limited. *Implantation of a humeral component alone,* without a glenoid component, may be the more sensible and preferred choice rather than leaving the glenoid component unsupported by bone. This is, however, the only possible alternative when the glenoid is too frail or defective to support any type of fixation device. In these cases, the coracoid process can be found free floating, since its attachment to the scapula has been worn away. Burkhead has proposed to use the capsule or a fascialata graft to resurface the glenoid in certain circumstances [16]. This *interposition arthroplasty* may be a salvage procedure in some young patients.

Potential Complications of Glenoid Resurfacing

Knowledge of the potential complications of glenoid resurfacing should help the surgeons to prevent and avoid them because most of them are related to a poor surgical technique.

Poor Positioning of the Glenoid Component

Poor orientation of the glenoid component is possible (Fig. 17) either in the vertical plane (excessive superior or inferior tilt) or in the horizontal plane (excessive anterior or posterior tilt).

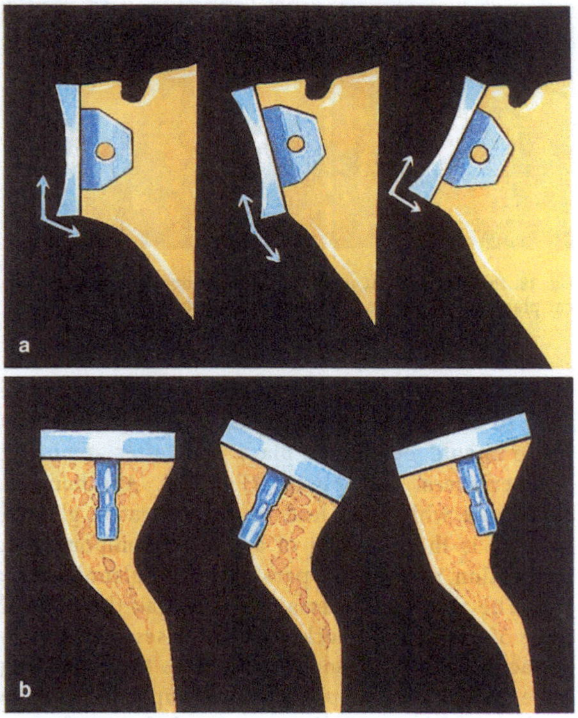

Fig. 17. Poor orientation of the glenoid component in the vertical plane (**a**) or in the horizontal plane (**b**)

Poor placement of the glenoid component is also possible either in the vertical plane (too low or too high) or in the horizontal plane (too anterior or too posterior; Fig. 18).

Careful preoperative radiological planning and meticulous surgical technique should avoid this complication.

Intraoperative Glenoid Fractures

In case of significant and asymmetrical glenoid wear, misplacement of the drill bit outside the medullary canal can occur leading to perforation

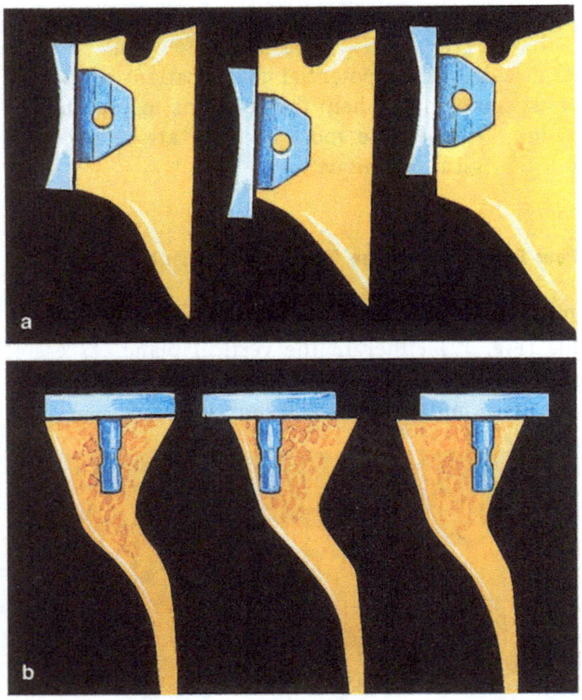

Fig. 18. Poor placement of the glenoid component in the vertical plane (**a**) or in the horizontal plane (**b**)

of the cortex. A glenoid orientation guide may be used to ensure correct orientation of the drill. This guide should be put in place only after removing the peripheral osteophytes (Fig. 7a). Another circumstance which can lead to intraoperative glenoid fracture is the insertion of a glenoid component in a direction not strictly parallel to the glenoid bone slot. The abnormal lever arm may break the cortical bone of the glenoid neck. In these cases, glenoid resurfacing is often abandoned because the remaining bone does not supply enough support for the implant and bone quality may preclude satisfactory fixation of the fragments. Finally, use of a multiple pegs glenoid component may lead to fragmentation of the glenoid bone stock and intra operative fractures [58]. Cofield has reported on patients with intraoperative glenoid fractures and has emphasized that pain relief was not as predictable for these hemiarthroplasty patients compared to a typical patients with a total shoulder arthroplasty [20].

Neuro-vascular Injury

The incidence of neurologic complications after total shoulder arthroplasty has been evaluated to be 4% in a series of 417 patients by Lynch et al. [36]. These authors assumed that injury to the brachial plexus occurred in their patients by traction because most of the deficits were partial and incomplete. They also found that postarthroplasty neurologic complications were related to a deltopectoral sparing approach, the use of methotrexate in rheumatoid patients and a longer operative time. In fact, positioning during total shoulder arthroplasty seems to be the main cause of neurologic deficits. Cadaveric studies and strain gauge testing have demonstrated that an arm placed in 90° of abduction, external rotation and slight extension produces traction on the plexus and that slight flexion of the shoulder relieves this traction. In rheumatoid arthritis the fascial structures are often of poor quality and may be responsible for traction injuries of the brachial plexus during preparation of the glenoid. Moreover, posterior dislocation of the humerus for glenoid preparation may increase stretching of the brachial plexus. It has been also reported that penetration of a drill through the posterior cortex of the scapula may lead to cement extrusion: the suprascapular nerve and its branches can be injured by the thermal reaction of the bone cement [23]. Fortunately, in most cases prognosis for neurologic recovery is good [36]. It is our experience that three precautions should be taken to avoid neuro-vascular injury: (a) isolate and protect the axillary nerve; (b) support the arm horizontally while dislocating the humerus posteriorly during exposure of the glenoid; (c) avoid osteotomy of the coracoid to stay on the lateral side of the conjoint tendon ("the safe side") and not to dissect on the medial side ("the suicide") [37].

Instability and Secondary Rotator Cuff Tears

In the majority of cases, the development of instability following shoulder arthroplasty is multifactorial and attributable to technical errors. It is often related to secondary cuff tears and more specifically to subscapularis stretching.

Anterior instability is often associated with subscapularis ruptures: use of a too big prosthetic head or of a thick metal-backed glenoid component with insufficient reaming of the glenoid surface will stress the suture line and repair process in the subscapularis tendon. This will lead to secondary subscapularis tear with anterior instability. Suture of the subscapularis tendon using non-absorbable sutures should avoid secondary subscapularis tears.

Superior instability. In the same way, overtightening of the supraspinatus because of a big head or a thick glenoid component may explain the frequency of proximal migration of the humeral component observed after total shoulder arthroplasty. Glenoid reaming should be adapted to the depth of the glenoid component which should be minimised. Conservation of the coraco-acromial ligament should avoid antero-superior instability. Any lateralisations of the joint line will lead to tightening of the soft tissue (with potential cuff tears) and increased forces across the glenoid (with potential glenoid loosening).

Posterior instability is frequently associated with a glenoid component which is retroverted with more than 20° or with posterior capsular stretching. Restoration of the normal offset and reorientation of the glenoid and/or posterior capsular stretching should avoid posterior instability.

Precise and meticulous surgical technique should avoid this problem by: (a) correctly orientating both the humeral and glenoid components; (b) obtaining stable and solid primary component fixation; (c) restoring correct soft tissue balancing in both the horizontal and the vertical planes.

Component Failure and Polyethylene-Metal Dissociation

Breaks of polyethylene components have been reported [25, 51] but has not been observed in our series. The most common cause of glenoid component failure is inadequate bone support for the glenoid component [14, 52]. As previously mentioned, the use of cement build-up in cases of glenoid deficiency is no longer recommended.

Polyethylene component dissociation from metal back tray has been reported by ourselves, Cofield [21] and Burkhead [15]. Polyethylene-metal dissociation may be prevented by: (a) use a of a reliable interlock between the polyethylene insert and the metal tray, (b) attaining joint stability at the time of surgery, (c) avoiding joint overtensioning which may cause stretching of the subscapularis repair. The two cases reported by Cofield as well as our own cases had severely stretched their subscapularis repair and had anterior and posterior translocation of the humeral component on the glenoid surface [21].

Component Loosening

In a recent report on total shoulder arthroplasty revision the incidence of glenoid loosening was 28% for failed unconstrained implant [57]. Recently, Torchia and Cofield [54] reported the results of eighty-nine total shoulder arthroplasties with a long-term following of twelve years (range 5–17 years). Eighty-four percent of the glenoid components have developed lucent lines and 44% demonstrated definitive radiographic loosening. Moreover, loosening of the glenoid implant was associated with pain (p=0.0001). The causes of glenoid loosening are thought to be multifactorial and include: (a) poor quality and deficient bone stock, (b) poor quality and deficient soft tissue allowing asymmetric shearing forces on the glenoid component either in the vertical or horizontal planes, (c) technical limitations of glenoid preparation and fixation. Prevention of glenoid loosening include: (a) Correct vertical orientation of the glenoid and cuff repair to avoid the vertical rocking horse phenomenon of loosening in the presence of rotator cuff deficiency and (b) Correct horizontal orientation of the glenoid and soft tissue balancing to avoid the horizontal rocking horse phenomenon in the presence of antero-posterior instability. Finally, use of a more anatomical humeral component may be a potential advantage: the correct spatial positioning of the humeral head relative to the humerus results in "bony balancing" which should result in normal glenohumeral kinematics, normal tensioning of soft tissues and decrease abnormal eccentric loads on the glenoid component [13].

Conclusion

Glenoid resurfacing is technically demanding but has become easier because of a better knowledge of normal glenoid anatomy and the patterns of glenoid loss as well as better instrumentation and better design of glenoid components. Technical errors include inadequate glenoid exposure, inadequate removing of peripheral osteophytes, inadequate reaming (excessive or insufficient), component malalignment, poor cementing technique and poor soft-tissue reconstruction and balancing. All these technical errors lead to poor orientation, insufficient bone support and/or overtightened glenohumeral joint. Training the shoulder surgeons in the techniques of glenoid resurfacing is of paramount importance.

References

1. Aliabadi P, Weissman BN (1994) Radiology of total shoulder arthroplasty. In: Friedman RJ (ed) Arthroplasty of the shoulder. Thieme Medical, New York, pp 53–69
2. Amstutz HC, Sew Hoy AL, Clarke IC (1981) UCLA Anatomic total shoulder. Clin Orthop 155:7–20
3. Badet R, Boileau P, Noël E, Walch G (1995) Arthrography and computed arthrotomography study of seventy patients with primary glenohumeral osteoarthritis. Rev Rhum 62(9):555–562

4. Barrett WP, Franklin JL, Jackins SE, Wyss CR, Matsen FA (1987) Total shoulder arthroplasty. J Bone Joint Surg 69Am:865–872
5. Barrett WP, Thornhill TS, Thomas WH, Gebhart EM, Sledge CB (1989) Nonconstrained total shoulder arthroplasty in patients with polyarticular rheumatoid arthritis. J Arthroplasty 4:91–96
6. Bell SN, Gschwend N (1986) Clinical experience with total arthroplasty and hemiarthroplasty of the shoulder using the Neer prosthesis. Int Orthop 10:217–222
7. Bigliani LU, Weinstein DM, Glasgow MT et al (1995) Glenohumeral arthroplasty for arthritis after instability surgery. J Shoulder Elbow Surg 4:87
8. Boyd AD, Thornhill TS, Thomas WH, Scott RD, Sledge CB (1990) Total shoulder replacement vs. hemiarthroplasty: indications for glenoid resurfacing. J Arthroplasty 5:329–336
9. Boyd AD, Thornhill TS, Ewald FC, Scott RD, Sledge CB (1991) Post operative humeral migration in total shoulder replacement: incidence and significance. J Arthroplasty 6:341–337
10. Boyd AD, Thornhill TS (1994) Glenoid resurfacing in shoulder arthroplasty. In: Friedman RJ (ed) Arthroplasty of the shoulder. Thieme, New York, pp 306–316
11. Boileau P, Walch G, Liotard JP, Noel E (1994) Neer shoulder prosthesis: results related to the etiology. Rev Rhum 61:539–547
12. Boileau P, Walch G (1997) Glenoid slope in osteoarthritic and rheumatoid shoulders before and after arthroplasty. J Shoulder Elbow Surg 6:194–195
13. Boileau P, Walch G (1997) The three-dimensional geometry of the proximal humerus. Implications for surgical technique and prosthetic design. J Bone Joint Surg 79Br:857–865
14. Brems JJ (1993) The glenoid component in total shoulder arthroplasty. J Shoulder Elbow Surg 2(1):47–54
15. Burkhead WZ (1994) Cementless shoulder arthroplasty. In: Friedman RJ (ed) Arthroplasty of the shouder. Thieme, New York, pp 281–305
16. Burkhead WZ, Hutton KS (1995) Biologic resurfacing of the glenoid with hemiarthroplasty of the shoulder. J Shoulder Elbow Surg 4:263
17. Clayton ML, Ferlic DC, Jeffers PD (1982) Prosthetic arthroplasties of the shoulder. Clin Orthop 164:184–191
18. Cofield RH (1984) Total shoulder arthroplasty with the Neer prosthesis. J Bone Joint Surg 66A:899–906
19. Cofield RH (1990) Degenerative and arthritic problems of the glenohumeral joint. In: Rockwood CR, Matsen FA (eds) The shoulder. Saunders, Philadelphia, pp 678–742
20. Cofield RH, Edgerton BC (1990) Total shoulder arthroplasty: complications and revision surgery. Instuct Course Lect 39:449–462
21. Cofield RH, Daly J (1992) Total shoulder arthroplasty with a tissue-ingrowth glenoid component. J Shoulder Elbow Surg 1:77–85
22. Cofield RH (1994) Uncemented total shoulder arthroplasty: a review. Clin Orthop 307:86–93
23. Collins DN, Harryman DT II, Lippitt SB, Jackins SE, Matsen FA III (1991) The technique of glenohumeral arthroplasty. Techn Orthop 6:43–59
24. Collins DN, Tencer A, Sidles J, Matsen FA III (1992) Edge displacement and deformation of glenoid components in response to eccentric loading. J Bone Joint Surg 74Am:501–507
25. Connor PM, Flatow EL (1997) Surgical considerations of bony deficiency in total shoulder arthroplasty. In: Warner JJP, Iannotti JP, Gerber C (eds) Complex and revisions problems in shoulder surgery. Lippincot-Raven, Philadelphia, pp 339–354
26. Engelbrecht E, Stellbring G (1976) Total Shoulder endoprosthese Modell "St Georg." Chirurg 47:525–530
27. Figgie HE III, Inglis AE, Golberg VM, Ranawat CS, Figgie MP, Wile JM (1988) An analysis of factors affecting the long term results of total shoulder arthroplasty in inflammatory arthritis. J Arthrop 3:123–130
28. Franklin JL, Jackins SE, Matsen FA (1987) Glenoid loosening in total shoulder arthroplasty: an association with rotator cuff deficiency. J Arthroplasty 3:39–46
29. Friedman RJ, Hawthorne KB, Genez BM (1992) The use of computerized tomography in the measurement of the glenoid version. J Bone Joint Surg Am 74:1032–1037
30. Glasson JM, Djurasovic M, Levine WN, Pollock RG, Flatow EL, Bigliani LU (1996) Hemiarthroplasty for glenohumeral osteoarthritis in patients with an intact rotator cuff: results correlated to degree of glenoid wear. Presented at the American Academy of Orthopaedics Surgeons, annual meeting, Atlanta, Georgia, USA
31. Harryman DT, Sidles JA, Harris SL, Lippitt SB, Matsen FA (1995) The effect of articular conformity and the size of the humeral head component on laxity and motion after gleno-humeral arthroplasty. J Bone Joint Surg Am 77:555–564
32. Harryman DT, Sidles JA, Clark JM, McQuade KS, Matsen FA (1990) Translation of the humeral head on the glenoid with passive gleno-humeral motion. J Bone Joint Surg Am 72A(9):1334–1343
33. Hawkins RJ, Bell RH, Jallay B (1989) Total shoulder arthroplasty Clin Orthop 242:188–194
34. Hawkins RJ, Angelo RL (1990) Glenohumeral osteoarthritis: a late complication of Putti-Platt repair. J Bone Joint Surg Am 72:1193
35. Kelly IG (1994) Unconstrained shoulder arthroplasty in rheumatoid arthritis. Clin Orthop 307:94
36. Lynch NM, Cofield RH, Silbert PL Hermann RC (1996) Neurologic complications after total shoulder arthroplasty. J Shoulder Elbow Surg 5:53–61
37. Matsen FA III, Lippit SB, Sidles JA, Harryman RJ (1994) Practical evaluation and management of the shoulder. Saunders, Philadelphia
38. Moeckel BH, Altchek DW, Warren RF, Wickiewicz TL, Dines DM (1993) Instability of the shoulder after arthroplasty. J Bone Joint Surg Am 75:492–497
39. Morrison DS (1993) Glenoid deficiency in total shouder arthroplasty. In: Bigliani LU (ed) Complications in shoulder surgery. Baltimore, Williams and Wilkins, pp 73–80
40. Muladji AB, Beddow FH, Lamb GHR (1994) CT measurement of glenoid erosion in arthritis. J Bone Joint Surg 76Br:384–388
41. Namba RS, Thornhill TS (1995) Posterior capsulorrhaphy in total shoulder arthroplasty. Clin Orthop 313:135–139
42. Neer CS, Watson KC, Stanton FJ (1982) Recent experience in total shoulder replacement. J Bone Joint Surg Am 64:319–337

43. Neer CS, Kirby RM (1982) Revision of humeral head and total shoulder arthroplasty. Clin Orthop 170:189–195
44. Neer CS, Craig EV, Fukuda H (1983) Cuff-tear arthroplathy. J Bone Joint Surg Am 65:1232
45. Neer CS, Morrison D (1988) Glenoid bone grafting in total shoulder arthroplasty. J Bone Joint Surg Am 70:1154
46. Neer CS (1990) Glenohumeral arthroplasty. In: Neer CS (ed) Shoulder reconstruction. Saunders, Philadelphia, pp 146–271
47. Norris BL, Lachiewicz PF (1996) Modern cement technique and the survivorship of total shoulder arthroplasty. Clin Orthop 328:76–85
48. O'Driscoll SW, Wright TM, Cofield RH (1993) Radiographic analysis of the glenoid component in total shoulder arthroplasty. J Shoulder Elbow Surg 2:S13
49. Orr TE, Carter DR, Shurmann DJ (1988) Stress analyses of glenoid component designs. Clin Orthop 232:217–224
50. Pollock RG, Deliz ED, McIlveen SJ et al (1992) Prosthetic replacement in rotator cuff deficient shoulders. J Shoulder Elbow Surg 1:173–186
51. Rodosky MW, Bigliani LU (1994) Surgical treatment of non-constrained glenoid component failure. Oper Techn Orthop 4:226–236
52. Rodosky MW, Bigliani LU (1996) Indications for glenoid resurfacing in shoulder arthroplasty. J Shoulder Elbow Surg 5:231–248
53. Sneppen O, Fruensgaard S, Johannsen HV, Olsen BS, Söjberg JO, Andersen HH (1996) Total shoulder replacement in rheumatoid arthritis: proximal migration and loosening. J Shoulder Elbow Surg 5:47–52
54. Torchia ME, Cofield RH, Settergren CR (1997) Total schoulder arthroplathy with the Neer prosthesis: long term results. J Shoulder and Elbow Surg 6; 6:495–505
55. Wilde AH, Borden LS, Brems JJ (1984) Experience with the Neer total shoulder replacement. In: Bateman JE, Welsh RP (eds) Surgery of the shoulder. Mosby, St Louis, pp 224–228
56. Walch G, Boileau P, Riand N (1997) Morphological study of the glenoid in primary glenohumral osteoarthritis. J Shoulder Elbow Surg 6:226 (abstract 22)
57. Wirth MA, Rockwood CA (1994) Complications of shoulder arthroplasty. Clin Orthop 307:47
58. Wirth MA, Basamania C, Rockwood CA Jr (1994) Fixation of glenoid component: Keel versus pegs. Oper Tech Orthop 4:218–225
59. Young SW, Lazarus MD, Harryman DT (1996) Practical guidelines to safe surgery about the subscapularis. J Shoulder Elbow Surg 6:467–470

Cemented Glenoid Component: Results in Osteoarthritis and Rheumatoid Arthritis

D. Molé, O. Roche, N. Riand, C. Lévigne, and G. Walch

Summary

This prospective multicentric radiographic analysis examined 146 cemented glenoid components implanted in 109 cases of osteoarthritis (OA) and 37 cases of rheumatoid arthritis (RA) with an average follow-up of 20 months (12–48). The glenoid component was all polyethylene, pear shaped, available in three sizes, with a flat back and fixed by means of a cemented keel. The radiolucent line score (RLL score) was used to quantify the lucent lines and evaluate their progression. A radiographic loosening of the glenoid component (complete lucent line of more than 2 mm and/or RLL score >12) was present in 9% of cases (19% in RA and 6% in OA). Neither continuous lucent lines (51%) nor loosening (9%) was correlated with the functional result, but both were correlated with upward migration of the humeral head. By contrast, progressing lucent lines, present in 31% of cases, were correlated with a worsening of the functional result. The glenoid component tended to be positioned too low (21%), with a superior tilt (12%), with an inferior tilt (17%) and or with excessive retroversion. This study emphasizes the technical difficulties of implantation of a glenoid component (exposure, preparation of the bone, cementing) and the limitations of cemented polyethylene component.

Introduction

The contemporary history of total shoulder arthroplasty only truly began in 1974 with Neer's study of the glenoid component [16, 17]. The promising results achieved in hemi-arthroplasty for fractures, encouraged a widening of the indications for degenerative and inflammatory conditions. Neer recommended the use of a polyethylene glenoid component stressing that, despite the increase in operating time, the functional results of arthroplasty for orthopaedic indications were improved. Since then, numerous studies have confirmed these findings [1, 2, 7, 20, 22].

However, the insertion of the glenoid component can be a source of difficulties and complications. The lack of bone stock limits the fixation possibilities (Fig. 1); exposure of the glenoid is often difficult due to capsulo-ligamentous retraction; the mechanical forces are increased with compressive forces maximal at 90° of lateral elevation equivalent to body weight or seven to ten times arm weight [18]. There are frequent evolving complications, but these are usually only radiographic; the level of lucent lines varies depending on the study from 30%–89% [2, 4, 7, 8, 14, 16, 21, 22]; the level of loosening varies between 0% and 12% [8, 14] in the medium-term but increases with follow-up [8]. These complications are often asymptomatic and the level of revision shoulder arthroplasty is small even though glenoid loosening is the most frequent cause for surgical revision. These numerous complications have led to some abandoning the use of the glenoid component.

The goal of this study was to analyse the conditions in which the glenoid prosthesis was inserted, its effect on the functional outcome and its radiographic appearance at follow-up, using the results from several centres but with just one type of prosthesis: the Aequalis Total Shoulder System (Tornier). The glenoid component is in polyethylene and is

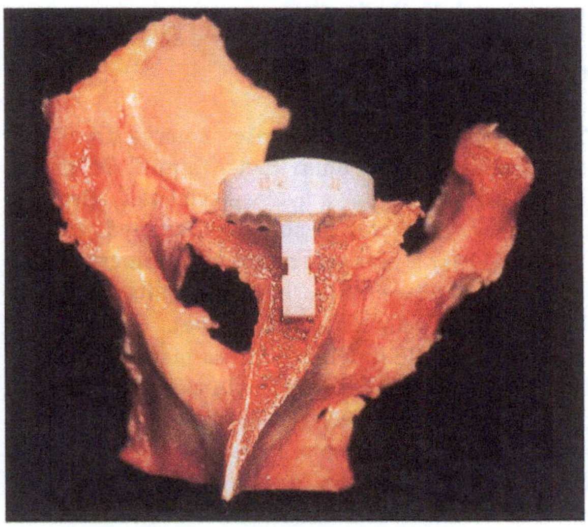

Fig. 1. Frontal anatomical cut with a glenoid in position. Note the brevity of the cancellous pyramid available for fixation and the risks of keel divergence

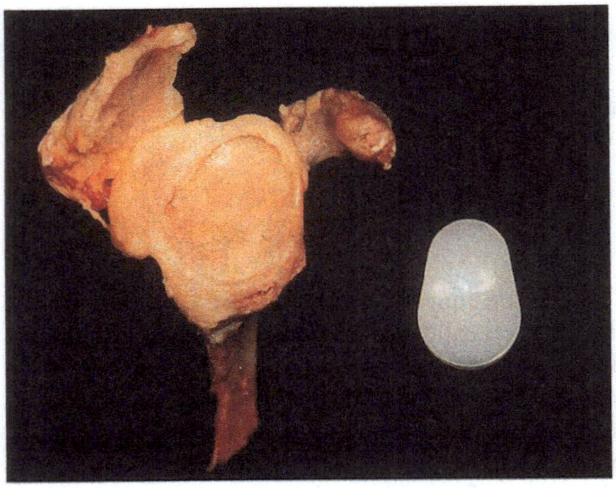

Fig. 2. Pear shape of the polyethylene glenoid adapted to the anatomy of the implantation surface. Comparison of the glenoid anatomy and the implant

cemented, it is pear shaped (Fig. 2), available in three sizes (small, medium and large) and is fixed by means of a perforated keel. We limited this study to cases of osteoathritis (OA) and rheumatoid arthritis (RA) as these two aetiologies are the most common and the number of cases involved allows statistical analysis to be carried out and reliable deductions to be made. We did not ignore the differences in the two pathologies, but nonetheless they do appear to be comparable with regards to the local conditions and their short and medium-term evolution.

Material and Methods

Material

The series consists of 205 cases coming from the 14 hospitals in this multi-centre study. Of these, 163 (79 %) had a polyethylene, cemented glenoid; in 20 cases (10 %) no glenoid was inserted, and in 22 cases (11 %) a new generation of uncemented glenoid was used (see Walch et al., "Results of a New Uncemented Prosthesis", this volume).

There was little difference in the material used in the two aetiologies. Of the 155 OA cases a cemented glenoid was used in 121 (77 %); half of these were medium-sized components; the glenoid was not resurfaced in 9 % and an uncemented glenoid was inserted in 14 %. Of the 50 rheumatoid cases 42 (84 %) had a cemented glenoid, which was the small component in 57 %; the glenoid was not resurfaced in 6 cases (12 %), and an uncemented glenoid was used in 2 (4 %).

Functional Evaluation

All the patients were seen with an average follow-up of 20 months (12–48). A comparative functional evaluation was made between the patients who did not have glenoid resurfacing and those who received a cemented implant. This was done using the Constant score normalised for age and sex [10].

Radiographic Evaluation

All the patients had an AP radiograph taken at follow-up. As with Brems [7], we were, however, faced with the problem of the quality and accuracy of the radiograph which needed to be perfectly square on to the glenoid component to allow analysis of its position and cementing. Overall the radiographic assessment was made on only 146 cases (109 OA and 37 RA). The following criteria were analysed:

The Position of the Glenoid Implant

- A subjective judgement of its position in relation to the equator of the bony glenoid: high, central or low.
- Inclination measured by the inclination angle (Fig. 3): the angle between the vertical plane of the glenoid plateau and the line joining the inferior part of the bony glenoid and the crossing point between the spine of the scapula and the

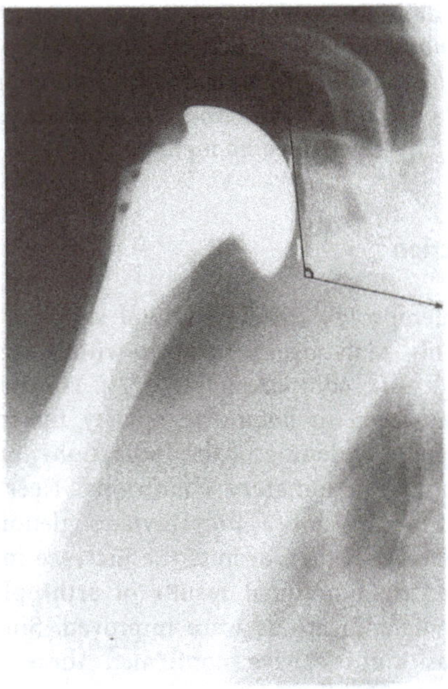

Fig. 3. Measurement of the frontal glenoid inclination angle between the superior and inferior edges of the implant and the lateral border of the scapular at the crossing point with the ribs

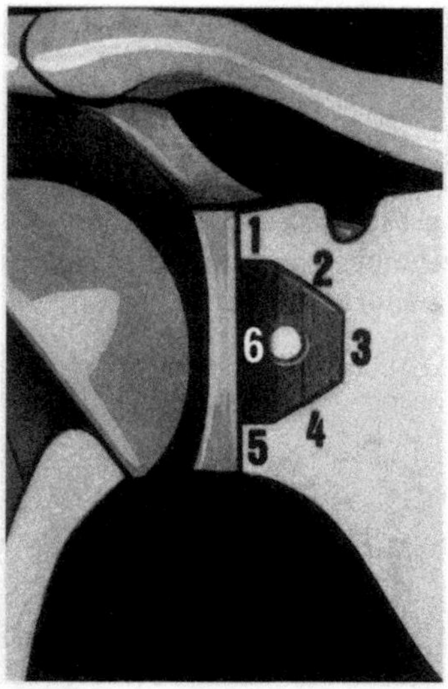

ZONES \ POINTS	< 1 mm (1 point)	1–2 mm (2 points)	> 2 mm (3 points)	RLL SCORE (18 points)
1		x		2
2	x			1
3	x			1
4	x			1
5		x		2
6		x		2

Total = 9/18

Fig. 4. Position of the six zones for measuring lucent lines and example of evaluation of the radio-lucent line (RLL) score (score = 9/18 in this case)

ribs. The glenoid prosthesis was considered as normally inclined when the angle was between the normal limits, established from radiographs of unaffected shoulders, of 90°–120°. The glenoid was inclined upwards when the angle was less than 90° and inclined downwards when the angle was greater than 120°.

Lucent Lines. Their presence was assessed by a single impartial examiner (N.R.) who was not part of the group of surgeons supplying cases for the study. Their position was established using the six zones (Fig. 4) corresponding to numbers 1, 5 and 6 for the upper, lower and middle parts of the tray and to zones 2, 3 and 4 around the periphery of the keel. Their thickness was measured in three grades; grade 1=less than 1 mm, grade 2=between 1 and 2 mm and grade 3=greater than 2 mm. We also calculated the *radiolucent line score (RLL score)* using the six zones and three grades for each patient. This is the sum of each zone involved multiplied by its grade giving a maximum of 18 (Fig. 4). The component is arbitrarily considered as being loose if the score is greater than 12. The relevance of the presence of a lucent line was established by establishing a correlation between the RLL score and the Constant score. In 71 patients for whom successive radiographs were available we were able to judge the evolution of the lucent lines. They were considered to be progressive when the RLL score increased with time, whether this was due to an increased number of zones becoming affected or an increase in the thickness of the existing lines or both.

Statistical Analysis

A statistical analysis was made by Dr. Adeleine of the medical data-processing laboratory of the Civil Hospitals of Lyon on a Compas 386 computer with SPSS software. The statistical test used for the qualitative variables was the χ^2 test and contingency tables with analysis of the residuals. For the quantitative variables, an analysis of variance was used with Scheffe's method of multiple comparison.

Results

Functional Evaluation

The Constant score normalised for age and sex was 92.3 where a glenoid was used (n=163) and was 78.4 where the glenoid was not resurfaced (n=20). This difference was statistically significant and occurred equally in OA (96.8 vs. 81) and in RA (78.7 vs. 70.5).

Radiographic Positioning of the Glenoid Component

Vertical centering proved to be rather approximate, bearing witness to the technical difficulties in exposure. The glenoid was judged to be central in 75% (80% in OA and 61% in RA), high in 4% (2% OA and 9% RA) and low in 21% (18% OA and 30% RA; Fig. 5).

Frontal inclination determined by measuring the angle between the glenoid prosthesis and the scapular spine was only within normal limits in 71%

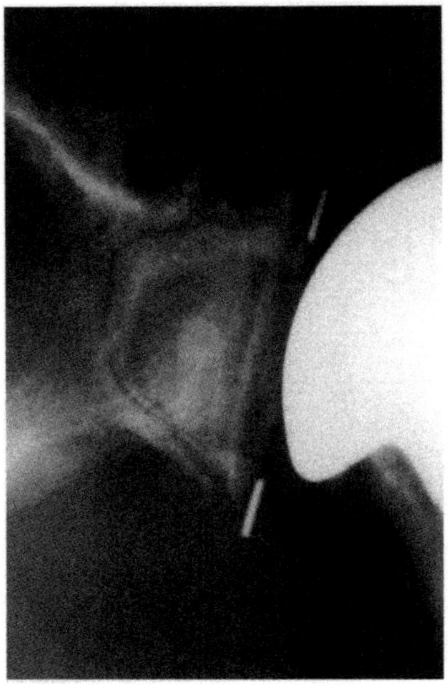

Fig. 5. Low glenoid. Note the inferior offset of the metal insert

(75% in OA and 64% in RA; Fig. 6). The glenoid was inclined downwards and outwards (open angle >120°) in 17% (14% OA and 23% in RA) and inclined upwards and outwards in 12% (11% in OA and 13% in RA).

In the absence of sufficient numbers of reproducible and reliable lateral radiographs we were not able to judge centering and inclination horizontal to the glenoid. Several examples, however, allow us to predict an increased risk of a posterior inclination of the glenoid implant when the glenoid is retroverted or worn posteriorly (Fig. 7). It is always possible to pierce the anterior cortex of the glenoid neck with the keel of the prosthesis, but this does not seem to have any mechanical or functional consequences with at least a short-term follow-up.

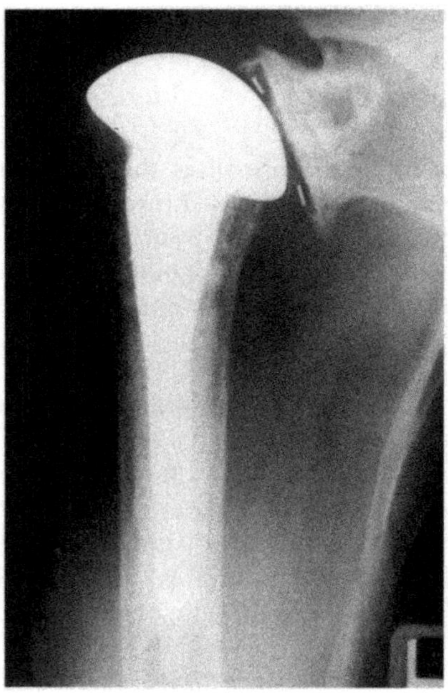

Fig. 6. Abnormal frontal glenoid inclination. The implant is orientated downwards and outwards

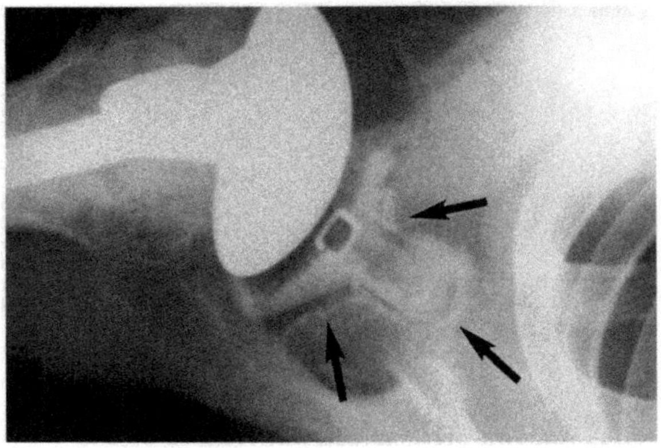

Fig. 7. Axillary view. Glenoid positioned with posterior tilt with perforation of the anterior cortex of the glenoid neck by the keel

Radiographic Lucent Lines

At review RLL were present, without detailing their spread or thickness, in 92% of cases (91% in OA and 97% in RA).

The division into the six zones of bone-implant contact (Table 1) shows that the lucencies occurred, in order of frequency, in the lower part of the glenoid (90.4%), the middle part of the tray (88.4%), the upper part of the glenoid (81.5%) and the keel with the same gradient of frequency in both aetiologies. The lucent lines appeared to be continuous for the whole length of the implant in 51% of cases (48% in OA and 61% in RA).

The thickness of the lucent line varied depending on its position. The division of grades depending on

Table 1. Frequency of RLL by zone and aetiology

	OA (*n*=109)		RA (*n*=37)		Total (*n*=146)	
Zone	*n*	%	*n*	%	*n*	%
1	84	77	35	95	119	81.5
2	62	57	29	78	91	62.3
3	61	56	24	65	85	58.2
4	76	70	25	68	101	69.1
5	97	89	35	95	132	90.4
6	93	85	36	97	129	88.4

Table 2. Size of Radio lucent lines (RLL) by zone (percentages)

Zone	Grade 1 (<1 mm)	Grade 2 (1–2 mm)	Grade 3 (>2 mm)	Total
1	63.0	14.3	4.2	81.5
2	49.3	9.9	3.1	62.3
3	46.6	8.4	3.1	58.2
4	56.9	8.4	3.8	69.1
5	56.9	21	12.5	90.4
6	59.8	21.9	6.7	88.4

Table 3. Radio lucent lines (RLL) score by aetiology (percentages)

RLL score	OA	RA	Global
<6	64	62	64
6–12	30	19	27
>12	6	19	9
Mean/18	5.96	7.30	6.29

the zones affected (Table 2) shows that it is in zones 1 and 5 (upper and lower parts of the glenoid) and in zone 6 (tray) that the greatest number of lucent lines thicker than 1 mm are to be found.

The RLL score (Table 3) was 6.29 out of 18 on average and was slightly higher in RA than in OA, which is evidence of the greater fragility of the cementing in this condition. A score greater than or equal to 12 is considered as being equivalent to loosening and the rate of loosening was 9 % (19 % in RA and 6 % in OA) or 13 cases. There were two migrations of the implant or 1.4 % of the total series (one for each pathology), and only one case was revised with simple removal of the component (a revision for glenoid loosening rate of 0.7 %).

Correlations

This large series allowed an extensive search into factors predicting the outcome of lucent lines. The review data records the main points of the preoperative state, the intervention, and the clinical and radiographic information at follow-up. All these were correlated with the lucent line score without demonstrating any apparent influence. A closer analysis dividing the six zones, always showed a correlation between vertical centering of the humeral head at follow-up with lucency in zone 5 (inferior). Whatever the aetiology concerned the lucent line was absent or less than 1 mm in 68 of the 98 cases where the head remained central (70 %) and in 19 of the 36 heads which had migrated upwards at follow-up (53 %). The lucent line was between 1 and 2 mm or greater than 2 mm in 30 % of cases where the head was central, in 47 % of those where the head had migrated upwards (p=0.02). Note that, conversely, the difference was not statistically significant in an analysis of rotator cuff tears.

The presence, distribution and thickness of a radiographic para-glenoid lucent line at follow-up had no effect on the functional result. The average Constant score varied only very slightly depending on the RLL score (Table 4).

The 71 % of patients who had successive radiographs allowed the evolution of the lucent lines with time to be judged. The lucency was progressive in 22 cases (31 %: 29 % in OA and 35 % in RA): they were stable with time in 49 patients (69 %). Progression is statistically correlated as having a prejudicial effect on the functional result. The average Constant score was 85.2 where there was a progressive lucency (92.4 in OA and 78.8 in RA) but was 96.9 when this was stable (99.6 in OA and 88.2 in RA).

Table 4. Functional impairment by Radio lucent lines (RLL) score

RLL score	Pain/15	Constant score
<6 (64 %)	12.8	95.8
6–12 (27 %)	12.5	92.5
>12 (9 %)	12.7	89.7

Discussion

Total Versus Hemiarthroplasty

The use of a glenoid component when carrying out a shoulder replacement is technically demanding, increasing the operating time and exposing the patient to the risks and complications specific to the glenoid. It is however, necessary for reestablishing the gleno-humeral lever arms, which is needed to get a good functional result [11]. This series confirms that the functional results achieved with a total arthroplasty are better than with a hemi-arthroplasty [4, 5]. The results are superior for all the parameters of the functional outcome (pain, mobility) and occur in both the aetiologies studied (OA and RA). Despite that, for some authors, the difference is only apparent in RA with the results being the same in OA [5]. The results obtained after a hemi-arthroplasty are, however, satisfactory with an average, adjusted Constant score of 78.4 %. This justifies not using a glenoid implant when the operative conditions or morphology merit this decision even if the insertion of a glenoid component seems necessary with this anatomical prosthesis to give the maximal outcome (Constant score of 92.3).

Any comparative conclusion must be tempered by the fact that this is a retrospective study. A bias may exist in this study because the choice between a hemi- and a total shoulder arthroplasty was dependent on the severity of the cases. In RA a hemiarthroplasty was sometimes chosen because of the severity of the destruction of the glenoid. Preoperative glenoid destruction more than the absence of glenoid component may explain the less favourable results observed in this aetiology. In OA the surgeon chosen a hemiarthroplasty in two different circumstances: in case of destruction of the glenoid bone stock because it was technically impossible or in case of where the glenoid erosion was judged to be minimal. The prognostic is obviously different in these two situations.

Radiographic Positioning of the Glenoid Component

Radiographic analysis of the position of the glenoid component confirms the technical difficulties in its implantation and allows the specific risks to be stressed. *In the frontal plane*, the prosthesis was centered vertically with regard to the equator of the glenoid in only 75 % of cases. There was a tendency to positioning the implant to low (21 %) and more often in RA. The reason for this is no doubt a fault in exposing the upper part of the glenoid. The risk is that the stabilising effect on the keel coming from the upper part of the cancellous pyramid and the floor of the coracoid will be lost. The vertical positioning has no effect on function or on the radiographic congruency of the gleno-humeral joint.

Radiographic determination of the frontal inclination of the glenoid is difficult. Brems [7] stressed the non-reproducibility of the radiographic views which differed depending on the rotation of the thorax or the upper limb, pain and muscular contraction and the angle of the beam [3]. Standardisation of the radiographic techniques using large format radiographs and metal markers [3] would seem necessary to precisely analyse this inclination which certainly has some effect on the AP stability of the prosthetic joint and on the future appearance of lucent lines. We used the angle between the prosthesis and the lateral border of the scapula which can be criticised as being unvalidated. However, it does do away with just relying on a subjective impression.

Muladji [15] and Boileau [3] were interested in the variation of the site of wear on the glenoid as seen on the vertical plane, with relation to the aetiology. These authors agree that in RA there is a preference for superior wear whereas in OA Muladji judges the wear to be central, and Boileau suggests that it is central and inferior. In our series the radiographic study at follow-up refocused our attention on position because the glenoid appeared to be correctly aligned in only 71 % of the cases. In 12 % the glenoid was inclined upwards which may be linked to a preferential superior erosion. This position is, for Boileau [3] the least favourable as, with time, it exposes the prosthesis to eccentration of the humeral head and sub-acromial impingement. In 17 % the glenoid was abnormally inclined downwards and outwards: this may be due to technical difficulties with the exposure in the same way that results in a low glenoid.

The inferior part of the glenoid is easier to expose, and the reamers are more easily positioned and therefore can be used more aggressively here. In RA errors in frontal inclination of the glenoid component are more frequent than in OA and also have a greater consequence due to the fact that the cuff is a less effective stabiliser in that condition. Sneppen [21] recorded that 51 % had upward migration of the humeral component after 7 years and judged this eccentricity as being responsible for 40 % of glenoid loosenings. Shoulder arthroplasty, as with other joint replacement, requires a detailed preoperative appreciation of the shape of the glenoid and proper planning of the surgical intervention.

In the horizontal plane, we did not have the necessary radiographic information to assess the position and inclination of the glenoid component. Our knowledge of the preponderance of posterior wear, all aetiologies combined [15, 19, 20], the frequency with which excessive retroversion causes susceptibility to OA [12] and the few examples available to us with lateral radiography or preoperative computed tomography show that the risk is unequivocally for excessive posterior inclination. This may be accompanied by perforation of the anterior cortex by the keel and cement [19, 20]. It should not go unacknowledged and equally justifies preoperative computed tomography and systematic preoperative planning as well as the surgical control of the anterior face of the neck of the glenoid. It has not yet been shown that excessive posterior retroversion carries an increased risk of postoperative posterior subluxation of the humeral head or of glenoid loosening.

Lucent Lines

The assessment of the lucent lines is the principle step in the radiographic analysis of the glenoid component. The definition of a lucent line is currently limited to a radiographic one: a black and radiotransparent line situated, as a rule, at the bone-cement interface [7, 16, 22]. Arthrography has not shown any diffusion of the contrast medium into the lucency [14]. Between 69% and 94% of lucent lines are present on the immediate postoperative radiographs which indicates a fault in the cementing and the persistence of a layer of haematoma at the interface. In contrast, the presence of a lucent line around the keel, in continuity throughout the interface, with a thickness greater than 2 mm and showing progression [21] may lead to glenoid loosening [2, 7, 21, 22]. The frequency of para-glenoid lucencies is assessed in different ways in the literature [8] giving proportions between 30% [16] and 89% [22].

In our study a lucent line was judged as being present in 92% of cases using a standardised interpretation made by one examiner different from the surgeons. These differences are more due to the hardness of the interpretation or the type of implant, technique or aetiology. The glenoid components used in this series were flat, and we must emphasized that all the prosthesis cases were implanted without ancillary material for the glenoid. The reamers, actually used to flatten the glenoid were not available at the beginning of our experience, and we had to use a burr. Consequently the surface of the bone was probably not as flat as required to allow perfect contact between the implant and the glenoid [9]. This is an important point which could explain the rate of radiolucency specially under the flange (Fig. 8).

The site of the lucent lines has already been described by Wilde [22] using three zones (tray, proximal and distal sections of the keel) and by Franklin [14] using five classes (site and thickness). We defined six zones within which the presence of a lucent line would seem to have a different mechanical effect: zone 1 is the upper pole of the tray where exposure can be difficult and the bone quality mediocre, zones 2–4 correspond to the keel – the principle fixation sites, zone 5 corresponds to the lower part of the glenoid which is easily exposed and of good mechanical quality but does undergo forces in tilting [14], finally zone 6 corresponds to the middle part of the tray directly above the keel.

The lucent lines were continuous in 51% of the cases in this series, which is about a middle value of continuous lucent lines as described in the literature (36%) for Barrett [2], 41% for Brems [7], 60% for Sneppen [21] and 68% for Wilde [22]). Whenever the lucent line is not in continuity, the main zones affected are 1, 5 and 6 (Fig. 8) where a lucency was present in almost all of the cases (Table 1). This may bring into question the use of cement on the tray when the layer of cement here is thinner when the reaming has been properly carried out and the glenoid properly applied to the bone surface [9]. The gradient of elasticity between polyethylene, cement and sub-chondral bone means that the apparition of a lucent line is almost inevitable. Wilde [22] emphasised the presence of a lucent line in zone 6 on the postoperative radiographs in 75% of cases.

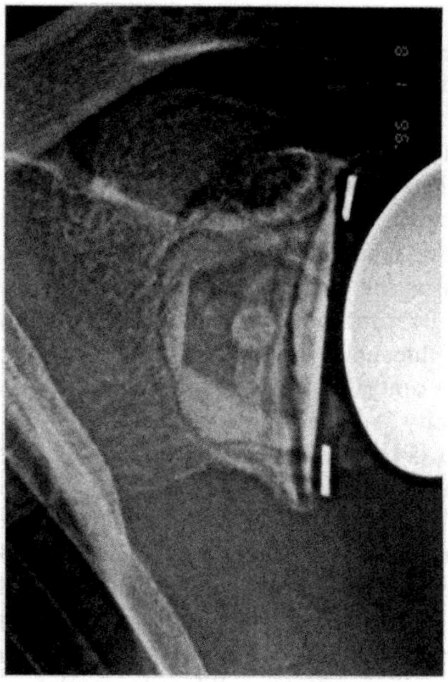

Fig. 8. Continuous lucent line throughout the length of the implant (RLL score 13). Note the size of the lucency in zone 6

The thickness of the lucent line, admittedly measured in an approximate way, is an important criteria in assessing its significance [7]. In agreement with most authors we differentiated three grades of thickness and it was in zone 5 (inferior) that we most often found substantial lucencies with thickness greater than 1 or 2 mm (grade 2 and 3).

The Radio Lucent Lines Score

The RLL score (0–18) is a numeric assessment of the importance of the radiographic lucency and includes its spread and thickness. It corresponds to the addition of the thickness gradings (0=no lucency, 1=less than 1 mm, 2=between 1 and 2 mm and 3=greater than 2 mm) for each of the zones where a line is present (Fig. 4). The score is zero where there is no lucency and is 18 where there is a continuous lucency greater than 2 mm thick. The average score in this series was 6.29. The RA score was 7.3 and greater than the 5.96 in OA which translates as a greater susceptibility to loosening in this pathology as already reported by others [21]. The quantification of the lucent lines using the RLL score is of triple interest in allowing statistical research into predictive factors and their correlation with radiographic and clinical findings, in analysing the progression of lucencies and their effect and in defining the level of loosening.

There was no apparent correlation between the RLL score and the preoperative data, the surgical findings or the clinical or radiographic signs at follow-up. By contrast, we found a statistically raised level of lucencies in zone 5 when there was an error in centralising the prosthesis and a superior eccentricity of the humeral head seen at review. Franklin [14] and Barrett [2] established a relationship between cuff tears and glenoid lucencies linked to the "rocking-horse effect" on the glenoid caused by an ascending humeral head. However, Boyd [6] and Sneppen [21] found that the state of the cuff had no influence on glenoid loosening. Despite its size our series did not allow us to conclude. The existence of a cuff tear did not correlate with the RLL scores nor with the presence of a lucency in the inferior zone. Superior humeral migration is sometimes independent of the state of the cuff and may be caused by glenoid tilt rather than causing it.

The lucent lines appeared to be progressive in 31 % of cases of the patients who had sequential radiographs for analysis. This progression is accompanied by a significant prejudicial effect on the functional result. Boyd [4] and Sneppen [21] have already stressed the absence of a radiographic or clinical correlation between lucent lines and functional outcome. The overall analysis of our series supports this impression. However, a distinction should be made between progressive and non-progressive lucent lines as the former are accompanied by a worsening in the clinical result and may be translated towards glenoid loosening.

Glenoid Loosening

Glenoid loosening is the principle complication in total shoulder arthroplasty and one of the most frequent causes of revision [7, 8]. The risk of loosening is the major deciding factor in the use of a glenoid component, in its design and fixation. However, the level of loosening is described in different ways whether one looks at the radiographic appearance or the clinical signs. Assessed by the size of the glenoid lucent line and without any radiographic-clinical correlation the level of loosening was evaluated as 12 % by Boyd [4], at 38.6 % by Brems [7] in a meta-analysis of 1413 prostheses with a follow-up greater than 5 years, at 44 % by Cofield [8] in the series with the longest follow-up of about 10 years. This level is high and seems to progress even if loosening is a long way from meaning that they require a systematic revision. In fact the level of revision for glenoid loosening is established at 1.9 % by Cofield [8] in a meta-analysis of 1459 prostheses, at 2.9 % by Brems [7] and at 5.3 % by Cofield in the oldest series. Glenoid loosening is therefore a frequent complication but is usually well tolerated [21]. In our series we arbitrarily decided that radiographic glenoid loosening occurred when the RLL score was greater than 12. The level was 9 % but the follow-up time is short. The use of the RLL score allows accurate analysis of progression with time. Currently there is no correlation between radiographic glenoid loosening and the functional result (Table 4). In 2 cases (1.4 %) the glenoid implant has migrated and only one patient (0.7 %) has undergone revision for glenoid loosening.

Conclusion

The glenoid component is the weak link in shoulder arthroplasty. In this series, as in others, the results for total arthroplasty were better than for hemiarthroplasty. However, whether it is for OA or RA, if the local conditions are unfavourable to its insertion then the glenoid can be dispensed with and the results remain acceptable.

The result is in part conditioned by the technique of implantation. Stringent preoperative planning should avoid errors in insertion especially those of centering the implant (risk of a low glenoid) and in horizontal inclination (risk of posterior tilt). In the horizontal plane the risk is of posterior inclination where there is predominant posterior wear and a knowledge of the shape of the glenoid allows the keel to be positioned properly and usually by preferential anterior reaming avoid the need for a bone graft which was required only once in this series.

Lucent lines were more frequent than in other series due to the severity of the radiographic analysis giving an average RLL score of 6.29 which is equivalent to a continuous lucent line of 1 mm. We could not demonstrate any predictive element in the presence of lucent lines. As with others, although we did not analyse our immediate postoperative radiographs. We believe that a number of these lucencies are already present as the patient leaves operating room and the technique of exposure, reaming and cementing all have to be considered. The use of the RLL score seems to be useful in quantifying the lucent lines and evaluating their progression. Loosening appears to be rare (9 %) and with no clinical presentation. In contrast, in 31 % of the cases with sequential radiographs, the lucency was the site of a worrying progression which does correlate with a worsening of the functional result.

This series is limited by the short follow-up (20 months) and can be considered as a preliminary report. At this stage the results of the glenoid prosthesis are good and certainly superior to those with hemi-arthroplasty but must still face the test of time. The frequency of radiographic lucent lines is worrying even though they have no clinical effect, except when they progress. A glenoid component is the preferred option but the cemented polyethylene implant has its limitations and the road is open for the use of other designs.

References

1. Amstutz HC, Sew Hoy AL, Clarke IC (1981) UCLA Anatomic total shoulder. Clin Orthop 155:7–20
2. Barrett WP, Franklin JL, Jackins SE, Wyss CR, Matsen FA (1987) Total shoulder arthroplasty. J Bone Joint Surg Am 69:965–972
3. Boileau P, Walch G (1997) Glenoid slope in osteoarthritic and rheumatoid shoulders before and after arthroplasty. J Shoulder Elbow Surg 6:194–195
4. Boyd AD, Thornhill TS (1994) Glenoid resurfacing in shoulder arthroplasty. In: Friedman RJ (ed) Arthroplasty of the shoulder. Thieme Medical, New York
5. Boyd AD, Thornhill TS, Thomas WH, Scott RD, Sledge CB (1990) Total shoulder replacement versus hemiarthroplasty: Indications for glenoid resurfacing. J Arthroplasty 5:329–336
6. Boyd AD, Thornhill TS, Ewald FC, Scott RD, Sledge CB (1991) Post operative humeral migration in total shoulder replacement: incidence and significance. J Arthroplasty 6:341–337
7. Brems J (1993) The glenoid component in total shoulder arthroplasty. J Elbow Surg 2:47–54
8. Cofield RH (1994) Long term results with the Neer prosthesis. Presented at the annual SECEC Meeting, Barcelona
9. Collins D, Tencer A, Sidles J, Matsen FA (1992) Edge displacement and deformation of glenoid components in response to eccentric loading. J Bone Joint Surg Am 74:501–507
10. Constant CR, Murley AH (1987) A clinical method of functional assessment of the shoulder. Clin Orthop 214:160–4
11. Engelbrecht E, Stellbring G (1976) Total Shulter endoprosthese Modell "St Georg." Chirurg 47:525–530
12. Figgie HE, Inglis AE, Goldberg VM et al (1988) An analysis of factors affecting the long term results of total shoulder arthroplasty in inflammatory arthritis. J Arthroplasty 3:123–130
13. Friedman RJ, Hawthorne KB, Genez BM (1992) The use of computerized tomography in the measurement of the glenoid version. J Bone Joint Surg Am 74:1032–1037
14. Franklin JL, Barrett WP, Jackins SE, Matsen FA (1988) Glenoid loosening in total shoulder arthroplasty. J Arthroplasty 3:39–46
15. Muladji AB, Beddow FH, Lamb GHR (1994) Ct measurement of glenoid erosion in arthritis. J Bone Joint Surg Br 76:384–388
16. Neer CS (1974) Replacement arthroplasty for glenohumeral osteoarthritis. J Bone Joint Surg Am 56:1–13
17. Neer CS, Watson KC, Stanton FJ (1982) Recent experience in total shoulder replacement. J Bone Joint Surg Am 64:319–337
18. Poppen NK, Walker PS (1978) Forces at the glenohumeral joint in abduction. Clin Orthop 135:165–170
19. Rodosky MW, Bigliani LU (1994) Surgical treatment of non-constrained glenoid component failure. Oper Techn Orthop 4:226–236
20. Rodosky MW, Bigliani LU (1996) Indications for glenoid resurfacing in shoulder arthroplasty. J Shoulder Elbow Surg 5:231–248
21. Sneppen O, Fruensgaard S, Johannsen HV, Olsen BS, Söjberg JO, Andersen HH (1996) Total shoulder replacement in rheumatoid arthritis: proximal migration and loosening. J Shoulder Elbow Surg 5:47–52
22. Wilde AH, Borden LS, Brems JJ (1984) Experience with the Neer total shoulder replacement. In: Bateman JE, Welsh RP (eds) Surgery of the shoulder. Mosby, St. Louis, pp 224–228

Results of a New Uncemented Glenoid Component

G. Walch, P. Boileau, and N. Riand

Summary

We report preliminary results using a new uncemented component: the Aequalis metal-backed glenoid (Tornier). The originality of this implant lies in a new anchorage device that uses an expanded screw system. There are two such screws which insert through the tray, and each consists of three hooked leaflets that open progressively into the cancellous bone as the screw thread is turned. The two main advantages of this implant are: (a) a strong primary bone fixation which allows a secondary bone ingrowth in the metal tray; (b) a minimum thickness of metal for the tray, avoiding lateralisation and overstuffing of the joint. We operated on 15 shoulders in 15 patients (9 osteoarthritis, 3 posttraumatic arthritis, 2 rheumatoid arthritis, and 1 osteonecrosis) with this new uncemented glenoid component and reviewed the results at a minimum 2-year follow-up (average 25.9 months). The absolute Constant score increased from 18.7 points (10–32 points) to 69.4 points postoperatively (49–82 points). All the glenoid components were osteointegrated without lucent lines, except in two cases (14 %). We report one complication: an early traumatic disassociation after anterior dislocation with rupture of the subscapularis 6 weeks postoperation. This series compares favourably with other published series and justifies our continuing with the component.

Introduction

Long-term fixation of prosthesis to bone remains a dream for orthopaedic surgeons. Cementless fixation for arthroplasty is not a new concept and has been used in the hip and the knee for many years. However, experience with cementless fixation for shoulder arthroplasty remains limited [2, 4–6, 8, 9].

Due to the disappointingly high percentage of lucent lines seen with the cemented Neer glenoid component in our experience, we developed an uncemented glenoid prosthesis with a porous surface to encourage bony ingrowth.

Design Rationale

The prosthesis consists of two parts: metal tray and polyethylene insert. The metal tray is flat backed with an hydroxyapatite coating (Fig. 1). The surface is made in diamond-shaped points with a depth of 0.15 mm and point separation of 1 mm. The tray is 3 mm thick, and this depth has been reduced to the minimum possible to avoid creating excess tension on the cuff and to prevent lateralisation of the articular surface. This was possible due to a new anchorage device which uses an expanding screw system that does not have the thick head required with a normal screw. There are two such screws which insert through the tray, and each consists of three hooked leaflets that open progressively into the cancellous bone as the screw-thread is turned. Their role is to provide primary component stability until biological fixation occurs as the hydroxyapatite surface integrates with the underlying bone. The second part of the implant is the polyethylene insert which click-fits onto the tray and is 4 mm deep at its central point (Fig. 2). The thickness of the glenoid component is 7 mm in total (3 mm of metal tray and 4 mm of polyethylene).

The prosthesis is available in three sizes (small, medium and large) which have increasing radii of curvature to adapt to the different sizes of humeral head. The radii of curvature are greater than those of the humeral heads and leave the surgeon the option to select any glenoid component regardless

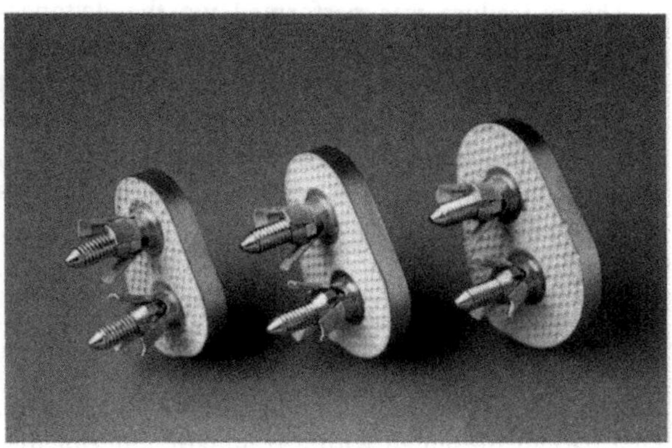

Fig. 1. Hydroxyapatite-coated metal tray available in three sizes

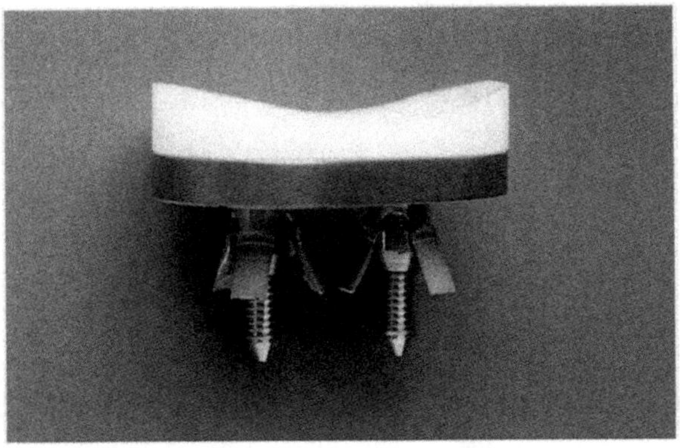

Fig. 2. Glenoid prosthesis with polyethylene insert and expansion screws

of the humeral head size. Even the smallest glenoid can be matched with the largest head.

Clinical Experience

Between December 1993 and April 1994, the two senior authors (P.B. and G.W.) implanted 15 components in 15 patients. There were 9 cases of osteoarthritis, 3 of posttraumatic arthritis, 2 of rheumatoid arthritis and 1 of avascular necrosis. There were 13 women and 2 men with an average age of 70.4 years (57–86). The dominant side was involved in 63 %.

The average preoperative absolute Constant score was 18.7 points (10–32) and the normalised average was 26 % (14 %–45 %). Preoperative passive anterior elevation was 93.6° (70°–150°). Actively this was 77° (30°–150°) and external rotation was 0° (–20° to 20°). The supraspinatus tendon was unaffected in 11 cases, was partially ruptured in 1 and had a full thickness tear in 3. Associated interventions included an acromioplasty with a cuff repair, three tenodeses of the long head of biceps and one subscapularis Z-plasty.

The procedure was performed via the deltopectoral approach and using the Aequalis humeral component in all cases. The patients were followed up at 3, 6, 12 and 24 months. A Constant score was evaluated systematically, and AP radiographs in neutral, internal and external rotation and axillary views were taken.

Results

All the patients had a minimum follow-up of 2 years. One patient presented with a traumatic anterior dislocation which occurred while being positioned for an axillary view radiograph 6 weeks postoperatively. The relocation caused disassociation of the polyethylene insert and scratches on the humeral surface. The patient underwent revision surgery in which the entire prosthesis was changed and a cemented glenoid inserted. Thirteen patients were reviewed with radiographs 1 and 2 years postoperation; one was reviewed after 1 year with radiographs but sent back a questionnaire and a radiograph at the 2-year appointment. Fourteen patients were therefore available for the 2-year review. The average follow-up time was 25.8 months (24 to 29). The absolute Constant score was 69.4 points (49–82), and the normalised score for age and sex was 97.5 % (56 %–110 %). Nine patients were very satisfied and 5 were satisfied with the outcome.

On the radiographs taken after 24 months there were no humeral lucencies, but two glenoid lucent lines were observed (14 %). The first of these was apparent immediately postoperatively and was due to poor positioning of the tray because too much cancellous graft had been put between the tray and the prepared bony surface of the glenoid. The most recent radiographs taken at 27 months showed a progressive regression of this lucent line (Fig. 3). In the second case the lucent line became apparent on the 1-year radiographs in a patient who had required osteotomies of both tuberosities during an operation to treat the sequelae of a fracture. On the postoperative radiographs the greater tuberosity showed lysis, the head was subluxed upwards, and there was a lucent line beneath the metal tray (Fig. 4). This lucency had evolved on the 1- and 2-year postoperative radiographs. There were no other lucencies seen in the other 12 cases, and these demonstrated perfect integration with the metal tray (Fig. 5).

Discussion

The first unconstrained uncemented glenoid component was designed by English and MacNab in 1976. The component had a porous surface and two screws to give primary fixation while waiting for bony ingrowth. A polyethylene insert clicked onto the tray. Thirteen cases were reviewed in 1987 [2] by MacElwain who reported one patient with a loose glenoid and lucent lines around the screws, but the percentages were not given.

Since 1981 Cofield has been using an uncemented glenoid and between 1983 and 1986 he implanted 32 porous coated [3]. A central plug and two peripheral screws gave primary stability. The patients were reviewed at an average of 51 months (29–80). He reported two disassociations between the insert and the tray (6 %) as well as 26 % with incomplete

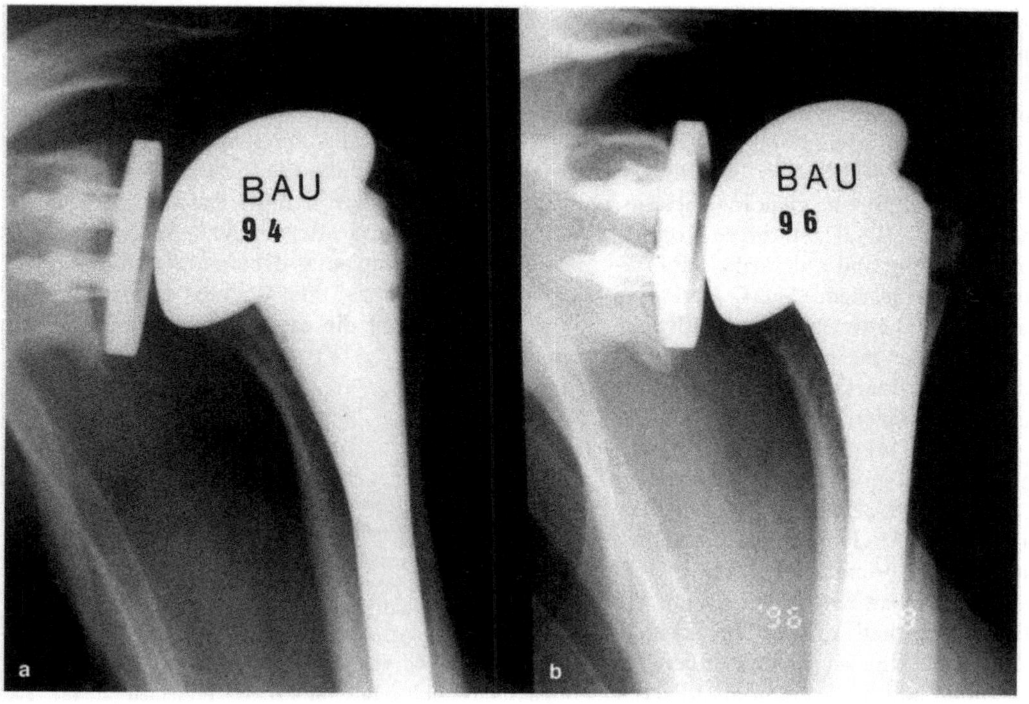

Fig. 3. Postoperative glenoid lucent line (**a**) which had disappeared on the 2-year radiograph (**b**)

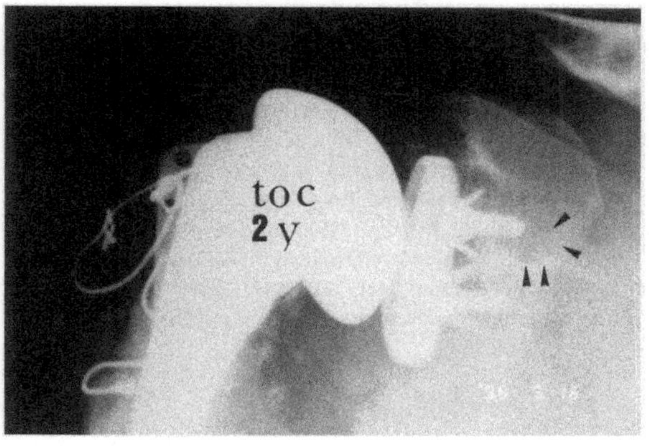

Fig. 4. Evolving glenoid lucent line

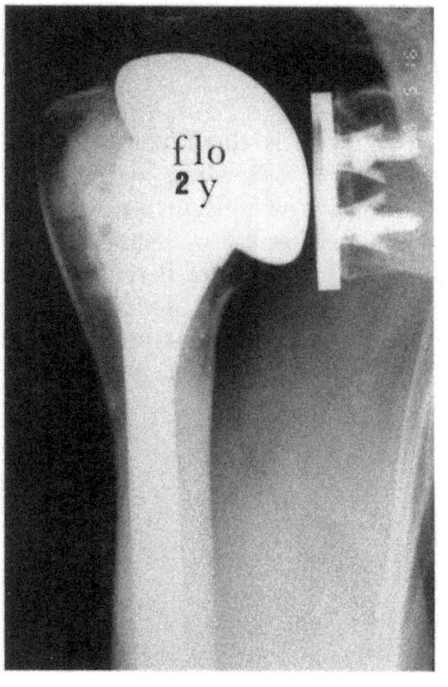

Fig. 5. Radiograph 2 years postoperation showing good integration with the metal tray

or interrupted lucent lines less than 1 mm, and 22 % with complete lucent lines of which 3 were greater than 1.5 mm and can therefore be considered as loose (9 %). He stopped using this implant in 1986 and modified the design. His second series using this modified implant ran from 1989 to 1993 and involved 180 cases [4]. With a 1- to 5-year follow-up he has reported two disassociations (1 %), three complete posterior erosions of the polyethylene insert (1.5 %) which required revision, six complete lucent lines (3 %) and one loose glenoid implant (0.5 %).

Copeland also uses an uncemented glenoid which originally was in polyethylene with a central plug. This was later modified to a conical plug and a metal back which press-fits into the glenoid. In 1990 the results for the polyethylene component only were reported and there were no loosenings at a 15-month follow-up [5].

Roper and Day have also designed an uncemented glenoid component with a central plug. Only 13 have been implanted without cement, but there appear to be only one loosening requiring revision after an average 5-year follow-up (minimum 1.5 years) [8].

The Select Shoulder was designed by Burkhead in 1987 and had various different glenoid implants. Eighty-nine uncemented, metal reinforced components with a porous coating and a primary stabilisation screw have been inserted. There were five reported disassociations between the polyethylene tray and the metal base in the first year, which led to it being taken off the market before the results in the other cases were known.

Martin and Thornhill [6] recently reported the results of an uncemented glenoid component (Kirschner II C) which has a plasma sprayed metal back and two screws to give primary stability. Between 1988 and 1991, 59 operations were carried out and followed-up with an average of 42 months (3–6 years). One patient had suffered breakage of the metal tray, and one of the screws and underwent revision while another had an asymptomatic screw breakage. In 29 % there was a non-evolving lucent line greater than 1.5 mm. There were no loosenings, migrations or polyethylene wear at this follow-up.

Conclusion

Although our series is small, consisting of only 15 cases with a short follow-up, we believe that the introduction of a new concept justifies the analysis of the preliminary results. A regular annual review is planned. It is unfortunate that the English-MacNab, Roper-Day and Select implants seem to have been forgotten about such that no benefit is gained by learning from any reported problems.

All our cases had a minimum 2-year follow-up, and we report one early traumatic disassociation (6 %) and two lucencies (14 %). This series compares favourably with other published series and justifies our continuing with the component. Only an annual review of our cases allows us to confirm that the results remain good with time. For the moment we can say that, 2 years after surgery, many polyethylene cemented implants demonstrate radiological lucent lines whereas this is only apparent in a small percentage of the cases with this uncemented implant.

References

1. Boileau P, Walch G, Noel E, Liotard JP (1994) Neer shoulder prosthesis. Outcome according to the shoulder disease. Rev Rhum Engl Ed 61:537–547
2. Burkhead W (1995) Cementless shoulder arthroplasty. In: Friedman RJ (ed) Arthroplasty of the shoulder. Thieme, Stuttgart, pp 281–305
3. Cofield RH (1994) Total shoulder arthroplasty: results complications and future directions. Presented at the 8th Annual Meeting of the European Society for Shoulder and Elbow Surgery. Barcelona, 16–18 June
4. Cofield RH, Daly PJ (1992) Total shoulder arthroplasty with a tissue-ingrowth glenoid component. J Shoulder Elbow Surg 1:77
5. Copeland S (1990) Cementless total shoulder replacement. In: Post M, Morrey BF, Hawkins RJ (eds) Surgery of the shoulder. St Louis, Mosby-Year Book, pp 289–297
6. Martin SD, Sledge CB, Thomas WH, Thornhill T (1996) Total shoulder arthrosplasty with an uncemented glenoid component. J Shoulder Elbow Surg 5:53
7. McElwain JP, English E (1987) The early results of porous-coated total shoulder arthroplasty. Clin Orthop 218:217
8. Roper BA, Paterson JMH, Day WH (1990) The Roper-Day total shoulder replacement. J Bone Joint Surg Br 72:694

Glenoid Resurfacing in Shoulder Arthroplasty: Pro's and Con's

G. Walch, P. Boileau, and I. Pozzi

Summary

This paper compares the results of hemiarthroplasty and total arthroplasty in the different aetiology. In fracture and stages III and IV avascular necrosis, a hemi-arthroplasty seems to be sufficient, while in stage V AVN, a total shoulder is preferred. In osteoarthritis with massive cuff tear and superior translation of the head, early loosening of the glenoid has been described due to the "rocking horse phenomenon". In our series 6 patients received a glenoid and 15 did not. We found no significant difference in the results at a follow-up of less than 2 years. However, taking into account the results in the literature, it seems preferable to perform a hemi-arthroplasty. In posttraumatic and primary osteoarthritis there is no definite answer. With glenoid resurfacing there is a better result in terms of pain relief (also found in our series) and no risk of long-term glenoid cartilage wear. The arguments against resurfacing the glenoid are the increase in operating time and the risks of component loosening. Although a hemi-arthroplasty can be inserted when there is a concave wear of the glenoid, it is better to resurface the glenoid when the wear is asymetrical or when the glenoid has a biconcave surface. In rheumatoid arthritis, the results for pain and mobility were better in our series, as in the literature, with a total arthroplasty. A total shoulder arthroplasty is recommended except where supero-medial erosion would compromise the positioning and stability of the glenoid component.

Introduction

The decision on whether to resurface the glenoid while performing a shoulder arthroplasty depends on the etiology and the clinical state of the glenoid. We report and compare the results of hemi and total arthroplasty in the different aetiologis.

Avascular Necrosis and Fractures

Following Neer's 40-years experience (1951) [15] most authors would suggest using a hemi-arthroplasty for these etiologis. Neer maintains that he never had to totalise a hemi-arthroplasty [16]. In the literature we have found no publication discussing revision for secondary glenoid erosion even though Boyd and Thornhill [4] reported definite glenoid erosion after 5 years. In our series of AVN, 11 patients with stage V disease had a glenoid implant and 23 with stages III and IV did not. We found no difference in the results for function or pain (Tables 1, 2). We therefore confirm the indication for performing a hemi-arthroplasty in stages III and IV AVN despite the long-term risk of glenoid wear. The modular prostheses actually allow a glenoid to be implanted if required without the need to remove the whole humeral component. In stage V necrosis where there is deterioration of the glenoid surface it is preferable to insert a total arthroplasty.

What criteria are used to determine the glenoid deterioration? Either the appearances on the AP radiographs in three rotations and the computed tomography arthrogram or the macroscopic appearance at operation can be used. In our opinion, it is

Table 1. Pain (out of 15 points) in total and hemi-arthroplasty

Aetiology	Total		Hemi		statistical
	n	Pain (Points)	*n*	Pain (Points)	significance (*P*)
Avascular necrosis (*n*=34)	11	13.2	23	12.9	<0.6
Rheumatoid arthritis (*n*=50)	44	12	6	10	<0.1
Primary gleno-humeral osteo-arthritis (*n*=154)	140	13.2	14	9.7	<0.02
Posttraumatic arthritis (*n*=65)	24	10.8	41	9.9	<0.3
Osteoarthritis with massive cuff tears (*n*=21)	6	11.6	15	10	<0.5
Entire series	225	12.7	99	10.6	<0.002

Table 2. Activities of daily living (out of 20 points) in total and hemi-arthroplasty

Aetiology	Total Arthroplasty *n*	ADL (Points)	Hemi Arthroplasty *n*	ADL (Points)	statistical significance (P)
Avascular necrosis (*n*=34)	11	15.6	23	15.5	<0.9
Rheumatoid arthritis (*n*=50)	44	15.6	6	13.5	<0.1
Primary gleno-humeral osteo-arthritis (*n*=154)	140	17	14	15	<0.02
Posttraumatic arthritis (*n*=65)	24	13.5	41	12	<0.1
Osteoarthritis with massive cuff tears (*n*=21)	6	11.6	15	11.2	<0.8
Entire series	225	16.2	99	13.2	<0.000

the preoperative imaging which should be analysed and which allows this decision to be made because the intra-operative appearances are always a somewhat similar, showing an off-white area which makes a true assessment of cartilage wear difficult. When the investigations show that the joint space remains present in all the rotations of the humeral head, it is preferable to insert a hemi-arthroplasty. On the other hand, when any of the three radiographic views or the CT scan show complete loss of articular cartilage in any part of the joint then glenoid resurfacing is desirable.

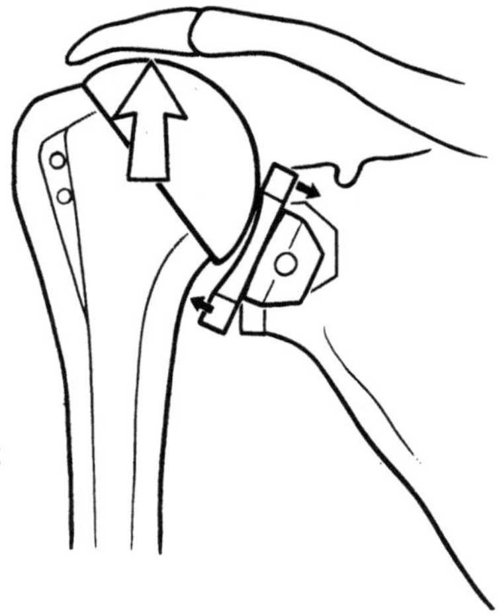

Fig. 1. Upward movement of the humeral head leading to the rocking horse effect on the glenoid causing loosening

Arthritis with Massive Cuff Tear

For nearly 10 years Barrett, Franklin and Matsen [1, 12] have shown that upward movement of the humerus causes the "rocking horse effect" of the head on the glenoid in the vertical plane leading to early loosening (Fig. 1). Boyd and Thornhill [4], however, did not find a close causal relationship. In our series 6 patients received a glenoid and 15 did not. There was no significant difference in either the clinical or radiographic results (Tables 3–5). However, the current recommendation is *not* to

Table 3. Active elevation of the shoulder in total and hemi-arthroplasty

Aetiology	Total Arthroplasty *n*	Active Elevation (Degrees)	Hemi Arthroplasty *n*	Active Elevation (Degrees)	statistical significance (*P*)
Avascular necrosis (*n*=34)	11	130	23	130	<0.9
Rheumatoid arthritis (*n*=50)	44	125	6	109	<0.2
Primary gleno-humeral osteo-arthritis (*n*=154)	140	144	14	130	<0.07
Posttraumatic arthritis (*n*=65)	24	111	41	88	<0.03
Osteoarthritis with massive cuff tears (*n*=21)	6	80	15	97	<0.3
Entire series	225	135	99	106	<0.000

Table 4. Strength (out of 25 points) in total and hemi-arthroplasty

Aetiology	Total Arthroplasty *n*	Strength (Points)	Hemi Arthroplasty *n*	Strength (Points)	statistical significance (*P*)
Avascular necrosis (*n*=34)	11	8.4	23	8.1	<0.8
Rheumatoid arthritis (*n*=50)	44	4.2	6	5	<0.6
Primary gleno-humeral osteo-arthritis (*n*=154)	140	8.1	14	6.2	<0.08
Posttraumatic arthritis (*n*=65)	24	7.4	41	7.3	<0.9
Osteoarthritis with massive cuff tears (*n*=21)	6	1.3	15	2.9	<0.2
Entire series	225	7.2	99	6.6	<0.3

Table 5. Objective results (adjusted Constant score) in totaland hemi-arthroplasty

Aetiology	Total Arthroplasty n	Total Arthroplasty Constant score (%)	Hemi Arthroplasty n	Hemi Arthroplasty Constant score (%)	statistical significance (*P*)
Avascular necrosis (*n*=34)	11	82.1	23	82.8	<0.9
Rheumatoid arthritis (*n*=50)	44	79	6	70	<0.2
Primary gleno-humeral osteo-arthritis (*n*=154)	140	96.8	14	81	<0.002
Posttraumatic arthritis (*n*=65)	24	69	41	65	<0.6
Osteoarthritis with massive cuff tears (*n*=21)	6	60	15	65	<0.5
Entire series	225	89	99	71	<0.000

insert a glenoid component when the humeral head has migrated upwards, and where there is no cuff.

Posttraumatic Arthritis and Primary Osteoarthritis

Here the choice is much more difficult and is more a question of habit than science. All the published work to date has shown that patients achieve identical ranges of movement, pain reduction and postoperative function with total and hemi-arthroplasties. However, Boyd et al. [4] have shown that after 5 years patients with a hemi-arthroplasty may start to suffer again, with their radiographs showing subchondral sclerosis and joint space narrowing especially at the upper pole of the glenoid. There is therefore a definite risk of progressive wear and pain in the glenoid in the long term which may require revision to a total shoulder. Nevertheless there are some elements which are against inserting a glenoid component straightaway: increasing the time and complexity of the procedure, the risk of intra-operative glenoid fracture as reported by Hawkins [14] and the risk of glenoid loosening as stressed by Barrett [1] and Cofield [9]. In a meta-analysis of the literature which covered nearly 1500 Neer total shoulder arthroplasties, Cofield [10] reported a level of glenoid lucent lines between 30, and 89 % of cases and obvious radiographic loosening of 0 %–12 %. The rate of revision for glenoid loosening was, however, very low, with Neer having revised less than 1 % of 1098 total shoulder prostheses [16].

In a meta-analysis of 1413 total shoulders Brems [7] reported 38.6 % with lucent lines, and 2.9 % of these were revised for glenoid loosening at an average follow-up of more than 5 years. It is therefore important to differentiate between glenoid lucent lines, minimal or asymptomatic radiographic loosening and loosening requiring revision. Brems [6] has shown that the glenoid lucency was present immediately postoperatively in 70 % of cases. Radiographic loosening can be defined as a progressing lucent line wider than 2 mm occurring around the keel. Barrett [1] states that lucent lines beneath the tray are not necessarily synonymous with loosening. Non-progressive lucent lines or lines less than 2 mm do not seem to have any clinical effect on either pain or mobility. Only time and long-tern follow-up of cemented glenoid components will allow confirmation that these lucencies are innocuous.

In our series (Tables 1–5) all the clinical parameters are in favour of total arthroplasty in osteoarthritis and posttraumatic arthritis, with statistically significant differences demonstrated for osteoarthritis but not for posttraumatic arthritis. Our experience has moved us towards performing a glenoid resurfacing whenever there is sufficient bone-stock. Some osteoarthritis cases have a glenoid that is so worn that the medullary canal has become too narrow to allow the keel of the prosthesis to be positioned.

A graft taken from the humeral head can be used to reconstruct the glenoid, but questions must be asked about its ability to integrate when one considers the difficulties in heading the graft and the poor quality of the bone itself. There would seem to be two groups of cases: if the glenoid is evenly worn and has retained a single concave surface (Fig. 2), it is preferable to insert a hemi-arthroplasty. If the glenoid has asymmetric wear and a biconcave sur-

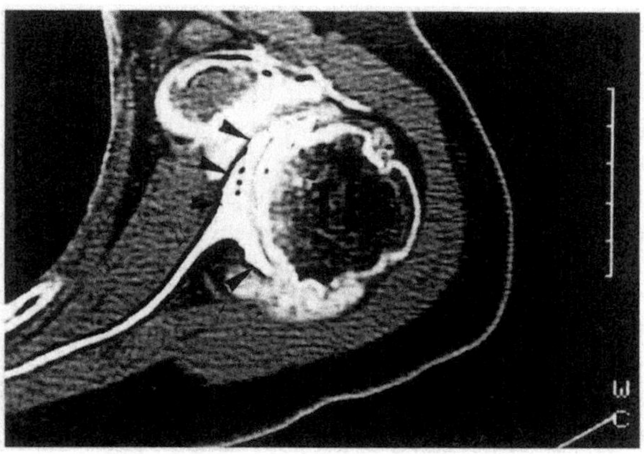

Fig. 2. Where there is uniform glenoid wear resulting in a single concavity then it is preferable to insert a hemi-arthroplasty

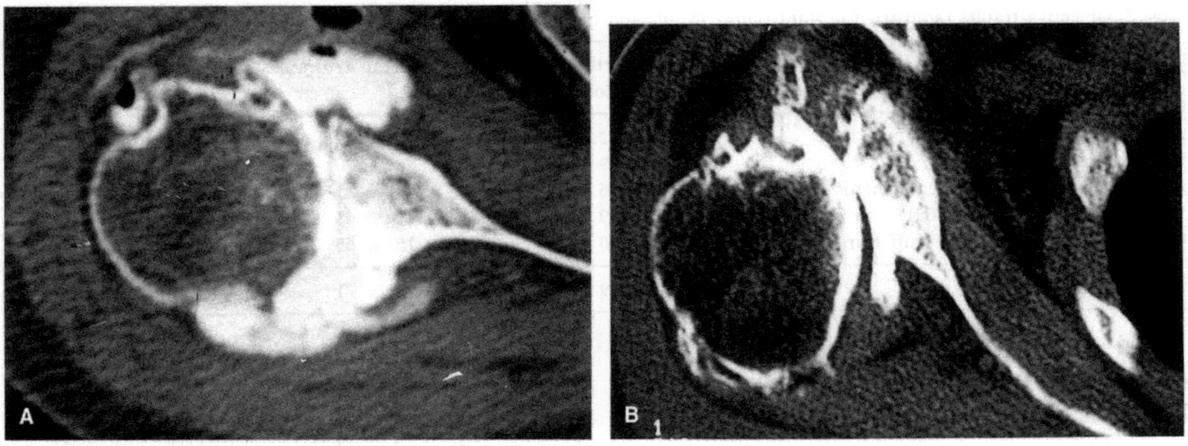

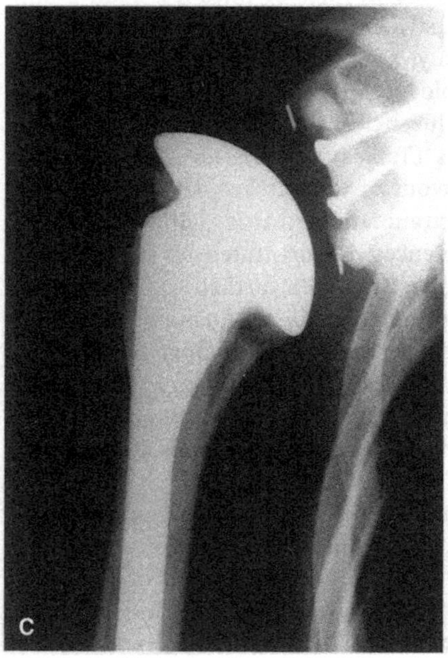

Fig. 3. Where there is moderate assymetrical wear (**A**) the anterior section should be flattened and a glenoid component inserted. If the wear is more significant (**B**), then it is better to reconstruct the glenoid with a graft (**C**)

face, it is necessary to resurface the glenoid either by using a burr to remove the anterior part in order to flatten it (Fig. 3A) or by inserting a posterior graft (Fig. 3B,C). This has been also the experience of Glasson et al. [13] who reported that the use of a hemi-arthroplasty appears to be more appropriate in patients with concentric glenoid.

Rheumatoid Arthritis

Many series reported in the literature [2–4, 8] have shown results slightly better overall for pain relief when using a total arthroplasty like we found in our study (Table 1). Mobility was also better (Table 2), with 125° of active anterior elevation with a glenoid as opposed to 109° without. The results in our and the other series are biased by the fact that the more severe lesions require a glenoid resurfacing because of the degree of glenoid wear. Boyd and Thornhill [5] advise a systematic resurfacing in patients with cartilaginous lesions related to the patients disease process and in inflammatory diseases in general. The failure that we suffered in a patient with systemic lupus erythematosis who underwent a hemi-arthroplasty confirms this opinion.

Major glenoid wear of the upper pole found in rheumatoid arthritis is often a contraindication because reconstruction of the glenoid using a graft is not logical in such cases and a hemi-arthroplasty is preferred. On the other hand, as described by Boyd and Thornhill, cuff tears (of moderate size or functional disability due to atrophy) are not contraindications to inserting a glenoid component because they have never observed loosening in rheumatoid arthritis due to the rocking horse mechanism as reported by Barrett [1] and Franklin [12].

Conclusion

Glenoid resurfacing is advised in posttraumatic arthritis and rheumatoid arthritis where the bonestock is sufficient. It is also advisable in primary osteoarthritis except where there is significant symmetrical wear eroding the medullary canal. Where the wear is asymmetrical it seems better to resurface the glenoid having either flattened the surface where the erosion is less severe or having inserted a posterior graft where the wear is more significant. In rheumatoid arthritis with marked supero-medial wear which compromises the stability of the glenoid component, a hemi-arthroplasty should be used. In cuff-tear arthritis and stage III and IV avascular necrosis a hemi-arthroplasty is recommended, but a total shoulder should be selected in stage V.

References

1. Barrett WP, Franklin JL, Jackins SE, Wyss CR, Matsen FA (1987) Total shoulder arthroplasty. J Bone Joint Surg 69A:865–872
2. Barrett WP, Thornhill TS, Thomas WH, Gebhart EM, Sledge CB (1989) Nonconstrained total shoulder arthroplasty in patients with polyarticular rheumatoid arthritis. J Arthroplasty 4:91–96
3. Bell SN, Gschwend N (1986) Clinical experience with total arthroplasty and hemiarthroplasty of the shoulder using the Neer prosthesis. Int Orthop 10:217–222
4. Boyd AD, Thornhill TS, Thomas WH, Scott RD, Sledge CB (1990) Total shoulder replacement vs hemiarthroplasty: Indications for glenoid resurfacing J Arthroplasty 5:329–336
5. Boyd AD, Thornhill TS (1994) Glenoid resurfacing in shoulder arthroplasty. In: Friedman RJ (ed) Arthroplasty of the shoulder. Thieme, Stuttgart, pp 306–316
6. Brems JJ, Wide AH, Borden LS, Boumphrey FRS (1986) Glenoid lucent lines (abstract). Orthop Trans 10:231
7. Brems JJ (1993) The glenoid component in total shoulder arthroplasty. J Shoulder Elbow Surg 2 (1):47–54
8. Clayton ML, Ferlic DC, Jeffers PD (1982) Prosthetic arthroplasties of the shoulder. Clin Orthop 164:184–191
9. Cofield RH (1984) Total shoulder arthroplasty with the Neer prosthesis. J. Bone Joint Surg Am 66:899–906
10. Cofield RH (1990) Degenerative and arthritic problems of the glenohumeral joint. In: Rockwood CR, Matsen FA (eds) The shoulder. Saunders, Philadelphia, pp 678–742
11. Constant CR, Murley AHG (1987) A clinical method of functionnal assessment of the shoulder. Clin Orthop 214:160–164
12. Franklin JL, Jackins SE, Matsen FA (1987) Glenoid loosening in total shoulder arthroplasty: an association with rotator cuff deficiency. Orthop Trans 11:446
13. Glasson JM, Djurasovic M, Levine WN, Pollock RG, Flatow EL, Bigliani LU (1996) Hemiarthroplasty for glenohumeral osteoarthritis in patients with an intact rotator cuff: results correlated to degree of glenoid wear. Presented at the Annual Meeting of the American Academy of Orthopaedics Surgeons, Atlanta
14. Hawkins RJ, Bell RH, Jallay B (1989) Total shoulder arthroplasty. Clin Orthop 242:188–194
15. Neer CS II (1955) Articular replacement of the humeral head. J Bone Joint Surg 37A:215–228
16. Neer CS (1990) Glenohumeral arthroplasty. In: Neer CS (ed) Shoulder reconstruction. Saunders, Philadelphia, pp 146–271

Section VI:

Multicentre Studies

The Aequalis Shoulder System

G. Walch and P. Boileau

Summary

The Aequalis Total Shoulder System is a complete adaptable and modular shoulder prosthesis. The design of this non-constrained shoulder arthroplasty is based on detailed investigations of the dimensions, the shape and the relations of the humeral proximal epiphysis and the glenoid. The goal of the Aequalis total shoulder arthroplasty is to adapt the prosthesis itself exactly to the individual anatomy and not to adapt the anatomy to the prosthesis. This is possible without multiplying the different components because of technological innovations. ***The humeral component*** *is constructed in titanium or chrome cobalt and is composed of three parts: three stems, four angular necks (125°, 130°, 135°, 140°) and ten sizes of humeral heads. An original technological system allows the variable orientation of the humeral articular surface to be respected in both the sagittal and the frontal planes. The obvious advantages of this adaptable shoulder arthroplasty are: the possibility to respect the inclination and the retroversion of each humerus, which are variable for each patient and even for both shoulders of a same patient, and the possibility to respect the medial and posterior offset of the articular head surface, without needing different prosthesis for the right and the left shoulder.* ***The glenoid component*** *is constructed of polyethylene and available in three sizes. A minimal thickness of polyethylene and a larger radius of curvature than the corresponding humeral head allows the physiological rolling and gliding mechanism of the joint. The various options are chosen very easily by the surgeon with the help of original guides. In addition to the* ***humeral and glenoid instrumentation,*** *there is a* ***fracture instrumentation*** *which allows for proper length and retroversion of the humerus to be restored.*

Introduction

The Aequalis shoulder prosthesis is a non-constrained gleno-humeral arthroplasty which has been developed over a ten year of cooperation period during which fundamental research work was combined with the expertise of the engineers at Tornier company [1–6, 11]. Its conception was based on the two principles which we feel as being essential in the goal of obtaining consistent clinical results: (a) to have a prosthesis which can perfectly match the anatomy of the shoulder due to the modularity and adaptability of the components; (b) to have instrumentation available to allow simple and reproducible insertion from one surgeon to the next.

Due to the availability of a range of sizes this three part implant (stem, neck and head) can be adapted to perfectly match the anatomy encountered rather than having to adapt the anatomy to match the prosthesis. The prosthesis is available either in titanium alloy or cobalt chrome depending on personal preference (Fig. 1).

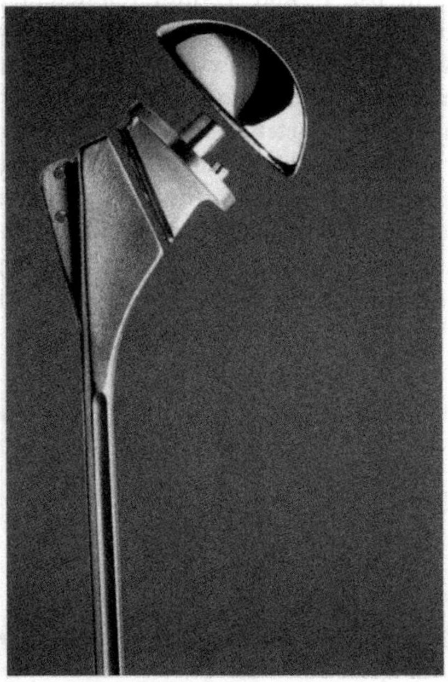

Fig. 1. The Aequalis prosthesis is composed of three sections; stem, neck and head

The Humeral Stem

After reviewing the various published studies we selected a cemented stem. In a review of the literature, Cofield [5] found that in 570 cases using a first-generation press-fit stem there was an unacceptable rate of loosening of 12.3 %, which compares unfavourably with the 0.8 % complication rate reported in a series of 730 cemented prostheses. Steward and Kelly [6] followed 37 cementless humeral prostheses for 9 years and found a 64 % migration rate. Torchia and Cofield [7] reported a 43 % migration rate in a series of 113 arthroplasties followed for between 5 and 17 years (mean 9.7 years). Not enough work has been published on implants with surfaces designed to encourage bone ingrowth to predict their future although Cofield has reported a 7 % migration rate in 73 implants followed for 31 months. Therefore the published literature clearly suggests that, at present, cemented humeral have a better outcome than uncemented ones. Furthermore, there are no established disadvantages in the use of cemented stems, and for these reasons we systematically cement the humeral component. Rotatory stability of the humeral component is achieved by optimal metaphyseal filling, an upper fin (which has two holes to allow reinsertion of the tuberosities in fracture cases) and, finally, anterior and posterior guide slots.

The humeral stems are 10.5 cm long and are available in 6-, 9- and 12-mm diameters (Fig. 2) for use in chronic cases, for example, osteoarthritis, rheumatoid arthritis, avascular necrosis, posttraumatic arthritis and cuff-tear arthropathy. The stem was deliberately shortened in order to better fit the cylinder of the proximal humeral canal before reaching the curvature change in the diaphysis. The humerus is in effect, S shaped with the upper curve situated between 10 and 15 cm from the greater tuberosity, and there is a risk from a longer stem of causing a fracture especially if the design tries to achieve maximal diaphyseal fill. It is also clear that as the humerus is shorter than the femur by 10–20 cm, the forces involved at the level of the shoulder are much smaller than those at the hip, and there is therefore no reason to have a stem of the same length as those in hip prostheses. However, there are 15 cm stems available in the 9- and 12-mm diameters for fresh fracture cases and for treating the sequelae of fractures, with a diaphyseal extension similar to those used in revision hip surgery.

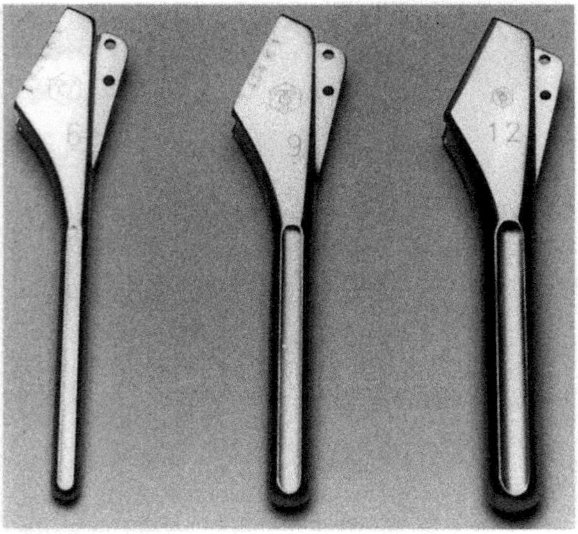

Fig. 2. Humeral stems are 10.5 cm long and are available in 6, 9, 12 mm diameters

The Humeral Head

Modularity comes from the availability of ten head sizes whose diameter and depth were determined from our basic anatomical studies. Each diameter has a corresponding thickness except for the largest 52 mm head diameters where there are two available thickness so as to better match the anatomical variations encountered. Matching the thickness and diameter of the articular surface is important in reestablishing the musculo-ligamentous balance of the shoulder and in maintaining the differences in radius of curvature between the glenoid and the humeral head. We did not want to have multiple different thickness available for each head diameter because this was not correlated with our anatomical studies [1–5].

We feel that the term 'soft-tissue balancing' should be restricted to the soft-tissues: posterior capsular release to recover a physiological posterior translation or posterior capsular plication in cases of chronic subluxation of the humeral head, anterior capsular release and subscapular lengthening to recover adequate external rotation. All these procedures allow the proper ligamentous and tendino-muscular balance and tensions to be reestablished. By matching one anatomical thickness for each diameter the humeral head is reconstituted with the correct spherical form and we call this 'bony balancing'. The association of bony and soft-tissue balancing leads to the more complete concept of 'anatomical balancing' which we advocate when carrying out a total shoulder arthroplasty.

The under surface of each head has an eccentric dial (Fig. 3) which has eight available positions to allow the articular head to be off-set both postero-anteriorly and medio-lateraly such that the humeral bone cut can be perfectly covered.

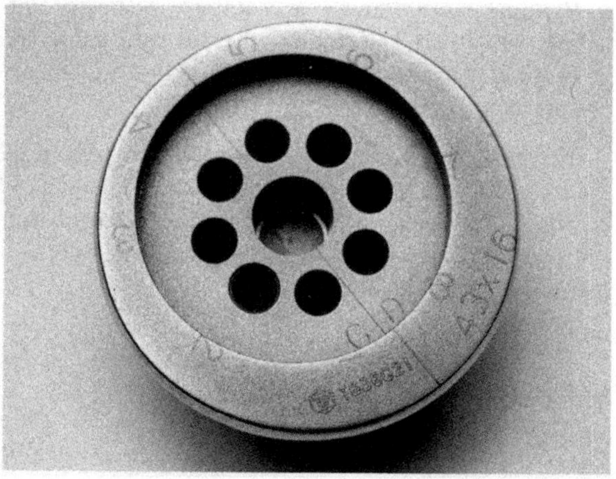

Fig. 3. Eccentric dial located on the under surface of the humeral head

The Neck

There are four necks available with 125°, 130°, 135° and 140° angles (Fig. 4) which allows the anatomical inclination of the humeral head in relation to the diaphysis to be matched in individual patients. The possibility of respecting the individual inclination of each humerus through this variable neck prosthesis also explains why we do not feel the necessity to have different thickness for the prosthetic head.

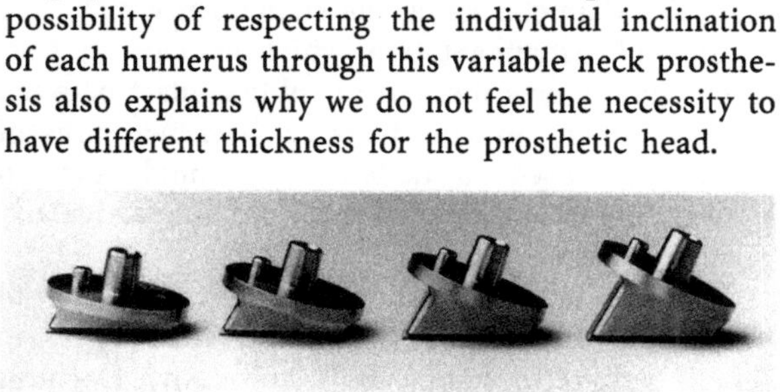

Fig. 4. Four necks available with 125°, 130°, 135°, and 140° angles

Assembly of the Prosthetic Components

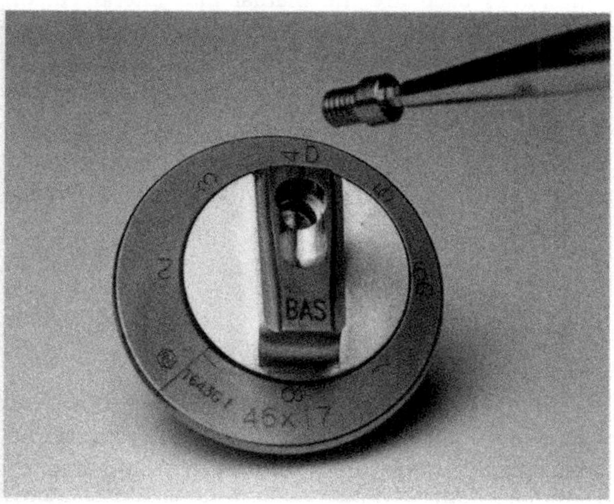

Fig. 5. The grub screw used to lock the neck onto the head

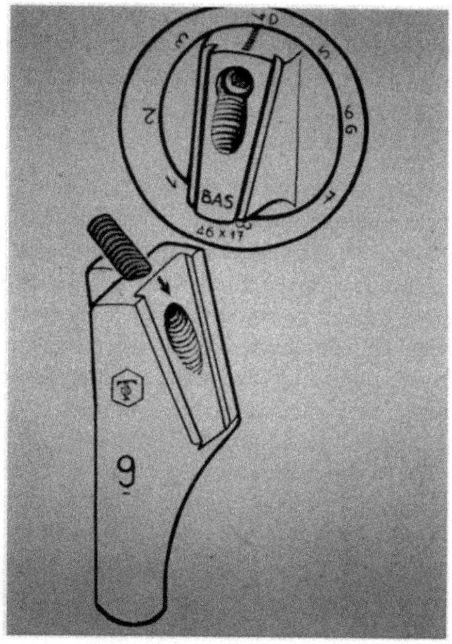

Fig. 6. Assembly of the neck onto the stem on the dovetail rail locked with a grub screw

The connection of the components has been designed taking into account that the shoulder is a very mobile joint:

- The head is fixed to the neck on a Morse taper locked with a grub screw. However, the Morse taper gives a disassembly force of 100 kg and is sufficient alone to stabilise the prosthesis (Fig. 5).
- The neck is then attached to the stem on a sliding dovetail rail and this is locked with a grub screw (Fig. 6).

The Glenoid Component

Three sizes of glenoid are available (Fig. 4). Each is characterised by its depth, height and radius of curvature. Anatomical studies of paired humerii and glenoids have allowed preferential combinations to be defined (Table 1).

Table 1. Preferential association between glenoid components and humeral components

Glenoid component	Humeral head component
Small	37/13.5 39/14 41/15
Medium	43/16 46/17
Large	48/18 50/16 and 50/19 52/19 and 52/23

We wanted to have minimal constraints between the head and the glenoid components and to leave the surgeon with all his options open. To achieve this, each articular head can be matched to each of the available glenoids.

There are two types of glenoid:

- All polyethylene with a flat or round back and a keel (Fig. 7). The keel is the same size for all the glenoids. This is for cemented use only.
- A metal backed component with a hydroxyapatite coating to encourage bony ingrowth and give definitive stability. The initial stability is achieved by two expansion screws which open out in the same way as hollow-wall fixing pegs. A 4-mm-deep polyethylene insert click fits onto the tray (Fig. 8).

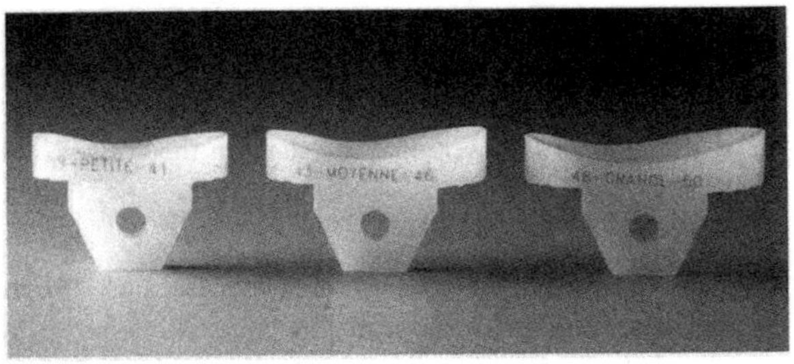

Fig. 7. The three sizes of polyethylene glenoid with flat-back and keel

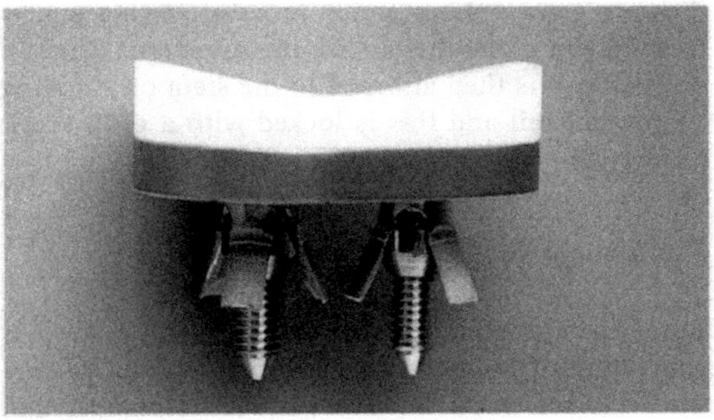

Fig. 8. Metal backed glenoid implant with expansion screws

Adaptability

The ability of the Aequalis system to adapt to each humerus is the result of the innovations included and these consist of:

- A variable inclination angle coming from the neck component which is selected intraoperatively by the surgeon using the inclination-retroversion guide.
- A variable retroversion selected in the same way using the trial.
- Variable medio-lateral and anterio-posterior offsets which are selected by the surgeon using the original eccentric dial system on the under surface of the head.

The ability to translate the articular surface in all planes means that the prosthesis can be adapted to all the pathological situations encountered and thus the proximal humerus can be reconstructed following the original anatomy.

Instrumentation

Three instrument sets have been developed to help surgeons in restoring the natural anatomy and in ensuring proper seating of the implants:

Humeral instrumentation, where the goal is to reconstruct the proximal humerus after having made the cut at the level of the anatomical neck or as near as possible to this important landmark. The principle is to define and then match these main measurements: head diameter, inclination angle, retroversion, postero-medial offset and humeral stem diameter using the components.

Glenoid instrumentation, which matches its pear shape and assures the best possible contact between the component and the bone surface. Two sizes of reamer are used to flatten the glenoid, and an angle-guide is available if required in particularly tight shoulders.

Fracture instrumentation, with the objective of positioning the prosthesis correctly with regard to length and retroversion. With tuberosity fractures the important landmarks from which measurements are made are lost. The principle here is to determine the length of the contralateral humerus preoperatively and to reproduce this, using a jig consisting of an arm support and a sliding ruler. The important landmarks used are the medial and lateral epicondyles at the elbow. Humeral retroversion is fixed using the protractor and allows the average of 20° to be matched. After having positioned and cemented the prosthesis in the correct position the surgeon can then pay particular attention to reconstructing the tuberosities and repairing the rotator cuff properly.

Conclusion

Following on from the monobloc Neer prosthesis which was the first generation of unconstrained arthroplasty, came the so-called second-generation shoulders, with variable head sizes. Now the Aequalis prosthesis can claim to be the third-generation, which in addition to being modular, allows the prosthesis to be adapted to each shoulder thanks to a series of innovations. The first Aequalis prosthesis was inserted in 1991, and the Aequalis group was set up in 1992 to follow the scientific development of the prosthesis. The initial group consisted of 12 French surgeons and has since been extended to include three other European surgeons. The goal has been to run multi-centre trials with data-sheets containing all the pre-, peri- and postoperative details completed for each patient and then collated on a central computer. The details of each case have been analysed and the results of various studies have lead to the production of this book.

References

1. Boileau P, Walch G, Liotard JP (1992) Cinéradiographic study of active elevation of the prothetic shoulder. J Orthop Surg 6:351–359
2. Boileau P, Walch G, Mazzoleni N, Urien JP (1993) In vitro study of humeral retrotorsion. J Shoulder Elbow Surg 2:512
3. Boileau P, Walch G (1994) The combined offset of the humeral sphere. J Shoulder Elbow Surg 3:21–6
4. Boileau P, Walch G (1995) Adaptabilité et modularité au cours des prothèses d'épaule. Acta Orthop Bel 61 [Suppl I]:49–61
5. Boileau P, Walch G (1996) Varus shoulder prosthesis: error or necessity? J Shoulder Elbow Surg 562:186
6. Boileau P, Walch G (1997) The three-dimensional Geometry of the proximal humerus: Duplications for surgical technique and prosthetic design. J Bone Joint Surg 79B 5:857–865
7. Cofield RH (1994) Uncemented total shoulder arthroplasty. A review. Clin Orthop 307:86–93
8. Stewart MPM, Kelly IG (1994) Seven to 13 years follow-up of the Neer total shoulder arthroplasty. Personnal communication, 8th meeting of the European Shoulder and Elbow Society. Barcelona, 16–18 June
9. Torchia ME, Cofield RH, Settergren CR (1994) Total shoulder arthroplasty with the Neer prosthesis: long term results. Presented at the 61st Annual Meeting of the American Academy of Orthopaedic Surgeons. New Orleans 24 February–1 March
10. O'Neill OR, Cofield RH (1993) Tissue ingrowth humeral component. Clinical and radiographic results of a new design. Presented at the 9th Open Meeting of the American Shoulder and Elbow Surgeons. San Francisco, February
11. Walch G, Boileau P (1992) Morphological study of the humeral proximal epiphysis. J Bone Joint Surg Br 74:14

An Overview of the Series

H. Mestdagh

Summary

To evaluate the early results of the Aequalis prosthesis, a prospective multicenter study was undertaken. The clinical and radiological results of the first 417 shoulder prostheses implanted have been evaluated with a minimum of 12 months of follow-up. Some details regarding the entire series are given here.

Patients

Between 1991 and 1994 the various teams participating in this study performed 417 Aequalis shoulder arthroplasties. After excluding tumours, the operative indications fell into the following three groups:

- Non-traumatic
  - Osteoarthritis 155
  - Rheumatoid arthritis 50
  - Atraumatic osteonecrosis 33
  - Osteoarthritis with massive cuff tear 21
- Traumatic
  - Fracture sequelae 71
  - Recent fractures 69
- Failed surgery
  - For instability 11
  - For rotator cuff disorder 7.

The average age of the patients was 63 years and this varied according to the etiology. Those with osteoarthritis with massive cuff tear averaged 72 years at the time of surgery whilst those with fracture malunions, rheumatoid arthritis and osteonecrosis were less than 60 years old.

There were 287 females and 133 males. The highest female preponderance was found in the rheumatoid population at 88.5 % and this was a little less so in osteoathritis (76 %), osteoarthritis with massive cuff tear (71 %) and recent fractures (76.5 %). Conversely there was a male preponderance in chronic posterior dislocations (67 %).

The dominant shoulder was involved in 58 %, the right in 41 % and 1 % were ambidextrous. The opposite shoulder was uninvolved in 56 %, had already undergone surgery in 14.5 % and was scheduled for surgery in 17 %. Bilateral involvement was seen mainly in the rheumatoid and osteoarthritis with massive cuff tear groups.

Operative Technique

There were 256 total shoulder replacements which amounted to about two-thirds of the procedures.

As a rule a hemiarthroplasty was inserted for recent fractures (97 %) and, to a lesser degree, in chronic posterior dislocations (83 %), osteoarthritis with massive cuff tear (71 %), avascular necrosis (68 %) and fracture malunions (63 %). Conversely a total shoulder was inserted for most of the osteoarthritis (91 %) and rheumatoid cases (88 %).

- A delto-pectoral approach was used in all cases except for 12 superior approaches and one posterior approach.
- The humeral prosthesis was cemented in 87 % of the cases. All recent fractures and fractures sequelae were cemented.
- The inclination angle, as restored using the neck implant, was 130° or 135° in nearly two-thirds of cases.
- The 9 mm humeral stem was used in more than half the cases.
- The most frequently used head sizes were the 43/16 and 46/17.
- Of the three glenoid implant sizes, the medium-sized one was used in nearly half the cases. However in the rheumatoid group there was a tendency towards using the small size.
- Probably because it was designed earlier the cemented polythene implant was used in 88 %.

A number of associated procedures were also performed:

- The subscapularis tendon was lengthened by juxtaglenoid capsulotomy in 60 % and by Z-plasty in 5 %.
- An acromioplasty was not carried out routinely and indeed was done in only 20 cases (5 %), most often in osteoarthritis and chronic posterior dislocations.

- Resection of the acromio-clavicular joint was even less common being carried out in only 10 cases (2.5 %) and almost exclusively in osteoarthritis and osteoarthritis with massive cuff tear.
- A cuff tear was repaired on 23 occasions (6 %), particularly in recent fractures and fracture malunions as well as in osteoarthritis with massive cuff tear. Tears were never repaired in the rheumatoid patients.
- The tendon of the long head of biceps was resected and tendonsed 21 times (5 %).
- Post-operatively the shoulder was only immobilised in 103 cases (25 %) but notably in two-thirds of the fracture cases.

Results

All patients were closely followed at 3, 6 months, at one year and then every year. An attempt was made to review all the operated patients with a minimum follow-up of 12 months and an average follow-up of 19 months. Overall the mean Constant score had increased from 6 (34 normalised) pre-operatively to 61 (81) after surgery. All the parameters improved: pain from 3 to 12, activities of daily living from 7 to 15, mobility from 12 to 27 and force from 3 to 7.

The average time to achieve a functional result was 7 months. This was shorter in avascular necrosis of the humeral head (6 months) and longer after fracture (9 months).

Section VII:
Primary Osteoarthritis

Primary Gleno-humeral Osteoarthritis: Clinical and Radiographic Classification

G. Walch, A. Boulahia, R. Badet, N. Riand, and J.F. Kempf

Summary

One hundred and fifty-one cases of primary gleno-humeral osteoarthritis were analysed clinically and radiographically with computed tomography. There were 76 % women and the mean age at operation was 66.8 years. Diagnosis was made only with true anteroposterior views of the shoulder which show the narrowing of the gleno-humeral joint and the presence of osteophytes. Arthrography showed a supraspinatus tear in 10 % of the cases which extended to the infraspinatus in 2.6 %. Glenoid retroversion averaged 15.4°. However, measurements of glenoid retroversion with computed tomography do not allow posterior wear to be distinguished from glenoid dysplasia. Posterior subluxation of the humeral head was observed in 45 % of the cases. We describe a classification of the glenoid morphology in three types: Type A (53.5 %) is characterised by an equal balance of forces acting on the glenoid and a centralised humeral head. Type B (39.5 %) has asymmetrical posterior force distribution on the glenoid and a posterior subluxation of the humeral head. Type C (5 %) is arbitrarily defined as glenoid retroversion greater than 25°. Posterior subluxation of the proximal humeral head was not correlated with either glenoid retroversion or humeral retroversion. However, subluxation of the humeral head may be responsible for the posterior glenoid erosion and the possible biconcave appearance of the glenoid observed in primary gleno-humeral osteoarthritis (Type B). The posterior subluxation of the humeral head may still be present after shoulder arthroplasty and may be responsible for glenoid loosening due to a "horizontal rocking horse effect".

Introduction

Primary gleno-humeral osteoarthritis is reported as being rare accounting for 3 % of arthritis cases. It has been well described in semiological terms [1, 4, 7, 12] but has often been confused with secondary arthritis particularly after massive rotator cuff tears. Primary gleno-humeral osteoarthritis was defined by Neer in 1974 [7] as consisting of: (a) limitation of gleno-humeral movement, (b) loss of joint space, (c) humeral head enlargement due to osteophytes, and (d) almost never having a cuff tear. Later the same author emphasised the importance of glenoid erosion which usually occurs posteriorly and can lead to chronic posterior subluxation of the head [9, 10].

The goal of the present study was to look for any epidemiological, clinical and radiological factors that could help to clarify the shoulders with primary gleno-humeral osteoarthritis.

Material and Methods

Our multi-centre study involved 151 shoulders in 141 patients [10 bilateral cases). Women were more frequently affected than men (76 % vs. 24 %). The right shoulder was affected in 60 % and the dominant side in 56 %. There was bilateral involvement in 43 % and 18.4 % had surgery on both shoulders. The average age at operation was 66.8 years (42–84).

The dominant clinical symptom was pain especially at night, with a mean Constant score of 3.2 out of 15. Limitation of movement was a consistent finding with a score of 14.1 out of 40. Passive anterior elevation was 104°; actively this was 88°, and external rotation with the elbow at the side was 8°. Shoulder function in the activities of daily living was also affected with a mean score of 7.3 out of 20. Force averaged 2 kg. The absolute Constant score was 28.7 points (4–72), and the normalised score was 39.4 % (58–95) Deltoid atrophy was present in 31 % of cases and infraspinatus atrophy in 36 %.

All the cases had a radiographic assessment of the shoulder consisting of true AP views (oblique in two planes) in three rotations plus an AP view of the contralateral shoulder. The opposite shoulder was unaffected in only 37.5 % of cases and had already undergone surgery with the insertion of a prosthesis in 18.4 %.

The loss of joint space was assessed on the plain radiographs (Fig. 1). It was judged to be total in 77 % and partial, between 2 and 5 mm of thickness, in 23 %. Osteophytes were always present and typi-

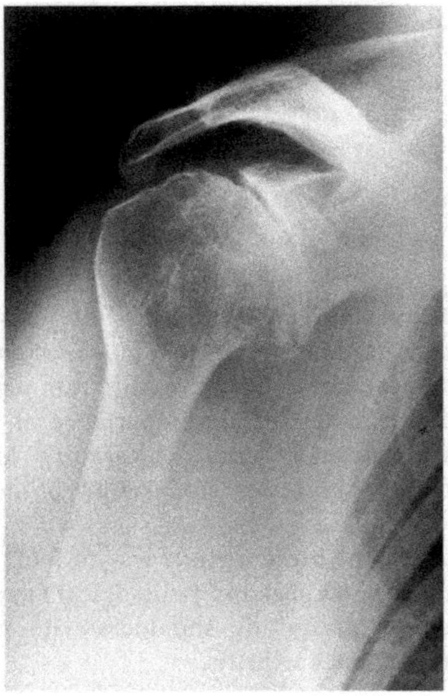

Fig. 1. Primary gleno-humeral arthritis with loss of joint space and peripheral osteophytes

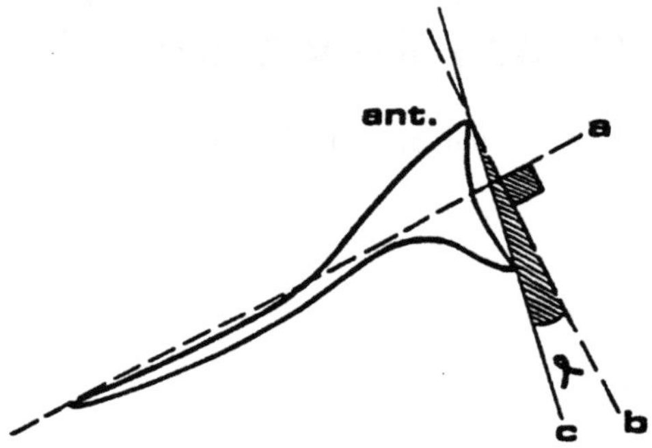

Fig. 2. Method used to measure glenoid version. *a* Axis of the blade of the scapula. *b* Line perpendicular to the blade of the scapula. *c* Line parallel to the anterior and posterior rims of the glenoid cavity. *Alpha*, glenoid retroversion angle

cally appeared as an inferior bell or droplet, but there was no relationship between the severity of the joint space loss and the osteophyte volume. Sub-chondral sclerosis was present in at least one of the two joint surfaces in 88 %. Loose bodies were found in 50 %.

The subacromial distance in neutral rotation defined as the distance between a line parallel to the inferior cortex of the acromial vault and a line at right angles to the highest point on the humeral head was greater or equal to 7 mm in 90 %. This criterion allowed the elimination of cases suffering from arthritis secondary to cuff tears.

An arthrogram was carried out in 84 cases and this demonstrated a partial rupture of the deep surface of supraspinatus in 6 % and a full thickness tear of supraspinatus in 10 %. A rupture involving infraspinatus was only found in 2.6 %. A computed tomographic (CT) arthrogram was carried out in 101 cases, and from these we were able to analyse and measure the glenoid retroversion, the position of the head in relation to the glenoid, the fatty degeneration of the cuff, the humeral retroversion and the glenoid morphology.

Glenoid Retroversion

Initially, this was measured using a system derived from that described by Friedman et al. [5]. The sagittal tilt of the glenoid cavity in relation to the long axis of the scapula was measured using the neutral axis (0° of tilt) perpendicular to the long axis of the scapula as a reference (Fig. 2). The plane of the CT section needed for this measurement (which is approximately in the middle of the glenoid cavity) is the first film on which the coracoid process is not visible. The angle of glenoid version is the acute angle delineated by the neutral axis and the long axis of the glenoid cavity. When glenoid version is exaggerated (retroversion) the posterior rim of the glenoid fossa is medial to the neutral axis and when glenoid version is decreased (anteversion) the anterior rim is medial to the neutral axis. When the axis of the glenoid fossa is superimposed on the neutral axis then the version is zero.

Position of the Head in Relation to the Glenoid

Subluxation of the head was measured using a technique derived from that described by Papilion [11]. A perpendicular line is drawn from the centre of a

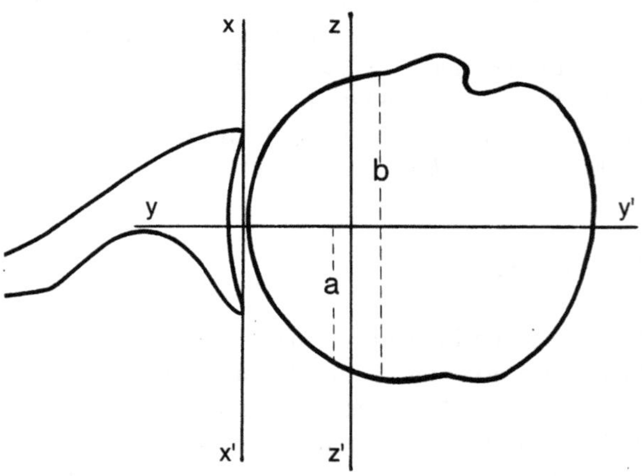

Fig. 3. *xx'*, Parallel to the glenoid surface; *yy'*, perpendicular to xx' passing through the midle of the glenoid; *zz'*, parallel to xx' passing through the medial third of the humeral head. The rations of subluxation is a/b

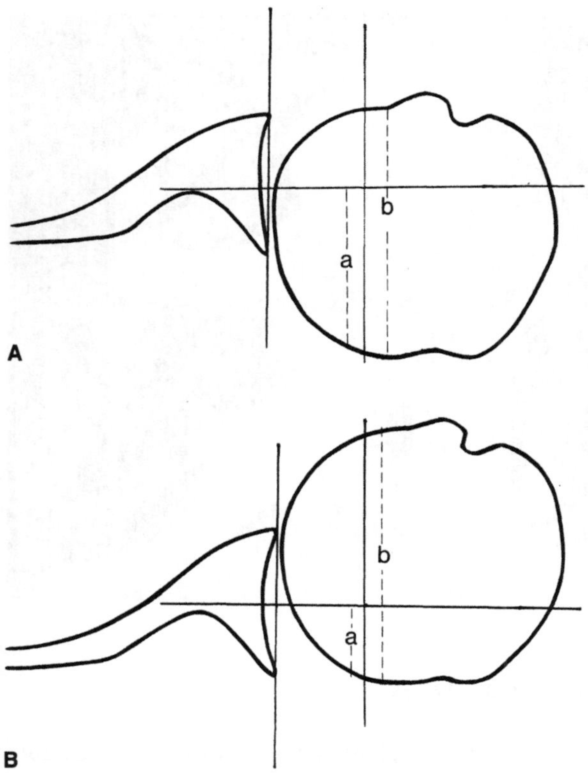

Fig. 4. A, a/b=4/6=66 %: posterior subluxation. **B**, a/b=2/6=33 %: anterior subluxation

line parallel to the glenoid surface, and then a line parallel to this is drawn passing through the medial third of the humeral head. On this last line the greatest diameter of the head is measured and the section posterior to the head. The ratio of subluxation is the ratio between the posterior section and the greatest head diameter (Fig. 3). When the ratio of subluxation is greater than 55 % the head is subluxed posteriorly and when it is less than 45 % the head is subluxed anteriorly (Fig. 4).

Fatty Degeneration of the Cuff

Fatty degeneration in the subscapularis and infraspinatus muscles was described according to Goutallier [4]. The degeneration was scored as 0 when there was no fat in the muscle, as 1 when there were fatty traces, as 2 when there was less fat than muscle, as 3 when fat equalled muscle and 4 when there was more fat than muscle (Figs. 5, 6).

Humeral Retroversion

Humeral retroversion was measured in the 50 cases in which the CT cuts included the inferior part of the humerus. The retroversion angle is formed between the superior epiphyseal axis (humeral head) and the inferior epiphyseal axis. The superior axis is determined on the CT cut where the coracoid disappears or on the one immediately below and corresponds to a right angle to the humeral head. We used the method of Bernageau and Godefroy [2], which is based on using the boundaries of the anatomical neck to define the superior epiphysis. The anatomical shape was often altered by the arthritis and the osteophytes which made the borders of the anatomical neck difficult to define. Starting from the bicipital groove the bony contours are followed anteriorly until the point where they ascend

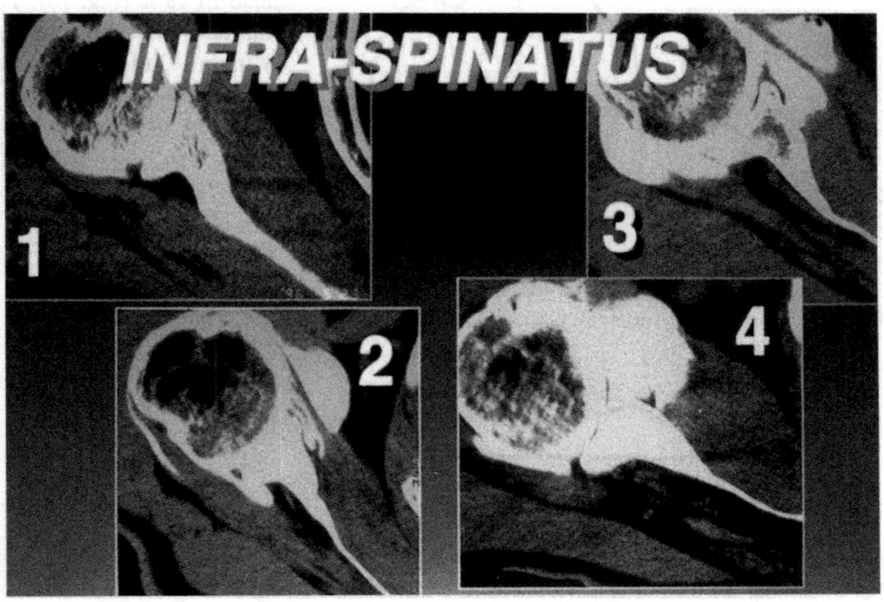

Fig. 5. Fatty degeneration of the infraspinatus muscle

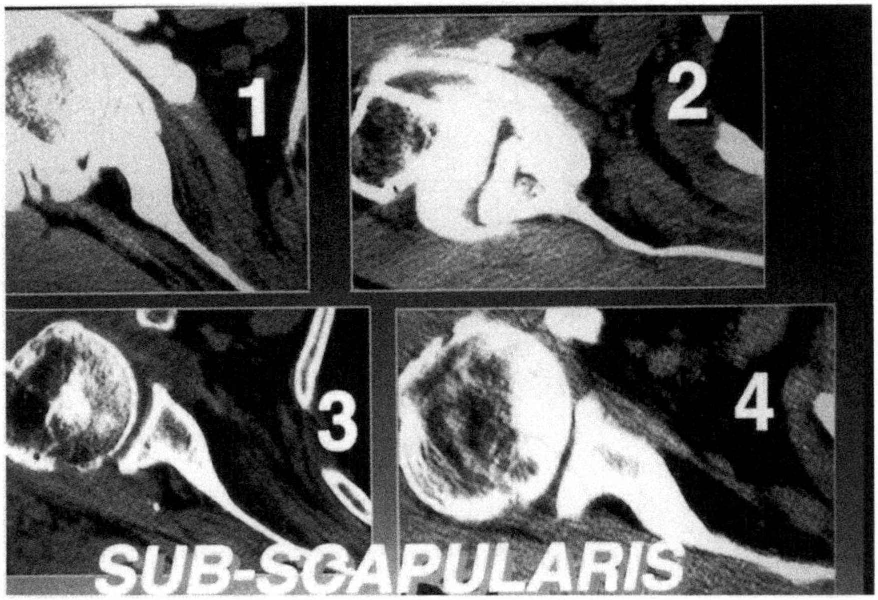

Fig. 6. Fatty degeneration of the subscapularis muscle

and which is by convention the anatomical neck. Posteriorly the same manoeuvre was carried out to find the limits between the head and the greater tuberosity. These two points are then joined by a line whose perpendicular defines the superior epiphyseal axis (Fig. 7). To define the inferior epiphyseal axis we selected as the reference axis the one used in practice, i.e. the palpable axis created by a line joining the medial and lateral epicondyles (Fig. 8).

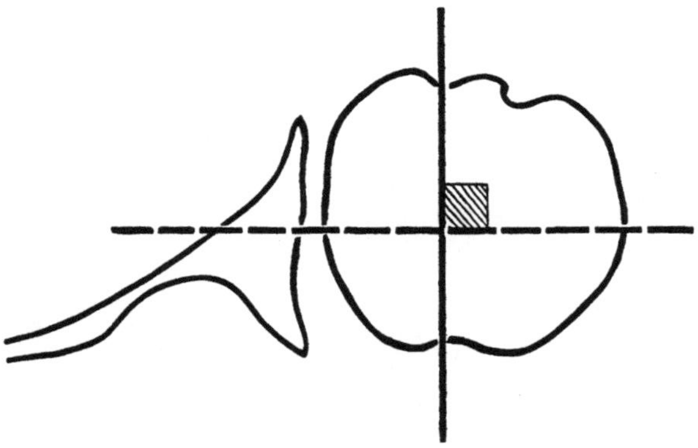

Fig. 7. Marking the superior epiphyseal axis

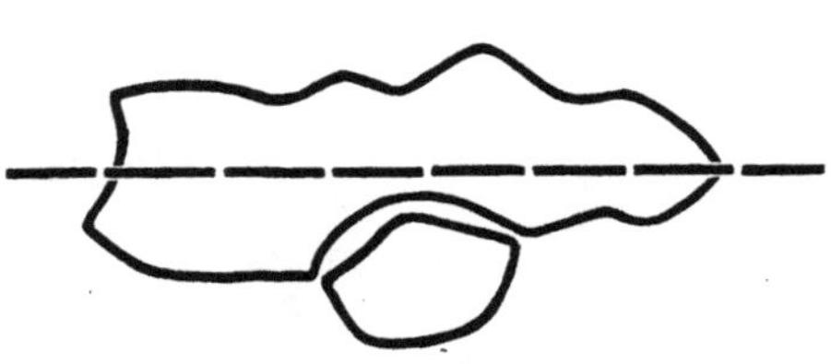

Fig. 8. Marking the inferior epiphyseal axis

Glenoid Morphology

The glenoid morphology was studied on the CT cuts to determine the arthritic wear, variations in retroversion and the distribution of forces.

Results

The mean glenoid retroversion was 15.4° with extremes of –4° to 44° (Fig. 9). The ratio of subluxation was 56.2 % with extremes of 35 %–80 %. Forty-five percent of cases displayed posterior subluxation and 6 % anterior subluxation with a centrally located head in 49 % (Fig. 10). There was either no or minimal fatty degeneration (stages 0, 1 and 2) of the subscapularis and infraspinatus in 89 % of cases and stage 3 and 4 in 11 %. For subscapularis there was stage 0.1 or 2 in 92 % and stage 3 or 4 in 8 % of cases. Mean humeral retroversion in the population

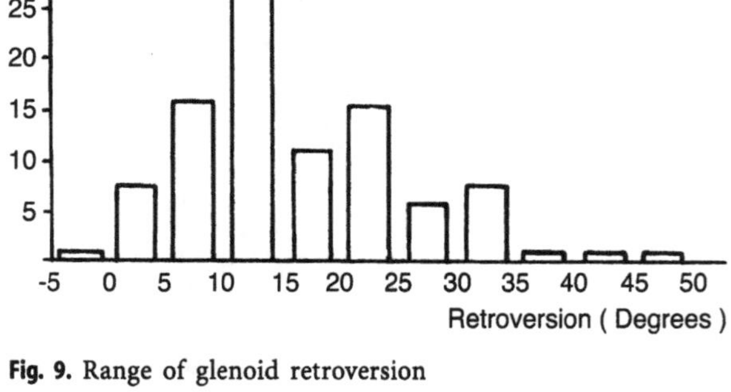

Fig. 9. Range of glenoid retroversion

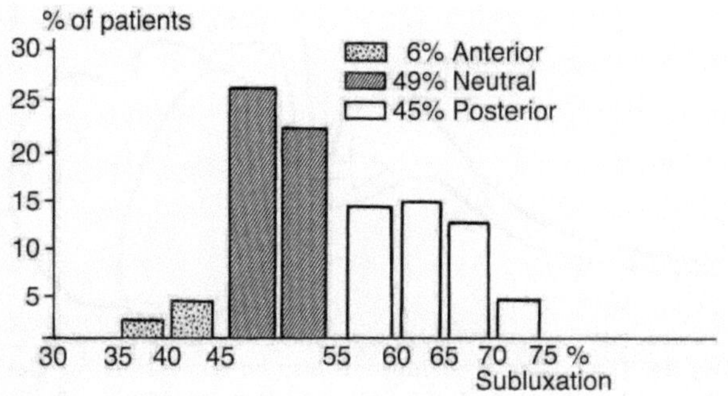

Fig. 10. Range of subluxation

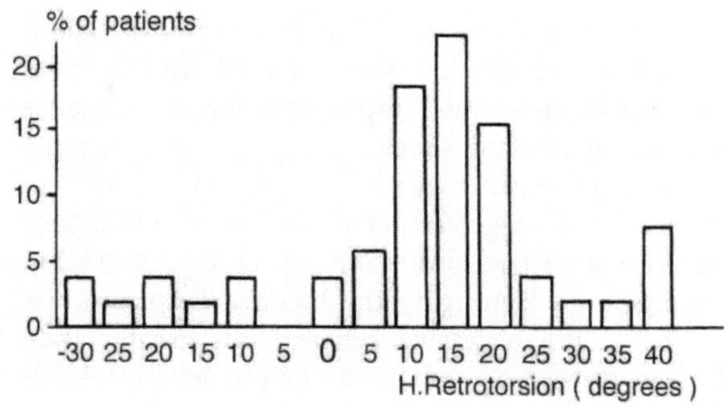

Fig. 11. Range of humeral retrotorsion

studied was 8.4° with extremes of −32° (anteversion) and +40° (retroversion; Fig. 11).

The glenoid morphology was described in three broad types (Fig. 12). *Type A* (53.5 %) was characterised by an equal balance of forces acting on the glenoid and a centralised head. Glenoid wear was either minor (type A1, 39.5 %) or major with significant central wear causing a glenoid cup (type A2, 14 %). *Type B* (39.5 %) had asymmetrical force distribution on the glenoid leading to either a loss of joint space (predominantly posterior), subchondral sclerosis (more marked on the posterior edge of the glenoid) and/or multiple posterior geodes (type B1, 12 %) or by a posterior cup which gave the appearance of a double concavity on the glenoid surface (type B2, 27.5 %). *Type C* (5 %) was arbitrarily defined as glenoid retroversion greater than 25° not due to arthritis erosion. There was no biconcavity and no central or posterior erosion. This retroversion was of primary dysplastic origin [13].

Clinical and Radiographic Correlations

The presence of clinical deltoid atrophy had an effect on active mobility with patients having 90° of active anterior elevation where there was no atrophy and only 72° where atrophy was present. Atrophy of infraspinatus also affected active anterior elevation (67° against 91°) and active external rotation (2.3° with atrophy against 10° without). Patients with a rupture of supraspinatus were older at 70.6 years than those without such a rupture whose average age was 65.9 years ($p<0.06$).

Supraspinatus rupture was correlated with infraspinatus atrophy ($p<0.01$), degeneration of infraspinatus ($p<0.009$) and degeneration of subscapularis ($p<0.01$).

Degeneration of infraspinatus influenced pain ($p<0.005$) and active mobility with only 61° of active elevation as compared with 93° where there was no degeneration ($p<0.004$). Subscapularis degeneration influenced pain ($p<0.05$) and reduced active elevation from 92° to 59° ($p<0.006$).

Posterior subluxation of the humeral head was not correlated with glenoid retroversion, humeral retrotorsion or fatty degeneration of the muscles of the cuff. We could find no element that explained this subluxation.

In type A there was usually no subluxation of the humeral head and the glenoid wear was symmetrical. The patients age increased linearly from type

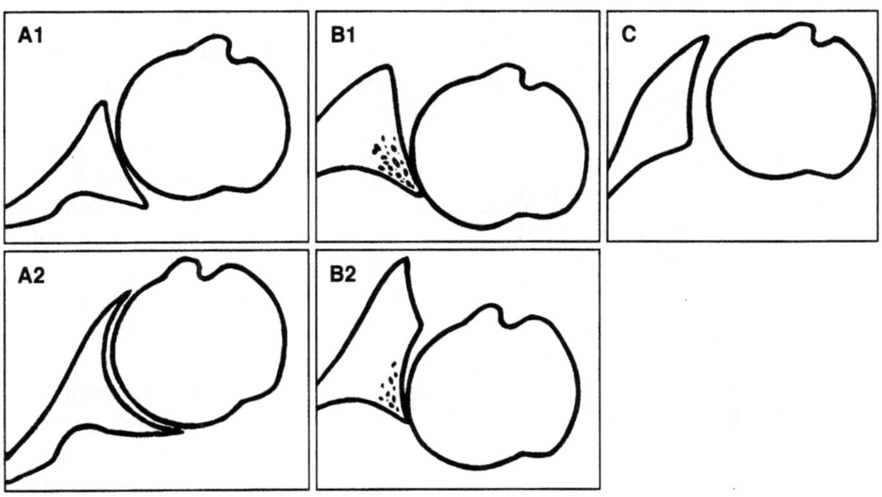

Fig. 12. Types of glenoid in primary gleno-humeral osteoarthritis (see text)

A1, at 62.3 years, to type A2 at 70.4 years. In type B the index of subluxation was increased, and the posterior subluxation was responsible for the changes observed in glenoid shape. The age of the patients increased from 62.9 years in type B1 to 69.7 in type B2. This suggests that this is an evolving process with a progression from B1 to B2 by erosion of the glenoid leading to the biconcave appearance. In type C the excessive retroversion greater than 25° was clearly of congenital origin with arthritis appearing relatively late because the average age at surgery was 61 years. This situation was fairly rare and was observed in 5% of the cases.

The type of glenoid was correlated with humeral head subluxation and this last link may be responsible for the posterior wear of the glenoid.

Discussion and Conclusion

The most important point revealed in this clinical and radiographic study is the relationship between posterior glenoid erosion, glenoid retroversion and subluxation of the humeral head.

The measurement of glenoid retroversion is inaccurate when there is posterior wear with a cup deformity because the measurement taken has to be a compromise between the primary retroversion and the wear retroversion (Fig. 13). This measurement does not take into account the difference between a congenital retroversion and a posterior erosion, clearly demonstrated by the double concavity deformity. Posterior subluxation existed in 45% of cases of primary osteoarthritis and was not due to excessive humeral retroversion because there was no statistical correlation between these two factors.

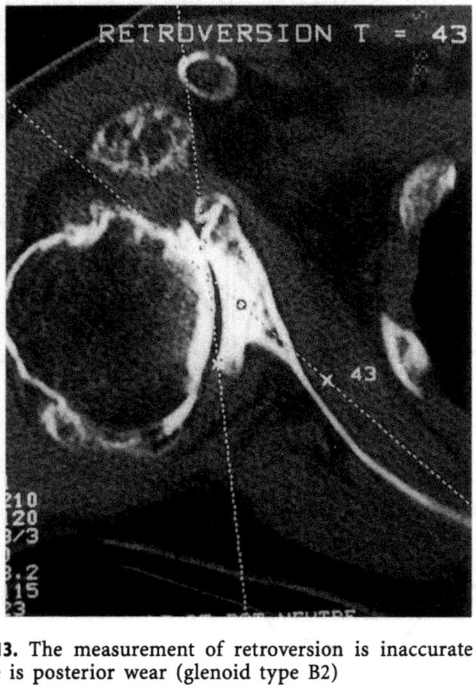

Fig. 13. The measurement of retroversion is inaccurate when there is posterior wear (glenoid type B2)

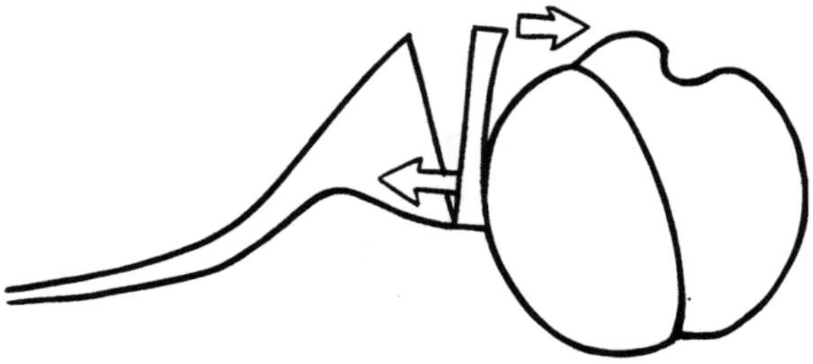

Fig. 14. The posterior subluxation may be responsible for glenoid loosening due to the rocking horse mechanism in the horizontal plane

On the other hand, subluxation of the humeral head was correlated with glenoid wear, and it is reasonable to suggest that the subluxation causes the wear. This presents a problem which must be emphasised: when one corrects the posterior glenoid wear (using a glenoid component with or without a graft) the subluxation is not corrected. This therefore leaves the risk of recurrence and may be responsible for glenoid loosening due to the "rocking horse" type mechanism described in the vertical plane by Franklin and Matsen [3]. In this case the deleterious effect occurs in the horizontal plane (Fig. 14). Can the development of future lucent lines be explained by this mechanism? Nor is humeral subluxation explained by humeral retroversion because no link was found between the two factors.

In our study the measurement of humeral retroversion, unlike that of subluxation and glenoid retroversion, had results for both inter and intra observer error which were poorly reproducible with a standard deviation of 11° between observers and 8.5° for the same observer. This poor reproducibility is explained by the arthritic changes which deform the normal landmarks of the anatomical neck.

Nonetheless, the absence of any correlation shows that it is probably a mistake to try to correct the posterior translation seen in some arthritis cases by changing humeral retroversion, i.e. positioning the prosthesis in anteversion instead of the inherent degree of retroversion.

If subluxation cannot be explained by any bony or muscular factors then why does it occur? We feel it is important to carry out a CT scan study of gleno-humeral osteoarthritis to try to find the cause so that it can be effectively corrected when inserting a total shoulder arthroplasty.

References

1. Badet R, Walch G, Boileau P (1995) Arthrography and cumputed arthrotomography study of seventy patients with primary gleno-humeral osteoarthritis Rev Rhum 62:555–562
2. Bernageau J, Godefroy D (1986) Le scanner de l'épaule. Le scanner ostéoarticulaire. Morvan, Massare, Frija Vigot 171–178
3. Franklin JL, Barret WP, Jackins SE, Matsen FA (1988) Glenoid loosening in total shoulder arthoplasty. J Arthroplasty 3:39–46
4. Forestier J (1936) Pourquoi l'arthrose de l'épaule est-elle une rareté? Aix-les-Bains Médical 4:5
5. Friedman RJ, Hawthorne KB, Genez BM (1992) The use of computerized tomography in the measurement of glenoid version. J Bone Joint Şurg Am 74:1032–1037
6. Goutallier D, Postel JM, Bernageau J, Lavau L, Voisin MC (1994) Fatty muscle degeneration in cuff ruptures. Pre and post-operative evaluation by CT-scan. Clin Orthop 304:78–83
7. Martingay I (1956) Contribution à l'étude de l'arthrose de l'épaule. Thèse Méd., Paris
8. Neer CS (1974) Replacement arthroplasty for gleno-humeral osteoarthritis. J Bone Joint Surg Am 56:1–13
9. Neer CS, Watson KC, Stanton FJ (1982) Recent experience in total shoulder replacement. J Bone Joint Surg Am 64:319–337
10. Neer CS, Morrison DS (1988) Glenoid bone-grafting in total shoulder arthroplasty. J Bone Joint Surg Am 70:1154–1162
11. Papilion JA, Larry M (1992) Fluoroscopic evaluation for subtle shoulder instability. Am J Sports Med 20:548–551
12. Ravault PP, Vignon G, Lejeune E, Maitrepierre J, Exertier J (1962) L'arthrose de l'épaule ou omarthrose. A propos de 45 observations. Rev Lyonnaise Méd 11:615–624
13. Wirth MA, Lyons FR, Rockwood CA (1993) Hypoplasia of the glenoid. A review of sixteen patients. J Bone Joint Surg Am 75:1175–1184

Results of Shoulder Arthroplasty in Primary Gleno-humeral Osteoarthritis

J.F. Kempf, G. Walch, and F. Lacaze

Summary

This prospective multicentrer study involved 155 shoulder arthroplasties operated on for osteoarthritis. Mean age at surgery was 66.6 years. The average follow-up was 19.4 months (range 12–46 months). There was a full-thickness degenerative cuff tear in 12.5 % and an attempt to repair was made in only five cases. The average normalised Constant Score was 39.4 % preoperatively and 95.5 % at review. The results were excellent or good in 80.5 %, fair in 12.8 % and poor in only 6.7 %. Two of the 13 press-fit humeral components demonstrated progressive radiographic loosening, whereas no signs of loosening were found in the 142 cemented humeral components. Glenoid lucencies were present in 60 % of the cases, they were incomplete in 55 % and progressive in 15 %. Three glenoid were definitively loosed with signs of migration. We did not find any statistical correlation between the final results and a preoperative cuff tear, associated acromioplasty or associated lengthening of the subscapularis. Fourteen patients did not have a glenoid component inserted because the glenoid surface was judged to be only slightly eroded. The absence of a glenoid component significantly worsened the results: the Constant score fells from 97 % to 81 % in the absence of a glenoid. The poorest result observed with hemiarthroplasty was clearly related to progressive glenoid erosion. Total shoulder arthroplasty gives better functional result than hemiarthroplasty in osteoarthritis. However, loosening of the glenoid component remains a potential complication and long term radiographic control is necessary.

Introduction

Primary osteoarthritis has historically been the commonest degenerative condition affecting the shoulder for which Neer proposed the insertion of an unconstrained prosthesis in 1974 [10]. Conservation of bone stock and the presence of an "almost always intact rotator cuff", appeared to Neer to be the two essential criteria in achieving a good clinical result after shoulder arthroplasty (Fig. 1). Since then,

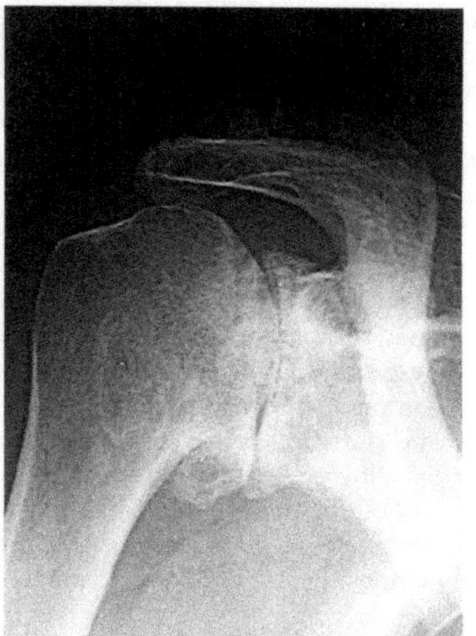

Fig. 1. Typical radiographic presentation of primary gleno-humeral osteoarthritis

there have been many series published in the literature which have confirmed these impressions and the initial results achieved by Neer [1, 2, 4, 5, 9, 11]. The level of reported complications in these series have always been low and have been particularly influenced by individual anatomical variations (combined cuff tears, posterior glenoid wear) and by variations in operative technique (replacing or not replacing the glenoid, cemented or uncemented humeral components) which have aroused disagreements between authors. This multicentre study involved 155 arthroplasties inserted in 14 different centres and reflects these anatomical and surgical variations with the goal being to analyse their effect on the final outcome.

Material and Methods

Methods

The system for reviewing the patients was the same in all the centres: the patients were recalled for a consultation which involved a history and clinical examination. The results were recorded using the Constant score which gives 15 points for pain, 20 for the activities of daily living, 40 for active mobility and 25 for strength, amounting to a total of 100 [7]. This total can be normalised for age and sex, using specially calculated tables, and this result is then expressed as a percentage for a normal shoulder in an individual of the same sex and age. The normalised Constant score is defined as excellent if it is 100 %, good from 86 % to 100 %, average from 51 % to 85 % and poor if less than 50 %. Radiographs in internal, neutral and external rotation and an axillary profile views were taken systematically. A statistical analysis was made by Dr. Adeleine of the medical data-processing laboratory of the Civil Hospitals of Lyon on a Compas 386 computer with SPSS software. The statistical test used for the qualitative variables was the χ^2 test, and contingency tables with analysis of the residuals. For the quantitative variables an analysis of variance was used with Scheffe's method of multiple comparison.

Patients

We were able to review 155 patients which had undergone the insertion of an Aequalis prosthesis with more than 1 year of follow-up, thanks to input from several centres and files were received from M. Basso, P. Boileau, J.P. Franceschi, C. Gerber, D. Goutallier, P. Habermeyer, J.F. Kempf, J.C. Le Huec, C. Levigne, H. Mestdagh, D. Molé, L. Nove-Josserand, J.C. Scheffer and G. Walch. The average follow-up was 19.4 months (12–49 months). In 75 % the patients were women, and the dominant arm was involved in 60 %. The average age was 66.6 years (24–84). The controlateral shoulder was pathological in 62 %. The patients were often inactive (25.2 %) or retired (62.8 %). Only 17 patients (12 %) were professionally active at the time of their operation. The preoperative Constant score was very mediocre at 28.7 points (normalised=39.4 %). All the elements of the score were reduced and, in particular, pain which had a score of only 3.3 out of 15; the activity level was 7.3 out of 20; mobility was 14 out of 40 and strength was 4 out of 25. On the preoperative clinical examination, there was no deltoid atrophy in 68.7 %, no supraspinatus atrophy in 62.5 % and no infraspinatus atrophy in 64 %. The state of the rotator cuff was assessed by preoperative computed tomographic (CT) arthrogram. The supraspinatus was the site of a partial rupture in 9 patients (6.6 %) and of a full-thickness tear in another 17 (12.5 %; Fig. 2). The infraspinatus was normal in 97 %. Fatty degeneration was assessed on CT using the Goutallier classification [8]: it was less than or equal to stage 2 (less fat tissue than muscle) in 90 % of the cases.

Surgical Technique

The operation was carried out via the delto-pectoral approach in the vast majority (95 %) of the cases.

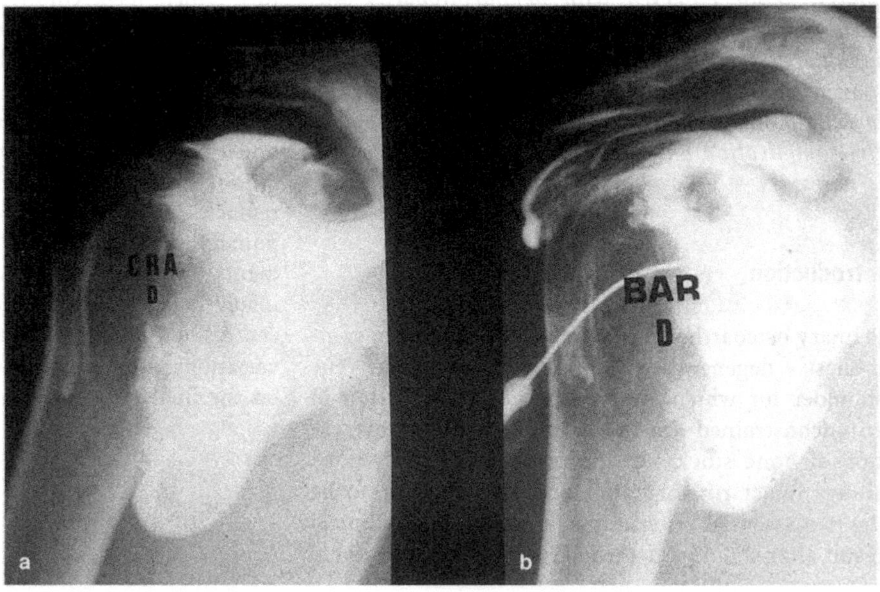

Fig. 2. a Typical negative arthrogram associated with osteoarthritis of the shoulder. **b** Rupure of the supraspinatus tendon occured in only 12.5 % of osteoarthritis

We recorded 7 trans-acromial superior approaches and one posterior approach. A procedure involving the subscapularis was frequently carried out: in 71 % of cases an anterior juxtaglenoid capsulotomy was performed, and in 5.8 % a Z-plasty tendon lengthening was done. An acromioplasty was performed in 11 patients, a tenodesis of the long head of biceps in 9 cases and resection of the lateral centimeter of the clavicle in 6. In only 5 cases of 17 full-thickness tear were attempts made to repair rotator cuff damage.

An Aequalis prosthesis was used in all cases. The humeral prosthesis had a 125° neck in 25.7 %, 130° in 34.2 %, 135° in 28.3 % and 140° in 11.8 %. The stem diameter was 6 mm in 10.5 %, 9 mm in 50.7 % and 12 mm in 38.8 %. All the available head sizes were used but the small sizes (39/14 and 41/15) were used in only 8 %. The stem was cemented in all cases except in 13 cases (8.8 %) where it was press-fitted. The overall humeral reconstruction was judged by the surgeon as being good in 88.5 % of cases, average in 9.4 % and poor in only 2.1 %. With regards to the glenoid implant, 14 patients (9.1 %) did not have a glenoid component inserted because the glenoid surface was judged to be only slightly eroded. There were 125 cemented glenoid implants (91.2 %) and 12 uncemented glenoid implants using the, new expansion screw glenoid (8.8 %). A small size glenoid component was used in 31.6 %, a medium sized component in 50 % and a large size in 18.4 %. External rotation elbow at the side at the end of the operation reached 28° from a preoperative average of 11°.

Postoperative Treatment

Immobilisation was not required in 72 % of the cases but, where it was seemed necessary by the surgeon, then a sling immobilising the arm in neutral rotation was used. Because our Health Care System has provision for inpatient rehabilitation, 117 patients (77 %) underwent rehabilitation in a specialist Centre for an average of 37 days.

Results

Constant Score

The postoperative absolute Constant score was an average of 69.8 points (Table 1). The normalised postoperative Constant score was 95.5 %, which is a value very close to normal when considered for age and sex. The increases achieved where particularly high for pain, which was 13 points out of 15 at review, activity, which was 16.9 points out of 20 and mobility, which was 32.1 points out of 40. Even force doubled its preoperative values: 2 kg preoperatively and 4 kg at review.

Mobility

Table 2 shows the values obtained for passive and active mobility in elevation, external rotation and internal rotation. There is a particularly clear post-

Table 1. Detailed Constant score

Constant score	Preoperative		Postoperative	Gain	Gain (%)
Pain (15 points)	3.3	⟶	13	+9.7	249
Activity (20 points)	7.3	⟶	16.9	+9.6	132
Mobility (40 points)	14	⟶	32.1	+18.1	129
Strength (25 points)	4	⟶	8	+4	100
Absolute Constant score (100 points)	28.7	⟶	69.8	+41.1	143
Normalised Constant score (%)	39.4 %	⟶	95.5 %	+56.1	142

Table 2. Results on mobility

Mobility	Preoperative		Postoperative	Gain
Passive anterior elevation	101°	⟶	151°	+50°
Active anterior elevation	88°	⟶	143°	+55°
Passive external rotation	11.5°	⟶	44°	+32.5°
Active external rotation	9°	⟶	41.5°	+32.5°
Active external rotation (90° abduction)	Na		71°	–
Internal rotation	Na		L3	–
Internal rotation (90° abduction)	Na		35°	–

Na, Nonavailable.

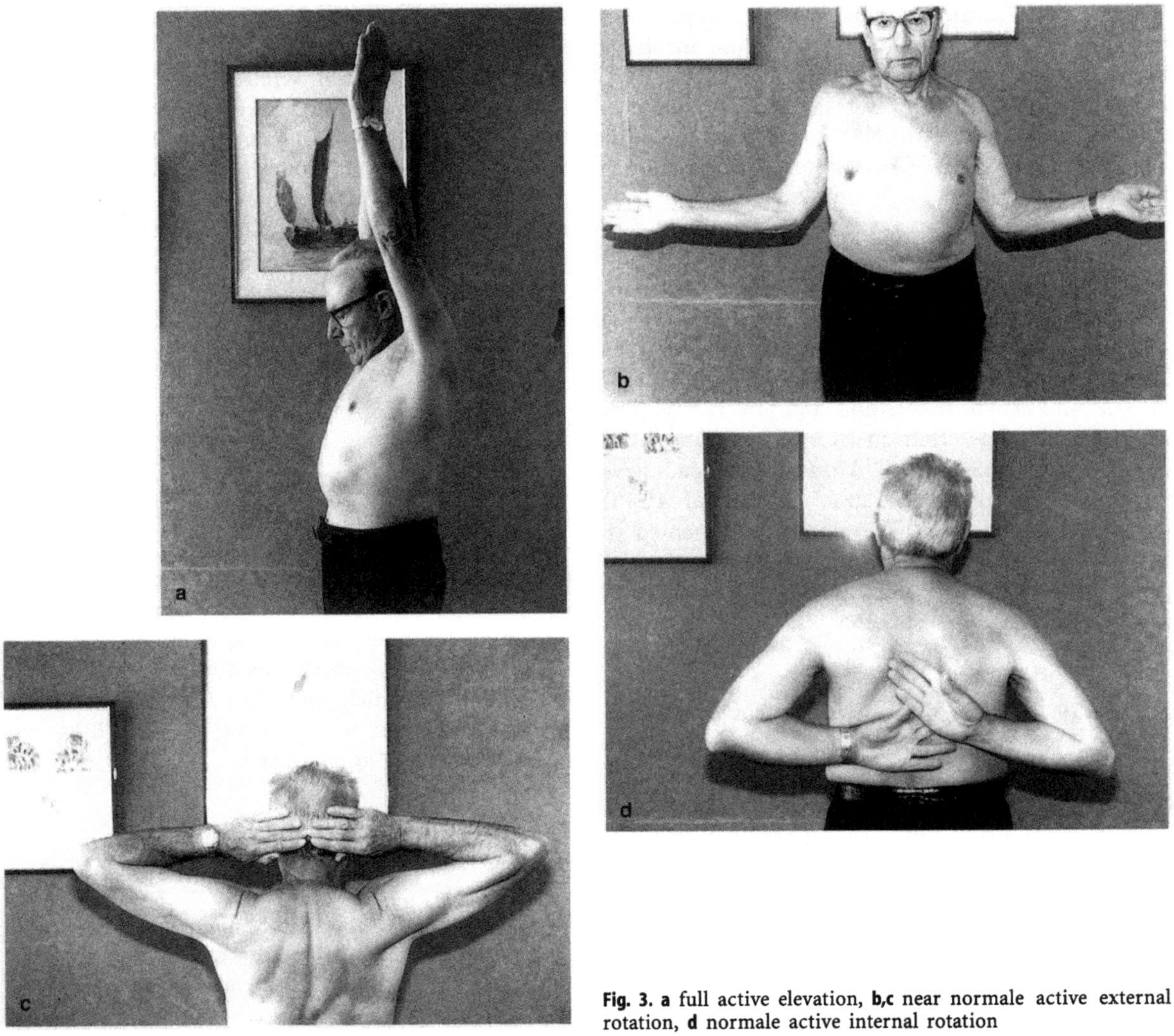

Fig. 3. a full active elevation, **b,c** near normale active external rotation, **d** normale active internal rotation

operative improvement in average anterior elevation which reached 151° passively and 143° actively: an improvement of 50 % on the preoperative levels. External rotation elbow at the side reached 44° passively and 41.5° actively on average postoperatively which was a gain of 32° in comparison to the preoperative values (Fig. 3).

Qualitative Objective Results

There was an excellent or good result in 80.5 % and an average result in 12.8 %. Only 10 patients (6.7 %), had a poor outcome. Amongst these poor results, one patient presented with glenoid loosening, two had a postoperative sympathetic reflex dystrophy and were very stiff at review, three patients over 80 years in age were more interested in their shoulders being rapidly pain free than in working to recover mobility and good function: their shoulders remained stiff at review. One patient did not have a glenoid component inserted despite having significant wear and complained of pain and functional limitation. One patient with work compensation did not want to return to work and in two cases no rational explication for the poor outcome could be discovered.

Subjective Results

The subjective results were also very satisfying with only 10 patients (6.6 %) disappointed. One patient was unhappy with the intervention and 92.7 % were either happy or very happy with their operation. The patients estimated the time required to achieve this result as being 6.6 months on average (1–24).

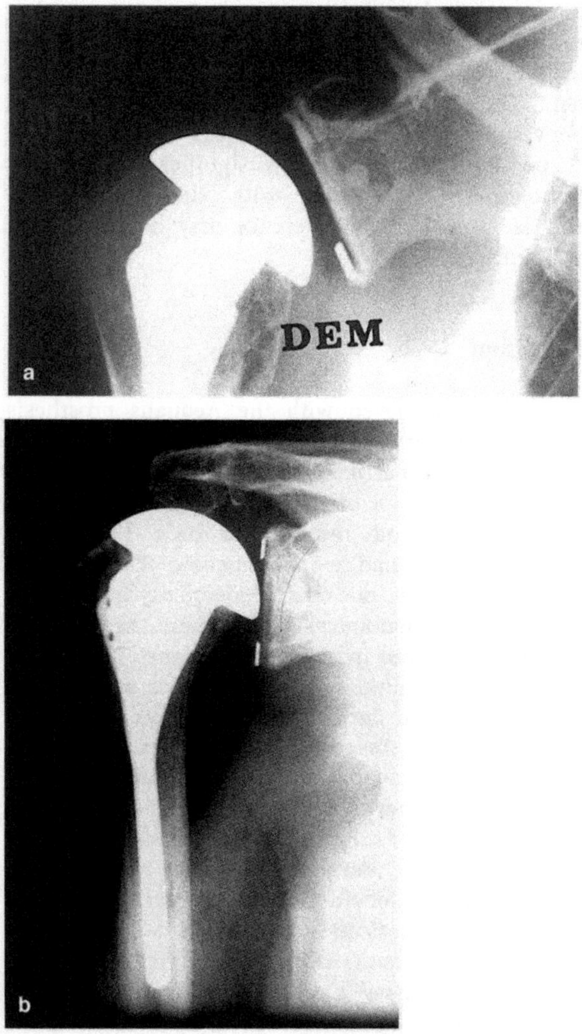

Fig. 4. a Good reconstruction of the proximal humeral epiphysis. **b** Aequalis prosthesis

Radiographic Results

Peri-prosthetic ossifications were found and considered as minimal in 18 patients (12.5 %) and only one patient presented with ossifications judged as significant. We recorded two humeral distal migration out of the 13 press-fitted humeral components and 9 humeral lucent lines (8.3 %) which were all incomplete and non-progressive. Glenoid lucencies were much more common than at the humeral level because only 47 cases (40 %) did not exhibit lucent lines. Of the 67 lines reported (60 %) they were incomplete in 55 % and progressive in only 15 % (Fig. 5). Three glenoids were loose with signs of migration. This complication is discussed in Chap. 43.

Complications and Revisions

Five per cent (10 cases) of the cases had a local complication. We recorded three humeral fractures, one infection, one haematoma and five neurological problems. Six patients (4 %) underwent revision; one for infection where the prosthesis had to be removed, one for totalisation of the hemi-arthroplasty, one to evacuate a haematoma and three for glenoid loosening. (A detailed analysis of these complications is presented by Mestdagh et al., "Intra- and Postoperative Complications of Shoulder Arthroplasty", in this volume).

Factors Effecting the Outcome

Statistical analysis was used to determine some predictable factors that could be associated with poor results.

Approach and Subscapularis Release or Lengthening. Seven patients were operated on via a superior transacromial approach. There was no significant difference between this and the delto-pectoral approach for any of the criteria studied. The only point worth mentioning was a slightly reduced average force after a superior approach. Procedures carried out on subscapularis such as Z-plasty elongation or an anterior releasing juxta-glenoid capsulotomy were carried out when the surgeon judged that external rotation was insufficient. These releasing procedures proved to make no difference because the 115 patients who underwent such a procedure had exactly comparable results to the 40 who did not, for all the criteria studied.

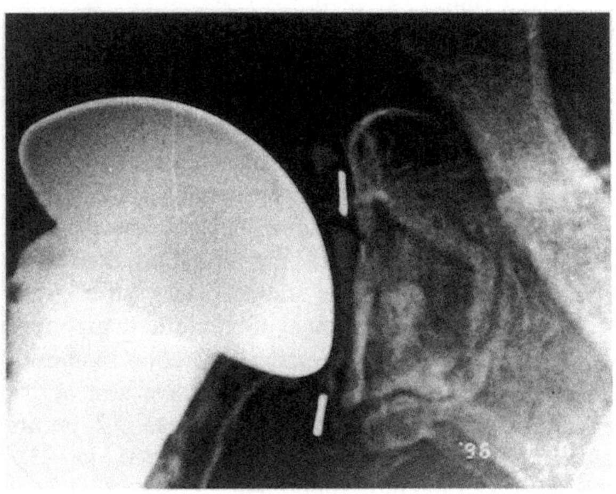

Fig. 5. Complete progressive radiolucent line

External rotation elbow at the side was 43.8° when there was a specific allied procedure and 45.8° when there was not.

The Influence of Procedures on the Rotator Cuff. Preoperative CT arthrograms demonstrated 17 full-thickness tears of the rotator cuff which were always limited to the supraspinatus and 9 partial ruptures of the deep surface of supraspinatus. Eleven patients had an acromioplasty and 5 had a cuff repair by direct suture at the same time as the main operation. Nine other patients had a tenotomy or tenodesis of the long head of biceps when it was judged pathological at the time of surgery. Although it was not statistically significant, cuff tear was shown to have a negative effect on the postoperative Constant score. The normalised score was 92.5% where there was a preoperative cuff tear and 96.5% in its absence ($p<0.2$). The result for force was the most significantly effected parameter with an average of 4 kg without a tear and 2 kg with a tear. Because of the multicentre nature of the study the disparate procedures carried out on the cuff makes it difficult to analyse their effect on the results. Surprisingly, in the midst of this group of 26 patients presenting with either a partial or full thickness tear of supraspinatus, we found no difference in the outcome whether or not there had been an acromioplasty (11 cases), a cuff repair (5 cases) or if the long head of biceps had been sacrificed (9 cases).

Factors Involving the Implant. The size of the head or the glenoid and the angle of the neck had no influence on the results, which is to be expected as the sizes where selected to anatomically reconstruct the humeral epiphysis. The size of the humeral stem did not affect the presence of lucent lines. On the other hand, if the stem was inserted uncemented, we found a clear increase in lucent lines with a rate of 44% as opposed to 5.3% when the stem was cemented (Fig. 6). We could not find any significant influence of the lucent line on the clinical outcome for any of the clinical criteria studied. However, the absence of a glenoid component significantly worsened the result at review (Fig. 7, Table 3). In the absence of a glenoid, the Constant score fell from 70.8–58.3 and the normalised score from 97% to 81%. The absence of glenoid component also significantly reduced external rotation in abduction, internal rotation and both passive and active anterior elevation. The pain score was 9.7 points without glenoid component as opposed to 13.7 points with a glenoid component.

Influence of Glenoid Shape. Table 4 shows the spread of hemi-arthroplasties and total arthroplasties as a function of glenoid shape. It does not seem that the surgeons were influenced by this element in making their decision to insert a glenoid component. The percentage of hemi-arthroplasties remains between 0% and 14% regardless of the glenoid shape. We did not find any significant clinical or radiographic differences with different glenoid shapes. This lack of difference may be because of the short follow-up.

Discussion

The results achieved with the Aequalis prosthesis used in primary osteoarthritis were encouraging: Even using the particularly stringent Constant scoring system, 80.5% of our patients achieved either excellent or good results and only 10 patients (6.7%) of them had a poor outcome. This is probably explained by the relative simplicity of this surgery in these anatomical forms where the head has remained centered in the vertical plane. The rotator cuff was nearly always intact, muscular atrophy was insignificant and fatty degeneration seen on the CT scan was rarely present. It is only particularly unfavourable anatomical conditions such as significant wear in an abnormally retroverted glenoid which act as a source of surgical difficulty and thus detract from the result. Other authors such as Neer [12, 13], Mansat [9] and Cofield [5, 6] also report satisfactory results for this indication in 84%–98% of cases. The quality of the results obtained in this multi-centre study, despite using a review scoring system which is more severe than those used by other authors, may also be explained by the quality of the implant used which allowed an anatomical reconstruction of the gleno-humeral joint in the vast majority of cases.

Repairing a cuff tear is advisable to limit further damage but not effecting a repair does not have an effect on the clinical outcome – at least in the short term. It seems that the humeral stem must be cemented in place. The results of this study very clearly shows that whenever possible the glenoid should be resurfaced. However, as with many other authors we found a high level of glenoid lucent lines which do not seem, at least for the moment, to lead to a high rate of loosening as this was only 2.2%, but, again, our follow-up is short. Improving the quality of the cementing and especially the use of an uncemented glenoid which has promising results (reported in another chapter) should allow further progress in this field.

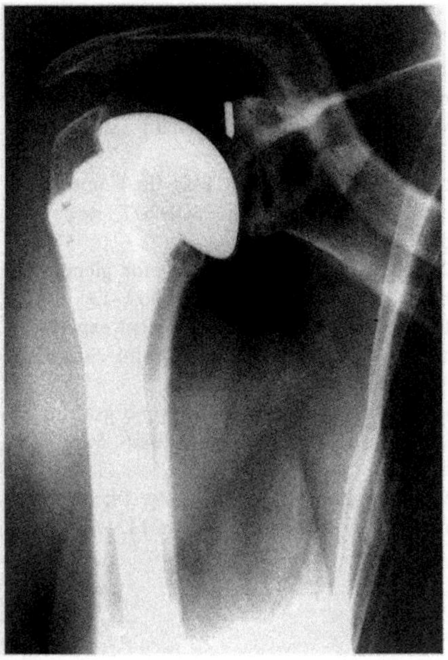

Fig. 6. Migration of a noncemented humeral stem

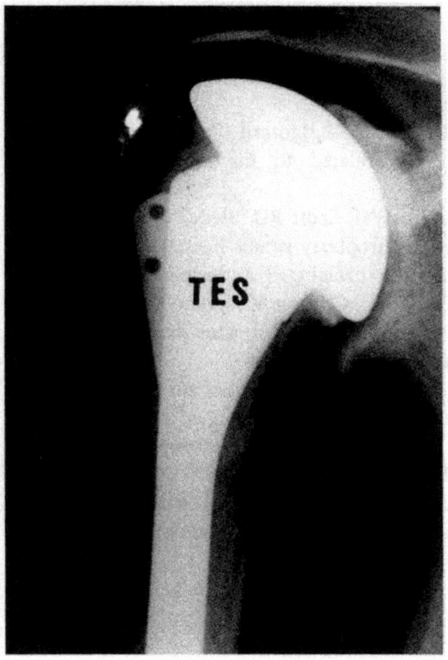

Fig. 7. Hemi-arthroplasty with glenoid erosion

Table 3. Results related to the type of prosthesis: total versus hemiarthroplasty

Results	Hemi-arthroplasty (*n*=14)	Total shoulder prosthesis (*n*=141)
Pain (15 points)	9.7	13.7
Activity (20 points)	15	17
Mobility (40 points)	27.3	32.7
Strength (25 points)	6.2	8.1
Absolute Constant score (100 points)	58.3	70.8
Normalised Constant score	81 %	96.9 %
Passive anterior elevation	135°	153°
Active anterior elevation	130°	144.8°

Table 4. Number of glenoid components implanted by glenoid morphology

		Hemi-arthroplasty	
Glenoid morphology	Total shoulder arthroplasty	*n*	%
A1 (*n*=40)	37	3	8 %
A2 (*n*=14)	12	2	14 %
B1 (*n*=12)	12	0	0 %
B2 (*n*=28)	25	3	11 %
C (*n*=5)	5	0	0 %
Nonavailable (*n*=56)	48	8	14 %

Conclusion

This multicentre study of 155 cases confirms that osteoarthritis is an excellent indication for a total shoulder arthroplasty. The quality of the results that we achieved may be due to the Aequalis prosthesis, which allows better and more accurate anatomical reconstruction of the gleno-humeral joint. We have also been able to confirm the anatomical and biomechanical principles on which the design of the prosthesis was based.

References

1. Barrett WP et al (1987) Total shoulder arthroplasty. J Bone Joint Surg Am 69:865
2. Boileau P, Walch G, Noel E, Liotard JP (1994) Neer shoulder prosthesis: Results related to the etiology. Rev Rhum 61:539–547
3. Boyd AD, Thomas WH, Scott RD, Sledge CB, Thornhill TS (1990) Shoulder arthroplasty versus hemiarthroplasty. Indication for glenoid resurfacing. J Arthroplasty 5:329–336
4. Brenner BC, Ferlic DC, Clayton ML, Dennis DA (1989) Survivorship of unconstrained total shoulder arthroplasty. J Bone Joint Surg Am 71:1289–1296
5. Cofield RH, Briggs BT (1979) Glenohumeral arthritis. J Bone Joint Surg Am 61:668–677
6. Cofield RH (1984) Total shoulder arthroplasty with Neer prosthesis. J Bone Joint Surg Am 66:899–906
7. Constant CR, Murley AHG (1987) A clinical method of functional assessement of the shoulder. Clin Orthop 214:160–164
8. Goutallier D, Postel JM, Bernageau J, Lavau L, Voisin MC (1994) Fatty muscle degeneration in cuff ruptures. Pre and post-operative evaluation by CT-scan. Clin Orthop 304: 78–83
9. Mansat M et al (1995) Résultats à plus de 5 ans de la prothèse d'épaule de Neer. Symp SOFCOT Rev Chir Orthop [Suppl II]:75–133
10. Neer CS (1974) Replacement arthroplasty for glenohumeral osteoarthritis. J Bone Joint Surg Am 56:1–13
11. Neer CS, Watson KC, Stanton FJ (1982) Recent experience in total shoulder arthroplasty. J Bone Joint Surg Am 64:319–337
12. Neer CS, Morrisson DS (1988) Glenoid bone grafting in total shoulder arthroplasty. J Bone Joint Surg Am 70:1154–1162
13. Neer CS (1990) Glenohumeral arthroplasty. In: Shoulder reconstruction. Saunders, Philadelphia, pp 143–271

Section VIII:

Rheumatoid Arthritis

The Role of Medical Synovectomy in Treatment of the Rheumatoid Shoulder

E. Noel, T. Thomas, E. Ollagnier, A. Constantin, J.G. Tebib, and M. Bouvier

Summary

The shoulder is often involved in rheumatoid. The rheumatoid pannus is specific for rheumatoid disease and is responsible for the erosive lesions which lead to the progressive destruction of the gleno-humeral joint. The goal of medical synovectomy is to destroy the pathological synovium in the hope that normal synovium will then regenerate. We carried out a retrospective study of 36 rheumatoid shoulders which had undergone at least one medical synovectomy. These shoulders were reviewed clinically using the Constant score and radiographically with a minimum follow-up of 2 years. On 30 occasions a radioactive synovectomy was performed using 2 mCi rhenium-186 and on six occasions, osmic acid was used. Thirty shoulders had one injection and six had two. The average delay between the onset of rheumatoid arthritis and the synovectomy was 7.3 years (1–24). Twenty-one shoulders (58 %) were greatly improved (7 cases) or improved (14) and 15 shoulders (42 %) remained unchanged (9) or were worse (6). The absolute Constant score was 59.7 points on average (16–93) and the normalised score averaged 81 % (18–116.5). There were no radiographic changes in comparison to the originals in 39.4 % of cases, but there was deterioration in 60.6 %. The best time to carry out the synovectomy is undeniably when the radiographic lesions are minimal (no radiological abnormality or only microcysts). Medical synovectomy has a place in the treatment of the rheumatoid shoulder but its results are closely linked to the timing of the intervention. It should not be considered as an isolated treatment but should be part of an overall treatment plan.

Introduction

The shoulder is often involved in rheumatoid arthritis and clinical signs may be present in between 50 and 90 % of cases [7]. This article does not discuss disease localised to the acromio-clavicular joint which, although common, does not present the same treatment problems. Shoulder involvement is often neglected and particularly so when it occurs on a background of multiple complaints where the priority is generally given to the weight-bearing joints. The usual treatment for shoulder pain due to rheumatoid arthritis is symptomatic using corticosteroid injections given under image intensifier control. However, the difficulty in proving the presence of a rheumatoid pannus in the shoulder may be the reason why inappropriate medical synovectomies are carried out.

Histologicaly, it is the rheumatoid pannus which is specific for rheumatoid disease and which is responsible for the erosive lesions which lead to the progressive destruction of the joint. The pannus which consists of lymphocytes, macrophages and monocytes, secretes inflammatory cytokines, proliferates and progressively invades the joint and then the sub-chondral bone (Fig. 1). During this evolution the radiographic appearances can range from an erosion at the level of the insertion of the synovium with the greater tuberosity (Fig. 2), through the appearance of large geodes in the humeral head (Fig. 3) to joint destruction (Fig. 4). Many radiographic classifications of rheumatoid arthritis damage have been proposed [11, 26, 29].

The primary goal in treating a rheumatoid shoulder is to avoid progression of the disease process towards destruction of the joint which can occur very rapidly (Fig. 5). In order to achieve this, the therapeutic measures which can be used are: *medical:* either with systemic medications which alter the disease process (gold salts, thiol derivatives, methotrexate etc.) or local treatments (steroid injections, chemical or radioactive synovectomies) and *surgical:* open or arthroscopic synovectomies or more radical procedures such as hemi- or total shoulder arthroplasty. Arthrodesis has currently been abandoned in rheumatoid arthritis.

We assessed the results of medical synovectomy in the rheumatoid shoulder and determine any factors which might influence its outcome. We carried out a retrospective study of 36 rheumatoid shoulders which had undergone at least one medical synovectomy. These shoulders were reviewed clinically using the Constant score [4] and radiographically with a minimum follow-up of 2 years.

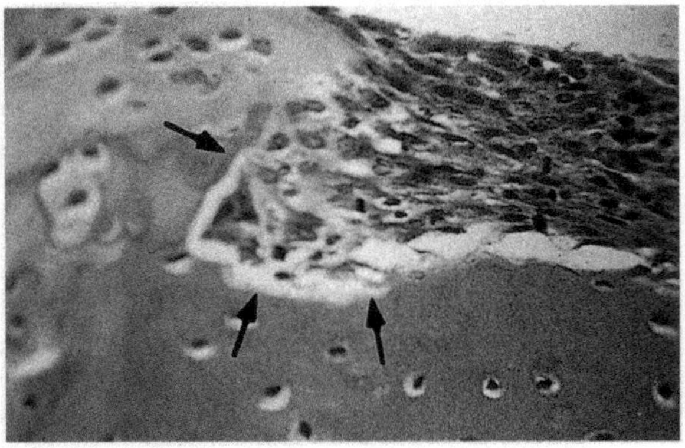

Fig. 1. Histological sections of rheumatoid pannus. (From Clinical Immunology, De Boeck University; J. Brostoff, G.K. Scadding, D. Male, Y.M. Roitt)

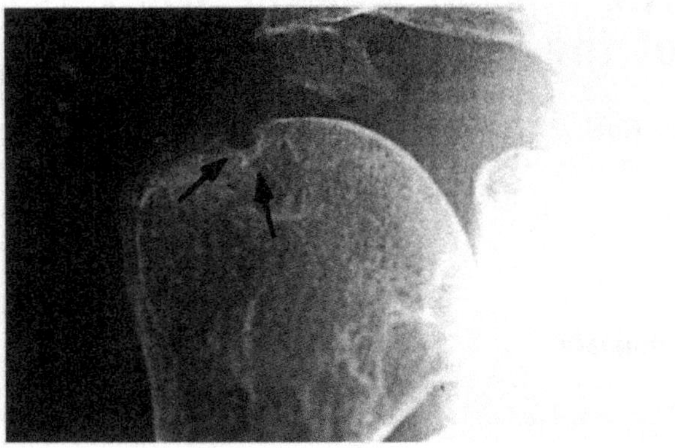

Fig. 2. Erosion at the greater tuberosity

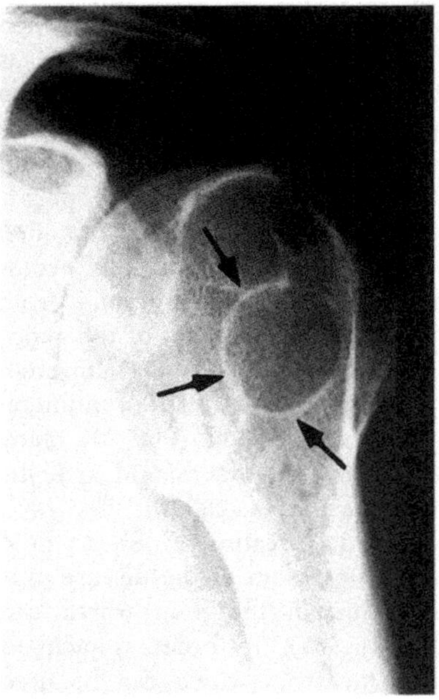

Fig. 3. A large geode in the humeral head

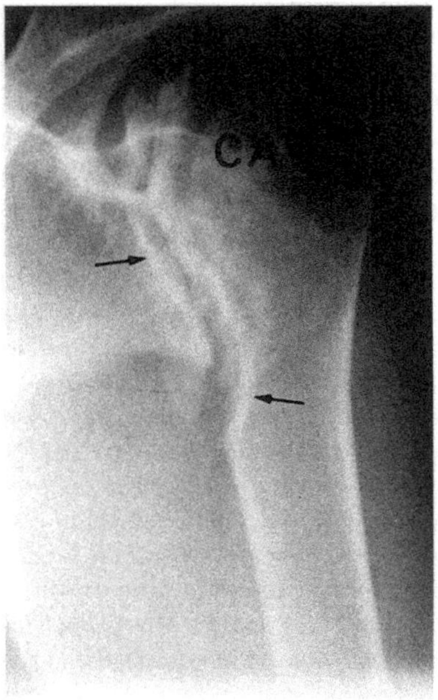

Fig. 4. Complete joint destruction

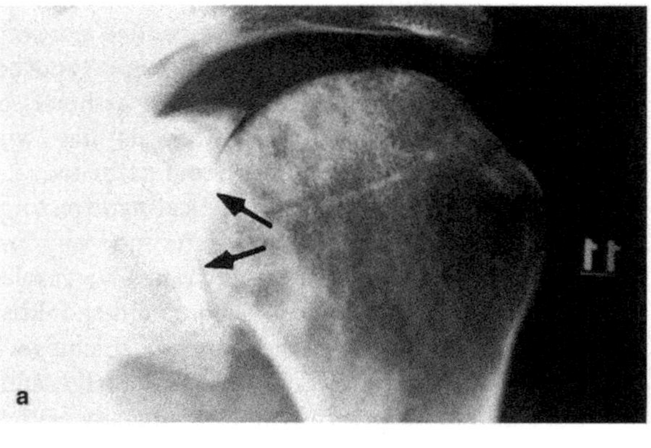

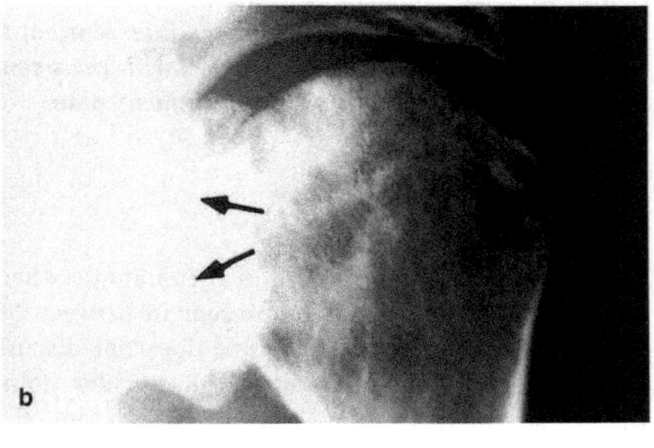

Fig. 5. a Loss of gleno-humeral joint space (April 1993). **b** Rapid deterioration in joint space narrowing in the same patient (February 1994)

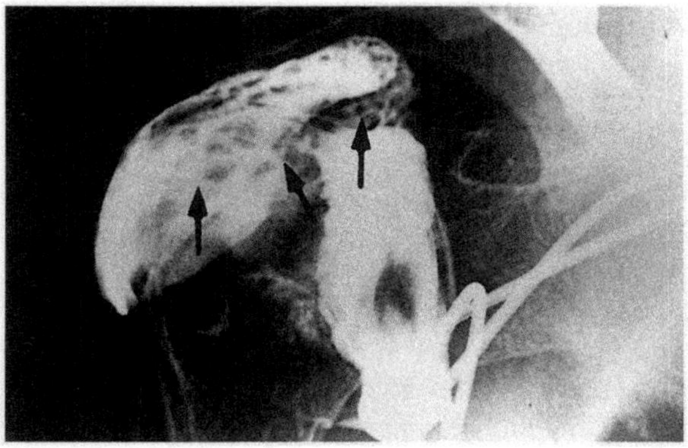

Fig. 6. Synovial proliferation in the sub-acromial bursa as shown on arthrography

Medical Synovectomy

Medical synovectomy has been used since 1951 with varying results [22]. The goal is to destroy the pathological synovium (Fig. 6) in the hope that normal synovium will then regenerate. In the knee such regeneration occurs 3–4 months after synovial destruction [25], but unfortunately the new synovium is frequently rapidly reaffected by the disease. A wide variety of products have been injected since 1951 (osmic acid, alkalising agents, radioactive substances – initially gold and then yttrium, rhenium and erbium). Today alkalising agents and gold are no longer used and erbium is reserved for the small joints. In the shoulder medical synovectomies are carried out using either osmic acid or radioactive yttrium-90 or rhenium-186.

Synovectomy Using Osmic Acid

Intra-articular injection of osmium tetroxide (osmic acid) has been used by the Scandinavians since 1951 [22], but extremely painful reactions led to the technique being abandoned for many years until the injections were given in combination with corticosteroid and local anaesthetic [2]. Osmium tetroxide has a strong affinity for lipids and coagulated proteins and acts by reducing the enzymatic activity of the synovium resulting after several weeks in synovial sclerosis. The side effects of osmic acid are mostly theoretical although it is indisputable that diffusion of the product outside the joint must be zealously avoided with the shoulder being strictly immobilised for 48 h after the injection. Despite the combined injection with xylocaine and corticosteroid there can still be a painful reaction in the hours following the injection and occasionally there is a transient febrile reaction on the evening following the injection.

A damaging action by osmic acid on the cartilage is not recognised by all authors although there is a persistent dark discolouration of the cartilage though without any definite macroscopic lesion appearing during the injection. However, there have been recorded cases of preexisting cartilaginous lesions being worsened. Electron microscopy has shown changes in the structure of the chondrocytes [14], but any clinical impact this might have is difficult to determine. The therapeutic effects of osmic acid have mainly been evaluated in the knee where uncontrolled trials have given about 50 % good results for a 6- to 12-month period. Controlled trials are rare [15–17] but in the knee they show that osmic acid gave better results than placebo or steroid and gave equivalent results to radioactive synovectomy with yttrium and surgical synovectomy at 1 year.

Radioactive Synovectomy

The use of radioactive products was developed more recently with Ansell [1] using radioactive gold in 1963 and yttrium-90 appeared in 1968. Gold 198 was abandoned because it gave off gamma radiation which, as opposed to beta radiation, passed beyond the joint. Yttrium is a pure beta emitter and rhenium is practically pure (72 % beta and 15 % gamma). In vitro the radioactive metal is fixed to a colloid and then injected into the joint. The colloid molecules have a very strong affinity for the synovial membrane and carry the radioactive product into the superficial cellular layers. The synoviocytes are therefore exposed to beta radiation which causes a progressive necrosis over the first month and then reaches to the deeper layers causing synovial fibrosis within 3 months. As a second stage, and in the cases giving the best results, a normal synovium regenerates. The average soft-tissue penetration varies with the product used [5]: for yttrium this is 3.6 mm while it is 1.2 mm for rhenium and 0.3 mm for erbium. It is therefore advised that yttrium is used for the knee and rhenium or yttrium for the shoulder, depending on the thickness of the pannus.

After the intra-articular injection, the majority of the radioactive material remains within the joint but the main risk is extra-articular diffusion. Some colloid particles may diffuse via the lymphatics (5 %–10 % of the initial activity) and certain authors [27] have shown that this can cause chromosomal abnormalities in the circulating lymphocytes. The importance of these abnormalities is debatable, but it seems to cause a multi-factorial chromosomal instability which disappears after 4–6 weeks. The carcinogenic and leukaemic risks after radioactive synovectomy are so rare as to be almost non-existent and these potential problems have already been investigated in hyperthyroidism treated with radioactive Iodine. It is therefore very important to use pure beta emitters and to strictly immobilise the joint after injection to minimise any diffusion of the colloid. Under these conditions, Lloyd [12] reported chromosomal lesions in 0.011 % of cases. It must also be mentioned that the toxicity of the radioactive products is directly related to the total injected dose given to the whole individual (the maximum dose varies between authors from 15–25 mCi). For the shoulder the injected dose is usually about 2–4 mCi rhenium or 1–2 mCi yttrium. When other joints are being injected at the same sitting the classic teaching is that not more than 10 mCi should be given on the same day to any one person.

The published series report on average 64 % favourable results when all joints and all products are taken into consideration, with the results being better when the treatment is carried out earlier. For yttrium controlled and uncontrolled trials have given good results which are generally better than 50 % at 6–12 months of follow-up. A meta-analysis carried out by Jones [8] showed a statistically significant superiority for yttrium over placebo and a tendency to its being better than corticosteroids.

Results of Medical Synovectomy in the Treatment of the Rheumatoid Shoulder: Analysis of the Literature

Very few studies allow these comparisons to be made. Sheppeard [23] compared osmic acid with yttrium and showed identical results (more than 50 % good results) at 1 year but better results with osmic acid at 3 years. Medical synovectomies have never given better results than surgical synovectomy beyond 1 year [8, 17].

Medical synovectomy is carried out much less frequently in the shoulder than in the knee, and it accounted for only 9.8 % of the cases in Schutte's series [24] and 4.1 % for radioactive and 1.3 % for osmic acid in Colcombets work. In the Rheumatological Department of Lyon (Prof. Bouvier), 662 joints affected with rheumatoid disease have received radioactive synovectomies since 1989 with the shoulder involved on 47 occasions (7.1 %).

The published literature contains very few references to the results of medical synovectomy in the rheumatoid shoulder:

- Schutte [24] followed 19 shoulders amongst 174 knees every 6 months for 3 years. The best results were achieved when the procedure was carried out during Steinbrocker stage I disease and when the disease was minimally active or was responding well to treatment. There was no reference to differences between sero-positive and sero-negative disease.
- Rau [21], in the same population, found 60 % with good results at 6 and 12 months, 54 % at 2 years and 50 % at 3 years. Repeating the synovectomy did not improve the outcome. The quality of the result was assessed on pain, joint swelling, mobility, steroid injections and inflammatory marker levels.
- Stucki [28] reported the results of 164 chemical synovectomies of which 82 were in rheumatoid patients (the others were in psoriatic arthropathy, spondyloarthropathy and chronic osteoarthritis). The results were good in about 50 % of the cases, were better for Larsen stage 0, 1 and 2 than for stage 3 [11] and were better for the knee and the elbow than the shoulder and ankle. This author believes that repeated synovectomies are bound to fail.
- Colombet [3] in his thesis recorded 47 % with good and very good results for the shoulder at 18 months. The percentage of good results dropped depending on the radiographic stage at which the intervention was carried out (61 %, 49 % and 23 % respectively for Steinbrocker stages I, II and II). This author did not find any difference between osmic acid and radioactive synovectomy.
- In 1989 Menkes [13], reporting on a 2- to 10-year follow-up, stated that the functional improvement was maintained in 51 % of cases while there were no radiographic changes in 53 % of the shoulders.

A Personal Series of 36 Rheumatoid Shoulders Treated by Medical Synovectomy

We carried out a retrospective study of 36 rheumatoid shoulders in 24 patients who underwent a medical synovectomy between 1975 and 1994 to look at their clinical and radiographic progression.

The patients came from the Rheumatology Department at Lyon (Prof. Bouvier) and from the Rheumatology Department of St. Etienne (Prof. Alexandre). These were patients reviewed between 15 November 1995 and 15 June 1996. The patients all had rheumatoid disease and had undergone either an osmic acid or radioactive synovectomy in at least one shoulder with a minimum follow-up of 24 months. For each shoulder there were AP radio-

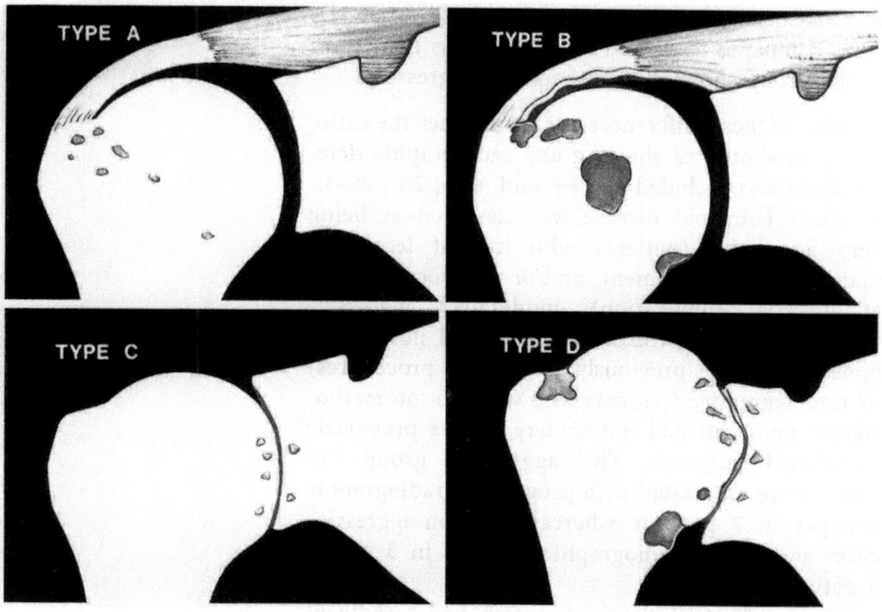

Fig. 7. The four distinct roentgenographic aspects of the rheumatoid shoulder according to Walch et al. *Type A*, Microcysts; *type B*, macrocysts; *type C*, joint space narrowing; *type D*, articular destruction

graphs in neutral rotation taken just before the synovectomy and the same view repeated at follow-up. During the review a subjective impression of the result was recorded as well as the Constant score for each shoulder. Any incomplete file was not included in the series.

The study population consisted of 24 patients (21 women and 3 men) with an average age at intervention of 52.7 years (24–71.5 years). The rheumatoid disease was sero-positive in 20 patients. The right shoulder was involved in 20 cases.

We used the classification described by Walch et al. to grade the cases radiographically before and after medical synovectomy. This classification distinguishes four distinct roentgenographic aspects (Fig. 7): type A, microcysts; type B, macrocysts; type C, joint space narrowing; and type D, articular destruction. We found the following distribution: no abnormality:24 %, radiographic type A:56 %, radiographic type B:24 %.

On 30 occasions a radioactive synovectomy was performed using 2 mCi rhenium-186 and on six occasions osmic acid was used. Thirty shoulders had one injection and six had two. The average delay between the onset of rheumatoid arthritis and the synovectomy was 7.3 years (1–24).

The average follow-up was 88.5 months (25–252 months) after the injection.

Results

Subjective Results. 21 shoulders were greatly improved (7 cases) or improved (14) amounting to 58 % of the population and 15 shoulders remained unchanged (9) or were worse (6) – 42 % of the population.

Constant Scores. The absolute scores were 59.7 points on average (16–93) and the normalised score averaged 81 % (18–116.5).

Radiographic Results. At review the Walch classification gave the following distribution: no abnormality 2.8 %, type A 33.3 %, type B 52.7 %, type C 5.6 % and type D 5.6 %. There were no radiographic changes in comparison to the originals in 39.4 % of cases, but there was deterioration in 60.6 % with this being scored as + (42.4 %), ++ (9.1 %) and +++ (9.1 %). When the shoulder had undergone two synovectomies the radiographic review showed deterioration more often (4 out of 6) than no change (2 out of 6). The population of shoulders which had significant radiographic worsening (++ or +++; 6 cases) was compared with that which showed no radiographic changes with time (13 cases).

- The average interval between the onset of rheumatoid arthritis and the date of the first synovectomy in the group with radiographic changes was longer at 11 years compared to 8.2 years.
- The average follow-up time after the synovectomy was also significantly longer at 117.5 months as compared to 87.5 months for this group.

- The Constant score was significantly lower at 32.5 as compared to 61 and was always less than 50 in the group showing radiographic progression.

None of these differences was found when the entire group of shoulders showing any radiographic deterioration was included (+, ++ and +++; 23 cases).

The rheumatoid disease was classified as being very aggressive (patients who had at least one major joint replacement and/or a procedure for atlanto-axial subluxation), moderately aggressive (patients on methotrexate but who had not undergone one of the previously mentioned procedures) or non-aggressive (patients who were not on methotrexate and who had not undergone the previously mentioned surgery). The aggressive group (11 cases) were associated with progressive radiographic changes in 7 patients whereas the non-aggressive cases showed no radiographic changes in 3 out of 4 patients.

The numbers of shoulders which had a radioactive synovectomy (30 cases) and those who had an osmic acid synovectomy (6 cases) where very unequal. However, if comparisons are to be made it seems that the results were a little better with osmic acid:

- 66.7 % had a satisfying subjective result with osmic acid whereas this level was 56.6 % for radioactive synovectomy.
- The absolute Constant score was 62.2 for osmic acid compared to 59.2 for radioactive synovectomy at review.
- At review the osmic acid group had 33.3 % with radiographic deterioration as compared to 63.4 % in the radioactive group.

However, it should be noted that the average time between the onset of the rheumatoid disease and the first synovectomy was 5 years with osmic acid and 7.8 years for a radioactive synovectomy. It should also be noted that the average follow-up time for osmic acid after the synovectomy was 131 months and this was only 80 months for the radioactive group.

Discussion

Although studies looking specifically at the rheumatoid shoulder are extremely rare, the findings made by analysing the pannus and the treatment results in the rheumatoid knee can generally be extrapolated to the shoulder. There is however, an important factor with the shoulder in that the rotator cuff, which is relatively frequently damaged in rheumatoid disease, has a very complicating effect.

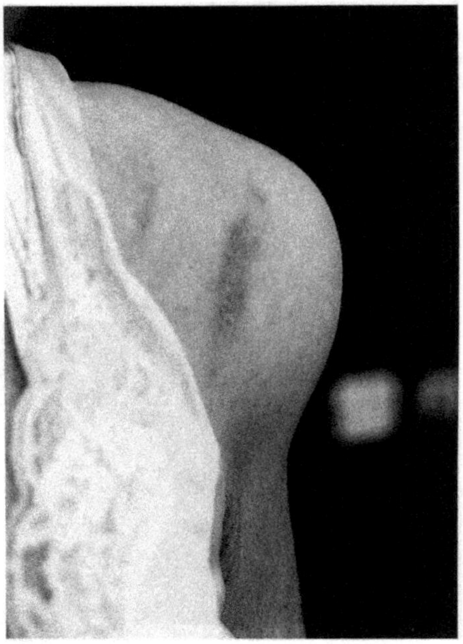

Fig. 8. Shoulder swelling due to a bursitis in a rheumatoid patient

In contrast to the knee, it can often be difficult to confirm clinically that the shoulder is affected by rheumatoid arthritis. An inflammatory type pain does not always imply rheumatoid arthritis and swelling of the shoulder is rarely evident clinically. When it does exist (Fig. 8), it indicates either a true arthritis, an arthritis with a bursitis indicating a cuff tear or an isolated bursitis indicating synovial metaplasia in the sub-acromial bursa. In the vast majority of cases the diagnosis of a rheumatoid shoulder can be suspected when there is a persistent inflammatory type pain localised to the joint in a patient known to have rheumatoid disease. A simple radiographic examination should always be done, and if this is totally normal, the only way to make the diagnosis of a rheumatoid shoulder is to use more sophisticated imaging techniques and particularly magnetic resonance imaging (MRI). This demonstrates any synovial pannus [10], its locality and volume, demonstrates any reactionary extravasation and shows up any cartilage damage as well as the state of the cuff [9].

Given the potentially deleterious side-effects of osmic acid and the cumulative toxicity of radioactive synovectomy, the indications for a medical synovectomy must be well justified (a positive diagnosis when the radiographs are normal and it is contraindicated when the radiographs show advanced disease). When there are good clinical indications, medical synovectomy plays an important role in the treatment of the rheumatoid shoulder. The choice of the type of synovectomy is based more on the potential complications of each rather than any evident superiority of one over the other even if certain tendencies seem to be apparent. The best time to carry out the synovectomy is undeniably when the radiographic lesions are minimal (no abnormality or Steinbrocker stage I or Walch type A).

Local treatments such as synovectomy should not be considered in isolation and should be part of an overall treatment programme dealing with the rheumatoid disease. Medical synovectomies have no effect on the systemic aspects of the disease and often fail if the disease is in a progressive or aggressive phase. They should therefore be suggested only when background treatment has been established and, when this has taken effect (this may take from weeks to month depending on the treatment used), it is then reasonable to carry out a medical synovectomy in the remaining inflamed joints.

If the disease fails to respond to treatment or if the pannus recurs locally the physician is presented with the problem of a failed synovectomy, where the percentage increases with the follow-up time. In these cases, it is necessary to consider alternative treatments and it is here that surgical synovectomy (arthroscopically) may have a place, except where there is a rapid deterioration in the radiographic changes.

Ostergaard [18] has shown that the volume of synovial pannus seems to act as a marker for the severity of the rheumatoid damage in a joint and it is therefore interesting to be able to follow its evolution. The same author [19] studied the effects of osmic acid on the rheumatoid pannus in 14 knees (8 rheumatoid and 6 juvenile arthritis cases) and showed that the reduction in volume of the pannus demonstrated on MRI 1 month afterwards correlated with the clinical results. The use of ultrasound was compared with MRI in arthritis of the knee (13 inflammatory knees of which 10 where rheumatoid) and was less good overall and in particular in looking at the synovial membrane and bony erosions [20].

Conclusion

Medical synovectomy has a place in the treatment of the rheumatoid shoulder but its results are closely linked to the timing of the intervention. It should not be considered as an isolated treatment but should be part of an overall treatment plan. If the conditions of injection are scrupulously adhered to, the complications are minimal. If the synovectomy fails, other therapeutic measures should be quickly considered, and among these surgery has an important place. Future prospective studies on the rheumatoid shoulder are advised (minimum 2 year follow-up after medical synovectomy, comparison between asmic acid and radioacive synovectromy or between medical and surgical synovectromy) with the results being analysed on the clinical and radiographic findings (radiographs and MRI). Such prospective studies should allow the optimal treatment modalities for the rheumatoid shoulder to be defined.

References

1. Ansell BM, Crook A, Mallard JR, Bywaters GL (1963) Evaluation of intraarticular colloidal gold Au 198 in the treatment of persistent knee effusions. Ann Rheum Dis 22: 435–439
2. Berglund K (1958) Communication sur l'emploi de l'acide osmique. Nord Med 60:1370
3. Colcombet P (1974) Les synoviorthèses dans le traitement de la polyarthrite rhumatoïde. Thèse Méd., Lyon, p 195
4. Constant CR, Murley AH (1987) Clinical method of functional assessment of the shoulder. Clin Orthop 214: 160–164
5. Cruz-Esteban C, Wilke WS (1995) Non surgical synovectomy. Baillieres Clin Rheumatol 9(4):787–801
6. Delbarre F (1968) La synoviorthèse (définition, buts et moyens) Rev Rhum 35:1–8
7. Ennevaara K (1967) Painful shoulder joint in rheumatoid arthritis: a clinical and radiological study of 200 cases with special reference to arthrography of gleno-humeral joint. Acta Rheum Scand 11:111–116
8. Jones G (1993) Yttrium synovectomy: A meta-analysis of the literature. Austr NZ J Med 23:272–275
9. Kieft GJ, Dijkmans BAC, Bloem JL, Kroon HM (1990) Magnetic resonance imaging of the shoulder in patients with rheumatoid arthritis. Ann Rheum Dis 49:7–11
10. König H, Siepper J, Wolf KJ (1990) Rheumatoid arthritis: evaluation of hypervascular and fibrous pannus with dynamic MR imaging enhanced with Gd-DTPA. Radiology 176:473–477
11. Larsen A, Dale K, Eek M (1977) Radiographic evaluation of rheumatoid arthritis and related conditions by standard reference films. Acta Radiol Diag 18:481–491
12. Lloyd DC, Reeder EJ (1978) Chromosome aberrations and intraarticular yttrium 90. Lancet II:617
13. Menkes CJ, Millet B (1989) Synoviorthesis of the shoulder joint in rheumatoid arthritis. Rheumatology (Basel) 12:46–51
14. Mitchell N, Laurin C, Shepard N (1973) The effect of osmium tetroxide and nitrogen mustard on normal articular cartilage. J Bone Joint Surg Br 55:814–821
15. Nissila M, Isomaki H, Koota K et al (1977) Osmic acid in rheumatoid synovitis I. Scand J Rheumatol 6:158–160
16. Nissila M, Isomaki H, Koota K et al (1977) Osmic acid in rheumatoid synovitis II. Scand J Rheumatol 6:111–112
17. Nissila M, Anttila P, Hamalainen M, Jalava S (1978) Comparison of chemical, radiation and surgical synovectomy for knee joint synovitis. Scand J Rheumatol 7:225–228

18. Ostergaard M, Gideon P, Henriksen O, Lorenzen I (1994) Synovial volume. a marker of disease severity in rheumatoid arthritis? Quantification by MRI. Scand J Rheumatol 23:197–202
19. Ostergaard M, Stoltenberg M, Gideon P, Wieslander S, Sonn-Holm S, Kryger P, Sonne M (1995) Effect of intraarticular osmic acid on synovial membrane volume and inflamation, determined by magnetic resonance imaging. Scand J Rheumatol 24:5–12
20. Ostergaard M, Court-Payen M, Gideon P, Wieslander S, Cortsen M, Lorenzen I, Henriksen O (1995) Ultrasonography in arthritis of the knee. A comparison with MR imaging. Acta Radiol 36(1):19–26
21. Rau U R, Schutte H (1983) Results of radiosynviorthesis with yttrium 90 in chronic synovitis: a long term prospective study. I. Total results and effect of local factors. Z Rheumatol 42:(5):265–270
22. Reiss G, Swensson A (1951) Intra-articular injections of osmic acid in painful joint affections. Acta Med Scand 259:27–32
23. Sheppeard H, Aldin A, Ward DJ (1981) Osmic acid versus yttrium 90 in rheumatoid synovitis of the knee. Scand J Rheumatol 10:234–236
24. Shutte H, Rau R (1983) Results of radiosynviorthesis with yttrium 90 in chronic synovitis: a long term prospective study. II. Effect of general disease parameters. Z Rheumatol 42, 5:271–279
25. Sim FH (1985) Synovial proliferative disorders: role of synovectomy. Arthroscopy 1:198–204
26. Steinbrocker O, Traeger CH, Batterman RC (1949) Therapeutic criteria in rheumatoid arthritis. JAMA 140:659–662
27. Stevenson AC, Bedford J, Hill AGS, Hill HFH (1971) Chromosome damage in patients treated with intraarticular injections of radioactive gold. Lancet 1:837–839
28. Stucki G, Bozzone P, Treuer E, Wassmer P, Felder M (1993) Efficacy and safety of radiation synovectomy with yttrium 90: a retrospective long-term analysis of 164 applications in 82 patients. Br J Rheumatol 32(5):383–386
29. Walch G, Noel E, Guier C, Frehel M (1990) Rheumatoid arthritis of the shoulder. A review of 250 patients. In: Post M, Morrey BF, Hawkins RJ (eds) Surgery of the shoulder. Mosby-Year Book, St. Louis, pp 267–269

Rheumatoid Arthritis of the Shoulder: Radiological Presentation and Results of Arthroplasty

C. Lévigne and J.P. Franceschi

Summary

Fifty rheumatoid shoulders (44 patients) treated with an Aequalis shoulder arthroplasty were reviewed with an mean follow-up of 20 months (12–45). Three radiographic forms were distinguished as defined on two criteria: the sphericity of the humeral head and upward migration of the head in relation to the glenoid. The three forms (similar to those described by Neer) do not have the same functional prognosis after insertion of a prosthesis. The ***"centered" (or dry) form*** *(36 %) occurs in patients with an average age of 58 years and is reminiscent of the radiographic appearance seen in osteoarthritis with a normal acromio-humeral distance (only 6 % of cuff tear). The main problem is stiffness, with a limited gain in active anterior elevation regardless of the preoperative range of movement (average elevation 123°, gain 24°). The* ***"destructive" (or wet) form*** *(19 %) characterised by destruction of the humeral head which loses its sphericity because of marginal erosion. It occurs in younger patients (average 47 years). The cuff is often damaged (33 % of cuff tear), and there is wear which rapidly involves all the articular surfaces. Paradoxically, the best functional results were seen in this destructive form, with an average in active anterior elevation of almost 70° (average 154° of active elevation, gain 68°). The* ***"ascending" (or resorptive) form*** *(41 %) characterised by upward migration of the humeral head which precedes superior glenoid wear in patients which are 61 years old. The frequent presence of a cuff tear (26 %) penalises postoperative recovery of active anterior elevation (average elevation 116°, gain 28°) and external rotation. Finally, 8 press-fit humeral components demonstrated progressive loosening with distal migration whereas no signs of loosening were found in the 42 cemented humeral components. A distal migration of the humeral component superior to 5 mm (6 cases) was clearly associated with decrease functional result. This emphasizes the necessity to cement the humeral component in the rheumatoid shoulder.*

Introduction

The shoulder is frequently involved in the natural history of rheumatoid arthritis, with authors reporting rates of between 60 % and 90 % [9, 15]. There are many published reports of the results of shoulder arthroplasty for this aetiology. Generally, the authors emphasise the quality of the results with regard to pain. On the other hand, the results for active movement and function appear to be less impressive especially if compared with those for osteoarthritis [2, 3, 13].

The degree of bony destruction of the articular surfaces and rotator cuff ruptures are the two essential factors which are reported to be detrimental to the result [1, 3, 7, 9–11, 13, 17, 18]. Moreover, these two factors play a part particularly when surgery is carried out late in the progression of the disease.

Taking into account the frequency of radiographic lucent lines around the cemented glenoid implant and the number of established loosenings, there is strongly divided opinion between those in favour of total shoulder replacement and those in favour of hemi-arthroplasty [1, 7, 10, 11, 13, 16–18]. Our study with its short follow-up of 20 months on average was not designed to settle this argument one way or the other. In this prospective study of 50 cases with follow-up of more than 1 year our main intention was to clarify the functional result that could reasonably be expected from a shoulder arthroplasty for rheumatoid arthritis and define any clinical or radiographic factors which might have a significant effect on the result.

Materials and Methods

Patients

Our multicentre study involved 44 patients (50 shoulders) operated on between 1992 and 1995. Six patients had undergone bilateral operations. The classic female predominance in rheumatoid arthritis was found with 88 % of females in the present study. The dominant shoulder was involved in 53 % of the cases. The disease had been active for between 1 and 30 years (11 years on average) and the average age at the time of surgery was 57 years (30–74 years). The preoperative Constant score adjusted for sex and age was, on average, 25.9% (11%–56%). The average pain score was 2.8 (0–8). Among these patients 81% could carry out activities only up to the horizontal level, 80% could not perform regular activities of daily living alone, and 90% could not use their arm at shoulder level. Average preoperative range of movement was 100° (30°–160°) of passive anterior elevation, 73° (20°–150°) of active anterior elevation and 11° (30°–70°) of external rotation elbow at the side. For the less disabled patients a rapid evolution in the radiographic criteria was the indication for surgery.

The Preoperative Radiographs

The preoperative radiographs were available for assessment in 47 cases. Glenoid wear was graded as *stage 1* when the sub-chondral bone was intact or minimally deformed, as *stage 2* when the wear reached the foot of the coracoid and as *stage 3* when it went beyond the foot of the coracoid (Fig. 1). Wear of the humeral head was graded as *stage 1* when the sub-chondral bone was intact or had micro-geodes, as *stage 2* when the anatomical neck was deformed by a notch greater than 10 mm and as *stage 3* when the head had lost its spherical form (Fig. 2).

Despite many attempts we found that quantifying glenoid or humeral wear by measurement was neither accurate nor reproducible. Glenoid wear was divided into 18 stage 1 (38%), 18 stage 2 (38%) and 11 stage 3 (24%). Head wear was divided into 33 stage 1 (70%), 5 stage 2 (11%) and 9 stage 3 (19%). All associations of stages between humeral wear and glenoid wear, were possible. However, glenoid wear was, nevertheless, often more marked than humeral wear in the same patient. The subacromial space, measured as the acromio-humeral distance on the AP radiograph in neutral rotation, averaged 6.3 mm (3–12 mm) preoperatively.

The State of the Rotator Cuff

The state of the rotator cuff was determined by a computed tomographic arthrogram in 60% of the cases, by magnetic resonance imaging in 12% and intra-operatively in the rest. The tears consisted of 7 complete supraspinatus ruptures (14%), 2 partial

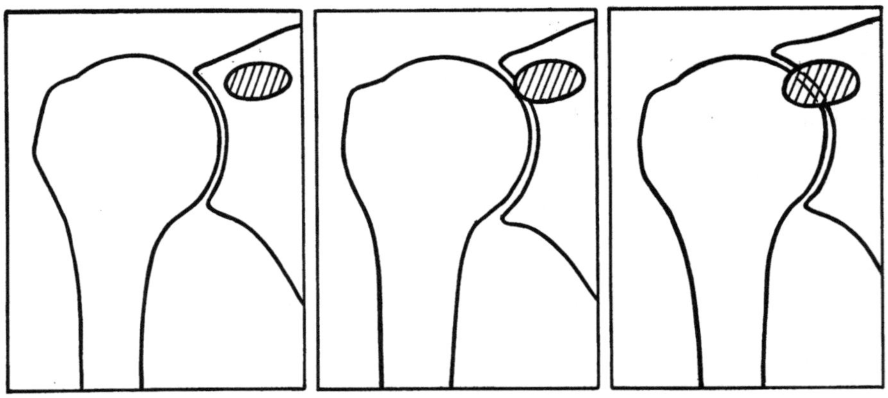

Fig. 1. Assessing glenoid wear in rheumatoid arthritis on true AP-view: stage 1, subchondral bone intact or minimally deformed; stage 2, wear reaching the foot of the coracoid; stage 3, wear beyond the foot of the coracoid

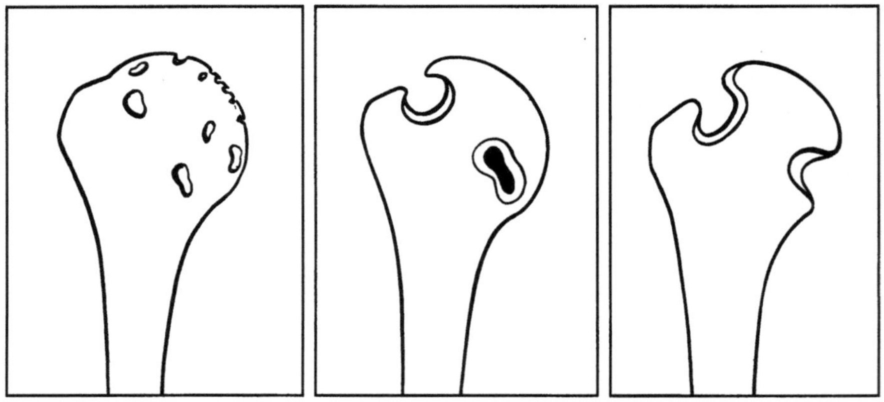

Fig. 2. Assessing humeral head wear in rheumatoid arthritis on true AP-view: stage 1, microgeodes; stage 2, Notch in the greater tuberosity; style 3, loss of spherical form

Table 1. Fatty degeneration of the infraspinatus in rheumatoid arthritis, as seen on computed tomography

Fatty degeneration of the infraspinatus	Number of shoulders	Percentage
Stage 0 (no fatty degeneration)	1	3 %
Stage 1 (the muscle contains some fatty streak)	12	39 %
Sage 2 (important fatty infiltration)	12	39 %
Stage 3 (as much fat than muscle present)	5	16 %
Stage 4 (more fat than muscle)	1	3 %

ruptures of the deep surface of supraspinatus (4 %) and there were 41 water-tight cuffs (82 %). Amongst the water-tight cuffs, more than half were assessed as very thin by the surgeon. Fatty degeneration of infraspinatus on computed tomography classified using the Bernageau and Goutallier system [8], was carried out in 31 shoulders (62 %) and is summarized in Table 1.

Surgical Technique

In each case the operation was carried out by a surgeon from the multi-centre group who specialises in shoulder surgery and had been trained in using the implant so as to limit any unexpected problems arising from not following the technical details. In all but one case, where a superior transacromial approach was used, the deltopectoral approach was used. The operation included a vertical division of sub-scapularis, resutured at the end of the procedure following a juxtaglenoid capsulotomy in 75 % of the cases and without preliminary release in 25 %. A glenoid component was inserted in 44 cases: cemented in 41 (82 %) and uncemented, using the expansion screw system, in 3 cases (6 %). In 6 cases (12 %) a hemi-arthroplasty was carried out. The humeral implant was cemented in 84 % and uncemented in 16 % (8 shoulders). The Aequalis prosthesis (Tornier) was used in all cases. The intervention was judged by the surgeon as very satisfactory in 68 %, satisfactory in 28 % and unsatisfactory in 4 % of the cases. One perioperative humeral fracture, which required immediate internal fixation with a plate, was recorded but this did not affect the postoperative recovery or the final result.

Postoperative Treatment

Postoperative rehabilitation began immediately in all cases. One shoulder was placed on principle in an abduction pillow and 6 shoulders (12 %) in a neutral rotation brace. Postoperative rehabilitation was at a specialist centre for 72 % of the patients, with an average stay of 30 days.

Review

All the patients were seen with a minimum follow-up of 12 months (average 20 months). The evaluation consisted of a history and clinical examination to establish the Constant score [4] and the subjective result. The minimum radiographic examination consisted of a lateral view of the scapula and an AP view in neutral rotation which allowed the following parameters to be analysed: the acromio-humeral distance (in millimetres), the position of the glenoid component (vertical centering, size, inclination, lateral offset), the position of the humeral component and the existence of lucent lines around the two implants. All the clinical and radiographic information was recorded on proformas which were then subjected to statistical analysis to look for any significant correlations. The χ^2 test was used for qualitative variables and the Scheffe's method of multiple comparison was used for quantitative variables.

A New Radiological Classification

By examining the different preoperative radiographic appearances and particularly by analysing the radiographic history of the many patients followed regularly since their initial diagnosis, we were able to distinguish *three radiographic forms* as defined on two criteria: the sphericity of the humeral head and upward migration of the head in relation to the glenoid.

The "Ascending" Form. This was the most frequent occurring in 19 cases in our series (41 %; Fig. 3). It is characterised by upward migration of the humeral head which precedes glenoid wear. The head retains its sphericity throughout the evolution. Narrowing of the joint space occurs at the superior pole of the glenoid followed by localised wear at this level, which progressively destroys the sub-chondral bone and gives the glenoid a sinusoidal appearance on the AP radiograph. The humeral head retains its sphericity but migrates upwards, inwards and backwards under the spine of the scapula. It ascends and medialises. At a more evolved stage the surgical neck of the humerus comes into contact with the

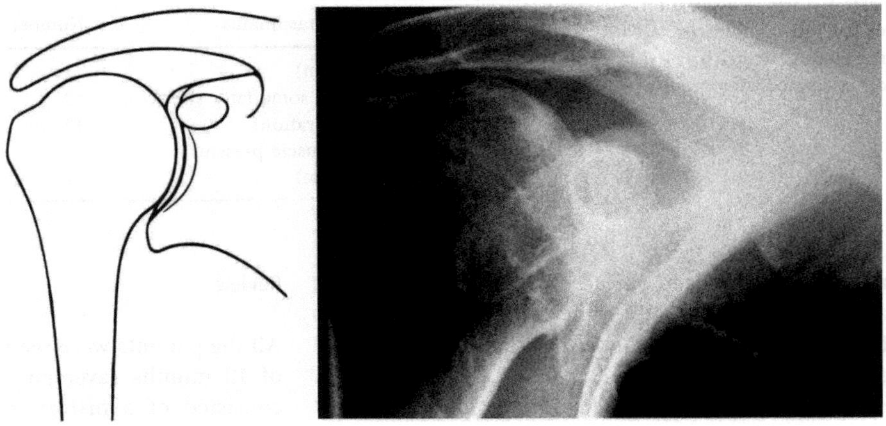

Fig. 3. The ascending form of rheumatoid arthritis

inferior border of the glenoid which leaves an imprint and creates the classical notch on the medial surface of the surgical neck.

The "Centered" Form. This was almost as frequent, occurring in 17 cases in our series (36%; Fig. 4). It is characterised by the absence of upward migration of the humeral head and a progress, uniform wear of the glenoid throughout its height. The humeral head retains its sphericity but pushes into the glenoid like an "egg into an egg-cup". This form is reminiscent of the appearance seen in osteoarthritis and may be accompanied by marginal osteophytes at the superior and inferior poles of the glenoid. The progressive medialisation of the humeral head is followed in time by a reduction in the acromio-humeral distance.

The "Destructive" Form. This is less frequent occurring in 9 cases (19%; Fig. 5). It is characterised by destruction of the humeral head which loses its sphericity. Wear occurs at the level of the anatomical neck producing a characteristic notch which progressively wears away at the circumference of the neck to give it a 'champagne cork' appearance. This very aggressive form of rheumatoid arthritis destroys the glenoid simultaneously. Some of the cases did not display a loss of joint space due to the articular incongruity.

The epidemiological, clinical and radiological factors related with these three forms are shown in Table 2. Apart from these, two cases were judged as unclassifiable (4%). These were two shoulders in the same patient who presented with massive erosion of the inferior pole of the glenoid and the pillar of the scapula with a significant increase in the subacromial space.

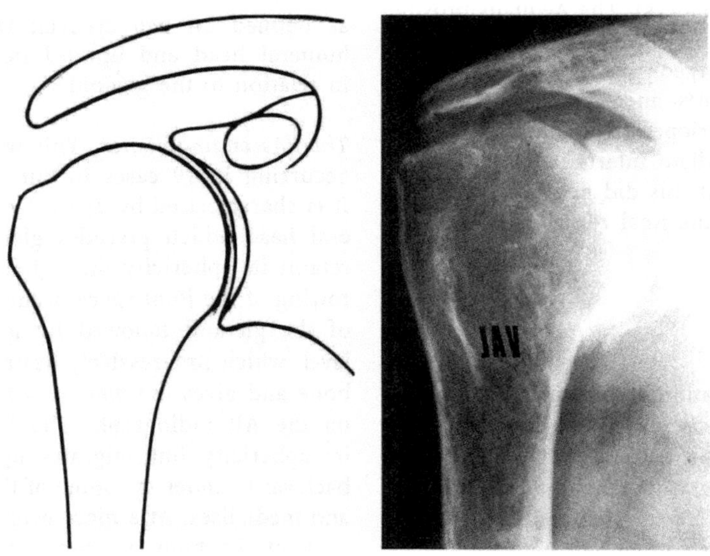

Fig. 4. The centered form of rheumatoid arthritis

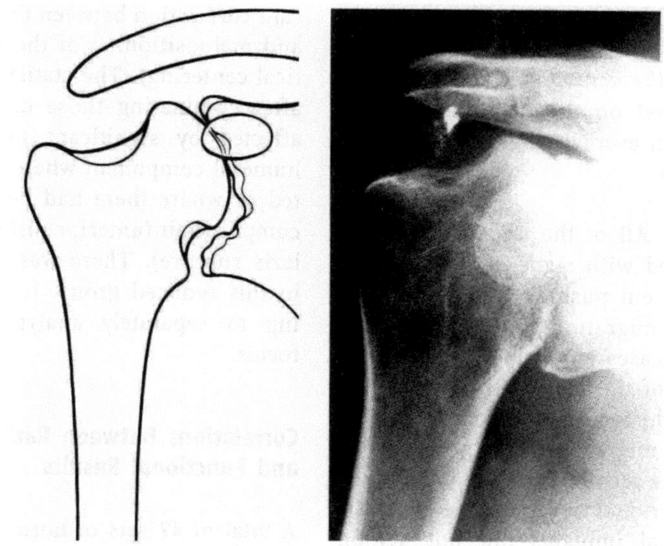

Fig. 5. The destructive form of rheumatoid arthritis

Table 2. Pre and Postoperative detailed Constant scores for the entire series

Constant score	Pre-operative		Post-operative	Gain
Pain (15 points)	2.8	→	11.8	+ 9
Activity (20 points)	5.5	→	15.1	+ 9.6
Mobility (40 points)	9.8	→	27	+17.2
Strength (25 points)	1.5	→	4.2	+ 2.7
Constant score (100 points)	19.8	→	58.2	+38.4
Normalised Constant score (%)	25.9	→	77.8	+51.9

Results of Shoulder Arthroplasty in Rheumatoid Arthritis

Overall results of the series of 50 shoulder arthroplasties were assessed after an average follow-up of 20 months (12–45) and are summarized in Table 2.

Complications

Early complications amounted to one anterior dislocation due to rupture of sub-scapularis which required reoperation and one postoperative posterior dislocation which required relocation under anaesthesia and which led to complete loosening of the glenoid. Three (6 %) bruised circumflex nerves were reported but these were transitory and did not affect the final result.

Clinical Results

Subjectively, 70 % of the patients were very happy, 24 % were happy and 6 % were disappointed. The three disappointed patients were the two who had had dislocations and one who had subsidence of an uncemented humeral component. The Constant score increased from 19.8 points preoperatively to 58.2 points postoperatively: an increase of a 38.4 points. The normalised Constant score increased from 25.9 % to 77.8 %: an increase of 51.9 %. The increase for each criteria is shown in Table 3. Active anterior elevation averaged 122° – an increase of 49°. External rotation elbow at the side averaged 38° – a gain of 27°. The patients estimated the average rehabilitation time as 7.5 months (2–24).

Statistical analysis revealed only one significant correlation between the age of the patient at the time of surgery and the increase in active anterior elevation ($p<0.01$), with younger patients achieving a greater gain in this movement. On the other hand, there was no significant relationship with the duration of disease, the preoperative Constant score or preoperative active anterior elevation. Nor was any statistically significant correlation found between the clinical result expressed as the Constant score or active anterior elevation and the different preoperative radiographic parameters (acromiohumeral distance, cuff rupture, fatty degeneration of infraspinatus, glenoid wear, humeral wear or malposition of the components).

Radiographic Results

The distance between the acromion and the humeral component as measured on the AP radiograph in neutral rotation was on average 6.7 mm with a negligible gain of 0.3 mm.

The Humeral Implant. All of the uncemented humeral implants presented with signs of distal migration of the humeral stem pushing into the flare of the diaphysis. This migration was greater than 5 mm in 6 of the 8 cases and less than 5 mm in the other two. Many of the patients presented with true bony lysis at the inferior extremity of the implant. When the migration was greater than 5 mm (6 cases) it was accompanied by an evolving decrease in the functional level of the shoulder. The cemented humeral implants did not demonstrate lucent lines in 92% of the cases and no cemented humeral component was loose. Three patients showed a lucent line around the stem at the cement-bone interface whose evolution has not yet been determined. One case presented with evolving bony resorption beneath the head which may be due to a foreign body reaction around degradation particles.

The Glenoid Implant. The three metal backed, uncemented glenoids did not show any lucencies. Amongst the cemented glenoids, analysis showed there to be lucent lines at the cement-bone interface in 97%. This lucent line was often very thin, less than 1 mm, and occurred preferentially in zones 1, 5, and 6, i.e. beneath the tray of the implant (Fig. 6). Six glenoids were considered as loose due to a significant or evolving lucent line. The assessment criteria are detailed in a separate study (see Molé et al. "Cemented Glenoid Component: Results in Osteoarthritis and Rheumatoid Arthritis", this volume). One glenoid component presented with true migration (a case of early posterior dislocation with closed reduction). In total, of the 38 glenoid implants which underwent radiographic analysis, 3% showed migration, 16% were loose, 78% had lucent lines and only 3% were without any abnormality. We were not able to demonstrate any statistically significant correlation between the existence of a lucent line and malpositioning of the implant (inclination, vertical centering). The statistical analysis was repeated after eliminating those cases where the result was affected by significant migration (5 mm) of the humeral component where this had not been cemented or where there had been an early postoperative complication (anterior dislocation due to sub-scapularis rupture). There was no significant correlation in this reduced group. It therefore seemed interesting to separately analyse the three radiographic forms.

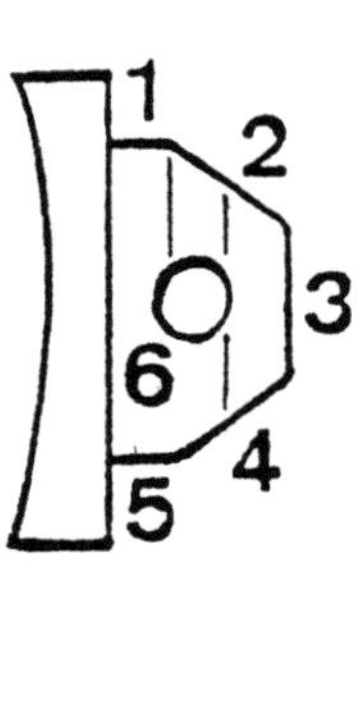

Fig. 6. Zones of lucent lines around the glenoid implant

Correlations Between Radiographic Forms and Functional Results

A total of 47 sets of notes were available. Two cases were judged to be unclassifiable and 7 cases were excluded as before due to non-specific complications (distal migration greater than 5 mm with an ucemented humeral component, anterior dislocation due to rupture of sub-scapularis). The analysis was therefore carried out on 38 patients (Table 3).

Ascending Form

At an average follow-up of 21 months the normalised Constant score had increased by 47 points (28–75), active anterior elevation had risen by 28° (89°–116°) and external rotation elbow at the side by 27° (7°–34°). On the radiographic analysis the acromio-humeral distance was only negligibly modified with a gain of 0.5 mm.

Centered Form

At an average follow-up of 23 months the normalised Constant score had increased by 52 points (26–78), active anterior elevation had risen by 24° (99°–123°) and external rotation elbow at the side by 36° (7°–41°). On the radiographic analysis the acromio-humeral distance had increased by 1.5 mm (6.7–8.2).

Destructive Form

At an average follow-up of 19 months the normalised Constant score had increased by 62 points (24–86), active anterior elevation had risen by 68° (78°–154°) and external rotation elbow at the side by 20° (24°–44°). On the radiographic analysis the acromio-humeral distance remained unchanged at 6.1 mm.

Table 3. Epidemiology, pre- and postoperative results for the three radiographic forms of rheumatoid shoulders

	Ascending form (resorptive)	Centered form (dry)	Destructive from (wet)
Number (frequency)	n=16 (41 %)	n=14 (36 %)	n=8 (19 %)
Age at operation	61 years	58 years	47 years
Anterior active elevation (pre- and postop.)	89°→116° (+28°)	99°→123° (+24°)	78°→154° (+68°)
External rotation (pre- and postop.)	7°→34° (+27°)	7°→41° (+34°)	24°→44° (+20°)
Cuff tear	26 %	6 %	33 %
Glenoid wear	+ (sup. and post.)	± (central)	++ (global)
A-H distance (mm) (pre- and postop.)	6.2→6.7 (+0.5)	6.7→8.2 (+1.5)	6.1→6.1 (0)
Absolute Constant score (pre- and postop)	28→75 (+47)	26→78 (+52)	24→86 (+62)

Statistical analysis of the different factors by radiographic form revealed a significant statistical difference concerning active anterior elevation which was clearly improved in the destructive form (154°) when compared with the centered form (123°) or the ascending form (116°). There also was a significant difference in the acromio-humeral distance: the increase of 1.5 mm in the centered form was significantly better than in the destructive and ascending forms.

Discussion

Why a New Series?

Many series on the results of shoulder arthroplasty in rheumatoid arthritis have already been published and have put the accent on two main points: (a) The frequency of lucent lines around the cemented glenoid implant, increasing with follow-up, which raises fears of increasing loosening with time and explains why certain surgeons prefer to perform a hemiarthroplasty rather than a total arthroplasty. The short average follow-up in our series does not allow us to make a creditable analyse of this parameter. (b) A modest functional improvement in comparison to that obtained in osteoarthritis. The analysis of this fact and of the prognostic value of preoperative clinical and radiographic factors constituted the main goals of this study.

This series seemed particularly useful for such an analysis because the cases all used the same prosthesis inserted in a standard manner which would, naturally, diminish the influence of technical or technological elements on the results. Finally, this series can be distinguished from the others because the decision to operate was generally made earlier and depended equally on clinical factors and radiographic factors such as reduction in joint space, which has been demonstrated to mark the turning point in the disease [19].

The Sub-acromial Space in Rheumatoid Arthritis

Contrary to the usual correlations found in classical cuff tear pathologies between reduction in the acromio-humeral distance and the frequency of a cuff tear, this series showed no such correlation between these two factors.

In our series 18 % of the cases presented with a supraspinatus cuff tear and 82 % had a watertight cuff. The sub-acromial distances in the two groups were 6.4 mm and 6.3 mm respectively. Moreover, 22 cases had a sub-acromial distance less than or equal to 5 mm and only 18 % had a cuff tear. This is fairly specific to inflammatory disorders in which the cuff thins without rupturing as discussed by other authors [14, 18].

We also analysed the sub-acromial distance in relation to fatty degeneration of the infraspinatus. It was 6.6 mm in stage 1, 5.4 mm in stage 2, 5.2 mm in stage 3 and 3 mm in the only stage 4 case. The small number of cases in each group does not allow for statistical validation.

Why a New Classification?

Many classifications have already been suggested and are regularly used in rheumatoid arthritis. Larsen [12] describes six stages (0–5) based on the level of the 'destructive lesions' and narrowing of the gleno-humeral joint space. Our series consisted of 74% at stage 4 and 26% at stage 5. However, this classification, used mostly in rheumatology, suffers from a lack of discrimination between stages 3, 4 and 5 which correspond to 'destructive lesions of average size, severe or major'. Moreover, this classification implies an inevitable evolution from one stage to the next which we were not always able to prove during radiographic follow-up of our patients.

Crossan and Vallance [5] described a five-stage classification which is quite close to that of Larsen but stresses the importance of humeral head sphericity which is preserved for a long time and the subacromial distance which was correlated with the state of the rotator cuff.

Walch and Noel [19] in an attempt to simplify the classification and to determine the criteria which had prognostic value, proposed a four-stage classification, emphasising stage C, characterised by narrowing of the gleno-humeral joint space. This stage marks the turning point in the disease evolution and the insertion of a prosthesis should be suggested at this time. In fact the passage to stage D, characterised by destructive lesions of the glenoid and/or the humerus and/or the rotator cuff is rapid (on average 2 years) and compromises the functional result of an arthroplasty.

In our series we had 65% in stage C and 35% in stage D, but the distinction between stages C and D is often difficult. Moreover the radiographic signs and their evolution did not seem the same in all the patients affected by rheumatoid arthritis as there were many different radiographic types.

Neer [14] had already made this point in describing four forms: a *dry form* with sub-chondral geodes, loss of joint space and, sometimes, osteophytes; a *wet form with* erosion of the articular surfaces which become frayed; a *resorptive form* which is characterised by severe wear and centralisation of the head (which explains the clinical appearance of these shoulders as 'Bourgogne wine-bottle shaped' as opposed to the normal 'Bordeaux wine-bottle shape') and a final form reported by Kelly [11] which is characterised by major destruction of the glenoid and the humeral head with contact between the humeral diaphysis and the inferior pole of the glenoid.

The classification derived from this study has similarities to that described by Neer. The *ascending form* characterised by upward migration of the humeral head which retains its sphericity and superior wear of the glenoid with a sinusoidal appearance corresponds to *Neer's resorptive form*. The *centered form*, with certain appearances in common with osteoarthritis, corresponds to *Neer's dry form:* the "egg in the egg-cup". Finally, the *destructive form* characterised by destruction of the humeral head into a 'champagne cork', corresponds to *Neer's wet form* (Fig. 7).

For us, this classification presents several interesting points (table 3):

- Epidemiologically the destructive form attacks younger patients (47 years on average) than the central (58 years) and ascending forms (61 years; $p<0.01$). The duration of the disease is not shorter but its onset is earlier than in the other forms.
- Clinically the functional handicap and pain were equal in all three types. Active anterior elevation was comparable in all three forms but passive movement was better conserved in the destructive

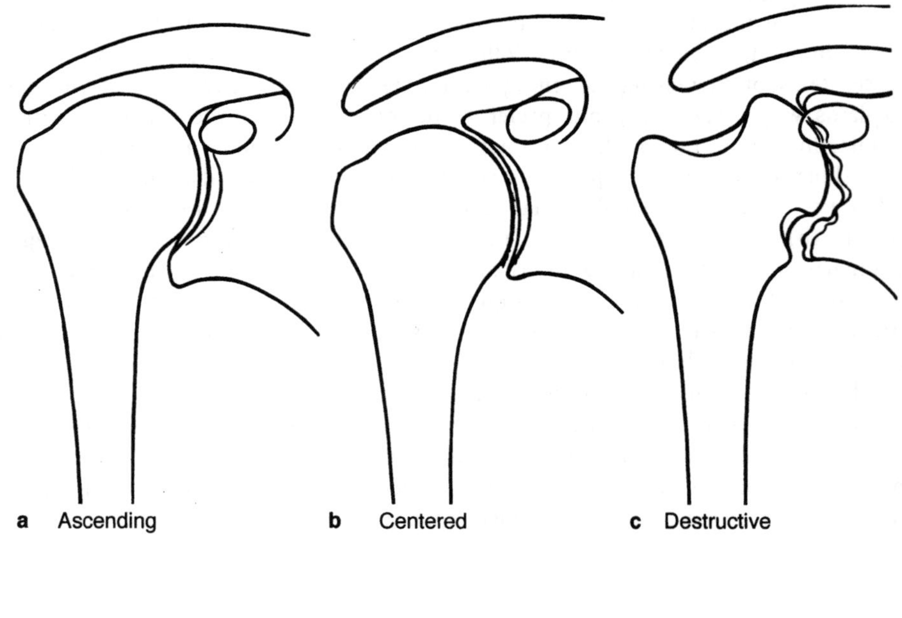

Fig. 7 a–c. The radiographic presentation of the rheumatoid shoulder. **a** Ascending. **b** Centered. **c** Destructive form: in anterior elevation as much as in external rotation (Table 2).

- In terms of their evolution, the three forms differed with regard to the rotator cuff, the glenoid and the humeral head.

The percentage of supraspinatous *cuff tears* was 33 % in the destructive form, 26 % in the ascending form and only 6 % in the centered form. This illustrates the aggressiveness of the disease on the cuff in the destructive forms. In the ascending form, where the sub-acromial space is the narrowest (average 5.7 mm), one would have expected a high rate of cuff tears. In reality, it is the thinness of the cuff, which has been noted by most of the surgeons. Our findings agree perfectly with those of Kelly [11]. The study of fatty degeneration of infra-spinatous showed that the muscle is completely unaffected in the centered form (92 % less than or equal to stage 2). This was a little less in the ascending (77 % less than or equal to stage 2) and the destructive forms (66 % less than or equal to stage 2). The differences were not significant.

The glenoid wear and topography progression were very different in the three forms. It occurs superiorly and posteriorly in the ascending form; it remains central in both vertical and transverse planes in the centered form and has a slow progression: in our series no erosion had passed beyond the foot of the coracoid (stage 3) and only 47 % had reached stage 2. On the other hand, in the destructive form, glenoid wear was very significant passing beyond the foot of the coracoid in 78 % of the cases with disordered topography throughout the glenoid.

The humeral head characteristics make up part of the criteria of the classification. It retains its sphericity throughout the evolution of the centered and ascending forms while it is rapidly destroyed in the destructive form.

These particular characteristics in the natural history of the wear of the humeral head and the glenoid allow us to state that these are three different forms and not three stages in the evolution of one form.

- Technically, the centered form did not generally pose any problem for fixation of the components but as these patients are often very stiff, exposure and preparation of the glenoid can be difficult. The ascending form can present technical problems in achieving uniform pressure on the glenoid component due to the postero-superior bony defect. There is a problem of glenoid bone stock in the destructive form as well as in making the humeral cut because the large notch in the anatomical neck alters the usual landmarks. One needs to go by the position of the supraspinatus.
- The three forms do not have the same functional prognosis after insertion of a prosthesis. Paradoxically, the best functional results were seen in the *destructive form* with an increase in active anterior elevation of almost 70°. This functional improvement is independent of the level of bony wear which may be either in the glenoid or the humerus. The presence of a cuff tear does not necessarily worsen the outcome but the only bad functional result came in a patient who had a large cuff tear with stage 2 fatty degeneration and, particularly, atrophy of supraspinatus and sub-scapularis. It seems essential to us that in this form one should not wait for a cuff tear to occur before intervening. With regards to external rotation, the increase was fairly small at 19°, but this movement had been relatively well preserved preoperatively.

The gain in active anterior elevation in the *centered form* was only 24° and this was relatively constant regardless of the preoperative range of movement. The central forms are certainly less aggressive than the destructive form especially with regard to the cuff and the sub-chondral bone but contrary to that form, the functional result is strictly dependent on the preoperative stiffness. This is an important element of the therapeutic indications. There was a statistically significant increase in the acromio-humeral distance. This occurred as if the progressive ascendance of the humeral head during the preoperative phase was due more to medialisation of the head than to any change in the rotator cuff. One can imagine that relateralising the joint line to its original position will retighten the cuff and restore the sub-acromial space.

In the *ascending form* the increase in active anterior elevation was smaller at 28° but there were major differences between patients. The acromio-humeral distance did not change significantly. On the other hand, the state of the cuff did seem to play an important role: 12 cases did not have a cuff tear and had an average increase of 38° and 4 cases with a supraspinatus tear recorded no increase in active anterior elevation. We did not find any effect related to the glenoid wear or to malpositioning of the glenoid component which in this group often had a superior inclination due to the postero-superior defect. In this group the prosthesis could not allow recentering of the humeral head which remained in a high position. The average increase in external rotation of 27° was dependent on the state of the cuff. Where there was no cuff tear the average gain was 33°, but this dropped to only 13° in the four cases where there was a cuff tear. It is therefore clear that in the ascending form the presence of a cuff tear penalises postoperative recovery of active anterior elevation and external rotation.

Conclusion

In the final analysis, this classification, based strictly on radiographic criteria, seems to be a useful element in evaluating the potential evolution of each patient, of warning of possible technical difficulties and of making a prognosis of outcome after arthroplasty. The ascending form occurs most frequently and the joint space narrowing may evolve rapidly and cause problems due to the postero-superior glenoid wear and thinning of the rotator cuff. The centered form occurs almost as frequently and although the bony wear occurs very slowly, this form causes a particular problem with stiffness. The destructive form occurs in younger patients and its aggressive nature means that the cuff is often damaged and that there is wear which rapidly involves all the articular surfaces.

Whatever the radiographic form the appearance of joint space narrowing, whether diffuse or localised and especially when in the upper part of the glenoid, must be considered as the turning point in the natural history of the disease and at this stage a shoulder arthroplasty should be considered.

References

1. Barrett NP, Thornhill TS, Thomas WH, Gebhart EM, Sledge CB (1989) Non constrained total shoulder arthroplasty in patients with polyarticular rheumatoid arthritis. J Arthroplasty 4:91–96
2. Bell SN, Gschwend N (1986) Clinical experience with total arthroplasty and hemiarthroplasty of the shoulder using the Neer prosthesis. Int Orthop 10:217–222
3. Cofield RH (1984) Total shoulder arthroplasty with the Neer prosthesis. J Bone Joint Surg Am 66:899–906
4. Constant CR, Murley AHG (1987) A clinical method of functional assessment of the shoulder. Clin Orthop 124:160–164
5. Crossan JF, Vallance R (1982) The shoulder joint in rheumatoid arthritis. In: Bayley J, Kessel L (eds) Shoulder surgery. Springer, Berlin Heidelberg New York
6. Friedman RJ, Thornhill TS, Thomas WH, Sledge CB (1989) Non constrained total shoulder replacement in patients who have rheumatoid arthritis and class IV function. J Bone Joint Surg Am 71:494–498
7. Friedman RJ (1993) Total shoulder arthroplasty in rheumatoid arthritis. In: Friedman RJ (ed) Arthroplasty of the shoulder. Thieme Medical, New York, pp 158–169
8. Goutallier D, Postel JM, Bernageau J, Lavau L, Voisin MC (1994) Fatty muscle degeneration in cuff ruptures: pre and postoperative evaluation by CT-scan. Clin Orthop 308:78–83
9. Gschwend N, Kentsch A (1984) Surgery of the rheumatoid shoulder. In: Bateman JE, Welsh RP (eds) Surgery of the shoulder. Mosby, St. Louis, pp 269–280
10. Kelly IG, Foster RS, Fischer WD (1987) Neer total shoulder replacement in rheumatoid arthritis. J Bone Joint Surg Br 69:723–726
11. Kelly IG (1994) Unconstrained shoulder arthroplasty in rheumatoid arthritis. Clin Orthop 307:94–102
12. Larsen A, Dale K, Eek M (1977) Radiographic evaluation of rheumatoid arthritis and related conditions by standard reference films. Acta Radiol Diagn 18:481–491
13. Neer CS, Watson KC, Stanton FJ (1982) Recent experience in total shoulder replacement. J Bone Joint Surg Am 64:319–337
14. Neer CS (1990) Shoulder reconstruction. Saunders, Philadelphia, pp 216–222
15. Petersson CJ (1986) Painful shoulder in patients with rheumatoid arthritis. Scand J Rheumatol 15:275. 279
16. Redfern TR, Hardinge K (1990) Hemiarthroplasty for the rheumatoid shoulder. In: Post M, Morrey BF, Hawkins RJ (eds) Surgery of the shoulder. Mosby-Year Book, St. Louis, pp 270–272
17. Sneppen O, Fruensgaard S, Johannsen HV, Olsen BS, Sojbjerg JO, Andersen NH (1996) Total shoulder replacement in rheumatoid arthritis: proximal migration and loosening. J Shoulder Elbow Surg 5:47–52
18. Thomas BJ, Amstutz HC, Cracchiolo A (1991) Shoulder arthroplasty for Rheumatoid Arthritis. Clin Orthop 265:125–128
19. Walch G, Noel E, Guier C, Frehel M (1990) Rheumatoid arthritis of the shoulder: A review of 250 patients. In: Post M, Morrey BF, Hawkins RJ (eds) Surgery of the shoulder. Mosby-Year Book, St. Louis, pp 267–269

Section IX:

Atraumatic Avascular Necrosis of the Humeral Head

Conservative Treatment of Atraumatic Avascular Necrosis of the Humeral Head

F. Kelberine, J.L. Grauer, and P. Hardy

Summary

We report the results of a multicentric study of 43 a traumatic vascular necrosis (AVN) of the humeral head treated conservatively either with a medical treatment, with arthroscopy or with core decompression. In the first group of 35 cases of AVN medically treated, the average Constant score was 53 points (14–100) with 1–11 years follow-up. This results were correlated with the subjective results which was excellent in 7, good in 7, moderate in 7 and poor in 14. Tolerance of AVN can persist in the long term up to 10 years. Deterioration can be progressive or sudden and occurs 3–4 years after the diagnostic of necrosis. Factors of poor prognosis are the widespread of necrosis and the aggravation of the necrotic staging, according to Cruess, whatever the initial stage is. In a second group of 7 cases, AVN was treated by arthroscopic excision of a intra-articular loose body which revealed the disease. With 2–10 years of follow-up, the Constant score was 78 points (63–90). Also, there were advanced anatomical lesions; all the patients were satisfied or very satisfied. Finally, one case of core decompression with bone graft failed with deterioration in the anatomical lesion. However, the Constant score was 72 points with 7 years of follow-up. A review of the literature confirms the limited place of this technique. This study confirms the absence of any prognostic value in the initial stage of the lesion at diagnostic of AVN and the value of arthroscopic treatment for removing loose body.

Introduction

Regardless of aetiology, avascular necrosis of the humeral head is an excellent indication for a shoulder arthroplasty as soon as it causes a functional disability. The diagnosis is often made when the destruction is at an advanced phase, which justifies the insertion of a prosthesis. Despite its progressive onset and a long history of symptoms [5, 6, 19, 26], head necrosis is rarely considered as a diagnosis and certainly remains underestimated [10]. Is it possible to make an earlier diagnosis and instigate treatment which would delay the time to prosthetic surgery? There are few studies reporting on the evolution and prognostic indicators which lead to the need for surgery [4, 7, 22, 25]. The aim of our study was to carry out a retrospective, multi-centre analysis of the epidemiological, clinical and radiographic characteristics of atraumatic necrosis of the humeral head treated conservatively and to compare these with the data in the literature. Three treatments were used in this series: symptomatic, arthroscopic (removal of the loose fragments) and finally decompressive forage. Each group was examined separately. We also tried to trace the natural history of avascular necrosis of the humeral head and to assess the factors which allow for short, medium or long-term tolerance of the condition and to detect any elements which lead to decompensation of this tolerance.

Materials and Methods

We reviewed 47 sets of notes from 12 centres; of these, 36 were complete and included 43 cases of avascular necroses of numeral head treated conservatively with three different treatments: 35 were treated medically, 7 had a therapeutic arthroscopy and there was one decompressive forage. (The data were provided by the following collaborators: M. Basso, Hyères; T. Boyer and H. Dorfman, Paris; P. Hardy, Paris; C. Dromer, Toulouse; R. Gallice, Aix-en-Provence; J.-L. Grauer and F. Kelberine, Aix-en-Provence; D. Molé, Nancy; J. Nizard, Nantes; E. Noel, Lyon; L. Noné-Josserand and G. Walch, Lyon; P. Ouaniche, Toulon; Y. Rozand, Grenoble.)

Medical Treatment

Group 1 consisted of 29 patients with an average age of 43 years (16–77) with a balanced sex ratio (15 men and 14 women) and the following age distribution: 10 years or under, 1; 11–20 years, 3; 21–30 years 9; 31–40 years, 5; 41–50 years, 4; 51–60 years, 3; 61–70 years. Frequently another joint demonstrated necrosis: femoral head in 19 cases, femoral condyle in 2, talar dome once and the contralateral shoulder in 11 (of which 5 could not be included in the study due to incomplete data). Of the 35 shoulders, 20 were right-sided and dominant and 15 were left-sided and non-dominant.

The activity level was recorded in 33 cases and on the occupational front remained moderate two times out of three (4 heavy manual, 6 manual, 12 part-time and 11 not working) but was poor with regard to sporting level (1 competitive, 2 hobby, 1 occasional and 29 sedentary). Three patients had suffered work-related injuries.

The aetiology of the AVN was attributed to the use of corticosteroids in 50% and other causes: steroids, 16; alcohol, 3; lupus disease, 2; metabolic, 2; arthritis, 1; osteoarthrosis, 1; sickle cell disease, 1; irradiation, 1; surgery, 1; idiopathic, 7. 20% in 3 patients the use of crutches for another injury caused decompensation of their tolerance to the AVN.

The initial presenting symptom was pain on 27 occasions: this was severe (0–5 on the Constant score) for 2 patients, moderate for 10 (5–10 points) and minimal for 15 (greater than 10). There was a progressive onset of symptoms in 24 out of 27 cases. In 10 cases there was associated stiffness but the severity, characteristics and any passive or active involvement was not detailed in this retrospective study; so, in 6 cases, this led to an initial mis-diagnosis of 5 frozen shoulders and 1 full-thickness cuff tear (the repair of which did not improve the symptoms; Fig. 1). In 8 cases the lesion was an incidental finding.

The initial diagnosis was based on the standard radiographs. We studied the stage of evolution of the necrosis using the Cruess modification of the Arlet and Ficat classification [5]:

- Stage I: normal radiograph
- Stage II: sub-chondral condensation or cyst
- Stage III: spheric egg shell
- Stage IV: nonspheric humeral head
- Stage V: osteoarthritis.

There were 3 stage I (where the diagnosis was made on complimentary investigations, e.g. magnetic resonance imaging (MRI) or bone scan]), 9 stage II, 6 stage III, 14 stage IV and 3 stage V. We also assessed the spread of the necrosis on the AP radiograph in neutral rotation by dividing the head into upper, middle and lower thirds. There was necrosis involving one third in 6 cases (4 upper and 2 middle), involving two thirds in 15 cases (14 upper and 1 lower) and involving the entire head in 14 cases (Fig. 2). Finally, we noted the presence of 4 free osteocartillaginous fragments, 4 inferior osteophytes without loss of the joint-space and the conservation of a section of the upper part of the head in 50% regardless of the stage and spread of the lesion (Fig. 2).

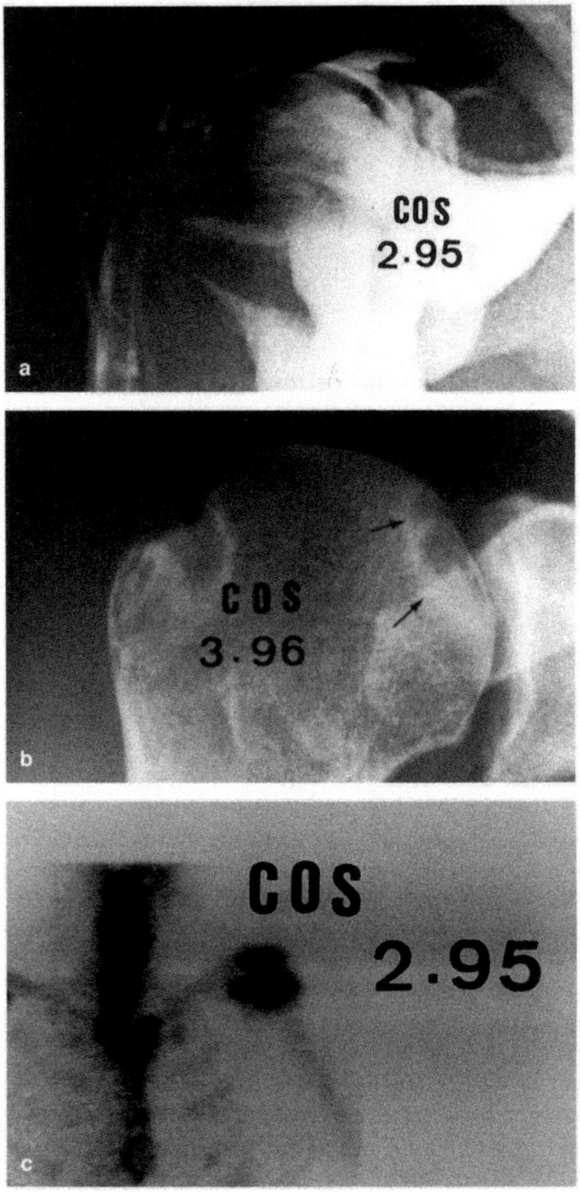

Fig. 1. Female with right-sided shoulder pain. **a** Cuff tear shown on arthrogram (*wide arrow*). **b** persistent pain 8 months after cuff repair. Stage III necrosis of the middle third (*narrow arrows*) which was demonstrated. **c** by preoperative bone-scan showing subacromial and head changes

In this group, where some cases had an 11 year follow-up, the inconsistency and variety in the use of complimentary investigations (6 computed tomography, 8 bone scans, 5 arthrography and 5 MRI) means no interpretation of the information they gave could be made. This was the same with the symptomatic treatments used, which is why this group allowed us to assess the natural history of

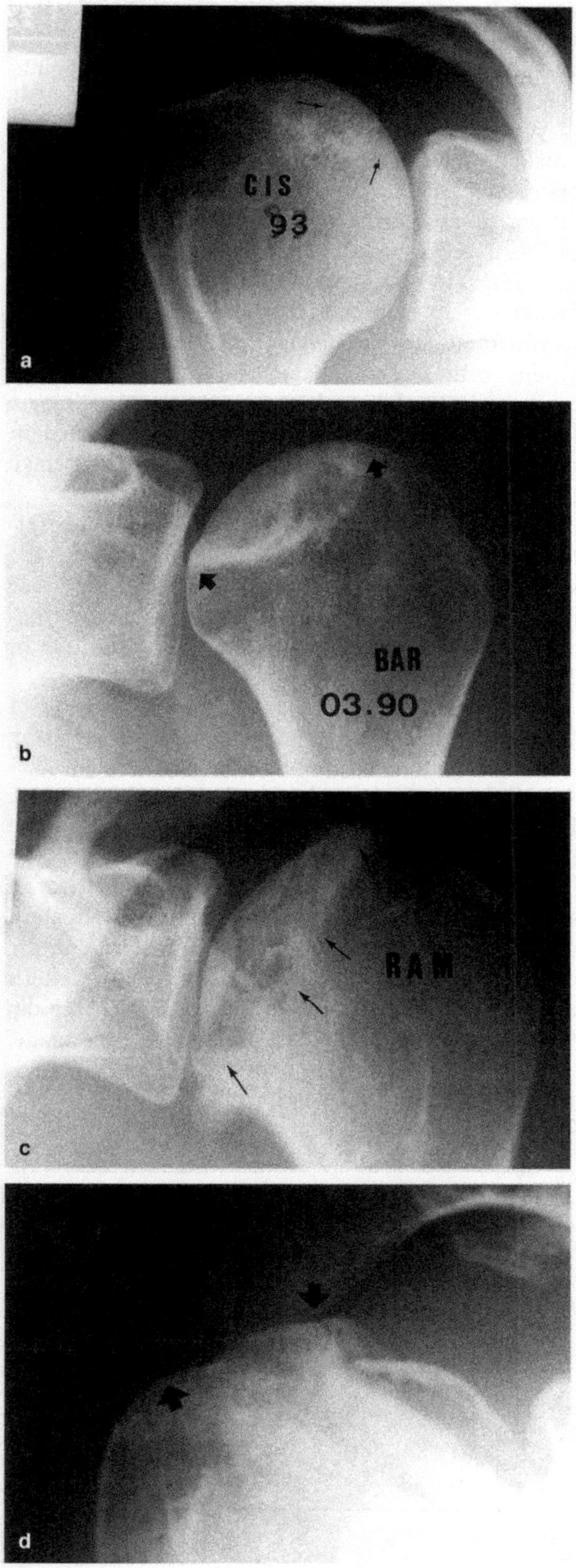

Fig. 2. a. Stage I avascular necrosis. **b** Stage II AVN. **c** Stage IV AVN (*narrow arrows*) with conservation of a superior 'cobblestone' (*wide arrow*) and a loose body. **d** Collapse of the humeral head with conservation of the superior 'cobblestone' (*downward arrow*) medial to the greater tuberosity (*upward arrow*)

AVN. The medical treatments (excluding analgesics) in the 43 patients were: nonsteroidal anti-inflammatories, 6; rehabilitation, 7; intra-articular infiltrations, 5; physiotherapy, 5; unknown, 20.

Arthroscopic Treatment

Group 2 consisted of 6 patients with an average age of 42 years (43–49) with a female predominance: 5 women, whose AVN was a consequence of steroid use, and 1 man whose aetiology was alcohol abuse. All were employed (1 heavy manual, 3 manual and 3 part-time), and 5 played sport (4 as a hobby and 1 occasionally). 2 patients were work injuried.

Multifocal involvement was also frequent: 3 femoral head and 2 femoral condylar necroses and 4 contra-lateral humeral necroses (one of which was treated arthroscopically). Of these 7 shoulders, 4 were right-sided and dominant and 3 where left and non-dominant. Moderate (5–10) or severe pain (0–5) was always the presenting symptom and occurred acutely in 6 of the 7 cases and with 'cracking' in 6 of the 7.

Radiographically, the AVN involved the whole of the head in 2 cases, two-thirds in 2 and one-third in 3. There were stage III lesions in 1, stage IV in 5 and stage V in 1. In all cases there was a loose fragment which was the deciding factor in performing an arthroscopy for its removal. The cartilaginous edges were also debrided without touching the bed of the defect (Fig. 3).

Core Decompression

There was only one case of decompressive forage in a stage 3 AVN involving the upper two-thirds of the head in a young, active, male dentist. There was multi-focal necrosis involving both hips and the opposite shoulder, as a result of corticosteroid therapy. The intervention was done by the delto-pectoral approach and involved making an anterior window to carry out the head forage and the insertion of a cancellous iliac bone-graft.

Results

At follow-up, the results were recorded using the Constant scoring system (which is given as the absolute value) and the subjective assessment from the patient. Standard radiographs were used to judge the anatomical evolution of the lesion.

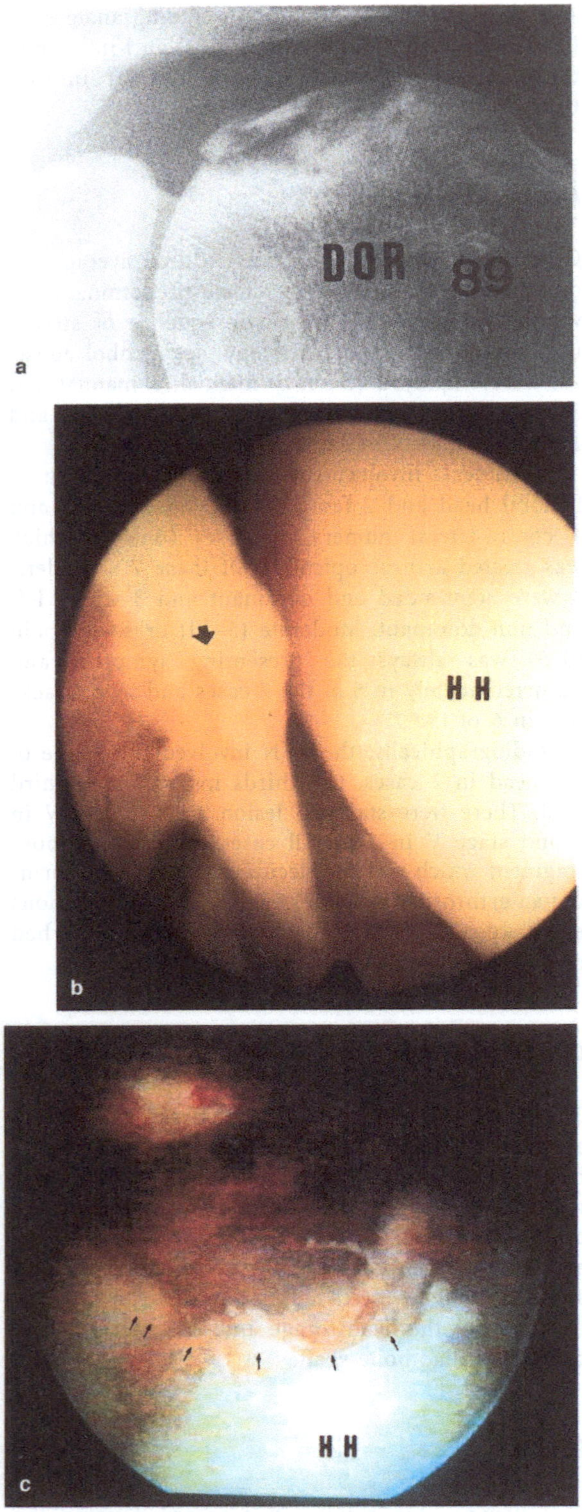

Fig. 3. a Loose body in stage IV AVN. **b** Arthroscopic view of loose body (*wide arrow*). **c** Arthroscopic view of the cephalic defect (*fine arrows*)

Medical Treatment

The mean overall Constant score was 52.6 points (14–100) an average follow-up of 47 months (1–11 years). Seven patients were very satisfied, 7 were satisfied, 7 were moderately pleased and 14 had a poor result. There was a very close correlation between the patients subjective opinion of their result and the Constant score with a coefficient of correlation of 0.84 (Fig. 4). We therefore analysed the different parameters in each of the four subjective groups.

We found no significant difference between the groups with regard to age, sex, presenting symptoms, uni- or bilateral involvement or aetiology. Involvement of the dominant arm, work related in my activity level of the patient and the initial stage of the lesion were not prognostic factors.

In contrast, the spread of the initial lesion (although not statistically significant because of the small numbers involved) did seem to be a clear prognostic factor. Widespread initial necrosis, especially if global, gave a poor outcome regardless of its stage.

The second prejudicial factor is a worsening of the anatomical stage which represents an evolving necrosis (again independent of the initial stage). Eleven of the 14 poor results occurred in this context. However, static anatomical staging or radiographic improvement did not signify a good result.

The third prognostic element was the delay in evolution of the AVN. Our groups were equal in age, sex and type of lesion. The analysis of the delay in evolution allowed us to establish a pattern of evolution. The poor results occurred rapidly (32±16.5 months) after the diagnosis was made.

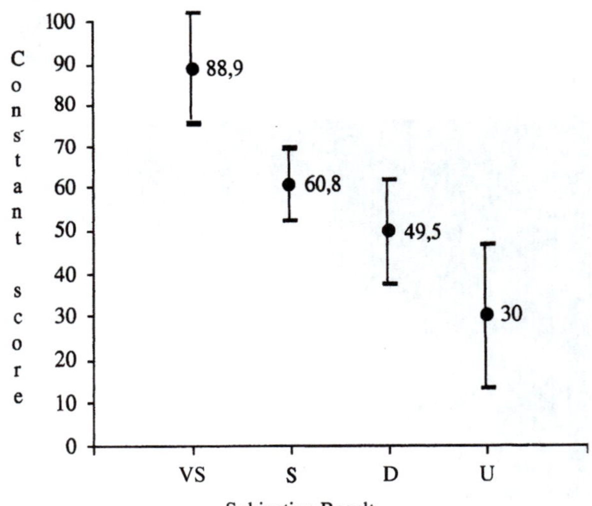

Fig. 4. Correlation between the patient's subjective assessement and the Constant Score. *Symbol*, mean value plus standard deviation; *VS*, very satisfied; *S*, satisfied; *D*, disappointed; *U*, unhappy

However, in the short term, symptomatic treatment could obtain a good result (29.3±15.4 months) where the evolution should be towards a moderate, but acceptable, medium-term result (55.6±23.8 months) or towards an excellent, and sustainable, long-term result (85.7±38.5 months).

The change from a moderate, tolerated result (Constant score of 49.5 points±12) to a poor, non-tolerated outcome (Constant score of 30 points±16.5) occurred between 32 and 48 months after the diagnosis. There was a reduction in functional score in all four parameters but especially in pain which dropped from 7.2 to 2.3 on average. Clinical decompensation was accompanied by renewed crepitus in 10 of the 14 cases and 11 of these 14 patients presented with radiographic worsening of the necrosis.

Of the 35 patients, 14 required secondary surgery; this occurred in 13 of the 14 with poor subjective results and in one with a moderate subjective result (despite a Constant score of 35) who presented with a loose body. The intervention was arthroscopic removal of a loose body on 4 occasions and arthroplasty on 10. The arthroplasty was for stage IV or V AVN in 8 cases and for stage II in 2 cases.

Arthroscopic Treatment

Group 2 had an average follow-up of 62 months (2–10 years). The overall Constant score was 77.7 points on average (63–90). Patients considered their condition as excellent in 5 cases and satisfactory in 2. Functional result was independent of the anatomical evolution, in that two showed radiographic deterioration, three remained stable and two were partly filled (Figs. 5, 6).

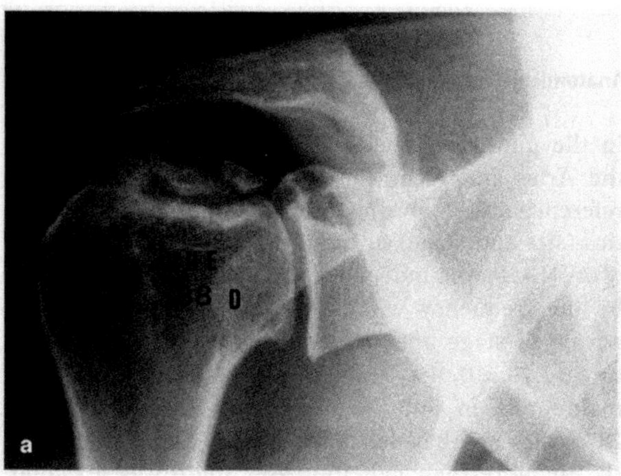

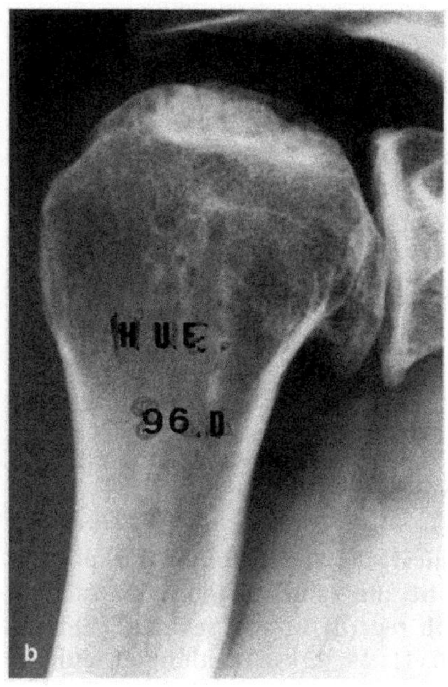

Fig. 5. Example of evolution after arthroscopic treatment. **a** Radiograph before arthroscopy: large sequestration. **b** Radiograph 8 years postoperation: evolution to osteoarthritis (Constant score=90)

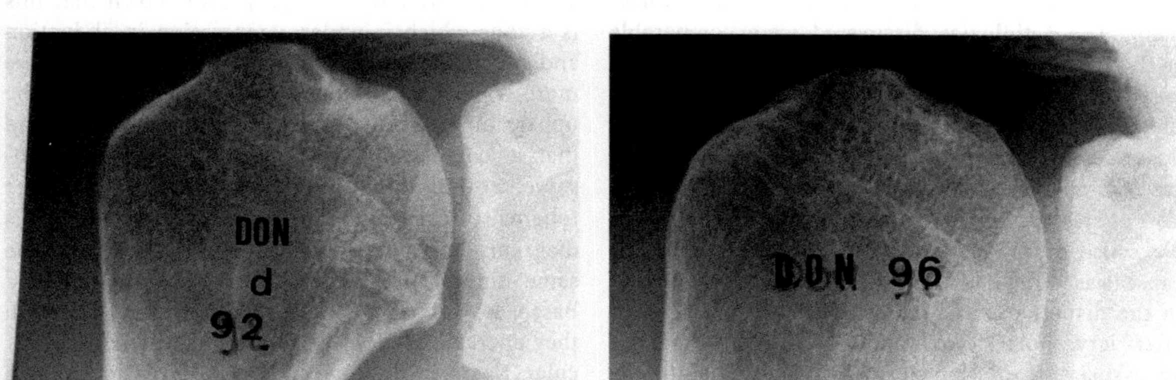

Fig. 6. Another example of evolution after arthroscopic treatment. **a** Radiograph done the day of arthroscopy: AVN stage IV. **b** Radiograph 4 years postoperation: partial improvement

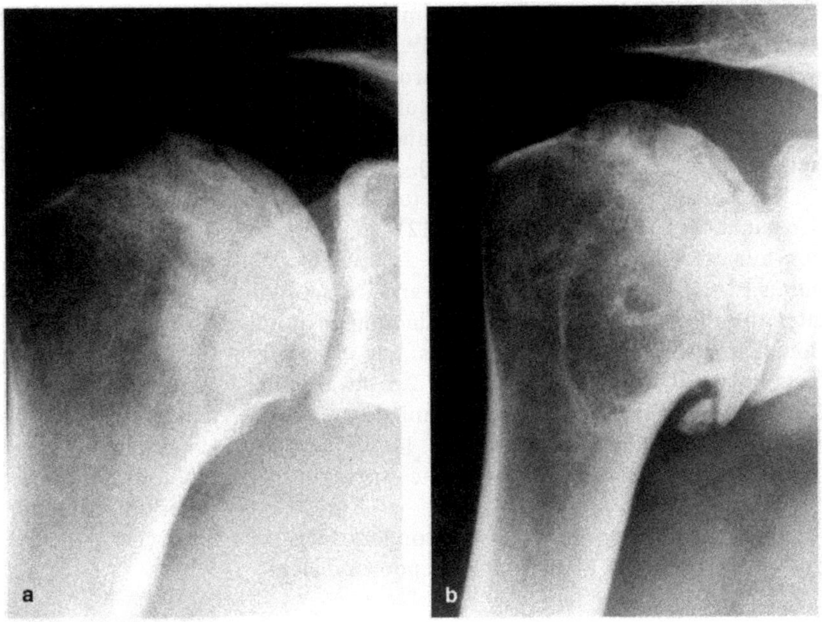

Fig. 7. Example of evolution after core decompression. **a** Preoperative radiograph: AVN stage III. **b** Radiograph 7 years after core decompression and graft: evolution to ostroarthritis.

Core Decompression

Group 3 patient was reviewed at 7 years. Despite a Constant score of 72 points the patient considered the result as poor and the radiographs showed a deterioration in the anatomical lesion (Fig. 7).

Discussion

Epidemiological Characteristics

The epidemiological characteristics of our population seemed to be the same as those reported in the literature with regards to age, sex, side and dominance [2, 5, 10, 11, 19, 23]. As with other authors, we found frequent bilateral or multifocal involvement. The aetiologies discovered were comparable to those reported by Cofield [2], Cruess [3], Frostick and Wallace [10], Gazielly [11] and Neer [23], with the most common factor being long-term, or high-dose use of corticosteroids. We did not have any cases of necrosis following just intra-articular injection of steroids which has been proposed as a possible cause of AVN by Laroche [20]. Sometimes the cause was difficult to uncover as it may have been in the distant past, as in dysbaric necrosis [27], or after very short steroid treatments [26]. It may be an association of elements which gives rise to the potential for necrosis [1].

Anatomical Characteristics

In the published series, the Cruess modification of the Arlet and Ficat classification serves [5] as the reference for analysing the anatomical characteristics (site and stage) of the necrosis. The presentation of AVN remains independent of its stage as is shown by the frequency with which lesions present at an advanced stage both in our series and in the literature [2, 8, 10, 19, 25]. Sphericity of the head was maintained in only 46.5 % of our cases, and only 28 % did not have a loose body (12 stages I and II). In more than half the cases there was articular incongruence with a sunken sequestrum (44.1 %) and 4 cases had arthritis (9.3 %). Preferential localisation to the upper third of the articular surface is classic. Inman and Salter [17] have shown that this is a zone which is under compression in abduction and functional anterior elevation. When the AVN is more widespread it almost always spreads from the upper third. Finally, in half of the cases we found that a 'cobblestone' of articular surface was conserved at the summit of the head close to the greater tuberosity. This was reproduced by Neer [23] in his diagrams without actually being described. The same finding was made by Nové-Josserand and Basso in almost all of the AVN cases on which they operated (see Nové-Josserand and Basso, "Avascular Necrosis of the Humeral Head: Clinical and Radiological Classification" and Basso and L. Nové-Josserand, "Results of Shoulder Arthroplasty for Avascular Necrosis of the Humeral Head", this volume). This healthy zone corresponds to a section which is not vascularised by the anterior circumflex artery as described by Gerber, Schneeberger and Vinh [12].

Natural History of AVN of the Humeral Head

The natural history of AVN of the humeral head has rarely been studied [7, 25]. We have tried to establish a pattern of functional evolution based on these cases and, in particular, on the group 1 patients treated medically. An analysis of the variation in tolerance to AVN was carried out using the subjective results which were closely correlated with the Constant scores. The diagnosis of AVN is often an incidental finding and illustrates the frequency with which it is tolerated initially, as reported in the literature [3, 4, 6, 10, 13, 21, 27]. As with Van Blarcom [27] and Dines [7], we believe that this tolerance can persist, and even improve, in the long-term up to about 10 years. It may, of course, also deteriorate progressively giving altered but tolerable function as shown by some of the AVN cases diagnosed at mid-term. A poorly tolerated AVN reveals sometimes suddenly the disease. However, sometimes there is a change from a tolerated necrosis to one causing a functional handicap and this seems an essential point. As already noted by Dines [7], Gazielly [11] and Rutherford [25], this critical step occurred, in our series, between 3 and 4 years after the diagnosis of necrosis and so there is justification for regular review for this period of time. It occurs with a frank clinical decompensation and a drop in the Constant score of 30 points, which is very close to the 27 and 24 point drops reported by Nové-Josserand in this publication and by Gazielly [11] in their series of AVN cases treated by arthroplasty. As with Cofield [2], Neer [23] and Rutherford [25], our patients with a poor functional outcome all ended up by undergoing surgery. The deterioration, although usually progressive, can also be rapid when it may be associated with cracking or blocking of the shoulder, which corresponds to anatomical collapse of the head with the liberation of a loose body. It should be noted that groups 2 and 3 fit perfectly into this pattern of evolution where poor tolerance, whether of progressive or acute origin, leads to surgical intervention.

Factors Affecting Tolerance in AVN of the Humeral Head Treated Medically

Humeral head necrosis due to thalassaemia [6, 21, 28] or of dysbaric origin [13, 27] did not occur in our series but generally have a best prognosis. In contrast, as with Neer [23], Gazielly [11] and Cofield [2], we did not find any prognostic factors linked to patient status. Moreover, as with Cruess [3], we report decompensation in the tolerance to AVN due to the use of crutches as part of the treatment for a pathology effecting the lower limbs.

The stage of necrosis was considered by Rutherford [25] as being a prejudicial factor and he attributed the 5 poor results in 16 cases with a 4.5-year follow-up, to those with stage IV and V. In 66 cases with a 9-year follow-up, Dines [7] recorded 36 poor results in stages III to V. Cruess [4] reported 8 excellent results with stage I or II AVN in 16 cases but another 6 good results in patients with more advanced AVN. In our series, the different stages of necrosis were divided amongst the different subjective result groups. In our opinion this is independent of the AVN stage at the time of diagnosis. The fact that there can be perfect tolerance of advanced head necrosis supports this argument.

In contrast, the presence of widespread necrosis was clearly a prejudicial factor and corresponded with an absence of "weightbearing area". A deterioration in the anatomical stage at follow-up was a significant factor reflecting evolution of the AVN which had lost its established, balanced state. These two elements remain independent of the initial stage which, to our knowledge, has not been considered previously in the literature.

The Place of Medical Treatment

The diversity of medical treatments used in the group 1 patients does not allow their efficacy to be assessed. The different series in the literature analysed the spontaneous evolution of AVN rather than the effectiveness of its treatment which was not detailed [3, 4, 7, 25, 26]. For these authors, the early stages of necrosis (I and II) clearly responded well to antalgics. Non-steroidal anti-inflammatories used as antalgics and infiltrations represent symptomatic treatment which have no effect on preventing the evolution of the necrosis. Some authors stress the importance of rehabilitation with the aim of reducing the compressive forces acting on the pathological zone in abduction [2, 23].

The Place of Conservative Surgical Treatment is Very Specific

Arthroscopy seems to be the treatment of choice in a specific, active patients whose AVN is "no symptomatic" prior to an acute decompensation. Arthroscopic removal of the loose body achieved 2 good and 5 excellent long-term results in our series: once again independent of the initial stage of the lesion and of the size of the fragment, including stage V cases which sooner or later probably require arthroplasty. Several sporadic cases have been published: Hamada [14] with regard to osteochondritis, and Fleega [9], Hayes [15], Isakawa [18] and Petrini [24] on AVN. The clinical presentation was always characterised by an acute incident with blockage of the joint and removal of the fragment (combined with débridement for Fleega) always gave a satisfactory result.

Decompressive forage is supported by the results obtained by forage of the femoral head and the work of Hungerford [16] who notes that the ischaemia is due to a compartment syndrome secondary to a pressure increase in the bone marrow. Mont et al. [22] followed 30 cases for 5 years and stated that decompression of the humeral head gave 22 good or very good results in stage I or II disease but without detailing the symptoms which justified the intervention and 3 months. The eight failures, in this series all occurred in stage III and IV disease. Other authors report only failures: 5 out of 6 for Dines [7], 1 out of 1 for Frostick and Wallace [10], 2 out of 2 for Neer [23] and our single case (although the stage was very advanced). Finally, Cofield [2], in a comparative study of 16 cases with a 4-year follow-up, reported identical results for each anatomical stage between forage and medical treatment. As with Greg and Walder [13], we believe that, in the absence of any proof of the effectiveness of this intervention in arresting the development of necrosis, there is no place for prophylactic surgery for AVN of the humeral head.

Anatomical reformation of the humeral head was reported by Cruess [4] and David [6] in thalassaemic necrosis after medical treatment. We noted 4 improvements or partial reformations (2 after arthroscopy and 2 after medical treatment) although these were not linked with an improvement in function.

The problem of diagnosis is not referred to very often in the literature. It is only a problem in progressive evolution with minimal pain. The association with stiffness, whose frequency has been reported by Cruess [3, 4], Neer [23] and Taylor [26], may the diagnosis more difficult. However, we still had 5 mis-diagnoses of frozen shoulder and in our retrospective series, stiffness was certainly underestimated, mainly due to faults in the data collected. It is for these reasons that passive stiffness combined with a moderate degree of pain should be investigated either by bone-scanning [13] or MRI [8, 23].

Conclusion

The frequent late diagnosis of AVN of the humeral head bears witness to how well it can be tolerated functionally. However, it evolves with time. While bearing in mind the limits of a retrospective, multi-centre study, the length of follow-up and the limited number of patients, this study has allowed us to propose a pattern of evolution of avascular necrosis of the humeral head.

The necrosis may remain asymptomatic over a long period, including those where there is severe anatomical damage confirming the absence of any prognostic value in the initial stage of the lesion at diagnosis.

Deterioration in the functional result logically leads on to surgical intervention. Poor tolerance may appear suddenly with collapse of the humeral head and/or release of a loose body. Arthroscopy has a specific place in these patients where removal of the fragment gives good results and restores a new equilibrium in the shoulder. There may be progressive decompensation which usually starts to occur about 3 years after the diagnosis.

The risk factors are the degree of spread of the necrosis at the time of diagnosis and any deterioration in its anatomical stage regardless of the initial stage. Such an upset in the state of equilibrium was, in our series, an indication for shoulder arthroplasty.

References

1. Chrysanthou CP (1978) Dysbaric osteonecrosis: etiological and pathogenic concepts. Clin Orthop 130:94–106
2. Cofield RH (1994) Osteonecrosis. In: Friedman RJ (ed) Arthroplasty of the shoulder. Thieme Medical, New York, pp 170–181
3. Cruess RL (1976) Steroid-induced avascular necrosis of the head of the humerus. Natural history and management. J Bone Joint Surg Br 58:313–317
4. Cruess RL (1978) Experience with steroid-induced avascular necrosis of the shoulder and etiologic considerations regarding osteonecrosis of the hip. Clin Orthop 130:86–93
5. Cruess RL (1986) Osteonecrosis of bone. Current concepts as to etiology and pathogenesis. Clin Orthop 208:30–39
6. David HG, Bridgman SA, Davies SC, Hine AL, Emery RJ (1993) The shoulder in sickle-cell disease J Bone Joint Surg Br 75:538–545
7. Dines DM, Warren RF, Pagnani MJ, Linsalata JC (1995) Osteonecrosis of the proximal humerus: natural history, long term follow up and radiographic predictors of outcome. VIII European Congress on Elbow and Shoulder Surgery, Barcelona, June
8. Dufour M, Romani M, Ghersi A, Ohresser E, Roux H (1991) Ostéonécroses aseptiques ou avasculaires. Feuillets Radiol 31:353–373

9. Fleega BA (1996) Avascular necrosis of the humeral head: a new treatment method based on arthroscopic minimum invasive mean. J Shoulder Elbow Surg 5 [Suppl 2]:S66
10. Frostick SP, Wallace WA (1989) Osteonecrosis of the humeral head. Baillière's Clin Rheumatol 3:651–667
11. Gazielly D, Thomas T, Bruyere G, Pasquier B, Grossetete JL (1993) Résultats de l'arthroplastie prothétique type Neer dans le traitement de l'ostéonecrose de la tête humérale. A propos de 25 cas opérés. Rev Chir Orthop [Suppl 1]: 99–105
12. Gerber C, Schneeberger AG, Vinh TS (1990) The arterial vascularization of the humeral head. J Bone Joint Surg Am 72:1486–1494
13. Gregg PJ, Walder DN (1986) Caisson disease of bone. Clin Orthop 210:43–54
14. Hamada S, Hamada M, Nishiue S, Doi T (1992) Osteochondris dissecans of the humeral head. Arthroscopy 8:132–137
15. Hayes JM (1989) Arthroscopic treatment of steroid-induced osteonecrosis of the humeral head. Arthroscopy 5:218–221
16. Hungerford DS (1981) Pathogenic considerations in ischemic necrosis of bone. Can J Surg 24:583–588
17. Inman VT, Saunder JB, Abott LC (1944) Observations on the function of the shoulder joint. J Bone Joint Surg 26A 26:1–30
18. Isikawa H, Ueba Y, Yonezawa T, Kurosaka M, Ohno O, Hirohata K (1988) Osteochondris dissecans of the shoulder in a tennis player. Am J Sport Med 16:547–550
19. Jacobs B (1978) Epidemiology of traumatic and nontraumatic osteonecrosis. Clin Orthop 130:51–67
20. Laroche M, Arlet J, Mazieres B (1989) Osteonecrosis of the femoral and humeral heads after intraarticular corticoid injections. J Rheumatol 17:549–551
21. Man S, Koren A (1993) Avascular necrosis of bones in children with sickle cell anemia. Pediatr Hematol Oncol 10:385–387
22. Mont MA, Maar DC, Urquhart MW, Lennox D, Hungerford DS (1993) Avascular necrosis of the humeral head treated by core decompression. J Bone Joint Surg Br 75:785–788
23. Neer CS (1990) Glenohumeral arthroplasty: avascular necrosis of the humeral head. In: Shoulder reconstruction. Saunders, Philadelphia, pp 194–202
24. Petrini A, Grassi G, Zaccaria CP (1984) Osteochondrite dissecante della testa omerale. Chir Org Mov 59:83–85
25. Rutherford CS, Cofield RH (1987) Osteonecrosis of the shoulder. Orthop Trans 11:239
26. Taylor LJ (1984) Multi-focal avascular necrosis after short-term high-dose steroid therapy. J Bone Joint Surg Br 66:431–433
27. Van Blarcom ST, Czarnecki DJ, Fueredi GA, Wenzel MS (1990) Does dysbaric osteonecrosis progress in the absence of further baric exposure. A 10-year radiologic follow-up of 15 patients. Am J Radiol 155:95–97
28. Wingate JK, Schiff CF, Friedman RJ (1996) Humeral head necrosis in sickle cell disease. J Shoulder Elbow Surg 5 [Suppl 2]:S18

Atraumatic Avascular Necrosis of the Humeral Head: Clinical and Radiographic Classification

L. Nové-Josserand and M. Basso

Summary

This retrospective study reports the clinical and radiographic appearances of 43 shoulders which were operated on for avascular necrosis (excluding posttraumatic AVN). The aetiologies were comparable to those in the literature. The most frequent cause after idiopathic necrosis was secondary to corticosteroid therapy. The overall clinical picture is unspecific and does not match the radiographic appearance. The natural history is variable. The radiographic appearance, described in five stages, is characteristic for the lesion. The necrosis always appeared in the same area of the upper part of the humeral head opposite the superior pole of the glenoid; areas of major mechanical forces. In all cases, except for radiation necrosis, the articular summit of the humeral head in contact with the greater tuberosity was conserved. This specific radiographic sign allows the particular clinico-radiographic form occurring in elderly women (over 70 years) which presents with rapid, massive collapse of the humeral head to be linked in with avascular necrosis. This form of necrosis is debatable in marking the border line limits with the rapidly destructive arthropathies. Radiation necrosis, occurring late after irradiation, is differentiated by its histology (no evidence of repair) and its radiographic appearance (generalised head necrosis and joint space narrowing).

Introduction

Avascular necrosis is defined histologically by the death of marrow and bone cells, clinically by a picture of pain and stiffening of the joint and radiographically by a characteristic evolution. Osteonecrosis may be primary or idiopathic, or occur secondary to a known cause, a systemic illness or after trauma or irradiation. In this chapter we have excluded posttraumatic osteonecrosis, which is discussed in the section on fracture sequalae and malunions. It is idiopathic necrosis which is of main interest to researchers as it remains incompletely understood.

Few basic studies have been carried out specifically on humeral necrosis and their radiographic and clinical appearances have allowed the observations made for necrosis of the hip to be extrapolated to the shoulder [9].

In general, the frequency of osteonecrosis is estimated as 1 in 1000 [19]. The upper femur is by far the most common site with the upper humerus and lower femur being affected about equally [9]. Rosenberg et al. suggested that one humerus was affected for every 19 femurs [31]. In certain populations, such as in carriers of thalassaemia, the incidence may be much greater [27]. Cruess reported 22 affected humeri in 111 cortiocosteroid induced osteonecroses [10].

There are two noteworthy elements [10]. The first is the frequency of bilateral osteonecrosis and the second is its multifocal character. Humeral necrosis is often associated with necrosis in the hip or in another site with the order of frequency being: femoral condyle, capitellum, scaphoid, semi-lunate and talus. It is worth recording that the majority of these sites consist of large cartilaginous coverings with a blood supply coming from the body of the bone. Only necrosis of the femoral condyles is difficult to explain from this vascular viewpoint.

Aetiology

There are different pathological situations which seem to favour the development of osteonecrosis and in some the relationship seems undebatable. Some pathologies such as Gaucher's disease are rare. Others occur more commonly and are associated with a large proportion of the recorded cases of humeral osteonecrosis. This is the case for osteonecrosis in patients with sickle-cell disease and thalassaemia S (Afro-Caribbean and Mediterranean basin populations) [12]. It is equally the case for osteonecrosis in patients treated with corticosteroids who usually form the largest group in the analysed series [10, 11, 14].

Osteonecrosis after corticosteroid therapy appears preferentially in subjects who have received steroids for long periods for chronic diseases (rheumatoid conditions, asthma, transplants etc). Cruess [9] did not observe any cases during 6-month periods of steroid treatment. However, osteonecrosis can equally well occur after short periods of treatment taken systemically [1, 30, 36] and even after intra-articular injections [22].

In other diseases, the link with osteonecrosis is less evident: acute pancreatitis, obesity, familial hyperlipidaemias, hyperuricaemia, hyperthyroidism and lupus [7]. Despite all searches for an aetiological connection, there still remain 20%–30% which are idiopathic and where no cause can be found.

Histopathology

Numerous studies have been carried out on the histology of these lesions [2, 9, 26, 34] but few have studied the pathological changes in the early disease stages [2, 34]. Most of the studies have concentrated on the femoral head, but there is nothing to suggest any difference in humeral osteonecrosis. All the biopsies show that the spread of the lesions seen in the femur occurs well beyond the radiographic epiphyseal line. This fact has been confirmed more recently by magnetic resonance imaging (MRI) which shows more widespread bony changes than suspected on the standard radiographs.

In the preradiographic stage, the findings of Saito et al. [34] agree with those of Arlet and Ficat [2]. There is always necrosis affecting the two components of cancellous bone: medullary and trabecular. In a core biopsy one finds, from superficial to deep:

A Subchondral bone with complete ischaemic necrosis (no visible cells) and no signs of reparation (no bony regeneration or vascular proliferation)
B Complete necrosis of the cancellous bone with some signs of reparation: new bone laid down on the dead trabeculae, early medullary fibrosis
C Cancellous bone with areas of complete and incomplete necrosis
D Normal cancellous bone beyond the necrotic zone.

In nearly all cases, areas of recent or old haemorrhage are found in the marrow. For Arlet and Ficat [2] 'haemorrhage is not necrosis but it may provoke or succeed it' and Saito et al. [34] consider it a central element in the formation of necrosis.

In the more evolved stages the notable anatomical feature is the significant attempt at tissue repair: vascular proliferation and the presence of undifferentiated mesenchymal cells followed by their differentiation into haemopoietic and bony tissues. Bony repair does not follow the same pathway in cancellous as in sub-chondral bone. In cancellous bone, the mesenchymal cells of the marrow differentiate into osteoblasts which lay down new bone onto the necrotic trabeculae causing the densities seen on radiographs. In the compact subchondral bone, it occurs by a sequence of osteoclastic resorption and new bone deposition: this is the classic "creeping substitution" where there is a loss of bone mass and weakness. This explains the site of the initial fracture with subchondral collapse due to the influence of mechanical forces.

The articular cartilage, partly nourished from synovial fluid, remains normal for a long time. However, cartilaginous flaps may form due to bony collapse in the same way as with foreign bodies.

The histological and clinical factors would suggest that the formation of osteonecrosis is not identical in all cases [9]: damage due to vascular insults alone in fractures, by successive crises in sickle-cell disease and by progressive phenomena in alcoholism and steroid therapy.

Mechanical factors play an important role in understanding bony collapse. The necrotic trabeculae lose some of their mechanical properties [19]: 70% of their elastic modulus and 50% of their tensile strength. The trabecular fractures accumulate in the zone of maximum force where they produce a macroscopic depression in the superomedial pole of the humeral head and the anterosuperior quadrant of the femoral head [9, 29]. It is worth noting that the necrosis is usually more serious and occurs more rapidly where there is preexisting bone loss such as in prolonged steroid therapy, alcoholism and in renal transplants.

Pathophysiology

An understanding of the pathological processes which lead to osteonecrosis is still incomplete. The exact cause of the interruption to the arteriolar blood supply is not known. Three main pathophysiological theories have been proposed but each can explain only some of the features seen.

Slowing or Interruption of the Capillary Circulation

Due to Intramedullary Tamponade. This is a well proven process which occurs early [2, 21, 37]. It may be the consequence of hypertrophy of adipocytes in the marrow as seen in humans on steroid treatment [9, 11]. The accumulation of cells in the marrow in Gaucher's disease may have the same effect. This hypothesis does not apply so well to other aetiologies (e.g. sickle cell disease, Caisson's disease). The cause and effect link between lipid abnormalities and cell necrosis on the one hand and intramedullary tamponade on the other is not clear. Bone forms an undeformable compartment so that any increase in pressure within it directly effects the flow in the vessels which cross it by increasing local resistance. This theory forms the basis for decompressive forage [2, 21].

Due to Intraosseous Micro-emboli. This may lead to necrosis initially in very localised areas and then becoming clinically significant due to the repetition of the release of emboli. Experimentally one can achieve subchondral deposits after injection with markers [17, 21, 26]. Clinically fat emboli are a plausible cause in alcoholism and similarly, by blockage of the micro-circulation with crystals in gout, by aggregates of abnormal cells in Sickle-cell disease and by gas bubbles in Caissons disease. The increase in intramedullary pressure may therefore be secondary to these phenomena.

Hyperlipidaemia. This disorder may play a role, and is manifest in certain familial forms and in abnormalities of lipid metabolism induced by steroid therapy.

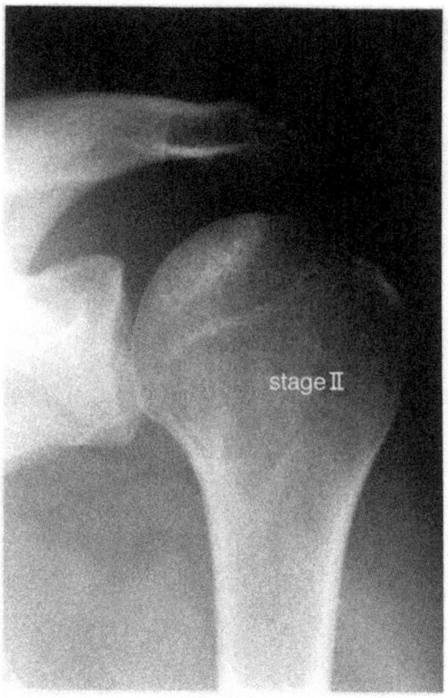

Fig. 1. Stage 2 osteonecrosis. A localised zone of osteoporosis at the superior pole of the humeral head surrounded by a dense border with the sclerosis indicating reparation in process

Venous Obstruction

This is obvious in the early disease stages [2, 21, 32, 37]. Pertrochanteric venography carried out via a needle in the greater trochanter demonstrates the characteristic elements: incomplete visualisation of the draining veins and stasis of the contrast in the metaphysis. These findings lend venography a significant value in diagnosis [2, 20] but still does not show whether there is a primary venous problem or if the obstruction is secondary to tamponade.

Arterial Insufficiency

This is the principle in posttraumatic necrosis. Arterial lesions secondary to the trauma (or to surgical intervention) lead to necrosis in areas where the blood supply comes from a terminal branch (anterior and posterior circumflex arteries) [16]. Although there are anastamoses these seem to be insufficient.

Radiographic Classification

It is essentially the radiographic appearance which is used in establishing the clinical classification. The classification of Marcus [25] is used in the English-speaking world, but it is that of Arlet and Ficat which acts as the worldwide reference [2]. Describing changes in the hip, it serves equally well for the humerus:

- Stage 1: A preradiographic stage: pain and stiffness with no radiographic changes. At this stage MRI is positive and shows non-specific bony changes.
- Stage 2: Abnormal images demonstrate the process of repair: diffuse osteoporosis of the contour of the head remains preserved (Fig. 1).
- In Stage 3: The characteristic osteonecrotic appearance with a triangle of mostly heterogeneous condensation is obvious. This stage is characterised by a subchondral fracture giving the 'crescent' sign. The characteristic site for this is the superomedial region of the head which is the contact area between the head and the glenoid at 90° of gleno-humeral abduction and the position of maximal compression. At this stage the joint line is preserved. There may be some loss of sphericity of the head with a flattering secondary to subchondral collapse (Figs. 2, 3).
- Stage 4: Characterised by extensive collapse and deformation of the humeral head. The cartilaginous envelope ruptured. The secondary mechanical changes act as the basis for arthritic changes (Fig. 4).
- Stage 5: Characterised by secondary destructive lesions crossing to the glenoid side of the joint (Fig. 5).

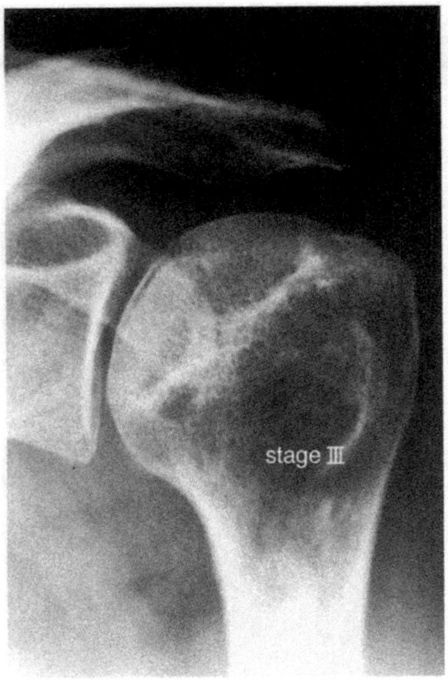

Fig. 2. Stage 3 osteonecrosis. Appearance of a crescent sign. This is a fracture of the necrotic sub-chondral bone. The humeral head retains its sphericity and the cartilage is normal at this stage

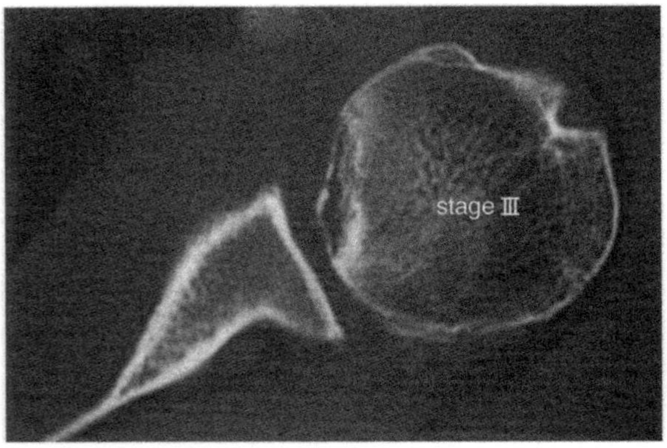

Fig. 3. The same lesion seen on CT scan. There is a sub-chondral space bordered by reactive bony condensation

The clinical picture is often non-characteristic. In contrast to femoral head necrosis it rarely presents with severe localised pain. The presentation of symptoms is generally more progressive with pain on movement and sometimes at rest and progressive stiffness. A little more specific are episodes of painful locking of the joint [18] or a painful, audible click from the joint due to a cartilaginous flap [10]. Cruess reports that loss of active movement often contrasts with preservation of passive movement over a long period [9–11].

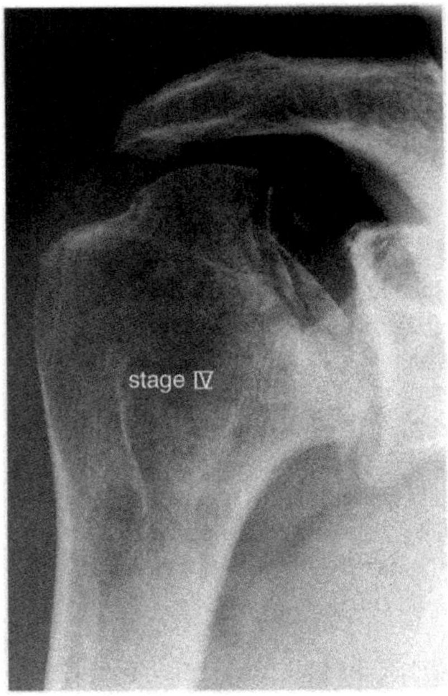

Fig. 4. Stage 4 osteonecrosis. Collapse of the humeral head which has lost its sphericity. This is a 66-year-old man with no specific antecedents who complained of 6 months of severe pain in his shoulder. Notice the major bony collapse opposite the upper pole of the glenoid, the characteristic sparing of the upper part of the humerus in contact with the greater tuberosity and the less significant bony condensation

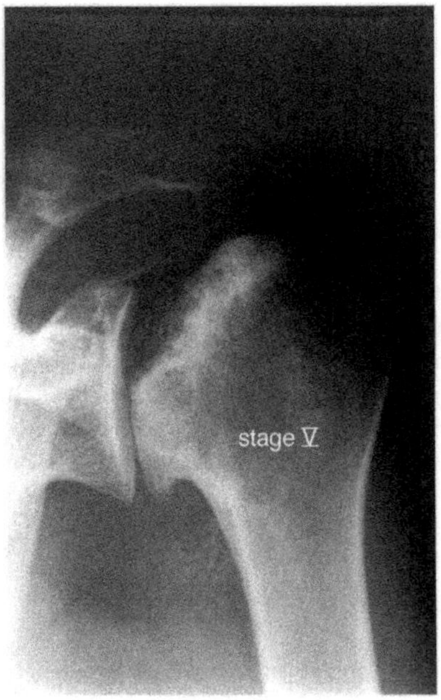

Fig. 5. Stage 5 osteonecrosis. There is a degenerative reaction of the inferior part of the gleno-humeral joint. This is a 43-year-old man with bilateral hip necrosis (operated) and shoulder necrosis (the contralateral shoulder is at stage 2)

An early diagnosis may be suspected clinically especially when there is an aetiological reason. Definitive diagnosis rests on MRI and bone scanning, where the images are less equivocal and reveal sub-clinical involvement in the controlateral shoulder in about half the cases [4, 19].

Materials and Methods

Our multicentre study was carried out on 43 shoulders (40 patients) which had received either a Neer prosthesis (10 cases) or an Aequalis prosthesis (33 cases) between 1989 and 1995. There were three bilateral cases. There were 27 females and 13 males. The average age at the time of surgery was 57 years and 10 months (33–90 years). The 14 patients aged over 70 made up 35% of our group. There were 24 right and 29 dominant shoulders.

The aetiologies were: idiopathic, 21; steroid treatment, 14 (of which 2 were on dialysis); alcoholism, 3; Gaucher's disease, 1; Caisson's disease, 1; colorectal haemorrhage, 1; radiotherapy, 2. In half the cases (20 patients) necrosis was isolated to the shoulder. The clinical results were based on the 35 cases with preoperative Constant scores and the radiographic results on all 43 cases.

Results

Using the radiographic classification we found 3 stage II, 2 stage III, 25 stage IV and 13 stage V cases.

On the clinical front (Table 1) the series, regardless of the radiographic stage, was characterised by poor scores in the subjective sections of the Constant score reflected as severe pain (average score 3.7±2.4) and a marked reduction in function (average score 6.7±2). Conversely, mobility diminished with the severity of the disease (average score 13±6, ranging from 19 in stage II, to 9 in stage V) (Table 2). We found no relationship between age and radiological stage.

The radiographic study showed that, apart from the two post radiotherapy cases, the necrotic area was always situated in the same area of the supero-medial section of the humeral head at a distance from the anatomical neck and always sparing the upper part of the humeral head at the greater tuberosity. From this point the necrosis extended distally over a variable distance.

We were able to describe a particular group of necrosis with massive head collapse occurring in females aged over 70 years (70–90). In these 9 cases the bony collapse did not affect the upper humeral head at the level of the greater tuberosity (Figs. 6, 7). In these cases the onset was severe and the evolution was rapid occurring over several months. At the time the shoulder was very painful (pain score 3±2.7), and mobility was severely limited (mobility score 5±3). The shoulder behaved as if paralysed. In 4 cases there was a massive cuff tear although it was intact in the other 5. In 4 cases the glenoid was damaged.

Discussion

Necrosis of the shoulder can occur at any age between 30 and 90. The aetiological factors were similar in our series to those in other published series notably in the French literature [15]. Regardless of the stage, pain was intense although there is some bias here as this is a retrospective series. Cruess [10, 11], Rutherford and Cofield [33] and Dines [13] have shown that the lesion can be well tolerated up to stage III. On the other hand, mobility diminishes as the radiographic stage worsens. This would appear logical for mechanical reasons as articular congruency is lost as the humeral head collapses.

Table 1. Preoperative Constant scores for the different radiographic stages

	Pain	Activity	Mobility	Force	Constant	Constant (adjusted)
Stage 2 (*n*=2)	4±1.4	9±3	19±1.4	4.5±0.7	36±3	47±13
Stage 3 (*n*=2)	1.5±2	7±1.5	13±4	1±1.4	22±6	27±3
Stage 4 (*n*=18)	4.6±2	7.5±2	15±6	4±3	31±10	39±12
Stage 5 (*n*=13)	2.8±2	5±2	9±5	1.5±2	18±9	24±11

Table 2. Preoperative and passive movement for the different radiographic stages

	Active anterior elevation	Passive anterior elevation	Active external rotation	Passive external rotation
Stage 2 (*n*=2)	100°	160°	55°	55°
Stage 3 (*n*=3)	75°±21°	90°	5°±7°	17°±3°
Stage 4 (*n*=18)	93°±42°	107°±37°	4°±19°	5°±15°
Stage 5 (*n*=13)	63°±47°	96°±44°	0°±14°	2°±14°

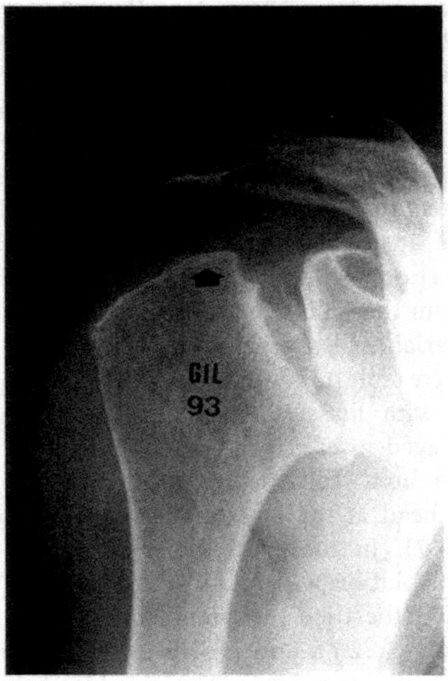

Fig. 6. Necrosis with massive collapse in a 90-year-old woman. The humeral head has disappeared except at the summit in contact with the greater tuberosity (a characteristic sign of osteonecrosis; *black arrow*). The sub-acromial space is maintained. The glenoid is affected at inferior pole by mechanical impaction

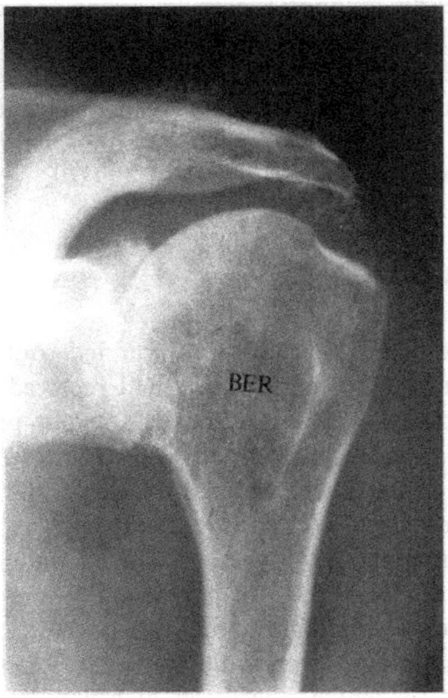

Fig. 7. Radionecrosis of the humeral head. There is overall damage to the head without sparing the upper part in contact with the greater tuberosity. There is a loss of the joint space

It is difficult to be exact about the time of onset and delay in evolution in this retrospective series. It seems though that there is a tendency towards stabilisation of the lesions associated with articular degradation in the younger and active patient (Fig. 5). As age increases so the humeral head deformation becomes larger, earlier with a true fracture opposite the upper pole of the glenoid. One should remember that the cancellous bone strength is poorer as well as regenerative power being weaker in the elderly patient (Fig. 4). In the younger patients the phenomenon of peripheral bone reparation, limiting the area of total necrosis, allows the lesion to stabilise.

In the literature there is little work on the natural history of humeral osteonecrosis [9–11, 13, 33]. The evolution has been shown to be variable and unpredictable both clinically and radiologically. Worsening seems to be the rule but is not always so, especially in the early stages. Cruess isolated a group who evolved towards a clinical and radiological stabilisation (minimally deformed head plus osteosclerosis). All the authors are in agreement in stating that stages IV and V are poorly tolerated and require surgical treatment [7, 9–11]. The effect of age of onset has not, however, been clarified.

The particular form with massive collapse occurring in elderly females leads to discussion about the border lines between humeral osteonecrosis and the various pictures of destructive arthropathies described by De Seze (senile haemorrhagic shoulder) [35], Neer (cuff tear arthropathy) [28], MacCarthy (Milwaukee shoulder) [24] and Lequesne (rapid destructive arthropathy) [23]. All these clinical scenarios concern elderly and particularly, female patients. The onset is severe and combines pain with marked functional impairment. The articular destruction is rapid and is part of the definition of Lequesne's rapidly destructive arthropathy. The cuff tear is a constant finding and a haemorrhagic extravasation is often found on aspiration. The common element in all these destructive arthropathies is osteolysis.

However, the clinico-radiological form which we described differs from these others on several points: the haemorrhagic extravasation was not mentioned in either the evolution or the surgical intervention; in 5 of our 9 cases, the rotator cuff was intact, and finally and most importantly, in our 9 cases we found an area of intact humeral head in contact with the greater tuberosity as in all the classical humeral osteonecrosis cases. Everything occurs as if the necrosis appears in the usual place in the humeral head but, for an unknown reason rapidly extends throughout the head without affecting the area in contact with the greater tuberosity. Massive necrosis with major collapse releases bony material into the joint triggering an inflammatory reaction and causing real turmoil in the joint giving no chance for any reparation. Damage to the glenoid seems to be mechanical and secondary to the disappearance of the humeral head. Careful examination of the published pictures have shown that a certain number of cases labelled under various headings, bear a striking resemblance to osteonecrosis with massive collapse [3, 6, 23, 24, 28, 35]. Finally, advanced age does not mean that the patient has this form with massive collapse because we have found patients over 70 presenting with classical osteonecrosis.

Postradiotherapy cases form a particular group. They are not a true avascular necrosis. The lesion secondary to radiation involves all the humeral head (osteoporosis) and histology confirms bony necrosis without any signs of reparation. Loss of joint space bears witness to the cartilage damage. Neer mentions the technical problems, essentially due to the soft tissues, in these cases [29].

Conclusion

Avascular necrosis of the humeral head is the second most common site and its characteristics are the same as those described for the hip. The clinical picture is less specific in comparison to the radiographic presentation and clinico-radiographic agreement is not the rule. The evolution is unpredictable and probably depends on age, aetiology and mechanical factors.

We have described a particular form with massive collapse occurring in the elderly. Within the group of destructive shoulder arthropathies the characteristic radiographic appearance shows this form to be related to the necroses.

References

1. Anderson JM, Helm R (1982) Multiple joint osteonecrosis following short-term steroid therapy. J Bone Joint Surg Am 64:139–141
2. Arlet J, Ficat P (1968) Diagnostic de l'ostéo-nécrose fémoro-capitale primitive au stade I (stade pré-radiologique) Rev Chir Orthop 54:637–648
3. Bardin T, Fritz P (1992) Arthropathies destructrices de l'épaule. Ann Radiol 35:184–187
4. Basset LW, Gold RH, Reicher M, Bennet LR, Tooke SM (1987) Magnetic resonance imaging in the early diagnosis of ischemic necrosis of the femoral head. Clin Orthop 214:237–248
5. Benoit J, Got C, Hardy P, Videcoq P (1989) L'ostéonécrose de la tête fémorale chez le transplanté rénal. Rev Chir Orthop 75:216–227
6. Campion GV, MacCrae F, Alawan W, Wat I, Bradfield J, Dieppe P (1986) A Idiopathic destructive arthritis of the shoulder. J Bone Joint Surg Am 68:1913–1919
7. Cofield RH (1994) Osteonecrosis. In: Friedman RJ (ed) Arthroplasty of the shoulder. Thieme Medical, New York, pp 170
8. Constant CR, Murley AH (1987) A clinical method of functional assessment of the Shoulder. Clin Orthop 214:160–164
9. Cruess RL (1986) Osteonecrosis of bone: current concepts as to etiology and pathogenesis. Clin Orthop 208:30–39
10. Cruess RL (1985) Corticosteroid-induced osteonecrosis of the humeral head. Orthop Clin of North Am 4:789–796
11. Cruess RL (1976) Steroid-induced avascular necrosis of the head of the humerus. J Bone Joint Surg Br 58:313–317
12. David HG, Bridgman SA, Davies SC, Hine AL, Emery RJ (1993) The shoulder in sickle cell disease. J Bone Joint Surg Br 75:538–545
13. Dines DM, Warren RF, Pagnani MJ, Linsalata JC (1994) Osteonecrosis of the proximal humerus: natural history, long term natural history, long term follow-up and radiographic predictors of outcome. European Society for Surgery of the Soulder and the Elbow. 16–18 June, Barcelona
14. Fisher DE, Bickel WH (1971) Corticosteroid-induced avascular necrosis. A clinical study of 77 patients. J Bone Joint Surg Am 53:859–873
15. Gazielly F, Thomas T, Bruyere G, Pasquier B, Grossetete JL (1995) Résultats de l'arthroplastie prothétique type Neer dans les traitements de l'ostéonécrose de la tête humérale. Rev Chir Orthop 81 [Suppl II]:99–103
16. Gerber C, Schneeberger AG, Vinh TS (1990) The arterial vascularization of the humeral head. J Bone Joint Surg 72A 72:1486–1494
17. Gregg PJ, Stothard J, Walder DN (1979) Regional distribution of circulating microspheres in the rabbit femur. J Bone Joint Surg Br 61:381
18. Hayes JM (1989) Arthroscopic treatment of steroid-induced osteonecrosis of the humeral head. Arthroscopy 5:218–221
19. Hernigou P (1995) Ostéonécrose des épiphyses de l'adulte. In: Encycl. Méd. Chir., Appareil locomoteur, 14028-A-10, Editions Techniques, Paris, p 12
20. Hopson CN, Siverhus SW (1988) Ischemic necrosis of the femoral head. J Bone Joint Surg Am 70:1048–1051
21. Hungerford DS, Lennox DW (1985) The importance of increased intraosseous pressure in the development of osteonecrosis of the femoral head: implications for treatment. Orthop Clin North Am 16:635–654
22. Laroche M, Arlet J, Mazières B (1990) Osteonecrosis of the femoral and humeral heads after intraarticular corticosteroid injections. J Rheumatol 17:549–551
23. Lequesne M, Fallut M, Coulomb R, Magnet JL, Strauss J (1982) L'arthropathie destructrice rapide de l'épaule. Rev Rhumatisme 49:427–437
24. MacCarthy DJ, Halverson PB, Carrera GF, Brewer BJ, Kozin F (1981) Milwaukee shoulder: association of microspheroids containing hydroxyapatite crystals, active collagenase and neutral protease with rotator cuff defects. A clinical aspect. Arthritis Rheum 24:464–473
25. Marcus ND, Enneking WF, Massam RA (1973) The silent hip in idiopathic aseptic necrosis. J Bone Joint Surg Am 55:1351

26. Merle D'Aubigné R (1965) Idiopathic necrosis of the femoral head in adults. J Bone Joint Surg Br 47:612–633
27. Milner PF, Krauss AP, Sebes JI, Sleeper LA, Dukes KA, Emery SH, Bellevue R, Koshy M, Moohr JW, Smith J (1993) Osteonecrosis of the humeral head in sickle cell disease. Clin Orthop 289:136–143
28. Neer CS, Craig EV, Fukuda H (1983) Cuff tear arthropathy. J Bone Joint Surg Am 65:1232–1244
29. Neer CS (1990) Shoulder reconstruction. Saunders, Philadelphia
30. O'Brien PH, Mack GR (1992) Multifocal osteonecrosis after short-term. High-dose corticosteroid therapy. Clin Orthop 279:176–179
31. Rosenberg F, Kahn MF, Bensasson M, Dorfmann H, de Seze S (1972) L'ostéonécrose aseptique de la tête humérale. Rev Rhum 39:407–416
32. Ruffie R, Fournie A, Ayrolles C, Cuq P (1962) Résultats de la phlébographie pertrochanterienne dans les ostéonécroses primitives de la tête fémorale chez l'adulte. Rev Rhum 29:551
33. Rutherford CS, Cofield RJ (1987) Osteonecrosis of the shoulder. Orthop Trans 11:239
34. Saito S, Inoue A, Ono K (1987) Intramedullary haemorrhage as a possible cause of avascular necrosis of the femoral head. J Bone Joint Surg Br 69:346–351
35. Seze de S, Hubault A, Rampon S (1967) L'épaule sénile hémorragique. In: L'Actualité Rhumatologique. Expansion Scientifique (eds), Paris, p 107
36. Taylor LJ (1984) Multifocal avascular necrosis after short-term high-dose steroid therapy. A report of three cases. J Bone Joint Surg Br 66:431–433
37. Urquhart MW, Mont MA, Maar DC, Lennox DW, Krackow KA, Hungerford DS (1992) Results of core decompression for avascular necrosis of the humeral head. Orthop Trans 16:780

Results of Shoulder Arthroplasty for Atraumatic Avascular Necrosis of the Humeral Head

M. Basso and L. Nové-Josserand

Summary

Thirty-three shoulders (30 patients) with atraumatic avascular necrosis, operated on with an Aequalis shoulder arthroplasty between 1991 and 1994, were reviewed with an average follow-up of 18 months (minimum 12 months). There were 23 women and 7 men; at the time of surgery the average age was 57 years (35–81 years). Objectively the results were good with an average 40 point increase in the absolute Constant score (preoperative average 27 points, postoperative 67 points). The best results were observed in types II–IV necrosis (21 cases) with an absolute Constant score of 71 points (±12). In type V necrosis (12 cases) the results were less favourable, with an absolute Constant score of 62 points (±16). Total arthroplasty (8 cases) yielded slightly better results for pain improvement and for mobility than hemi-arthoplasty (4 cases) in these shoulders with glenoid erosion. Two sub-groups were identified: (a) radiation necrosis (2 cases), where the results were poor with persistent pain and reduced mobility; (b) complete humeral head necrosis in elderly women (4 cases), where the prosthesis resulted in a pain-free shoulder in all cases although the mobility remained limited especially where there was a cuff tear.

Introduction

A review of the literature reveals very few series specifically analysing the results of shoulder arthroplasty for atraumatic avascular osteonecrosis. This is presumably because of the small numbers performed for this etiology [7, 10, 12, 13, 15, 31, 37]. In a 1994 review Cofield [7] found that only 71 of 1250 arthroplasties had been carried out for osteonecrosis (5 %). Most of the series consisted of only a few cases of osteonecrosis, and these were not analysed separately: 3 in the 46 cases reported by Amstutz [38], 5 for Bade [39], 6 for Boyd [40] and 5 for Warren [41]. When the results for osteonecrosis are analysed separately, Cofield reported these as being good with 90 % having pain relief and achieving 75 % of the normal range of movement.

Nové-Josserand et al. (this volume) shown that there are many different clinical presentations and types of articular damage occurring in the osteonecrosis group. We report the results of 33 shoulders, which received either hemi or total arthroplasties, using these different criteria. Posttraumatic osteonecrosis was excluded from the present series.

Materials and Methods

Between 1990 and 1994, 33 shoulders in 30 patients with atraumatic avascular osteonecrosis of the upper humerus were operated on in the 12 centres participating in this study. There were 23 women and 7 men and 3 bilateral cases. The mean age at surgery was 57 years (35–81) and the average follow-up was 18 months (12–34). There was an equal division between sides (17 of 33 were right sided) and dominance (19 of the 33 were the dominant side).

The necrosis was staged according to the Cruess modification [9] of the Arlet and Ficat [2] classification, and there were 2 stage II, 1 stage III, 18 stage IV and 12 stage V cases. There were 22 hemi- and 11 total shoulder arthroplasties. In six cases there was a full-thickness cuff tear, which was repaired in three. The results were evaluated pre- and postoperatively using the Constant system [8].

Results

Overall Results

For the 33 shoulders the mean postoperative absolute Constant score was 67 points (85 % when adjusted for age and sex). This was an increase of 40 points and 51 % on the preoperative scores. Considering the four components of the Constant system individually, there was virtually always a reduction in pain, and the functional improvement was good reaching three-quarters of normal. However, the improvement in force was mediocre, being only one-third of normal (Table 1). Active anterior elevation was 134° on average and external rotation elbow at the side was 36°, which were increases of 51° and 30° on the respective preoperative scores (Table 2).

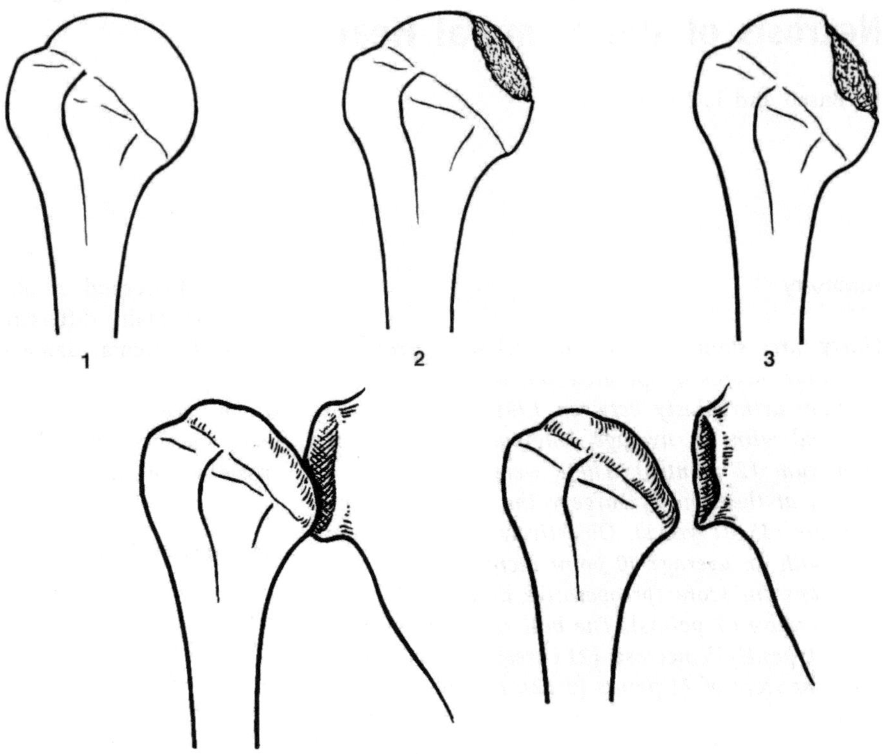

Fig. 1. Staging of humeral head necrosis: *Stage 1,* normal X-rays but marrow changes visible only on MRI; *stage 2,* sclerosis under the articular surface visible on plain X-rays; *stage 3,* subchondral fracture (crescent sign); *stage 4,* collapse of the humeral head articular surface; *stage 5,* secondary osteoarthritis with glenoid erosion

Table 1. Detailed Constant score for shoulder replacement in osteonecrosis

Constant score	Preoperative		Postoperative
Pain (1–15)	3.6±2.5	→	13±2.4
Activity (1–20)	7±2.3	→	16±3
Mobility (1–40)	13±6	→	30±7
Strength (1–25)	3.2±2.5	→	8±4.5
Absolute Constant score	27±11	→	67±14
Normalised Constant score (%)	34±14	→	85±15

Table 2. Results on mobility

Mobility	Preoperative		Postoperative
Passive anterior elevation	107°±41°	→	146°±26°
Active anterior elevation	83°±44°	→	134°±28°
Active external rotation	6°±21°	→	36°±23°
Passive external rotation	8°±19°	→	43°±21°

Results Depending on the State of the Glenoid

Did the state of the glenoid (uninvolved until stage V) have an effect on the results? The overall result was slightly less good in the stage V cases with preoperative Constant scores of 62 points (80 %) as compared with 71 points (89 %) for stages II–IV (Table 3). Active anterior elevation and external rotation were both reduced from 139° and 39° for the early stages as compared to 124° and 31° in stage V. However, the initial preoperative Constant scores were lower in stage V though they increased by virtually the same amount as in the other groups. Overall, the difference between stage V cases and the less severe stages becomes evident postoperatively.

Table 3. Functional Results correlated to the stage of necrosis

	AVN stages III, IV (*n*=21)			AVN stage V (*n*=12)		
Functional results	Preop.		Postop.	Preop.		Postop.
Active anterior elevation	91°±40°	→	139°±25°	67°±49°	→	124°±31°
Active external rotation	9°±24°	→	39°±23°	0°±14°	→	31°±21°
Absolute Constant score	31±10	→	71±12	19±10	→	62±16
Normalised Constant score (%)	39±12	→	89±15	24±12	→	80±15

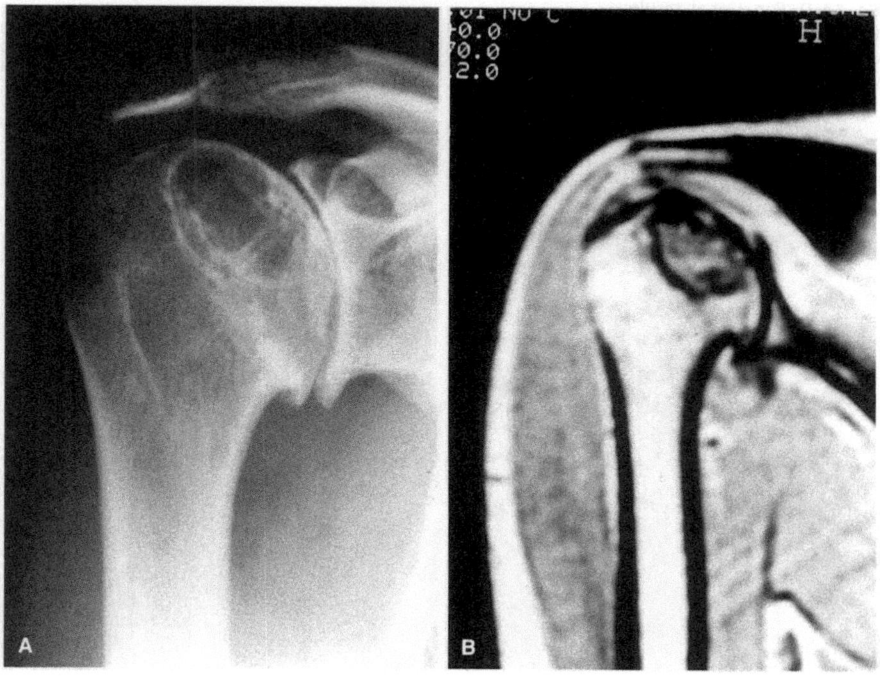

Fig. 2 A,B. Stage V atraumatic avascular necrosis as seen on. **A** AP-view. **B** MRI. (Notice the changes in the bone marrow)

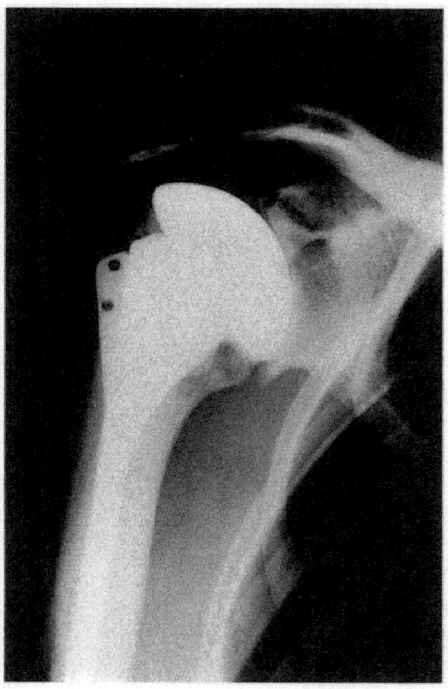

Fig. 3. Shoulder reconstruction with a hemi-arthroplasty was preferred in this young woman

Table 4. Effect of a glenoid prosthesis in stage V disease

Functional results in stage V	With glenoid (n=8)	Without glenoid (n=4)
Absolute Constant score	62±18	61±12
Normalised Constant score (%)	80±17	80±13
Active anterior elevation		
Preoperative	47°±36°	93°±60°
Postoperative	129°±35°	115°±24°
Active external rotation		
Preoperative	1.5°±15°	2.5°±17°
Postoperative	37°±19°	20°±23°

Effect of a Glenoid Prosthesis in Stage V Disease

The overall Constant score at review was identical with (62 points and 80%) and without a glenoid (61 points and 80%; Table 4). However, the implantation of a glenoid did have a beneficial effect in recovery of active mobility as those who had total arthroplasty achieved greater improvement in anterior elevation (129° vs. 115°) and external rotation (37° vs. 20°) although their preoperative elevation was considerably less (47° al 93°).

Results Depending on the State of The Cuff

There were six cases who presented with a cuff tear before their arthroplasty, and this group had a slightly poorer average Constant score (Table 5). Repairing the tear seemed to be beneficial because the three in whom the cuff was fixed achieved scores equal to the overall average (67 points) and much better than those in whom the tear was not repaired (51 points). However, it must be a repairable cuff-tear.

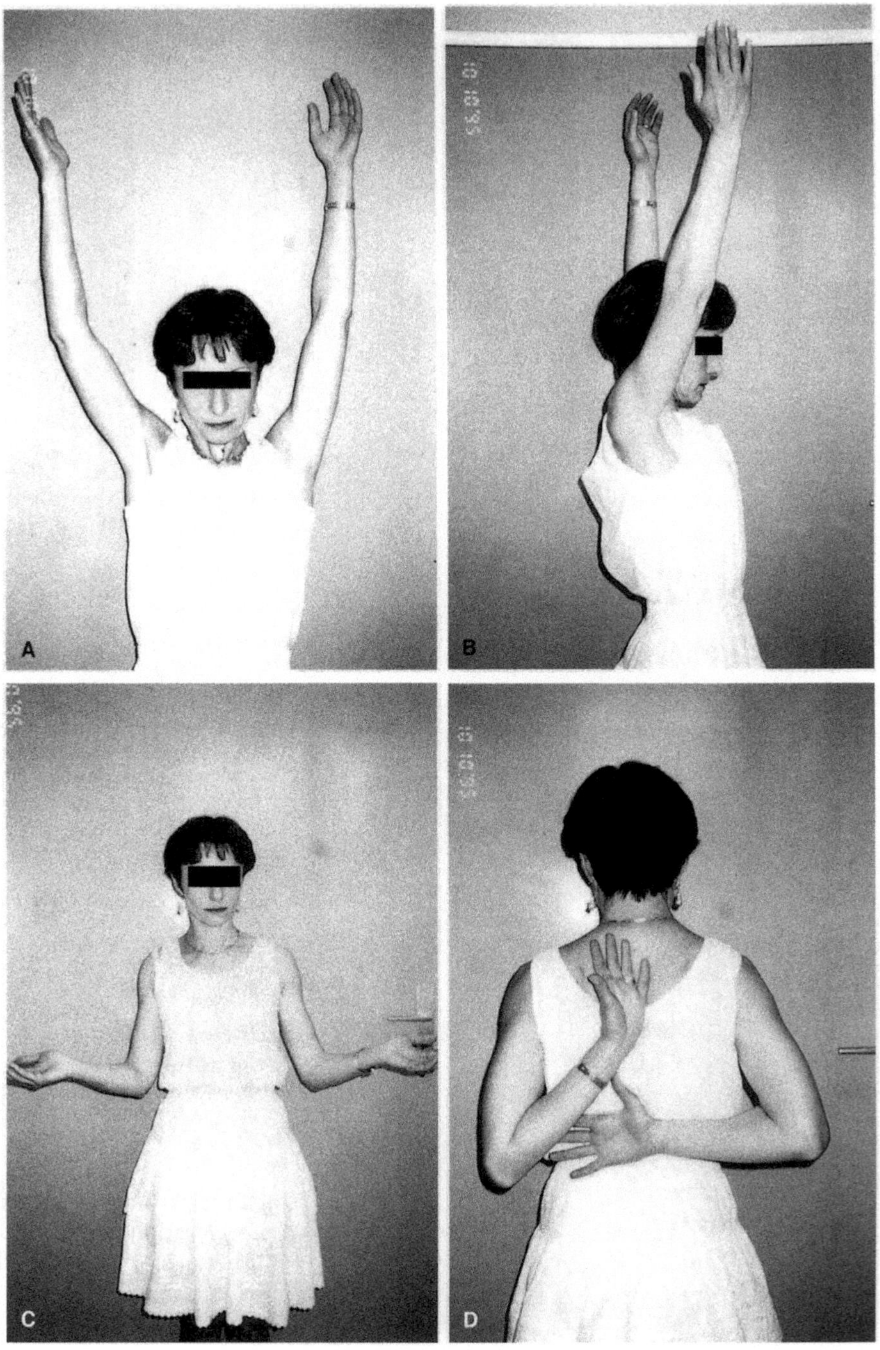

Fig. 4 A–D. Functional results with recovery of full activity at three years follow-up. (Same patient as in Figs. 2, 3)

Table 5. Results correlated with the state of the rotator cuff

Results		With cuff tear (n=6)	
	Without cuff tear (n=33)	Repaired (n=3)	Unrepaired (n=3)
Absolute Constant score	67±14	67	51
Normalised Constant score (%)	85±15	88	68

Results in the Osteonecrosis Encountered in the Elderly Females

This group was defined by Nové-Josserand (see pp 243 ff, this volume) as a particular group of necrosis with massive head collapse occurring in women aged over 70 years (70–90). There were four patients over 70 years old who made up this group of whom two had a hemi- and two a total shoulder arthroplasty. In two patients there was a massive cuff tear while the other two had intact cuffs. The average postoperative score of 56 points (84 %) in this group was only slightly inferior to the overall score despite the preoperative scores being considerably lower (13 and 20 % as compared to 27 and 34 %). Not surprisingly, the results were less good in the two cases with cuff tears, especially with regards to mobility which remained average.

Results Encountered in the Radionecrosis

It should be emphasised that two patients in the series presented with radionecrosis and in both cases the improvement in pain was disappointing, achieving only 8 out of 15 points, even though a reduction in pain is usually the first benefit in prosthetic surgery.

Subjective Results

The subjective results were determined by asking the patients if they were very satisfied, satisfied, disappointed or unhappy with the result of their surgery. The correlation with the Constant score is shown in Table 6.

Table 6. Subjective results correlated with the Constant score

Subjective results	*n*	Absolute Constant score	Normalised score (%)
Very satisfied	26	71	89
Satisfied	5	58	79
Disappointed	2	39	55
Unhappy	0	–	–

There were two disappointing results which occurred in a patient with radionecrosis following treatment for breast cancer who had a poor functional score and persistent pain and in a patient with poor postoperative mobility with fixed internal rotation after surgery for stage IV necrosis with a background of a CVA and complex neurological problems.

Professional Activity

Only eight of the patients aged less than 60 were working preoperatively and of these, five continued with the same job and three found other work. Four were only affected in the one shoulder while the other four had at least one other joint involved. Five other patients aged under 60 were on invalidity of whom 4 had bilateral shoulder and hip necrosis and the fifth was on renal dialysis.

Discussion

Taking into account the limitations imposed, it is possible to compare our results with those in the rare publications in the literature [7, 13, 15, 29, 33]. At the symposium organized by the French Orthopaedic and Traumatology Surgery Society (SOFCOT) in 1994 Gazielly et al. [15] reported a multicentre study of 23 idiopathic osteonecrosis cases operated on using a Neer II prosthesis, with a minimum 2-year follow-up and using the Constant scoring system. Cofield [17] reviewed 17 cases of arthroplasty for necrosis with over 4 years follow-up and reported 17 excellent or good results and excellent mobility (average abduction of 161° for the hemi-arthroplasties and 150° for the total arthroplasties, and 77° and 67° of external rotation, respectively). The SOFCOT series and ours were evaluated using the same scoring system allowing for easy comparison. The figures are shown in Table 7 and demonstrate that the initial scores were almost identical. Our postoperative scores were a little better with a 6-point and 10 % increase in the Constant scores.

Table 7. Comparative results of the SOFCOT and Aequalis series

Series	Absolute Constant score			Normalised Constant score (%)		
	Preop.	Postop.	Gain	Preop.	Postop.	Gain
SOFCOT (1994)	24	58	+34	30	71	+41
Aequalis (1996)	27	67	+40	34	85	+51

Conclusion

Our study demonstrates, that shoulder arthroplasty gives satisfactory results in idiopathic osteonecrosis of the proximal humerus. With regard to pain relief the results are excellent, and they are good for mobility with 75 % of the normal range being achieved. However, the results for improvement in force are mediocre reaching only one-third of normal.

It seems quite remarkable that each of the subgroups improved by about the same 40 points or 50 % on the Constant system, as did the overall group. The final score is therefore correlated to the starting point. The elderly female group actually improved from a very low starting point a little more than the average whereas the patients with a cuff tear achieved a slightly lower result.

References

1. Anderson JM, Helm R (1982) Multiple joint osteonecrosis following short-term steroid therapy. J Bone Joint Surg Am 64:139–141
2. Arlet J, Ficat P (1968) Diagnostic de l'ostéo-nécrose fémoro-capitale primitive au stade I (stade pré-radiologique). Rev Chir Orthop 54:637–648
3. Bardin T, Fritz P (1992) Arthropathies destructrices de l'épaule. Ann Radiol 35:184–187
4. Basset LW, Gold RH, Reicher M, Bennet LR, Tooke SM (1987) Magnetic resonance imaging in the early diagnosis of ischemic necrosis of the femoral head. Clin Orthop 214:237–248
5. Benoit J, Got C, Hardy P, Videcoq P (1989) L'ostéonécrose de la tête fémorale chez le transplanté rénal. Rev Chir Orthop 75:216–227
6. Campion GV, MacCrae F, Alawan W, Wat I, Bradfield J, Dieppe PA (1986) Idiopathic destructive arthritis of the shoulder. J Bone Joint Surg Am 68:1913–1919
7. Cofield RH (1994) Osteonecrosis. In: Friedman RJ (ed) Arthroplasty of the shoulder. Thieme, Stuttgart, pp 170
8. Constant CR, Murley AH (1987) A clinical method of functional assessment of the Shoulder. Clin Orthop 214:160–164
9. Cruess RL (1986) Osteonecrosis of bone: current concepts as to etiology and pathogenesis. Clin Orthop 208:30–39
10. Cruess RL (1985) Corticosteroid-induced osteonecrosis of the humeral head. Orthop Clin North Am 4:789–796
11. Cruess RL (1976) Steroid-induced avascular necrosis of the head of the humerus. J Bone Joint Surg Br 58:313–317
12. David HG, Bridgman SA, Davies SC, Hine AL, Emery RJ (1993) The shoulder in sickle cell disease. J Bone Joint Surg Br 75:538–545
13. Dines DM, Warren RF, Pagnani MJ, Linsalata JC (1994) Osteonecrosis of the proximal humerus: natural history, long term natural history, long term follow-up and radiographic predictors of outcome. Presented at the European Society for Surgery of the Soulder and the Elbow. 16–18 June, Barcelona
14. Fisher DE, Bickel WH (1971) Corticosteroid-induced avascular necrosis. A clinical study of 77 patients. J Bone Joint Surg Am 53:859–873
15. Gazielly F, Thomas T, Bruyere G, Pasquier B, Grossetete JL (1995) Résultats de l'arthroplastie prothétique type Neer dans les traitements de l'ostéonécrose de la tête humérale. Rev Chir Orthop 81 [Suppl II]:99–103
16. Gerber C, Schneeberger AG, Vinh TS (1990) The arterial vascularization of the humeral head. J Bone Joint Surg Am 72:1486–1494
17. Gregg PJ, Stothard J, Walder DN (1979) Regional distribution of circulating microspheres in the rabbit femur. J Bone Joint Surg Br 61:381
18. Hayes JM (1989) Arthroscopic treatment of steroid-induced osteonecrosis of the humeral head. Arthroscopy 5:218–221
19. Hernigou P (1995) Ostéonécrose des épiphyses de l'adulte. In: Encycl Méd Chir Appareil locomoteur. Techniques, Paris 14028-A-10:12
20. Hopson CN, Siverhus SW (1988) Ischemic necrosis of the femoral head. J Bone Joint Surg Am 70:1048–1051
21. Hungerford DS, Lennox DW (1985) The importance of increased intraosseous pressure in the development of osteonecrosis of the femoral head: implications for treatment. Orthop Clin North Am 16:635–654
22. Laroche M, Arlet J, Mazières B (1990) Osteonecrosis of the femoral and humeral heads after intraarticular corticosteroid injections. J Rheumatol 17:549–551
23. Lequesne M, Fallut M, Coulomb R, Magnet JL, Strauss J (1982) L'arthropathie destructrice rapide de l'épaule. Rev Rhumatisme 49:427–437
24. MacCarthy DJ, Halverson PB, Carrera GF, Brewer BJ, Kozin F (1981) Milwaukee shoulder: association of microspheroids containing hydroxyapatite crystals, active collagenase and neutral protease with rotator cuff defects. A clinical aspects. Arthritis Rheum 24:464–473
25. Marcus ND, Enneking WF, Massam RA (1973) The silent hip in idiopathic aseptic necrosis. J Bone Joint Surg Am 55:1351
26. Merle D'Aubigné R (1965) Idiopathic necrosis of the femoral head in adults. J Bone Joint Surg Br 47:612–633
27. Milner PF, Krauss AP, Sebes JI, Sleeper LA, Dukes KA, Emery SH, Bellevue R, Koshy M, Moohr JW, Smith J (1993) Osteonecrosis of the humeral head in sickle cell disease. Clin Orthop 289:136–143
28. Neer CS, Craig EV, Fukuda H (1983) Cuff tear arthropathy. J Bone Joint Surg Am 65:1232–1244
29. Neer CS (1990) Shoulder reconstruction. Saunders, Philadelphia
30. O'Brien TH, Mack GR (1992) Multifocal osteonecrosis after short-term. High-dose corticosteroid therapy. Clin Orthop 279:176–179
31. Rosenberg F, Kahn MF, Bensasson M, Dorfmann H, de Seze S (1972) L'ostéonécrose aseptique de la tête humérale. Rev Rhum 39:407–416
32. Ruffie R, Fournie A, Ayrolles C, Cuq P (1962) Résultats de la phlébographie pertrochanterienne dans les ostéonécroses primitives de la tête fémorale chez l'adulte. Rev Rhum 29:551
33. Rutherford CS, Cofield RJ (1987) Osteonecrosis of the shoulder. Orthop Trans 11:239

34. Saito S, Inoue A, Ono K (1987) Intramedullary haemorrhage as a possible cause of avascular necrosis of the femoral head. J Bone Joint Surg Br 69:346–351
35. Seze de S, Hubault A, Rampon S (1967) L'épaule sénile hémorragique. In: L'Actualité rhumatologique. Expansion Scientifique (eds), Paris, p 107
36. Taylor LJ (1984) Multifocal avascular necrosis after short-term high-dose steroid therapy. A report of three cases. J Bone Joint Surg Br 66:431–433
37. Urquhart MW, Mont MA, Maar DC, Lennox DW, Krackow KA, Hungerford DS (1992) Results of core decompression for avascular necrosis of the humeral head. Orthop Trans 16:780
38. Amstutz HC, Thomas BJ, Kabo N, Dinnan RW, Dorey F (1988) The DANA total shoulder arthroplasty. J Bone Joint Surg Am 70:1174–1182
39. Bade HA III., Warren RF, Ranawat CS, Inglis AE (1984) Long term results of Neer total shoulder replacement. In: Bateman JE, Welsh RP (eds), Surgery of the shoulder, Philadelphia, Be. Decker, p 294–302
40. Boyd AD, Thomas WA, Scott RD, Sledge CB, Thornhill TS (1990) Total shoulder arthroplasty versus hemiarthroplasty. J Arthroplasty 5:329–336
41. Warren RF, Ranawat CS, Inglis AE (1988) Total shoulder replacement. Indications and results of the Neer non-constrained prosthesis. Sem Arhtritis Rheum 17:232–245

Section X:

Osteoarthritis with Massive Cuff-Tear

Osteoarthritis with Massive Rotator Cuff-Tear: The Limitation of its Current Definitions

L. Favard, S. Lautmann, and P. Clement

Summary

Forty-six shoulders were analysed to define characteristic elements in order to better understand osteoarthritis with massive cuff-tear. The population presenting with this pathology is usually elderly (74 years) and female (80 %). The population can be subdivided into three groups: Group 1 (23 cases) have a progressive evolution of the shoulder towards acetabulisation. This consists of long-standing, evolving cuff-tears. This type corresponds to Neer's 'cuff-tear arthropathy'. Group 2 (9 cases) is distinctive and somewhat different from that of destructive arthropathies. This disorder corresponds to an osteoarthritis because of the centralized narrowing of the gleno-humeral joint. These arthropathies are particular in presenting with an associated unrepairable cuff-tear. In group 3 (14 cases) lysis and bone destruction are the dominant elements. In contrast to group 1, there are no signs of this having evolved from an old cuff-tear, and the cuff-tear is probably contemporary to, or has shortly preceded, the bony destruction. This group corresponds to rheumatological shoulders (senile haemorrhagic shoulder, Milwaukee shoulder, rapidly destructive arthropathy).

Introduction

In 1995 during the SOFCOT symposium [2] on shoulder prostheses, cuff-tear arthritis was defined as the association of a large rotator cuff-tear, upward migration of the humeral head, subacromial impingement and gleno-humeral cartilage wear. The same criterias are used in this study but with the added provision that not all the criterias need be present. In fact, any bony-cartilaginous damage combined with an unrepairable cuff-tear has been classified as an osteoarthritis with massive cuff-tear. It seemed interesting to us to analyse this somewhat disparate group of patients with the goal of trying to define any characterising elements in order to better treat patients and perhaps better understand osteoarthritis with massive cuff-tear.

Materials and Methods

The Aequalis prosthesis was used to treat 23 shoulders with osteoarthritis with massive cuff-tear, and the results are analysed in detail by Postel et al. ("Osteoarthritis with Massive Cuff-Tear: Results of an Unconstrained Shoulder Arthroplasty", this volume). However, in this study number of cases was insufficient to provide an precise idea of this pathology and we therefore added 23 cases of osteoarthritis with massive cuff-tear operated on by different surgeons using different prostheses. The common factor was that they were all in sufficient pain to justify this surgical intervention.

We analysed 46 shoulders. There were 9 men and 37 women. The right side was involved in 42 cases and the dominant side in 41 (90 %). The average age was 74.3 years (50–85). The controlateral shoulder, although much less painful, was damaged in 60 %.

The radiographs were analysed to assess the site and the degree of gleno-humeral joint wear, the subacromial height, changes in the shape of the head and the acromion and the presence of any bony lysis.

Results

All the shoulders had a massive cuff-tear that was confirmed intra-operatively. Gleno-humeral joint space narrowing was present and complete in 77 % of the patients, incomplete in 17 % and absent in 6 % (3 cases). It occurred at the upper part of the joint line in 73 %. Glenoid wear extended to the foot of the coracoid or further in 41 %. The average acromio-humeral joint space was 1.9 mm (0–7 mm). The humeral head was rounded-off with erosion of the tuberosities in 43 % and with signs of lysis in 41 %. The acromion had its shape altered by the imprint of the humeral head in 56 % and displayed lysis in 19 %. Regrouping these criteria yielded the following three groups:

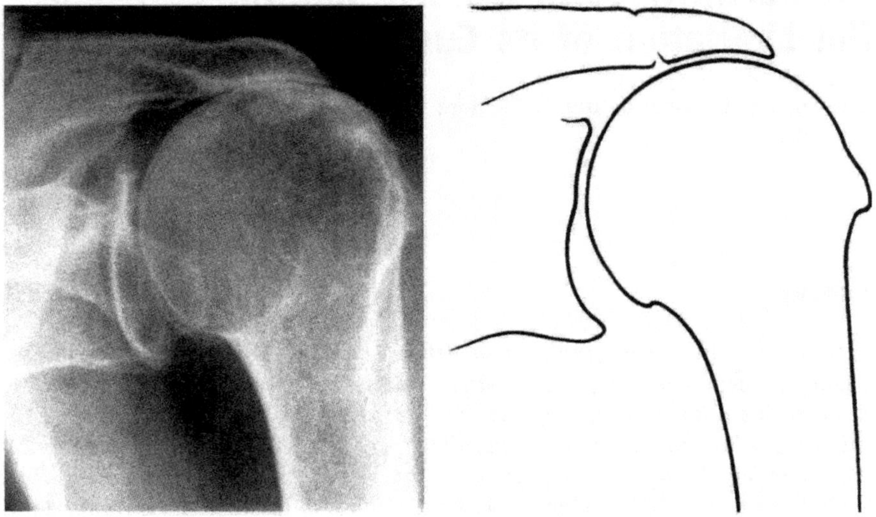

Fig. 1. Group 1. Superior gleno-humeral wear. Upward migration of the humeral head. Acromion modification with inferior concavity wear

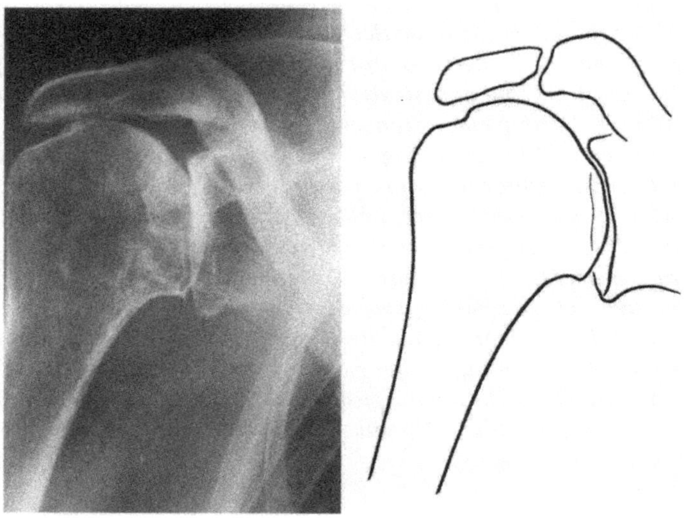

Fig. 2. Group 2. Central narrowing of the gleno-humeral joint. Little alteration in the shape of the acromion without humeral head imprint

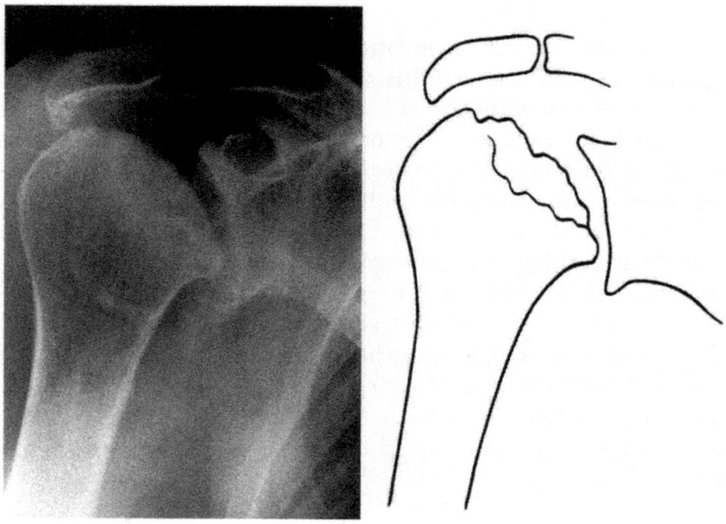

Fig. 3. Group 3. Lysis of either the humeral head or the acromion

Group 1 (Fig. 1). This included 23 cases (51%), or about half the shoulders studied. It is characterised by upward migration of the humeral head, superior gleno-humeral joint space narrowing, an acromion changed in shape due to the imprint of the humeral head and subacromial arthritis. Within this group 12 cases also presented with signs which precede the appearance of lysis or bony destruction.

Group 2 (Fig. 2). There were 9 cases (19%) in this group which is characterised by central gleno-humeral joint space narrowing and with little alteration in the shape of the acromion which does not have a humeral head imprint.

Group 3 (Fig. 3). This group contained 14 cases (30%) and is characterised by signs of bony destruction in the form of lysis of either the head or the acromion. The bony elements not affected by the lysis do not undergo any modification in their shape, for example, the greater tuberosity is not eroded and the acromion does not have a humeral head imprint. Gleno-humeral joint space narrowing is either minimal or non-existent.

There was no age difference between the three groups. The acromio-humeral joint space narrowing was significantly greater ($P<0.01$) in group 1 (1.3 mm on average) than in groups 3 (2.9 mm) and 2 (3.2 mm).

Discussion

The major criticism of this study is the lack of details of the natural history for every shoulder. Although they were all operated on, they did not all systematically undergo histological examination. Nonetheless, it does appear that cuff-tear arthritis is an arthropathy with a massive and generally unrepairable rotator cuff-tear. The population presenting with this pathology is usually elderly (74 years) and female (80%). The dominant side is virtually always damaged, but there is frequently contralateral involvement as well (60%). These findings agree with those recorded in the literature [3, 4, 8, 11].

The population can be subdivided into three groups (Figs. 1–3). The largest group is group 1 and it corresponds to the description given by Apoil [1] with progressive evolution of the shoulder towards acetabulisation. It consists of cuff-tears that evolve over long periods of time which explains how the bone slowly and progressively alters in shape as it adapts to the new position of the shoulder and results in a subacromial neo-articulation (Fig. 4). The wear is in the upper glenoid but can sometimes give the impression of an osteoarthritis. In fact, the wear is greater in the upper than in the lower pole of the glenoid. Thus the shoulder has the appearance of a hip (Fig. 1 and 4).

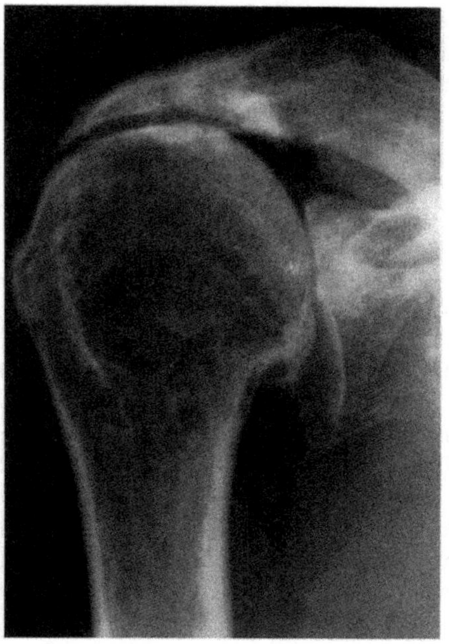

Fig. 4. Evolution of a long-tern rotator cuff-tear: hip appearance of the shoulder (group 1 shoulder with predominance of "mechanical factors")

Within this group some patients underwent a rapid and unfavourable course as evidenced on the radiographs which showed signs of destruction as concurrent phenomena became involved (Fig. 5).

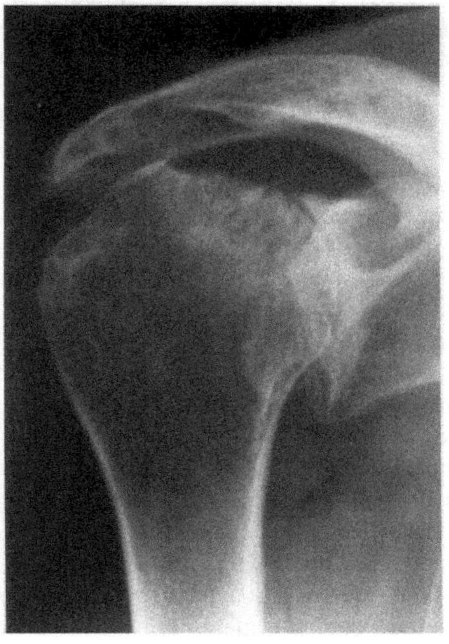

Fig. 5. Another exemple of group 1 shoulder but with begining of osteolysis

However, there are signs of prolonged damage before the acute episode occurred, such as superior glenoid wear and a subacromial headprint. Such bony changes are the result of old tears. On each occasion where a histological examination was carried out on these rapid decompensations occurring in old tears, a chondrocalcinosis was found. This natural history, and indeed this group in general, best approaches the description given by Neer [10] under the term "cuff-tear arthropathy".

From the clinical point of view this group poses the question of the cause of pain in a shoulder with a massive cuff tear which is usually well tolerated. In fact, the natural history of a cuff-tear can be simplified using the following model: when the rupture is new, the shoulder may be painful because of the subacromial impingement and the local inflammation. The acromio-humeral space is retained at this stage. Then it narrows progressively to become less than 7 mm, which represents a major tear, and the pain reappears when the tendon of the long head of biceps becomes the only element interposed between the head and the acromion. The space is now in approx. 5 mm [7]. Rupture, dislocation or division of the tendon of the long head of biceps results in a new painfree phase. The acromio-humeral space continues to narrow and a subacromial arthrosis then develops progressively. Usually the shoulder is pain free during this undoubtedly common stage [4, 6, 10].

At this point some shoulders become painful. If there are radiographic abnormalities such as lysis or changes in the bony structure, the shoulder falls into the group of destructive arthropathies, which explains the occurrence of pain. If there are no radiographic changes, perhaps some of the pain can be explained by the neo-articulation becoming arthritic in the same way a high congenital dislocation of the hip can start to cause discomfort when it is overused. Sometimes though the pain is due to the very earliest stages of a destructive arthropathy before the appearance of radiographic changes, which progress rapidly when they do appear. In every case the shoulders in group 1 are characterised by an old cuff-tear.

Group 2 is distinctive and somewhat different from the destructive arthropathies in general. It corresponds to "osteoarthritis" because of the overall gleno-humeral joint space narrowing. These arthropathies have the particularity of presenting with an associated unrepairable cuff tear, which has led surgeons to treat them as true cuff-tear arthritis. Moreover, these are definitely cuff-tear arthropathies because they combine gleno-humeral damage with an acromio-humeral distance of less than 7 mm. Nonetheless, it would appear that osteoarthritis is the primary etiology, and that the cuff-tear is a secondary occurrence.

The third group corresponds to "rheumatoid shoulders" with lysis and bone destruction being the dominant elements. In contrast to group 1 there are no signs of this having evolved from an old cuff-tear (Fig. 6). The cuff-tear must therefore be contemporary with or have occurred only shortly before the bony destructive phenomena, again in contrast to group 1. These shoulders correspond to the idiopathic destructive arthropathies [3], senile haemorrhagic shoulder [11], Milwaukee shoulder [9] and rapidly destructive arthropathy [8].

Finally, two theories have been proposed for the genesis of cuff-tear arthritis: one mechanical and one biochemical. Supporting the mechanical theory [4, 10], as defended by many orthopaedic surgeons and especially by Neer, are the facts that it affects the dominant side in elderly patients with worn glenoids, and that many of the shoulders have signs of a cuff-tear. This explains group 1. The biochemical theory [5] is favoured by the presence of crystals and enzymes in the synovial fluid, which might explain the bony destruction and cuff damage seen in the shoulders in group 3. The reality is very likely to be multifactorial: a background of an evolving rupture may favour the onset of biochemical phenomena and explain why some group 1 shoulders end up by developing into a destructive arthropathy.

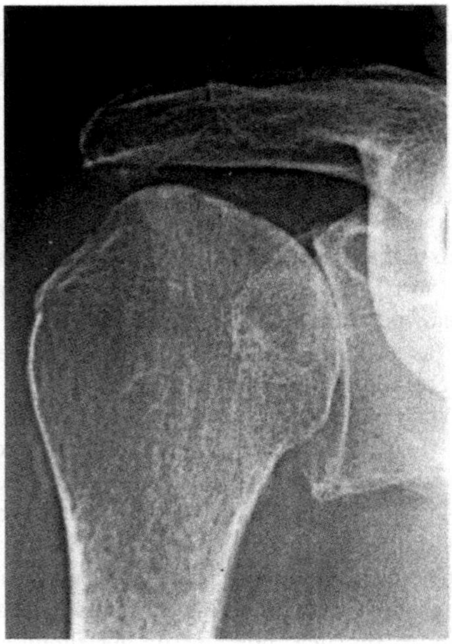

Fig. 6. Example of osteolysis without long-tern rotator cuff-tear. The acromion is not modified, and there is only little gleno-humeral narrowing (group 3 shoulder with predominance "biochemical factors")

On the other hand, the biochemical phenomena defended by some, and especially a microcrystaline origin for these arthropathies, have not been found by all authors [3], and the presence of crystals in the articular fluid does not mean that they are the cause of the joint destruction. They may just as easily be the consequence.

In conclusion, the group of cuff-tear arthritis crosses into the destructive arthropathy group. There is no unequivocal pathophysiological cause, and many questions still remain to be answered. Trying to answer these may help us to better treat these arthropathies.

References

1. Apoil A, Augereau B, Koechlin P (1988) Le vieillissement de l'épaule. Rev Chir Orthop 4:323–325
2. Apoil A, Candelier G, Collin M, Sautet A (1995) Prothèse de Neer dans l'omarthrose excentrée. Rev Chir Orthop [Suppl II]:115–119
3. Campion GV, McRae F, Alwan W, Watt I, Bradfield J, Dieppe PA (1988) Idiopathic destructive arthritis of the shoulder. Semin Arthritis Rheum 17:232–245
4. Caroit M, Labrousse C, Welfling J, Séze de M, Sèze de S (1964) Arthrose de l'épaule et détérioration de la coiffe des rotateurs. Rev Rhum 11:629–639
5. Dieppe PA, Doherty M, Macfarlane DG, Hutton CW, Watt I (1984) Apatite associated destructive arthritis. Br J Rheumatol 23:84–91
6. Edelson JG (1995) Patterns of degenerative change in the glenohumeral joint. J Bone Joint Surg Br 77:288–292
7. Hamada K, Fukuda H, Mikasa M, Kobayashi Y (1990) Roentgenographic findings in massive rotator cuff-tears. Clin Orthop 254:92–96
8. Lequesne M, Fallut M, Coulomb R, Magnet JL, Strauss J (1982) L'arthropathie destructrice rapide de l'épaule. Rev Rhum 49:427–437
9. MacCarthy DJ, Halverson PB, Carrera GF, Brewer BJ, Kozin F (1981) Milwaukee shoulder: association of microsheroids containing hydroxy apatite crystals, active collagenase and neutral protease with rotator cuff defects. I. Clinical aspects. Arthritis Rheum 24:464–473
10. Neer CS, Craig EV, Fukuda H (1983) Cuff-tear arthropathy. J Bone Joint Surg Am 65:1232–1244
11. Sèze de S, Hubault A, Rampon S (1967) L'épaule sénile hémorragique. In: L'Actualité rhumatologique. Expansion Scientifique Française (ed) Paris, pp 107–114

Rheumatological Management of Osteoarthritis with Massive Cuff-Tear

T. Schaeverbeke, J.C. Le Huec, and J. Dehais

Summary

Osteoarthritis with massive cuff-tear can be defined as the combination of glenohumeral osteoarthritis, characterised by narrowing of the gleno-humeral joint line with upward migration of the head, which can be demonstrated on an AP radiograph of the shoulder in neutral rotation by a reduction of the sub-acromial space to less than 7 mm. Osteoarthritis with massive cuff-tear usually presents with: inconsistent pain, severe episodes of shoulder stiffness affecting both active and passive movements and a functional disability, effecting all the activities of daily living. Various complications can occur with the evolution of a cuff-tear arthritis: a synovial fluid swelling, a spontaneous haemarthrosis (or "senile haemorrhagic shoulder"), the appearance of an acromiclavicular cyst. Medical treatment is purely symptomatic and varies depending on the clinical presentation. Pain can be treated by simple analgesics or by intra-articular steroid injections. Non-steroidal anti-inflammatory agents are not efficient here and are poorly tolerated in this elderly age group. A significant disability, secondary to joint stiffness, might lead to rehabilitation being suggested while realising that the chances of improving mobility are often small, and that any functional gain comes from adapting to the handicap.

Introduction

Massive rotator cuff-tears are often found in association with permanent proximal migration of the humeral head, and the resultant articular incongruency is responsible for the development of osteoarthritis. This relationship between massive cuff tears and osteoarthritis was well demonstrated by Caroit and De Seze in the early 1960s [1]. It is now established that can be the result of old massive cuff-tears. It is this particular form which is discussed in this chapter as it poses specific therapeutic problems.

Osteoarthritis with massive cuff-tear is defined as the combination of: (a) glenohumeral arthritis, characterised by loss of the joint space and the presence of osteophytes, usually at the inferior pole of the humeral head, with (b) superior migration of the humeral head, which is demonstrated on the antero-posterior radiograph in neutral rotation as an acromiohumeral distance of less than 7 mm.

The prevalence of cuff-tear arthritis is not accurately known but does appear to occur infrequently. Nove-Josserand systematically assessed 400 shoulders in a geriatric unit and found it in only 2% [2]. It is a pathology of those aged over 60.

Clinical Symptoms

Osteoarthritis with massive cuff-tear usually presents with:

- An insidious onset of pain which is episodic, of mechanical nature and rarely occurs at night. Various authors have reported the absence of any radiographic correlation such that significant changes on the radiographs may be associated with only minimal symptoms. The pain is sometimes due to the remaining intact long head of the biceps.
- Frequent episodes of severe shoulder stiffness which affects both the active and passive range of movements. The limitation is particularly apparent in anterior elevation and rotation. Moving the joint, including movements made with the elbow at the side, provokes painful "catching". This reduction in mobility seems to be as important as the loss of joint space and the sub-acromial impingement.
- An often significant functional impairment affecting all the activities of daily living such as personal hygiene, dressing, hair care, etc. This disability is linked to the loss of mobility and strength which occurs with a massive cuff tear.
- Atrophy of the supraspinatus and infraspinatus muscles which can be seen as a concavity in the supra and infraspinatus fossae.

Radiographic Appearance

The diagnosis of an osteoarthritis with massive cuff-tear can be made on the radiographs [3]. The classic signs of arthritis are seen as well as a reduction in the sub-acromial space (Fig. 1):

- Loss of the glenohumeral joint space is often moderate and occurs in the central section of the joint.
- Osteophytes: predominantly on the lower pole of the head. Although rarely seen on the glenoid side, they can equally well occur at its upper and lower poles.
- Sub-acromial sclerosis: on both sides of the joint.
- Sub-acromial space less than 7 mm.
- Acromio-tuberosity pseudo-arthropathy: this combines sclerotic osteophyte formation and erosion of the acromion and the tuberosities which can involve towards acetabulisation of the acromion.
- A humeral trough which is an erosion that can sometimes develop at the level of the humeral neck in some cases of osteoarthritis with proximal migration.

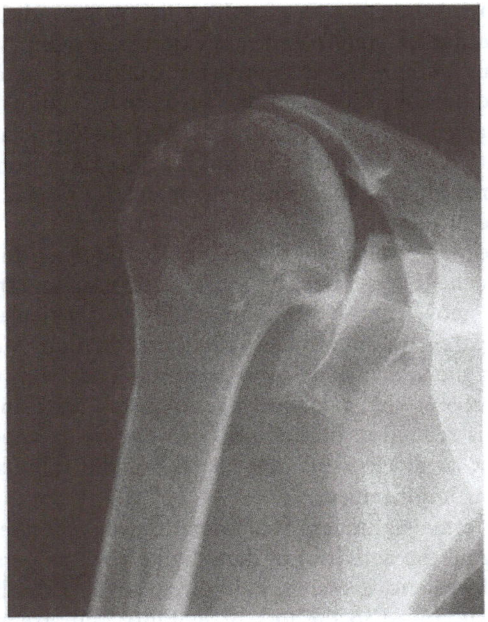

Fig. 1. Typical radiological aspect of osteoarthritis with massive cuff-tear

Natural History

The evolution of osteoarthritis with massive cuff-tear remains uncertain. Although it can be very well tolerated, as is classically described, the few published studies concerning the late evolution of massive cuff-tears (with or without arthritis) show that only 40 %–56 % of the patients have a functional shoulder [4–6]. The majority appear to develop chronic pain with an available degree of disability.

Clinical Presentation

Various events may occur during the evolution of osteoarthritis with massive cuff tear and different clinical presentation have been described in the literature:

- Acromio-clavicular cysts can appear which can occasionally be very large but are usually well tolerated as they cause little or no pain (Fig. 2). This may be visualised on the arthrography with the "geiser sign" described by Craig (Fig. 3).
- A reactive synovial effusion causing major swelling of the articulation, resulting in an acute exacerbation of pain and swelling in the antero-superior part of the shoulder. Aspiration reveals straw coloured synovial fluid.
- Spontaneous haemarthrosis giving the clinical scenario of the "senile haemorrhagic shoulder"

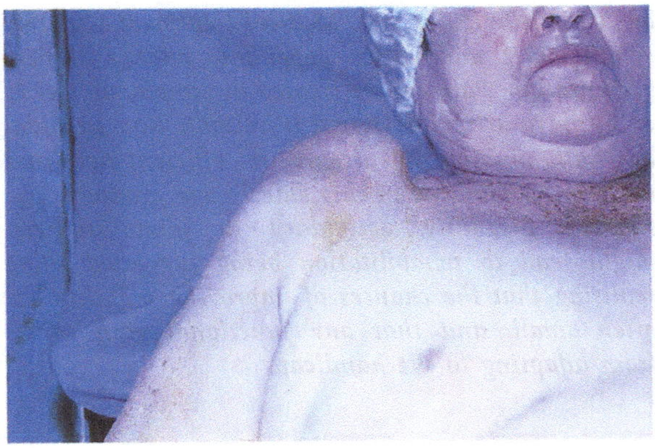

Fig. 2. Acromio-clavicular cyst

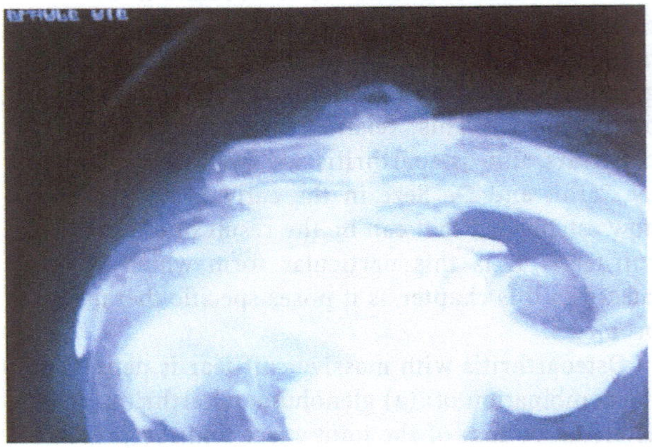

Fig. 3. The "geiser sign" with dye in the acromio-clavicular joint

[7]. This is a very rare complication of cuff-tear arthritis which presents with severe pain, significant swelling of the joint, which is red, warm and appears inflamed, and a total loss of function (Fig. 4). Occasionally bruising appears a few days afterwards in the anterior part of the upper limb. Aspiration reveals blood of varying hue depending on how much time has passed since the acute event. Sometimes the aspiration is a mixture of synovial fluid stained with blood. Many studies have commented on the frequent association with chondrocalcinosis [8], and this was found in more than half of our cases. Some authors have reported the frequent finding of crystals in the aspiration fluid: either calcium-pyrophosphate or apatite crystals. The major problem posed by these senile haemorrhagic shoulders is the frequency of recurrence and their resistance to medical treatment. The natural history is rapid destruction of the joint.

- 'Rapidly destructive shoulder', as described by Lequesne, is the parallel in the shoulder of rapidly destructive arthritis of the hip, and results in the loss of 25 % of the articular surface in less than 6 months [9]. This condition also has a frequent association with microcrystalline pathology [10].
- 'Milwaukee shoulder' was described by MacCarty and presents on a very similar, if not identical way, with a reactive synovial effusion, a massive cuff tear and a destructive arthropathy of the glenohumeral joint [11]. MacCarty, having detected the presence of microspheres of hydroxyapatite in the synovium and joint surfaces, proposed the following pathophysiological mechanism: the initial deposits of apatite into the synovium and capsule cause a synovitis which releases enzymes, particularly collagenases, leading to rupture of the cuff and the start of destructive arthropathy [12, 13]. In fact, it is not possible to state whether the presence of the crystals is the cause or the result of the bony destruction.
- 'Cuff tear arthropathy' as described by Neer is a destructive arthropathy following on from a long standing massive cuff tear [14].

This presentation can be summarised by saying that a small proportion of osteoarthritis with massive cuff-tear cases go on to a destructive arthropathy particularly when associated with a microcrystalline pathology. These destructive arthropathies present with very painful, acute swelling of either blood and articular fluid. They are characterised by recurrence of the swelling, the development of chronic pain and severe functional handicap.

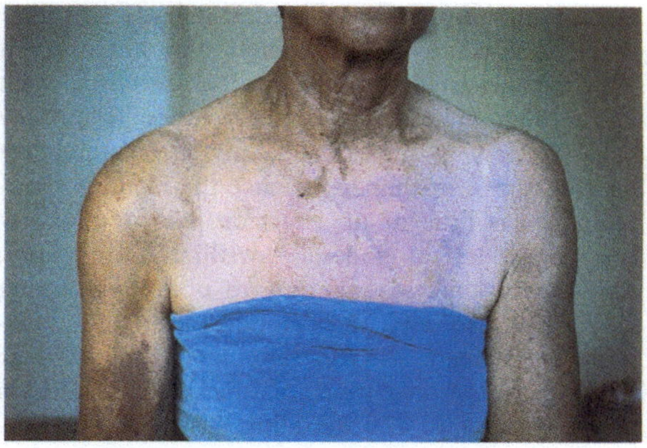

Fig. 4. "Senile haemorrhagic shoulder" with spontaneous haemarthrosis along the arm

Medical Treatment

Although the diagnosis of cuff-tear arthritis does not pose many problems, its treatment is very much more difficult. In fact, the proximal migration of the humeral head and the severe retraction of tendons as well as muscular atrophy mean that the surgical treatment is rarely employed except for tenotomy or tenodesis of the tendon of the long head of biceps when this is causing pain.

Medical treatment is purely symptomatic and varies depending on the clinical presentation.

Pain is treated with simple analgesics and intra-articular injection of steroids. Anti-inflammatory agents are not more efficacious here and are poorly tolerated in this age group.

The severe functional handicap, secondary to joint stiffness, may make the use of rehabilitation techniques reasonable, but it is recognised that the chance of improvement is limited and that any functional improvement usually comes from adapting to the handicap and the use of aids. However, there is no study which has satisfactorily assessed the results of rehabilitation for this indication.

Recurrent effusions, particularly in senile haemorrhagic shoulder, present a specific problem. Simple aspiration is invariably followed by the almost immediate recurrence of the fluid. Infiltration with steroids may dry up the effusion due to their sclerotic effect on the synovium. Some authors have suggested medical synovectomy. This treatment has a satisfactory effect on the effusion, which regresses and does not recur in 30 % of the cases after 6 months, but it has no effect on the pain or disability [16]. We carried out radioactive synovectomies using yttrium in seven cases with recurrent effusions (six haemarthroses and one synovial fluid) which failed to respond to intra-articular steroid injections. It should be noted that six of these patients has destructive chondrocalcinosis in other joints, particularly in the hands and knees. Each injection consisted of 2 mCi but had to be repeated in six of the patients up to three times, when they failed to dry up the effusion, giving a cumulative dose of 8 mCi. In our experience the medical synovectomy has little or no effect on pain or mobility and always left a moderate swelling in the joint. Any benefit took a long time to occur, presenting only after two and five months after the injection. These medical synovectomies do not appear to modify the evolution of the disease process towards a painful and disabling destructive arthropathy. Other authors have suggested using radiotherapy at anti-inflammatory dosages, but this therapeutic pathway has not been the subject of any evaluation.

References

1. Caroit M, Labrousse C, Wendling J, De Seze S (1964) Arthrose de l'épaule et détérioration de la coiffe des rotateurs (ruptures traumatiques et perforations trophiques de la coiffe des rotateurs). Rev Rhum 11:629–639
2. Novè Josserand Personal Communication, Lyon 1996
3. Hamada K, Fukuda H, Mikasa M, Kobayashi Y (1990) Roentgenographic findings in massive rotator cuff tears. A long term obsevation. Clin Orthop, 254:92–96
4. Caroit M, Rouaud JP, Texier T, Gaudouen Y, Delcambre B, Deloose F (1989) Le devenir des ruptures et des perforations complètes de la coiffe des rotateurs de l'épaule non opérées. Rev Rhum 56:815–821
5. Noë l E (1994) Les ruptures de la coiffe des rotateurs. Résultats du traitement conservateur. In: Simon L, Pellisiser J, Herisson C (eds) Actualités en rééducation fonctionnelle et réadaptation. Masson, Paris, pp 113–118
6. Bokor DJ, Hawkins RJ, Huckell GH, Angelo RL, Schickendantz MS (1993) Results of non operative management of full-thickness tears of the rotator cuff. Clin Orthop 294:103–110
7. Sèze de S, Hubault A, Rampon S (1967) L'épaule sénile hémorragique. In: L'Actualités rhumatologiques. Expansion Scientifique Française, Paris pp 107–114
8. Menkes CJ, Simon F, Chouraki M, Ecoffet M, Amor B, Delbarre F (1973) Les arthropathies destructrices de la chondrocalcinose. Rev Rhum 40:115–123
9. Lequesne M, Fallut M, Coulomb R, Magnet JL, Strauss J (1982) L'arthropatie destructrice rapide de l'épaule. Rev Rhum 49:427–437
10. Campion GV, McCrae F, Alwan W, Wat L, Bradfield J, Dieppe PA (1988) Idiopathic destructive arthritis of the shoulder. Semin Arthritis Rheum 17:232–245
11. McCarty DJ, Halverson PB, Carrera GF, Brewer BJ, Kozin F (1981) "Milwaukee shoulder" - assosiation of microspheroids containing hydroxyapatite crystals, active collagenese and neutral protease withrotator cuff defects. I. Clinical aspects. Arthritis Rheum 24:464–473
12. Halverson PB, Cheung HS, McCarty DJ, Garancis J, Mandel N (1981) "Milwaukee shoulder" - association of microspheroids containing hydroxyapatite crystals, active collagenese and neutral protease withrotator cuff defects. II. Synovial fluid studies. Arthritis Rheum 24:474–483
13 Garancis J, Cheung HS, Halverson PB, McCarty DJ (1981) "Milwaukee shoulder" - association of microspheroids containing hydroxyapatite crystals, active collagenese and neutral protease withrotator cuff defects. III. Morphologic and biochemical studies of an excised synovium showing chondromatosis. Arthritis Rheum, 24:484–491
14. Neer CS, Craig EV, Fukura H (1983) Cuff tear arthropathy. J Bone Joint Surg Am 65:1232–1244

Osteoarthritis with Massive Cuff-Tear: Results of an Unconstrained Shoulder Arthroplasty

J.M. Postel, J. Allain, L. Favard, and D. Goutallier

Summary

A total of 23 cases of arthroplasty for osteoarthritis with massive cuff tears were operated on between 1992 and 1995. Three patients died within 2 years of the arthroplasty leaving 20 patients which have been reviewed and X-rayed with at least 1 year follow-up, (average of 20 months). These patients were mostly elderly women, with an average age of 74 years. A hemi-arthroplasty was implanted in all patients except in six patients where a total shoulder arthroplasty was done. Overall, the average absolute Constant score had increased from 15.8 points (0–30) to 43.3 points (20–64) and the adjusted score from 20% (0%–59%) to 61% (29%–87%). Active forward elevation improved from an average of 57° preoperatively to an average of 98° postoperatively while active external rotation improved from 0° preoperatively to 24.5° postoperatively. About half the patients still had significant pain, and of these about one-half were disappointed with the operation. The use of a hemi-arthoplasty with an oversized head can be questioned in the light of this series and may be the reason for the pain. We now favour some laxity and avoid excessive tightness in prosthetic replacement for cuff-deficient shoulders. We observed one erosion of the acromion and one antero-superior migration of the humerus associated with an antero-superior approach leading to poor functional results. The changes seen with the glenoid components (complete lucent lines in two cases) confirms that it is not advised to implant a glenoid component when the cuff is severely damaged because of the "vertical rocking glenoid effect". On the whole, these elements confirm the caution with which unconstrained prosthetic arthroplasty should be indicated in this type of pathology.

Introduction

Association of a massive cuff-tear with destruction of the surface of the glenohumeral joint and/or erosion of the acromiohumeral joint may cause a painful and non-functional shoulder [1, 4, 5, 7, 11, 14, 16]. In most of these cuff-deficient shoulders, the head has migrated superiorly and has a new fulcrum under the coraco-acromial arch, and the surgical treatment remains a surgical challenge [17]. In these difficult pathological situations, unconstrained shoulder arthoplasty with or without cuff repair has been advocated with the recognition to be a "limited goal prosthesis" [1, 5, 10, 14, 16].

Unconstrained shoulder arthroplasty for osteoarthritis with massive cuff-tear is reported as giving good results with regard to pain relief, although the overall functional result remains average [1, 10, 14, 16]. However, because of the problems with fixation of the glenoid component some authors prefer to use a hemi-arthroplasty with the largest head size possible [10, 12, 14] while others favour the use of a constrained prosthesis [3, 6, 8, 15].

This series presents the short-term results achieved using a non-constrained shoulder arthroplasty, the Aequalis prosthesis, in the shoulders with disabling pain caused by the combination of an irreparable tear of the rotator cuff and destruction of the surface of the glenohumeral joint in the presence of a functional deltoid muscle.

Material and Methods

The patients selected had undergone shoulder arthroplasty for glenohumeral osteoarthritis associated with a massive cuff-tear (a tear always involving at least supraspinatus and infraspinatus). The acromiohumeral distance was 5 mm or less on the true AP view in neutral rotation, and there was inferior subacromial remodelling (Fig. 1). Twenty-three shoulders, operated on between 1992 and 1995, fulfilled these criteria. In seven of these the protuberances of the tuberosities had disappeared, and in five they were markedly reduced. In two cases the humeral head also demonstrate signs of lysis or collapse.

The patients were mostly elderly women (19 women and 4 men). Apart from two patients aged 50 and 53, whose radiographic appearances were exactly the same as for the rest of the group, all the patients were over 70 years old when they underwent surgery. The average age at operation was 74 years and the

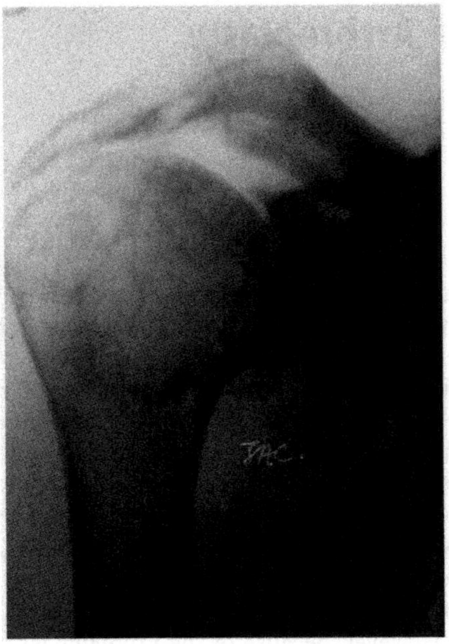

Fig. 1. Typical radiographic appearance of an osteoarthritis with massive cuff-tear showing a clear reduction in the subacromial distance and subacromial remodelling as well as the gleno-humeral narrowing

oldest patient was 85. The operated shoulder was the dominant one in 22 cases (21 right-sided dominant operations and two left-sided operations of which one was dominant).

On 22 occasions the delto-pectoral approach was used and on one occasion, the anterosuperior trans acromio-clavicular approach as described by Patte [13]. Acromioplasty was never performed. Instead, an effort was made to preserve the remnants of the coraco-acromial arch so that it acted as a superior stabilizer for the prosthesis. A massive deficiency of the cuff was found in each shoulder, involving the tendons of the supraspinatus, infraspinatus and sometimes the superior part of the subscapularis. Except in two cases, the cuff was judged to be irreparable because of the poor quality of the tissue and even with the use of mobilisation and transfer technique. Debridement of the rotator cuff alone was not considered sufficient treatment because of severe destruction of the gleno-humeral joint and/or acromio-humeral joint.

The subscapularis was released by a juxtaglenoid capsulotomy in eight patients and was lengthened in two patients by a coronal Z-plasty. The long head of the biceps was ruptured in 19 cases. In the 4 cases where it was present the long head of the biceps was cut or tenodesed after resection of the intra articular portion. Two cuff repairs were attempted but were judged as being unsatisfactory.

The humeral component of the Aequalis shoulder prosthesis was used in all of the shoulders. All the hemi-arthroplasties were cemented except one which was press-fitted. The prosthetic head used in the hemi-arthroplasties was the largest size available (50/19) on nine occasions and the 48/18 in four. The glenoid was resurfaced with a cemented polyethylene implant in six cases. Twelve of the 23 prostheses were inserted by the same surgeon (G.W.) and the rest by six different operators. The only operative complication recorded was a humeral diaphyseal fracture below the distal end of the prosthetic stem. This was reduced and fixed with screws.

Three patients died less than 2 years after surgery and one of these was due to undergo revision for persistent pain as a result of migration of the uncemented stem of a hemi-arthroplasty. All the other patients were reviewed with radiographs at more than 1 year. The average follow-up was 20 months and the longest was 31 months. For these 20 patients the pre- and postoperative shoulder function was evaluated using the Constant score [2].

Results

Functional Results

In all the cases the intervention was carried out as a pain relieving procedure ("limited goal prosthesis"). The average preoperative pain score was 2 out of 15 (0–6; Table 1). At review the pain had usually been improved with the average score reaching 10 (3–15). Nine patients (45%) still had significant pain with scores from 3 to 9 points, seven (35%) had moderate pain (scores of 10–13) and four (20%) were pain free. Three of the nine patients who still

Table 1. Detailed constant score for shoulder arthroplasty after osteoarthritis with massive cuff-tear

Constant score	Preoperative		Postoperative	Gain
Pain (15 points)	2	→	10	+ 8
Activity (20 points)	4.8	→	12.3	+ 7.5
Mobility (40 points)	7.6	→	18.8	+11.2
Strength (25 points)	1.4	→	2.3	+ 0.9
Absolute constant score (100 points)	15.8 (0–38)	→	43.4 (20–64)	+27.6
Normalized constant score (%)	20% (0–59%)	→	61.4% (29–87%)	+41.6%

had significant pain were disappointed by the operation, and one wanted further surgery.

Overall, the absolute Constant score increased from an average of 15.8 points (0–38) to 43.3 points (20–64) and the adjusted score from 20 % (0–59) to 61.4 % (29–87). The activities of daily living improved from 4.9 to 11.5 out of 20. Mobility increased from 7.6 to 18.8 out of 40. Active anterior elevation improved on average by 40° from 57° (0°–90°) to 98° (45°–160°). External rotation with the elbow at the side was 0° on average preoperatively (-40 to +30) and this reached 24.5° (-30 to +60) at follow-up. The force in the shoulder remained poor at 1.4 out of 25 preoperatively and only 2.3 postoperatively. Most of the patients reported improvement in the ability to perform the tasks of daily living as to comb their hair, to wash the opposite axilla, to perform perineal care, to use the hand at the level of the shoulder and to sleep on the affected side.

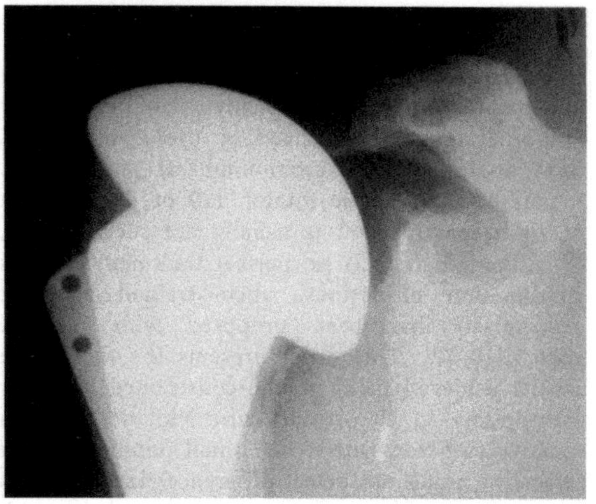

Fig. 2. Superior migration of the humeral component of a total arthroplasty carried out via the anterosuperior approach for osteoarthritis with massive cuff-tear

Radiographic Results

Apart from the distal migration of the press-fitted humeral component, there were few humeral changes seen with only one partial lucent line between cement and bone being observed. On the other hand, the radiographic changes in four glenoid components were more worrying: two showed complete lucent lines (at a follow-up of 25–31 months), one of which was evolving, associated with a poor functional result, one showed a suspected evolving inferior lucent line with a mediocre functional result and the last one showed a partial lucent line. One significant superior migration of the humeral prosthesis was observed after the antero-superior approach (Fig. 2) and one inferior acromial and glenoid erosion which evolved rapidly between the second and third postoperative years was noted (Fig. 3). There was no other notable wear of the glenoid occurring opposite to the humeral hemi-arthroplasties.

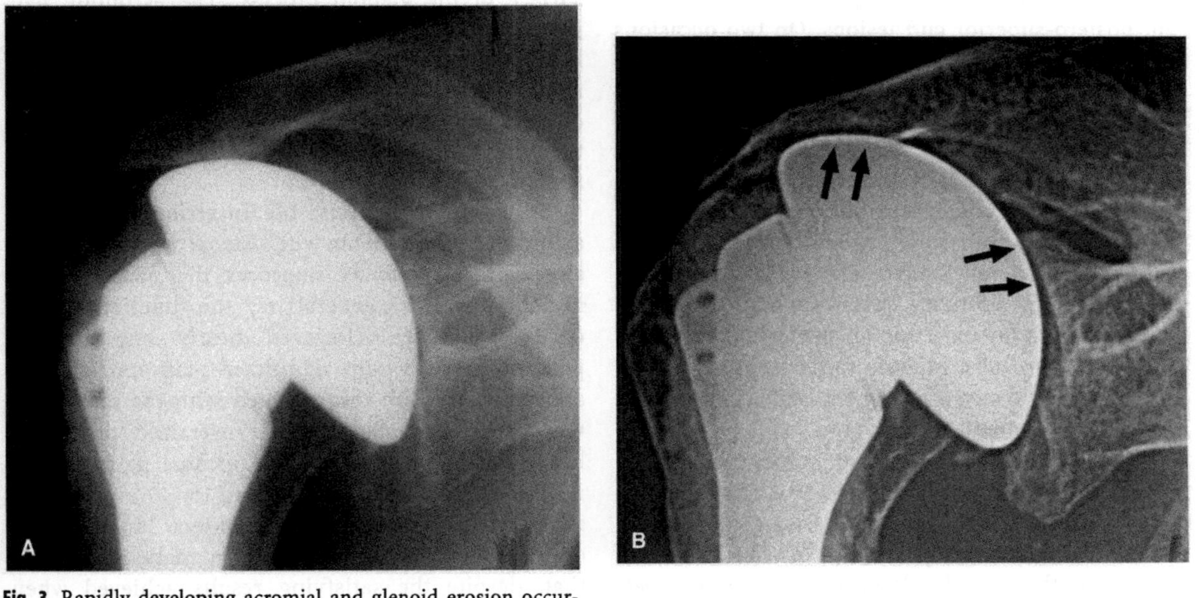

Fig. 3. Rapidly developing acromial and glenoid erosion occurring between the second (**A**) and third (**B**) postoperative years after a hemi-arthroplasty

Discussion

In the osteoarthritis with massive cuff tear, the pain and loss of function are usually related to erosion and/or lysis of the surface of the glenohumeral joint and/or of the acromiohumeral joint [4, 7]. Repair of a repairable rotator cuff or débridement of an irreparable cuff is usually not successful [1, 6]. Although there is no perfect treatment for this combination of lesions, unconstrained shoulder arthroplasty has been proposed with "limited goals" [10–12]. This series presents the short-term results achieved using a non-constrained shoulder arthroplasty in 20 osteoarthritic shoulders with a massive cuff-tear. Due to the small numbers in the series, we could not detect differences in the results with regards to the three types of osteoarthritis with massive cuff tear described by Favard et al. ("Osteoarthritis with Massive Rotator Cuff-Tear: The Limitation of its Current Definitions", this volume).

Because one antero-superior trans acromio-clavicular approach performed in the present series was associated with antero-superior migration of the humerus leading to a poor functional result, we recommend a deltopectoral approach. Those surgical approaches which include resecting the coracoacromial ligament, and which sacrifice the acromioclavicular joint (such as the anterosuperior approach) should be contra-indicated for this procedure. Care should be taken to maintain the coracoacromial ligamentous arch intact because it provides a superior buffer and stabilizer in these rotator cuff deficient shoulders [1, 14, 16].

All the operated shoulders presented with significant postero-superior cuff lesions. On two occasions these were repaired with difficulty and gave one satisfactory functional result (hemi-arthropasty with a postoperative pain score of 13, improved active elevation from 80° to 130° and external rotation from -10° to 50°) and one moderate result (total arthroplasty, pain free but with little mobility or function). In both these cases the state of the cuff at follow-up was not known. The subscapularis tendon is usually inferiorly retracted and should be divided at its bony insertion on the lesser tuberosity. This allows the subscapularis to be lengthen and to be superiorly transposed when reattached to the bone of the anatomical neck [14].

Pollock et al. recommend to implant a humeral component with a humeral head that should be as large as possible to fill the tuberosity-glenoid space and to avoid instability [14]. From the results of this series, the use of a large head remains debatable. Of the eight cases where the largest head size was used, five patients had a pain score less than 10, three reached 10 and none passed 10. We now believe that oversized prosthetic heads should not be used in these rotator cuff deficient shoulders. We agree with Arntz et al. that excessive tightness in these joints should be avoided [1]. To reach this goal these authors recommend placing the humeral component to allow 50% posterior subluxation of the prosthetic head on the glenoid and 90° of internal rotation of the abducted humerus [1]. Early migration of the one press fitted humeral stem observed in the present series favours the systematic cementing of the implant.

Franklin et al. have demonstrated an association between glenoid loosening in total shoulder arthroplasty and rotator cuff deficiency [5]. These authors and others pointed out the risk of loosening of the glenoid component because of eccentric shear forces occurring at the superior part of the glenoid component through a rocking motion at the joint [5, 9, 16]. The poor outcome seen with total shoulder arthroplasty in this series and the worrying lucent lines at the glenoid component interface confirm that it is not desirable to totalise an arthroplasty when the cuff has significant lesions. Furthermore, Pollock et al. observed in their series that the humeral hemiarthroplasty gained significantly more active elevation that the total replacement [14]. They felt that cuff repair was easier when a humeral head prosthesis alone was used because less lateralisation of the humerus occurred.

When implanting a hemi-arthoplasty for osteoarthritis with massive cuff-tear, the goal is that the prosthetic component articulates with the coraco-acromial complex as well as with some of the joint surface of the glenoid process. The acromion had generally resisted wear from the humeral prosthetic head, but the follow-up is short. However, the rapid appearance of an erosion under the acromion observed in one case shows a seed of doubt about the long-term tolerance of the acromion to wear from a hemi-arthroplasty.

In the final analysis, the insertion of a hemi-arthroplasty in patients with osteoarthritis and massive cuff tear usually improves the pain and the mobility and in a general way the functional value of the shoulder. However, nearly one-half the patients remains with significant pain and of these about one-half are disappointed with the operation. Our experience suggests that oversized prosthetic heads may be the reason for residual pain and we now favour some joint laxity and try to avoid tightness in these cuff-deficient shoulders. Finally, some of the radiographic changes seen make it possible that, despite the satisfying results achieved when the severity of the lesions treated is considered, these results may deteriorate with time. On the whole, these elements confirm the caution with which a prosthetic arthroplasty should be approached in this type of pathology. Although hemi-arthroplasty with or without partial rotator cuff reconstruction appears to be a possible alternative, the ideal procedure for these osteoarthitic shoulders with massive cuff-tears is yet to be determined.

References

1. Arntz G T, Jackins S, Matsen FAII (1993) Prosthetic replacement of the shoulder for the treatment of defects in the rotator cuff and the surface of the glenohumeral joint. J Bone Joint Surg Am 75:485–491
2. Constant CR, Murley AHG (1987) A clinical method of functional assessment of the shoulder. Clin Orthop 214:160–164
3. Coughlin MJ, Morris JM, West WF (1979) The semiconstrained total shoulder arthroplasty. J Bone Joint Surg Am 61:574–581
4. De Seze M (1967) L'épaule sénile hemorrhagique. L'Actualité Rheumatologique. Expansion Scientifique Française, Paris
5. Franklin JL, Barret WP, Jackins SE, Matsen FA (1988) Glenoid loosening in shoulder arthroplasty. Association with rotator cuff deficiency. J Arthroplasty 31:39–46
6. Grammont P, Trouilloud P, Laffay J P, Deries X (1987) Etude et réalisation d'une nouvelle prothèse d'épaule. Rhumatologie 39 (10):407–413
7. Lequesne M, Fallut M, Coulombe R et al. (1982) L'arthropathie destructive rapide de l'épaule. Rev Rhum Mal Osteoartic 49:427–437
8. Lettin AWF, Copeland SA, Scales JT (1982) The Stanmore total shoulder replacement. J Bone Joint Surg Br 64:47–51
9. Lohr JF, Cofield RH, Uhthof HK (1991) Glenoid component loosening in cuff-tear arthropathy. J Bone Joint Surg Am 73 [Suppl II]:106
10. Neer CS, Watson KC, Stanton FJ (1982) Recent experience in total shoulder replacement. J Bone Joint Surg Am 64:319–337
11. Neer CS, Craig EV, Fukuda H (1983) Cuff tear arthropathy. J Bone Joint Surg Am 65:1232–1244
12. Neer CS (1990) Glenohumeral arthroplasty. In: Shoulder Reconstruction. Sauders, Philadephia, pp-146–272
13. Patte D, Goutallier D (1985) Chirurgie de la coiffe des rotateurs. Enclycl Méd Chir Techniques Chirurgicales, Orthopédie Traumatologie 44, 285, 4.9.06
14. Pollock RG, Deliz EB, McIlveen, Flatow EL, Bigliani L (1992) Prosthetic replacement in rotator cuff-deficient shoulders J Shoulder Elbow Surg 1:173–186
15. Post M, Haskell SS, Jablon M (1983) Total shoulder replacement with a constrained prosthesis. J Bone Joint Surg Am 62:327–335
16. Williams GR, Rockwood CA (1994) Massive rotator cuff defects and gleno humeral arthritis. In: RJ Friedman (ed) Arthroplasty of the shoulder. Thieme, Stuttgart, pp 53–69
17. Weiner DS, Macnab I (1970) Superior migration of the humeral head. A radiological aid in the diagnosis of tears of the rotator cuff. J Bone Joint Surg Br 52:524–527

Section XI:

Acute Fractures of the Proximal Humerus

Anatomical and Pathological Classification of Proximal Humeral Fractures

J.C. Le Huec, P. Boileau, I. Hovorka, and R. Sinnerton

Summary

Classification of fractures of the proximal humerus is essential and should be taken into consideration when planning a surgical reconstruction. The Neer four-part classification for proximal humeral fractures remains the most useful and valuable classification used. In addition, some different variety of four-part fractures and head splitting fractures, as described by Duparc and Jakob, should be included in this classification. However, all classifications fail to consider three main problems that should be taken into consideration: (a) Poor intra- and interobserver reliability: the imprecise recognition of the fracture patterns is often due to the poor quality of the radiographs taken in emergency; computed tomography should be requested if there is any doubt over the fracture type. (b) Difficulty in assessing the displacement of the fracture: there is a tendency to underestimate or to overestimate the severity of some fractures. (c) Age, relevant to bone quality, is probably the most critical factor that should be taken into consideration and that is ignored in any classification; before deciding a treatment for a proximal humeral fractures surgeons should distinguish between young patients with good bone quality and old patients with poor bone quality and osteoporosis.

Introduction

Fractures of the proximal humerus are relatively frequent, making up 536 cases in a population of 53 000 followed over a 10-year period by Rose [21] and 565 cases in a population of 575 000 followed for 1 year by Kristiansen [13]. The fractures predominantly affect the female population (75 %) and the patients have an average age above 50 years [9, 13, 21]. In 90 % of cases the trauma involved is only moderate. The treatment for these fractures has undergone significant evolution, and precise knowledge of the anatomy and pathology specific to the different fracture patterns is essential in order to select the best treatment. Classification of fractures of the proximal humerus is essential and should be taken into consideration when planning a surgical reconstruction.

Blood Supply of the Proximal Humerus

Knowledge of the blood supply to bone is important when classifying fractures of the proximal humerus because it plays an important role in the chance for the fracture to consolidate, and it must be considered during the surgical approach. There are few anatomical studies of the blood supply. Apart from referring back to the classic works of Latarjet and Rouvière, we may quote more recent studies by Laing [14] and Moseley [16] which looked at the blood supply of the rotator cuff. Recently Gerber et al. [8] reported the results of an anatomical study of 29 cadavers. Brooks et al. [1] carried out an anatomical study of the blood supply after fractures.

The main arterial supply is the anterior circumflex artery, which is a constant feature. Its path reaches the level of the greater tuberosity in 20 % of cases, is higher in 6 % and lower in 74 % [8]. The artery passes horizontally, parallel to the inferior border of the glenoid and scapula. The artery gives off branches to the subscapularis in 65 % of cases and these do not supply bone. There are other constantly found branches which feed the proximal epiphysis and are found medial to the bicipital groove [1, 8]; these penetrate the anteromedial surface of the metaphysis or the diaphysis. Sometimes there is a single well-defined artery (28 %) coming off the anterior circumflex artery and spreading out at the anteromedial level of the humeral metaphysis. The anterior circumflex artery finally terminates in an anterolateral ascending branch, which is the essential nutrient artery to the superior extremity of the humerus [1, 8]. This is a constant branch and has a diameter varying of 0.5–1 mm. Its path is also constant and passes parallel to the inferior border of the glenoid in the same direction as the circumflex artery. It follows the line of the bicipital groove close to bone and gives off numerous branches in the sagittal and posterior planes. These are the most lateral terminal branches from this trunk and in some cases anastamose with vessels supplying the rotator cuff, as described by Moseley [16].

The posterior circumflex artery comes off the axillary artery, sometimes from a common trunk with the anterior circumflex artery (22 %). This vessel is always smaller and reaches the humerus at its medial edge, giving off terminal branches which feed upwards. Often two main branches can be seen among these terminal arteries (43 %) [1].

Angiographic studies carried out by Brooks [1] on subjects with a proximal humeral fracture yielded the following results:

- The anterolateral branch is rarely damaged in the initial trauma and is always found undamaged in anterior fracture dislocations.
- There are anastomoses between the anterior and posterior circumflex systems, between the anterior circumflex vessels and the acromiothoracic and subscapular vessels, and between the posterior circumflex vessels and the inferior scapular vessels.
- Vascular lesions, as demonstrated by blood pooling, are found in bony lesions where the fracture line passes in a plane parallel to the inferior border of the humeral head. These correspond to damage to the distal branches of the ascending anterolateral vessel.

Overall, the anatomical studies show the relative importance of the anterolateral branch of the anterior circumflex artery in the vascular supply of the metaphysis and upper diaphysis of the humerus [8]. Anastamoses with the supply to the cuff are rare [1, 8, 14, 16].

Angiographic studies carried out in fracture cases do not always demonstrate the same anatomical system. The anterolateral branch, adherent to the periosteum along the lateral border of the bicipital groove, should be the branch shown the most respect in the surgical approach and in manipulations to reduce fractures of the proximal humerus [1, 8]. The various fractures of the proximal humerus do not share the same high risk of head necrosis due to different traumatic damages to the vascular supply of the humeral head at the time of the injury.

Classification of Fractures of the Proximal Humerus

The Neer classification is based on the original ideas reported by Codman who made a significant contribution in 1934 when he divided proximal humeral fractures into four basic segments [4]. This author noted the different possible fracture lines at the head-diaphysis level and between the tuberosities along the anatomical line of epiphyseal union (Fig. 1). In Neer's four-part classification the parts

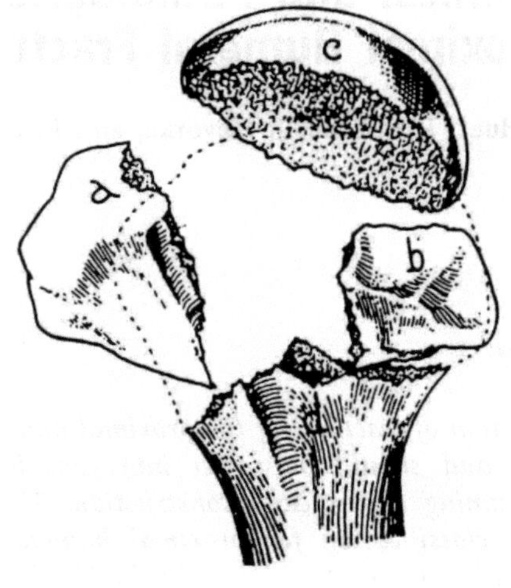

Fig. 1. Physiopathology of a four-part fractures according to Codman [4]

are the same as those described by Codman: the articular segment or humeral head, the greater tuberosity, the lesser tuberosity, and the diaphysis [18, 19]. When any of the four major segments is displaced over 1 cm or angulated more than 45°, the fracture is considered to be displaced. Fissure lines or hairline fractures are not to be considered displaced fragments. A fragment may have several undisplaced components that should not be considered separate fragments since they are in continuity and are held together by soft tissue. If those criteria are not met, and if the fragments are not displaced, the fracture should be considered as minimally displaced. Epidemiological studies have shown that 60 %–80 % of the proximal humeral fractures are minimally displaced [9, 13, 21].

In our opinion, the four-part classification remains a comprehensive system which integrates anatomy, biomechanics, and displacement of proximal humeral fractures. This classification is still the most useful and commonly used classification system. However, lack of precision concerning the different types of four-part fractures led us to integrate the works of other authors such as Duparc [6] or Jakob [11, 12]. The classification presented here has been slightly modified to include some subtypes or distinctive features that were felt to be important from both our clinical experience and the literature [5, 6, 9, 11, 12, 17].

Two-Part Fractures

Two-part fractures can be intra-articular (anatomical neck fractures) or extra-articular (surgical neck fractures, greater tuberosity fractures and lesser tuberosity fractures; Fig. 2).

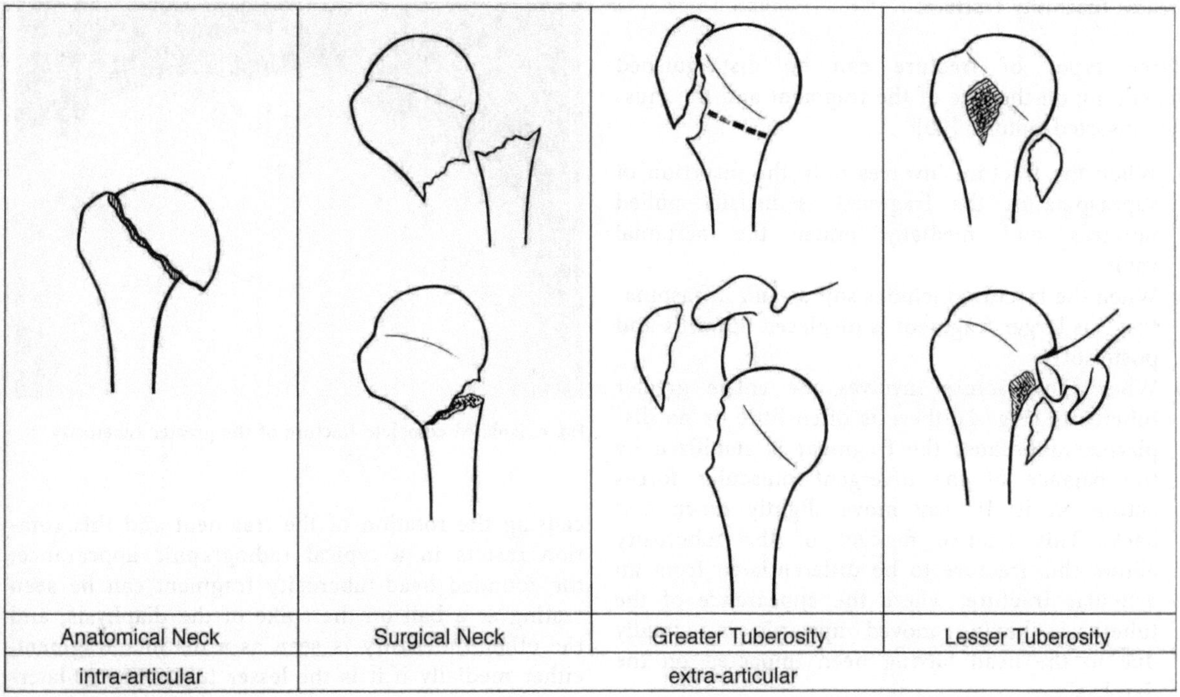

Fig. 2. The two-part fractures

Anatomical Neck Fractures

These fractures are extremely rare, being 0.3 % of all proximal humeral fractures [4, 19]. They are completely intra-articular and detach the humeral head at the level of the anatomical neck (Fig. 3), thus separating it from all vascular connections coming from the capsule. The tuberosities remain intact, but the head can be either impacted or loose. Although these fractures are rare, they have a very high rate of necrosis when displaced, and the treatment of choice is an arthroplasty in elderly patients. However, open reduction and internal fixation should be preferred in young patients because necrosis of the humeral head fragment may be well tolerated for many years.

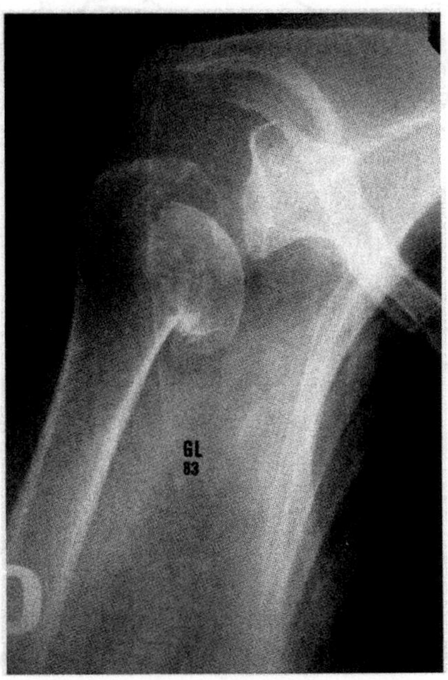

Fig. 3. Displaced anatomical neck fracture with a high risk of head necrosis

Surgical Neck Fractures

These usually occur at the level of the surgical neck, below the tuberosities but above the insertion of pectoralis major. Surgical neck fractures usually have a good prognosis when they are minimally displaced. However, they may have a poor prognosis when significantly displaced either because of nonunion or because of late humeral head necrosis. Surgical neck fractures require sometimes an open reduction because of interposition of soft tissue (long head of the biceps) and often an internal fixation because of unstable reduction.

Greater Tuberosity Fractures

Three types of fracture can be distinguished depending on the size of the fragment and the muscles inserted onto it [20]:

- When the fracture involves only the insertion of supraspinatus, the fragment is usually pulled upwards and medially under the acromial vault.
- When the fracture includes supra- and infraspinatus, this larger fragment is displaced upwards and posteriorly.
- When the fracture involves the entire greater tuberosity (Fig. 4), there is often little or no displacement because the fragment is stabilized by the balance of the divergent muscular forces acting on it. It may move slightly down and back. This relative descent of the tuberosity allows this fracture to be differentiated from an articular fracture, where the appearance of the tuberosity having moved upwards is actually due to the head having been impacted on the diaphysis.

The first two fracture types may cause pseudoparalysis of the shoulder, as seen in a cuff-tear, due to pain. Greater tuberosity fractures are often associated with an anterior dislocation: one should look for an anteroinferior glenoid fracture. When the greater tuberosity fragment remains displaced after reduction of the dislocation, these fractures should be treated using heavy nonabsorbable sutures or screw fixation.

Lesser Tuberosity Fractures

These occur much less frequently, involve the insertion of subscapularis and are displaced medially. They classically occur after a posterior dislocation as seen in seizures or electric shocks [17]. These fractures should be fixed when displaced to avoid subscapularis insufficiency.

Three-Part Fractures

These fractures are fairly common and do not always have a poor prognosis. They are often confused with four-part fractures due to difficulty in analyzing the radiographs. The fracture has one fragment consisting of the humeral head detached en bloc with one or other of the tuberosities, the diaphysis as the second fragment and the other tuberosity, free of all attachments, is the third fragment. The tuberosity which remains fixed to the head is responsible for causing the rotation of the fragment and this rotation results in a typical radiographic appearance; the rounded head-tuberosity fragment can be seen resting as a ball on the spike of the diaphysis, and the other tuberosity is seen as a distinct fragment, either medially if it is the lesser tuberosity or laterally if it is the greater tuberosity (Fig. 5). When displaced, these fractures are very difficult if not possible to reduce closed, but reduction is essential because they have good potential for consolidating with a good functional result on the condition that an anatomical reduction can be achieved. These fractures can be dislocated as shown in Fig. 5.

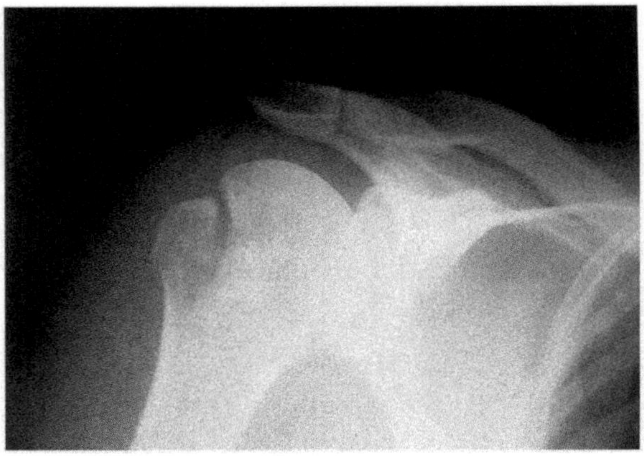

Fig. 4. Isolated complete fracture of the greater tuberosity

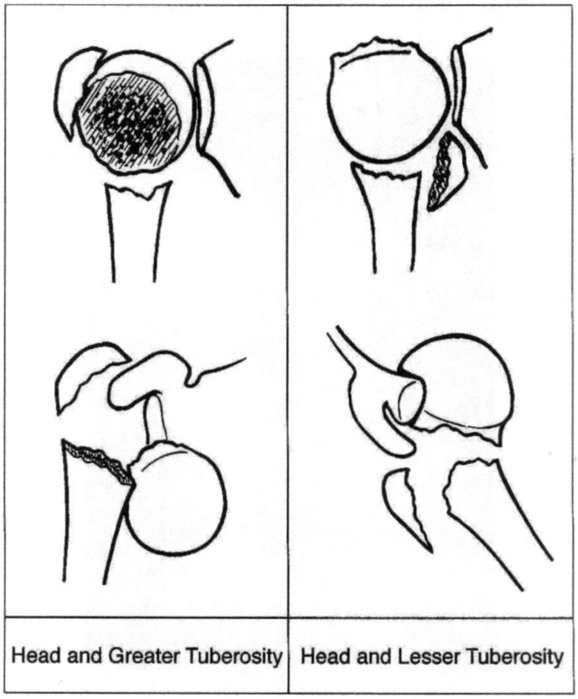

Fig. 5. The three-part fractures

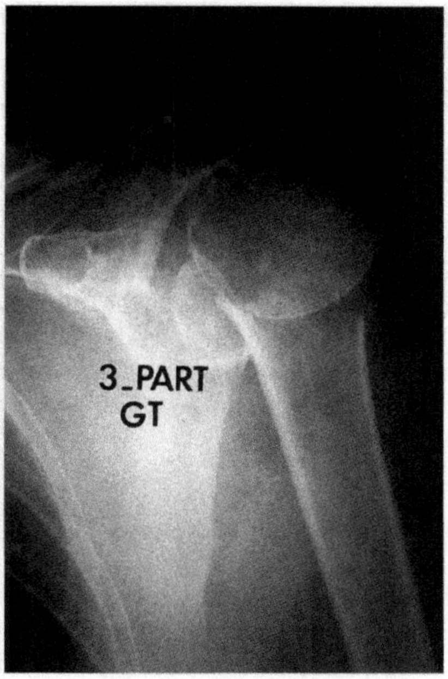

Fig. 6. Three-part fracture showing the "cup and ball" appearance with the greater tuberosity displaced posteriorly and medially

In *greater tuberosity three-part fracture* the head fragment faces backward because of the rotation provided by the lesser tuberosity which remains attached to the head. (Fig. 6). In *lesser tuberosity three-part fracture* the head fragment faces anteriorly due to the rotation by the greater tuberosity which is still attached to the head.

Four-Part Fractures

Four-part head-tuberosity fractures consist of the humeral head, the diaphysis and the two tuberosities. Taking into account the works of Duparc [6] and Jakob [11, 12], four subtypes can be distinguished depending on the degree of impaction of the head on the diaphysis and the presence or absence of dislocation of the head (Fig. 7).

Type 1 or Minimally Displaced Four-Part Fracture

The fracture divides the proximal humerus into four fragments, but they are minimally displaced with the head rotated less than 45°, and the separation between the tuberosities is less than 10 mm, as described by Jakob [11, 12]. They can be identified by the presence of a superior diastasis of the glenohumeral joint line (Fig. 8).

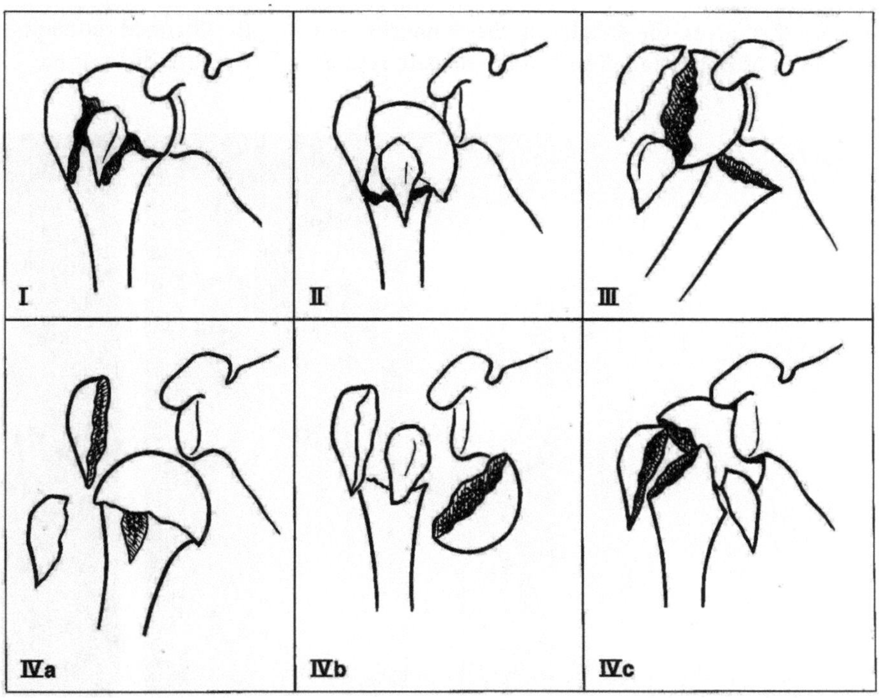

Fig. 7. The four-part fractures: *I*, nondisplaced; *II*, valgus or varus impacted; *III*, head centered with diaphysis medially displaced; *IVa*, inferior fracture dislocation; *IVb*, anterior fracture dislocation; *IVc*, posterior fracture dislocation

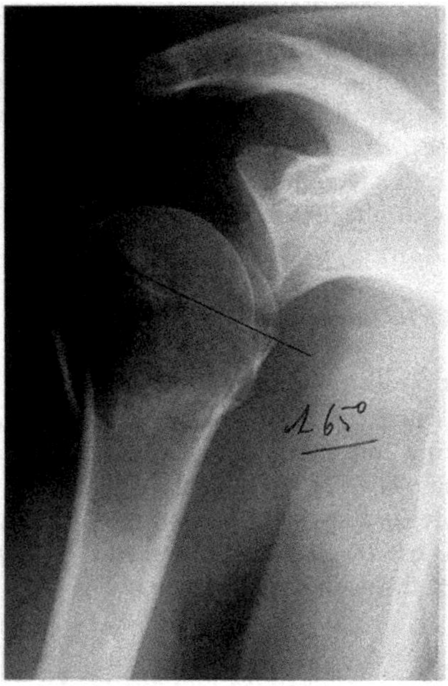

Fig. 8. Four-part head-tuberosity fracture impacted in slight valgus, type 1

Type 2 or Four-Part Impacted Fracture

The displacement is significant but the head remains impacted on the diaphysis. The distance between the upper pole of the impacted humeral head and the greater tuberosity is greater than 1 cm, and the head is rotated to more than 45° (Fig. 9). The important anatomical landmark is the greater tuberosity because this gives the height of the humerus and the degree of impaction. The head is usually rotated into valgus [12] with the fragment separating the tuberosities, but a varus rotation which has an even worse prognosis can also occur.

Type 3 or Four-Part Fracture with Diaphysis Displaced

The humeral head is free within the joint and completely disconnected from the tuberosities and the diaphysis. The diaphysis is usually displaced into the axilla with the head staying in place opposite the glenoid. There is an increased risk of necrosis. Computed tomography is useful in analyzing the position of the fragments.

Type 4 or Dislocated Four-Part Fracture

This subgroup has a dislocation associated with the fracture [5, 7] and the head may be displaced inferiorly anteriorly [24] or posteriorly [25], giving rise to two appearances:

- The head may remain impacted on the diaphysis but no longer opposite the glenoid. This is an aggravation of type 2 due to a much more violent force, and there is a significant risk of necrosis [10].
- On the other hand, the head may be loose and have been ejected from the joint while the tuberosities and diaphysis remain in a relatively anatomical position. The disimpaction of the head from the diaphysis may be due to the trauma or to ill-timed attempts at reducing an impacted fracture-dislocation.

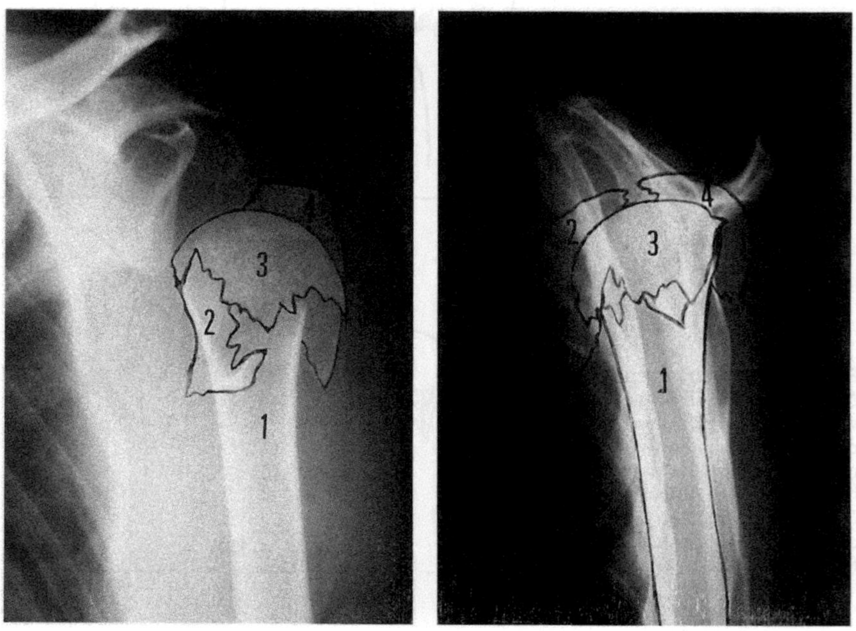

Fig. 9. Four-part head-tuberosity fracture impacted in valgus, type 2

There are two major threatening complications which can occur in four-part fractures: humeral head necrosis, which is often massive and has been recorded as occurring in all the types in all the series published [6, 10, 11], and malunions which, reproduce to varying degree the displacement seen in the type 2 fracture with horizontalization of the head and giving a false appearance of an ascending greater tuberosity.

Most authors agree that there are limited indications for internal fixation [6, 10, 12, 24] though this might be considered in type 2 fractures in young patients, since there is a high risk of necrosis, even though this may be well tolerated. For types 3 and 4 the insertion of an arthroplasty should be discussed.

Fractures of the Articular Surface

Impression Fractures

Small posterosuperior impression fractures are commonly observed with anterior dislocation, as described by Malgaigne and later by Hill and Sachs, and do not necessitate any surgical treatment. Larger anterior impression fractures usually result from posterior dislocation. Treatment depends on the age of the lesion and of the size of the head defect [25]. In a small (less than 20 % of the articular surface) and acute (less than 3 weeks) impression fracture, a closed reduction is usually successful and followed by immobilization in external rotation. In a larger impression fracture (less than 50 % of the articular surface), a subscapularis transfer, with or without the lesser tuberosity, is performed [15]. When 50 % of the head is impressed, shoulder arthroplasty is preferred (25).

Head-Splitting Fractures

This group of fractures was described by Duparc [6]. They are found only in traumatic dislocations of the shoulder and have the common starting point of the traumatic Hill-Sachs impaction lesion, which occurs during the dislocation and is situated at the junction of the greater tuberosity and the head – though occasionally more medially (Fig. 10). When the trauma is particularly violent, this lesion may initiate a fracture which heads towards the lateral metaphyseal cortex detaching the greater tuberosity. The tuberosity fracture is always complete but as a rule minimally displaced due to the balanced pull of the muscles acting on it. Less frequently the fracture isolates the head, as in a vertical fracture, where the fracture line starts at the upper border of the anatomical neck at the level of the impaction and travels vertically downwards towards the medial metaphyseal cortex. The lesser tuberosity remains attached to the head fragment and the greater tuberosity to the diaphysis. It is therefore a two-part fracture with one fragment consisting of the head and the lesser tuberosity and the second of the greater tuberosity and the diaphysis. It is possible to have a fracture in which the medial and lateral lines from the impaction can coexist. There is little risk of necrosis because the head retains a vascular supply from the capsule attached to its inferior spur: this is usually an indication for osteosynthesis.

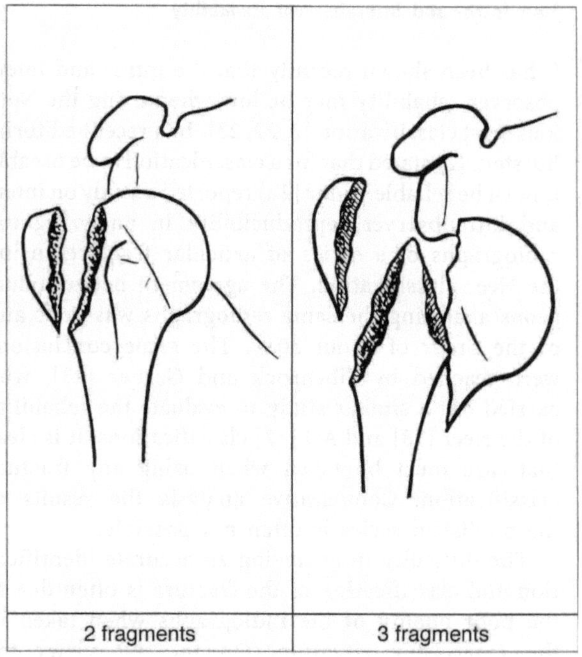

Fig. 10. Head-splitting fractures

Problems Encountered with Classification and Prognosis

The goal of a classification should be to allow therapeutic and prognostic guidelines. Neer's classification for proximal humeral fractures remains the most useful and valuable classification used because it gives a physiopathological concept of these fractures and is simple to memorize. However, this classification, as with any others, fails to consider three main problems that should be taken into consideration: the poor intra- and interobserver reliability, the difficulty in assessing displacement of the fractures (i.e., the potential head necrosis) and the osteoporotic quality of the bone in the elderly patients.

Poor Intra- and Interobserver Reliability

It has been shown recently that the intra- and interobserver reliability may be low when using the Neer four-part classification [2, 22, 23]. In a recent editorial Burstein [2] stated that for a classification to be useable it must be reliable. Sidor [22] reported a study on inter- and intraobserver reproducibility in analyzing the radiographs of a series of articular fractures using the Neer classification. The agreement between surgeons analyzing the same radiographs was poor and of the order of about 30%. The same conclusions were reached by Sibenrock and Gerber [23], who carried out a similar study to evaluate the reliability of the Neer [18] and AO [17] classifications. It is clear that care must be taken when using any fracture classification: Comparative analysis the results of the published series is often not possible.

The difficulty in achieving an accurate identification and classification of the fracture is often due to the poor quality of the radiographs when taken in the emergency situation. On the AP views the bony fragments are superimposed, thus making analysis very difficult [22, 23]. Transthoracic views are of little interest, and axillary views or Bernageau views are difficult to take properly. The "trauma series" of Neer is still the best initial method for diagnosing proximal humeral fractures. This consists of anteroposterior and lateral radiographs in the scapular plane and, if motion and pain permit, an axillary view [19, 23]. It is best to take good anteroposterior views, with gentle traction on the elbow to reduce the telescoping of the fragments and to ask for a lateral outlet view.

Computed tomography is an important adjunctive investigation [3] and should be requested when there is any doubt over the fracture classification and on every occasion when a prosthesis is being

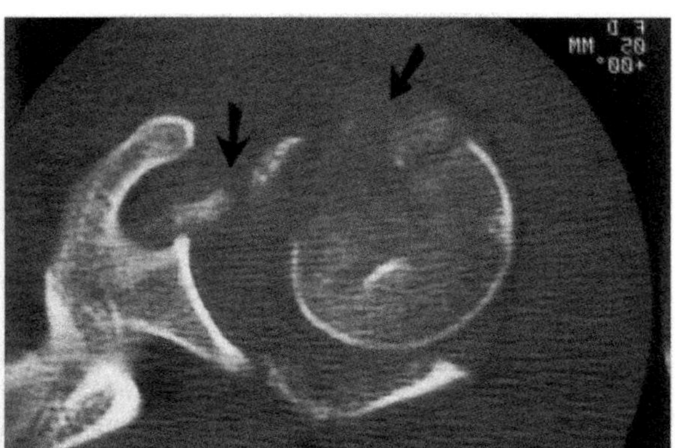

Fig. 11. Computed tomography allows the precise analysis of a four-part fracture: a fracture is involving the bicipital groove in this edge

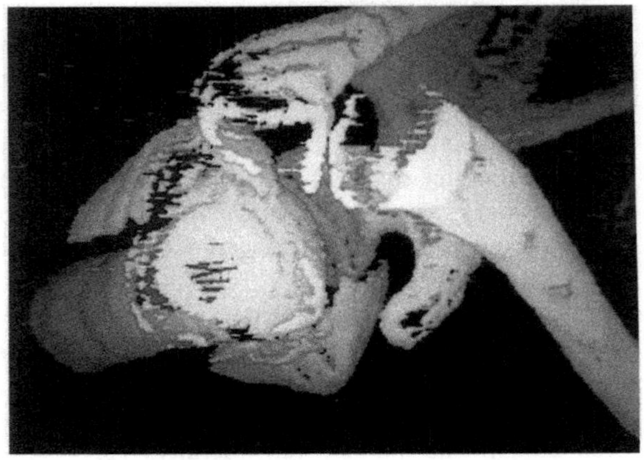

Fig. 12. Three-dimensional computed tomographic reconstruction shows that the main vertical fracture line is passing behind the bicipital groove

considered (Fig. 11). Three dimensional reconstruction is sometimes performed and allows a better analysis of the fracture lines and in particular allows the integrity of the bicipital groove to be assessed (Fig. 12). This is an essential landmark for carrying out an anatomical reconstruction of the tuberosities.

Finally, although it has been recently shown that the interobserver reliability of the Neer classification may be low, we believe that this classification remains valuable unless two conditions are respected: (a) two orthogonal views of the shoulder should be at least available. If possible the "trauma series" with a true AP view, a lateral view and an axillary view (or velpeau view) should be available. If not, computed tomography should be asked. (b) The definitive classification of the fracture can sometimes be made only intraoperatively by the surgeon himself.

Difficulty in Assessing the Displacement of the Fractures and the Potential Head Necrosis

Neer stated that only 20% of the fractures of the proximal humerus are displaced and need a surgical treatment. He gave two criteria to help the surgeons to classify the fracture as "displaced": 10 mm displacement and 45° angulation. There is no scientific confirmation that these criteria are those that should be used. These two criteria are not accurate enough to allow prediction of a potential osteonecrosis of the head segment or a poor functional result [7]. Furthermore, there may be a tendency to underestimate or overestimate the severity of some fractures. For instance, an "apparently nondisplaced" surgical neck fracture may lead to nonunion or necrosis of the humeral head. On the other hand, a "displaced" four-part valgus impacted fracture may be overestimated, leading to implant a shoulder prosthesis instead of performing an open reduction with internal fixation. The Neer classification inclines to the view that all displaced four-part fracture would benefit from a shoulder replacement. This is not necessarily true and is why the different types of four-part fractures and the head-splitting fractures should be included in the classification (Figs. 7, 10).

Osteoporosis

Finally, age, relevant to bone quality, is probably the most critical factor that should be taken into consideration when deciding a surgical treatment [7, 9, 21]. Horak reported that proximal humeral fractures increases with age and in females and have the same frequency as fractures of the proximal end of the femur [9]. Rose showed that proximal humeral fractures are the most common fracture of the humerus in the patients over 40 years of age and are primarily osteoporosis related, since the amount of trauma responsible for the fracture is significantly less in the older age group [21]. Both Rose and Horak reported that osteoporosis was a significant factor in these fractures [9, 21].

From a technical point of view, osteoporosis is synonymous with difficulty at the time of reduction and instability at the time of fixation. Osteoporosis is often ignored when deciding a surgical treatment of a displaced proximal humeral fracture. We believe that this prejudicial factor should be taken into account before planning any surgical treatment: a comminuted and unstable fracture in an elderly patient with osteoporotic bone does not have the same prognosis as a displaced fracture in a young patient with good bone quality. The goal of any treatment of fracture of the proximal humerus should be to reduce the tuberosities and especially the greater tuberosity to obtain an anatomical reconstruction. As emphasized by Gerber et al. [7, 8], osteonecrosis of the head fragment can be well tolerated unless the tuberosities are anatomically reduced and healed to the diaphysis.

Conclusion

Lack of consensus concerning fracture description and classification makes it difficult to evaluate treatment adequately. Although the four segments classification remains useful, surgeon's experience is needed to evaluate both the amount and tolerance of fragment's displacement and the bone quality. Bone osteoporosis in elderly patients is a critical factor that should be taken into account when choosing a surgical treatment.

References

1. Brooks CH, Revelli WJ, Heatley SW (1993) Vascularity of the humeral head after proximal humeral fractures. J Bone Joint Surg Br 75:132–136
2. Burstein AH (1992) Fracture classification system: do they work and are they useful. J Bone Joint Surg Am 75:12–13
3. Castagno AA, Shuman WP, Kilcoyne RF, Haynor DR, Morris ME, Matsen FA (1987) Complex fractures of the proximal humerus: role of CT in treatment. Radiology 165:759–752
4. Codman EA (1934) The shoulder, rupture of the supraspinatus tendon and other lesions in or about the subacromial bursa. In: The shoulder. Todd, Boston
5. DeMourgues G, Razemon JP, Leclair HP, Comtet JJ (1965) Les fractures-luxations de l'épaule. Rev Chir Orthop 51:151–165
6. Duparc J, Lagier A (1976) Les luxations-fractures de l'extrémité supérieure de l'humérus. Rev Chir Orthop 62:91–110
7. Gerber C et al (1990) Biological fixation of fractures. Arch Orthop Trauma Surg 109:295–303
8. Gerber C, Schneeberger AG, Vinh T (1990) The arterial vascularisation of the humeral head. An anatomical study. J Bone Joint Surg Am 72:1486–1494
9. Horak J, Nilson B (1975) Epidemiology of fractures of the upper end of the humerus. Clin Orthop 112:250–253
10. Huten D, Duparc J (1986) L'arthroplastie prothétique dans les traumatismes complexes récents et anciens de l'épaule. Rev Chir Orthop 72:517–529
11. Jakob RP, Kristiansen T, Mayo K, Ganz R, Mulle ME (1984) Classification and aspects of treatment of fractures of the proximal humerus. In: Bateman JE, Welsh RP (eds) Surgery of the shoulder. Mosby, St Louis/Decker, Toronto, pp 330–343
12. Jakob RP, Miniaci A, Anson PS et al (1991) Four part valgus impacted fractures of the proximal humerus. J Bone Joint Surg Br 73:295–298
13. Kristiansen B, Barford G, Bredesen J, Erin-Madsen J Grum B, Horsnaes MW, Aalberg JR (1987) Epidemiology of proximal humeral fractures. Acta Orthop Scand 58:75–77
14. Laing PG (1956) The arterial supply of the adult humerus. J Bone Joint Surg Am 38:1105–1116
15. Mac Maughlin HL (1952) Posterior dislocation of the shoulder. J Bone Joint Surg Am 34:584–590
16. Moseley HF, Goldie IAN (1936) The arterial pattern of the rotator cuff of the shoulder. J Bone Joint Surg Br 45:780–789
17. Muller ME, Nazarian S, Koch P (1987) Classification AO des fractures. Springer, Berlin Heidelberg New York
18. Neer CS (1970) Displaced proximal humeral fractures. I. Classification and evaluation J Bone Joint Surg Am 52:1077–1089
19. Neer CS, Brown TH, MacLaughlin HL (1953) Fracture of the head of the humerus with dislocation of the head fragment. Am J Surg 85:252–258
20. Olivier H, Dufour G, Duparc J (1976) Les fractures du trochiter. Rev Chir Orthop [Suppl] 62:113–118
21. Rose SH, Melton J, Morrey BF, Ilstrup DM, Riggs BL (1982) Epidemiologic features of humeral fractures. Clin Orthop 168:24–30

22. Sidor ML, Zuckerman JD, Lyon T, Cuomo F, Shoenberg N (1992) The Neer classification for proximal humeral fractures. J Bone Joint Surg Am 75:1745–1750
23. Siebenrock KA, Gerber C (1992) The reproductibility of classification of fractures of the proximal end of the humerus. J Bone Joint Surg Am 75:1751–1755
24. Vichard P (1988) Luxations-fractures de l'épaule. Conférence d'enseignement de la SOFCOT. Expansion Scientifique Française, Paris
25. Walch G, Boileau P, Martin B, Dejour H (1990) Unreduced posterior dislocations and fracture-dislocations of the shoulder French. J Orthop Surg 4(4):546–558

Therapeutic Indications in Fractures of the Proximal Humerus

H. Mestdagh

Summary

Although the precise radiographic analysis of the fractures of the proximal humerus allowed by modern imaging techniques has clarified the therapeutic indications, difficulties in interpretation do not make it any easier to choose the right technique from the many proposed. Classical open internal fixation has certainly yielded disappointing functional results, especially when performed with bulky implants not adapted to high fractures, comminutive fractures, and osteporotic bone. However, although it solves the difficult technical problems of reconstructing the proximal humerus, a prosthesis is not the universal solution to displaced fracture. Finally, the acute proximal humerus fractures for which a shoulder replacement is indicated are: (a) four-part displaced fractures and fracture-dislocations, (b) selected three-part fractures in elderly patients with osteopenic bone stock, (c) some head-splitting fractures, in which the articular segment is split with displacement, (d) some impression fractures involving about half or more of the articular surface.

Introduction

Fractures of the proximal humerus are very polymorphic occurring at all ages, covering many anatomical types, justifying many forms of treatment and having an unpredictable outcome. The precise radiographic analysis of the lesions available with modern imaging techniques has helped to clarify the therapeutic indications. By using the classifications of Neer [12] and Duparc [2], we can distinguish between nonarticular, infratuberosity fractures (with or without a tuberosity fracture) which have a favorable outcome and articular fractures and fracture dislocations which have a poorer outcome. One should always remenber that minimally displaced fractures, which represent about 80 % of upper humeral fractures, are amenable to simple treatment by early functional exercises. For the displaced fractures, the therapeutic option depends on the age of the patient and on the number of bone fragments detached.

Two-Part Fractures

Anatomical Neck Fractures

These are rare and are treated by K-wiring or transdeltoid percutaneous screw fixation in young patients or, occasionally in elderly patients, by hemiarthroplasty where there is a risk of necrosis [7].

Surgical Neck Fractures

These are the most common, and the outcome is usually good because the epiphysis remains vascularized by the capsular and muscle vessels.

Undisplaced or Minimally Displaced Fractures of the Surgical Neck

These are treated by immobilization with the elbow at the side in a Velpeau (or Dujarrier) type sling. If displaced, reduction should not be attempted at the risk of displacement or neurovascular damage.

Displaced Fractures of the Surgical Neck

These are difficult to reduce closed. In theory, reduction comprises the successive movements of traction, translation, and finally impaction of the diaphysis into the proximal fragment. The reduction may be unstable or impossible to achieve due to muscle interposition, and the functional result is often unsatisfactory [14]. Therefore whenever possible, the preferred treatment is percutaneous internal fixation – amounting to an augmented closed treatment. These types are an ideal indication for closed K-wiring using an ascending wire starting from the lateral side of the humeral metaphysis (Fig. 1A). More recently, intramedullary wiring has been recommended starting from the insertion zone of the deltoid [11], from the posterior surface of the humerus above the olecranon fossa [1], from the lateral epicondyle [20], or from the medial epicondyle [17]. In the two latter examples the subcutaneous

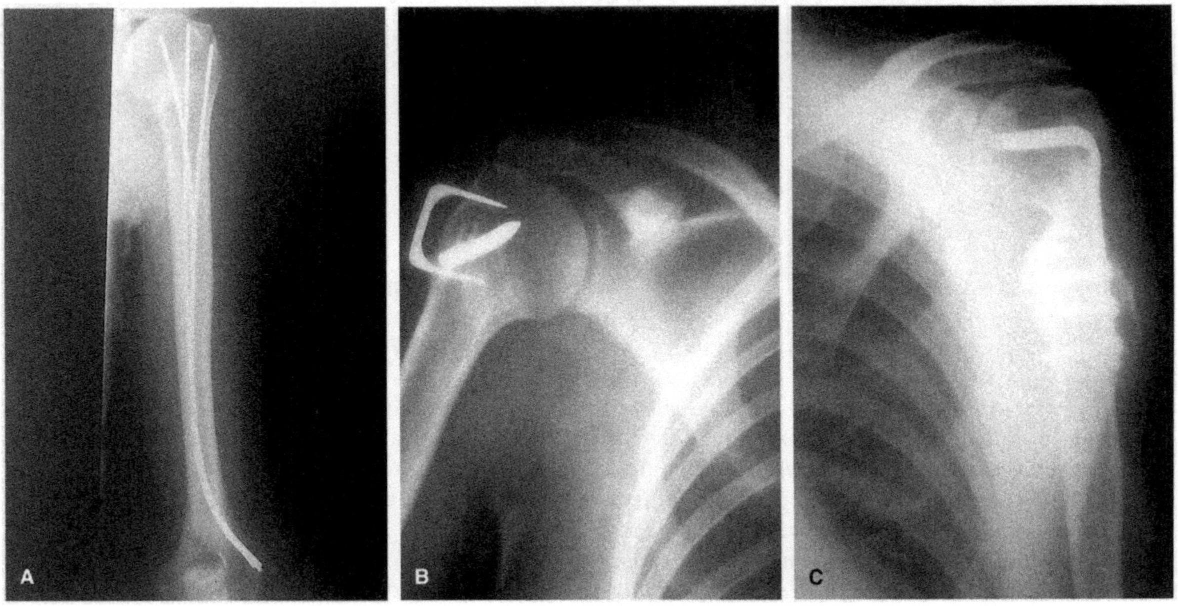

Fig. 1 A–C. Different types of osteosynthesis in displaced two-part surgical neck fractures: **A** Closed reduction and distal intramedullary nailing. **B** Stappling after open reduction. **C** Open reduction and internal fixation using a hooked (Milch) plate

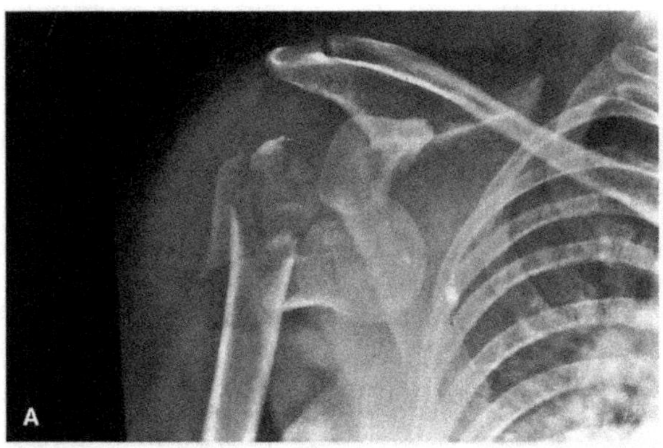

Fig. 2 A–C. Three-part greater tuberosity associated with anterior dislocation of the head fragment. **A** Before closed reduction. **B** After reduction and distal intramedullary nailing. **C** Complete healing associated with excellent functional result

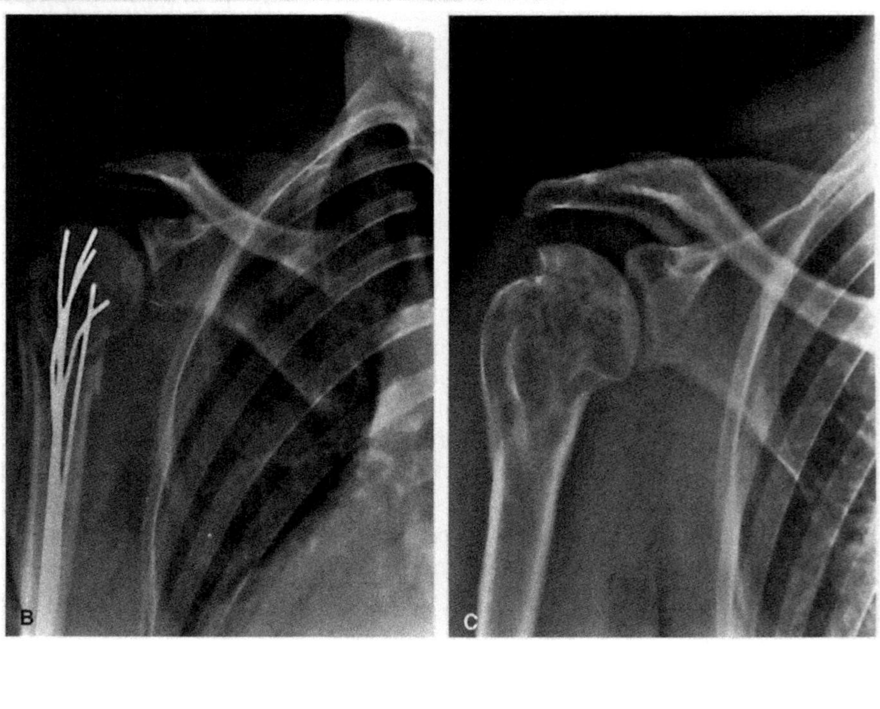

position of the ends of the wires runs a major risk of skin perforation or infection, and at the elbow level the wires may irritate the triceps and effect elbow movement. The Kapandji technique avoids these risks but cannot be applied to low or segmental fractures. Vichard has proposed fixation using two flexible nails inserted via the epicondyles. Hackethal stress the use of the maximum number of intermedullary wires to confer stability and avoid the need for immobilization.

Nailing is the second method of augmented closed reduction. There are numerous nails available, but none completely prevents rotation except a recent lockable new proximal nail (polarus nail). The Rush nail has little rotational control and the lockable Seidel nail is not suitable for high fractures. Moreover, if there is any secondary upward movement after impaction into the head, the nail may damage the cuff and cause subacromial impingement.

Open reduction and internal fixation does not have a good reputation. The least bulky materials (staples, screws, circlage) rarely afford a stable construction (Fig. 1B). In osteosynthesis with a plate the weak point is the poor grip of the screws in osteoporotic bone and an insufficient number of screws in high fractures. These problems may sometimes be overcome by a hooked (Milch) plate [16] (Fig. 1C).

The preference therefore must be for closed K-wiring where the reduction is unstable or where one wants to avoid immobilization, such as in polytrauma cases or the elderly patient in a poor general state.

Two-Part Surgical Neck Fracture Associated with Dislocation

Reduction can usually be achieved by gentle manipulation or prolonged traction [4]. In other cases closed intramedullary wiring is performed with the head dislocated, and then a careful reduction is carried out [11] (Fig. 2).

Greater Tuberosity Fractures

These fractures should be fixed when displaced using either nonabsorbable sutures or screws. An anterosuperior approach is preferred by most authors.

Lesser Tuberosity Fractures

These fractures are difficult to diagnose. Computed tomography may help by showing the displacement of the tuberosity fragment. A deltopectoral approach is useful to reduce and fix the bone fragment using sutures, staples, or screws.

Three-Part Fractures

Three-Part Greater Tuberosity Fractures

The treatment is decided on the displacement of the greater tuberosity and the diaphysis. Nonoperative treatment is justified only in undisplaced or minimally displaced greater tuberosity fractures. In the other cases internal fixation is always complex: nailing is difficult or impossible, and a plate must fix all three fragments. A combined fixation is often the "least bad" solution and consists of closed K-wiring of the infratuberosity fracture plus wiring or percutaneous screw fixation of simple fractures [13] and open intraosseous suture or (circlage wiring) in multifragmentary fractures of the greater tuberosity [1, 3, 6]. The difficulties encountered in reducing and fixing these fractures explains why some authors suggest hemiarthroplasty, at least in elderly patients.

Three-Part Lesser Tuberosity Fractures

While fixing the infratuberosity fracture, a displaced lesser tuberosity fracture may be reinserted using a screw or transosseous sutures.

Four-Part Fractures

These combine an intracapsular fracture line passing through the anatomical neck detaching the humeral head, with a vertical intertuberosity fracture line separating the two tuberosities. The humeral head is free of any attachments and runs a high risk of necrosis.

The therapeutic indications vary depending on the anatomical at type, as described by Duparc [2], but they remain controversial. Although the presence of a dislocation increases the risk of head necrosis, it is the type of fracture which defines the therapeutic approach (see J. C. Le Huec et al. Anatomical and Pathological Classification of proximal humeral fractures, this volume).

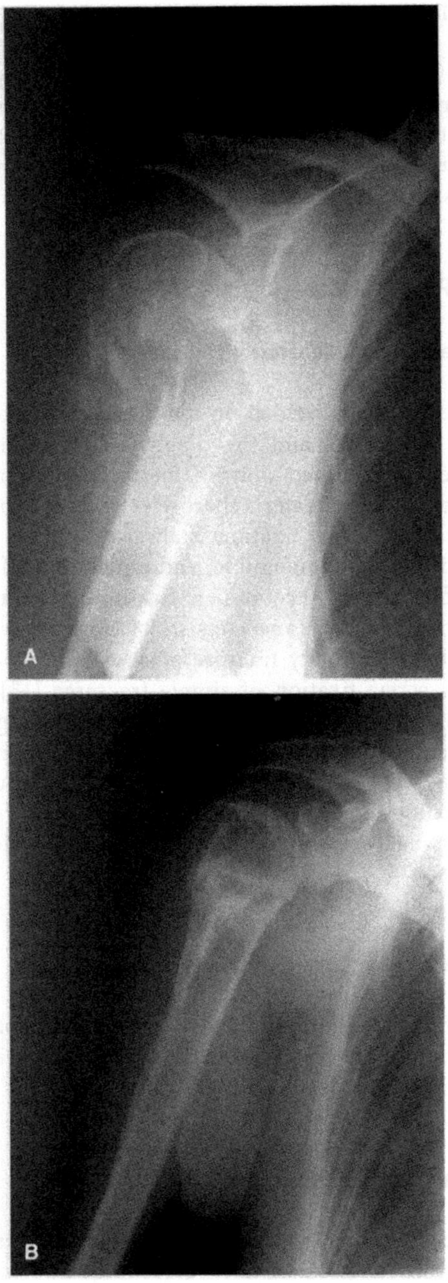

Fig. 3 A,B. Four-part fracture type 3. **A** Before closed reduction. **B** Good radiological and functional result after orthopedic treatment

Type 1 or Minimally Displaced Four-Part-Fracture

Four-part fractures with minimal displacement tend to consolidate if immobilized in a Velpeau (or Dujarrier) sling, but there is a risk of head necrosis. Reduction is not advised at the risk of displacement or neurovascular complications.

Type 2 or Four-Part Impacted Fracture

These fractures are displaced and impacted and may be treated nonoperatively but at the risk of a nonunion and head necrosis. Some authors [9] recommend a surgical approach to raise the humeral head and then reduce and fix the tuberosity. No method of internal fixation is satisfactory except perhaps the minimal fixations described by Jakob.

Type 3 or Four-Part-Fracture with Diaphysis Displaced

These are difficult to reduce. Plates are often not adapted to the size of the fragments and produce poor results, and intramedullary wiring does not hold. Transdeltoid percutaneous K-wiring plus 3–4 weeks of immobilization is recommended in the younger patient despite its difficulties and the significant risk of head necrosis or failure of the fixation (Fig. 3). In the elderly patient an arthroplasty might be preferred.

Type 4 or Dislocated Four-Part-Fracture

These are fractures associated with a dislocation of the head fragment which can be inferior (type 4a), anterior (type 4b), or posterior (type 4c). These fractures may be opened to achieve reduction, but this does not solve the difficulties of fixation (Fig. 5). This is the reason why some authors advocate a prosthesis as the definitive treatment even in the young [7].

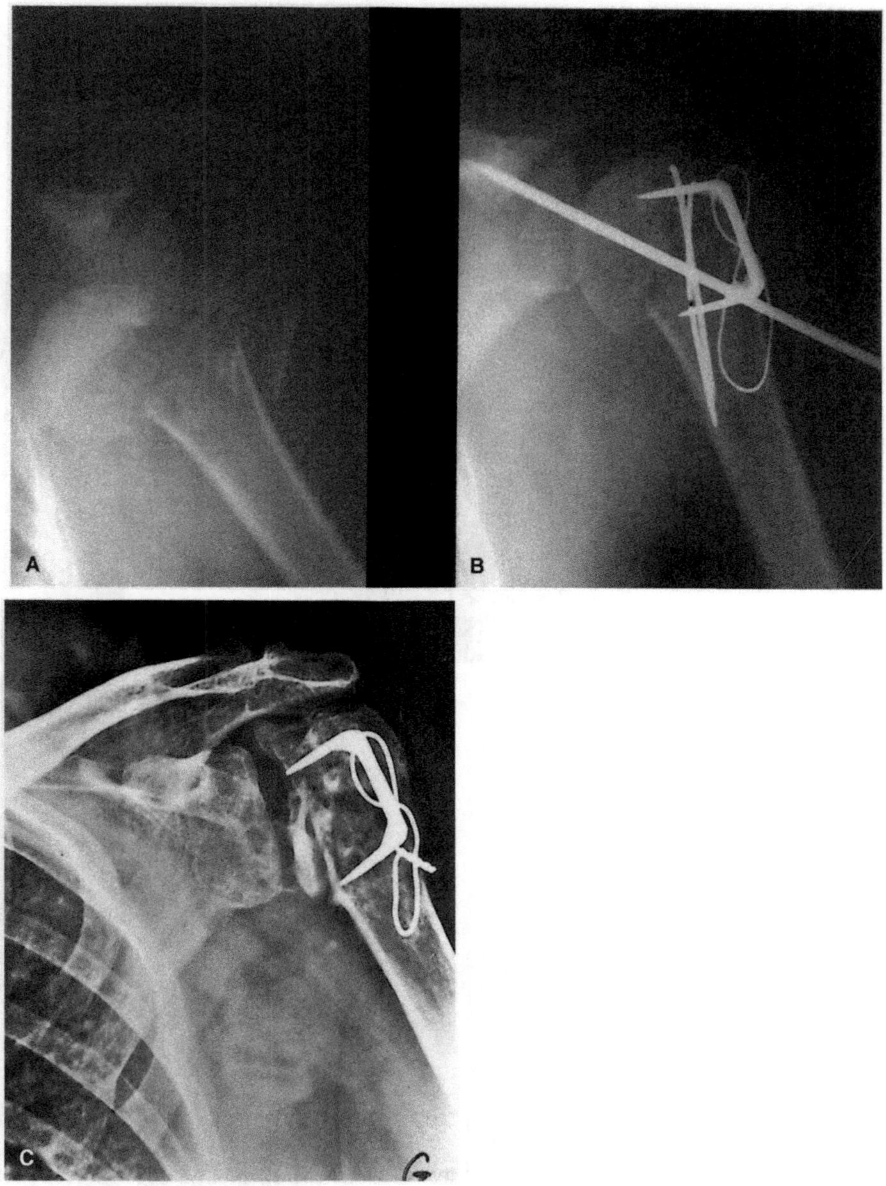

Fig. 4 A–C. Four-part fracture type 4 with posterior dislocation. **A** Preoperative AP view. **B** Open reduction and internal fixation. **C** Head necrosis with poor functional result

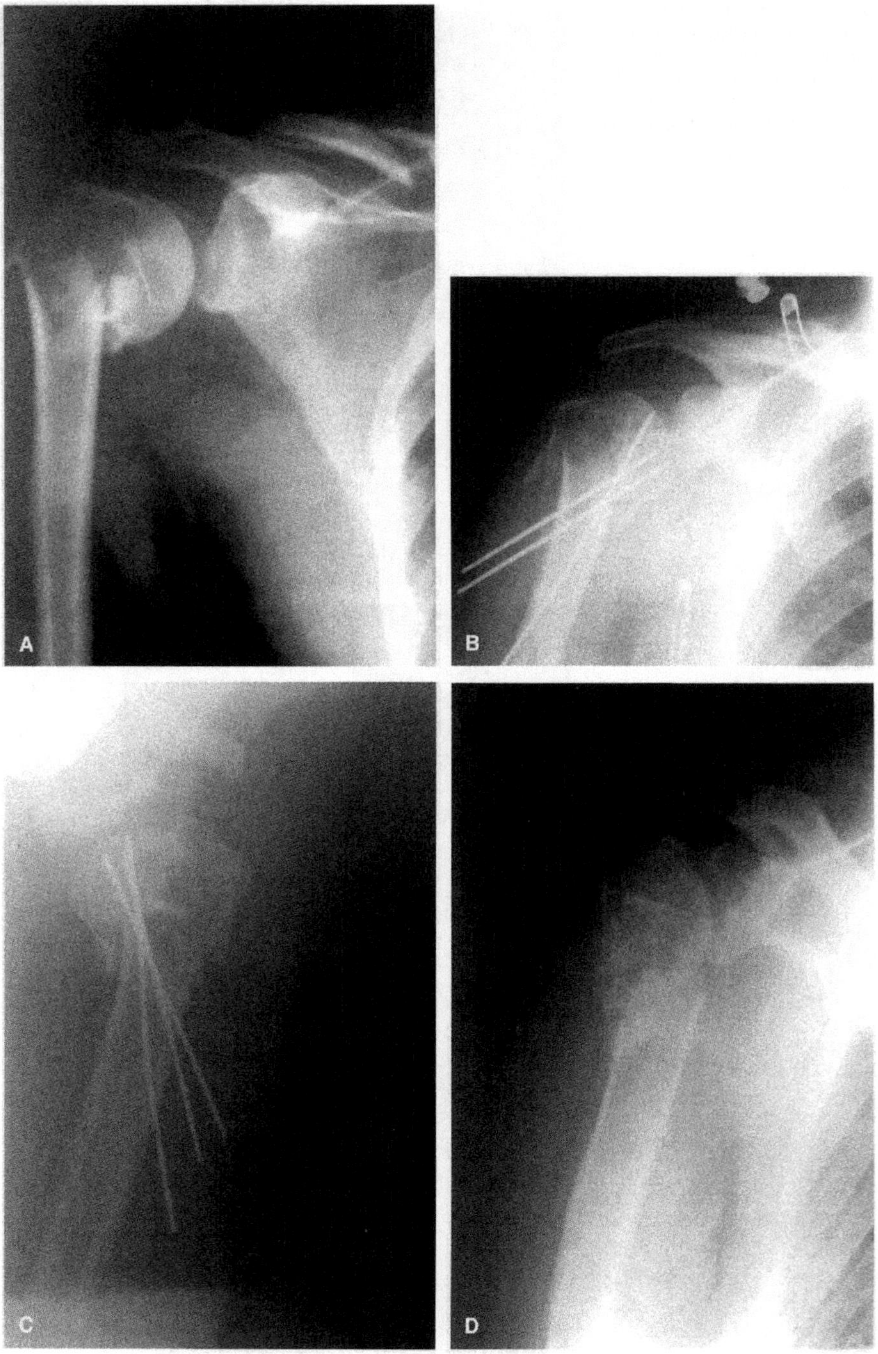

Fig. 5 A–D. Four-part head-splitting fracture. **A** Preoperative X-ray. **B** Closed, transdeltoid pinning. **C** Axillary view. **D** Despite malunion a good functional result was observed

Impacted or Head-Splitting Fractures

Impacted fractures are associated with an anterior or a posterior dislocation.

In anterior dislocations the head fracture is a completion of the Hill-Sachs lesion which may occur at the junction of the greater tuberosity and the head or within the head and taking off the lesser tuberosity. Reduction of dislocations with a Hill-Sachs lesion must be performed carefully, and the lesion in the head may need to be elevated and grafted, although it is usually well supported. A Hill-Sachs lesion complicated by a fracture requires reduction and fixation by screws or a plate.

In posterior dislocations the fracture starts in the reverse Hill-Sachs lesion and may detach one or more bony fragments. Similar care must be taken with these dislocations. In isolation the fracture impaction of the humeral head may be grafted or filled by a subscapularis or lesser tuberosity transfer. When more than a third of the articular surface is impacted, a prosthesis is recommended, especially in elderly patients. In a displaced fracture, internal fixation or a prosthesis are both justified. Head-splitting fractures are usually an indication for a shoulder replacement but closed reduction and internal fixation may be attempted in young people (Fig. 5 A–D).

Conclusion

The advent of modern imaging techniques has allowed a much better understanding of the fractures of the proximal humerus. Although a prosthesis may provide the technical answer to the difficult problems of reconstruction, it is not the universal solution to displaced fractures.

Classical open reduction and internal fixation have yielded disappointing results, especially when carried out with bulky implants which are not well adapted to high, multifragmentary fractures or osteoporotic bone.

Whenever possible, our preference undoubtedly lies in augmented closed treatment such as closed K-wiring. In more difficult cases, a combined procedure is proposed using transdeltoid screws or direct suture via a short deltopectoral incision in adjunct to the wiring. When postoperative immobilization is required, it should be as short as possible, and the use of an abduction splint in difficult cases helps functional recovery.

References

1. Apprill G, Boll P (1968) Le traitement des fractures du col de l'humérus par embrochage centro-médullaire sans ouverture du foyer de fracture. Rev Chir Orthop 54:657–666
2. Cofield RH (1986) Comminuted fractures of the proximal humerus. Clin Orthop 230:49–57
3. Duparc J, Langier A (1976) Les luxations fractures de l'extrémité supérieure de l'humérus. Rev Chir Orthop 62:91–110
4. Flatow EL, Cuomo F, Maday MG, Miller SR, Mac Ilveen SJ, Bigliani LU (1991) Open reduction an internal fixation of two-part displaced fractures of the greater tuberosity of the proximal part of the humerus. J Bone Joint Surg Am 73:1213–1218
5. Geneste R, Durandeau A, Gauzeri JM, Roy J (1980) Traitement des luxations-fractures de l'épaule. Rev Chir Orthop 6:383–386
6. Hackethal (1961) Die Bundelnagelung. Springer, Berlin Göttingen Heidelberg
7. Hawkins RJ, Bell RH, Gurr L (1986) The thre-part fracture of the proximal part of the humerus. J Bone Joint Surg Am 68:1410–1414
8. Hawkins RJ, Kiefer GN (1987) Internal fixation technique for proximal humeral fractures. Clin Orthop 223:77–85
9. Jaberg H, Jakob R (1992) Percutaneous stablization of unstable fracture of the humerus. J Bone Joint Surg Am 74:508–515
10. Jakob RP, Miniaci A, Anson PS, Jaberg H, Osterwalder A, Ganz R (1991) Four-part valgus impacted fractures of the proximal humerus. J Bone Joint Surg Br 73:295–298
11. Kapandji A (1989) L'ostéosynthèse par la technique des broches en palmiers des fractures du col chirurgical de l'humérus. Ann Chir Main 8:39–52
12. Mestdagh, Butruille Y, Tillie B, Bocquet F (1984) Résultats du traitement des fractures de l'extrémité supérieure de l'humérus par embrochage percutané. Ann Chir 38:5–13
13. Mestdagh H, Vigier P, Bocquet F, Butruille Y, Letendart J (1986) Résultats à long terme du traitement des fractures-luxations de l'extrémité supérieure de l'humérus. A propos de 64 cas. Rev Chir Orthop 72:132–135
14. Neer C II (1970) Displaced proximal humeral fractures. J Bone Joint Surg Am 52:1077–1103
15. Olivier H, Dufour G, Duparc J (1976) Les fractures du trochiter. Rev Chir Orthop 62:113–118
16. Paavolainen P, Bjorkenheim JM, Slatis P, Pankku P (1983) Operative treatment of severe proximal humeral fracture. Acta Orthop Scand 54:374–379
17. Rogez JM, Triclot P, Letanneur J (1978) Embrochage de l'humérus par voie interne sus-épitrochléene. J Chir 115:605–608
18. Svend-Hansen H (1974) Displaced proximal humeral fractures. Acta Orthop Scand 45:359–364
19. Vichard P, Bellanger P (1978) Traitement des fractures de l'extrémité supérieure de l'humérus par enclouage bipolaire ascendant avec clous élastiques. Nouv Presse Med 7:4041–4043
20. Vives P, Lestang M, Landi N, Robbe M (1976) Le traitement des fractures de l'extrémité supérieure de l'humérus par embrochage en faisceau par voie épicondylienne. Lille Chir 31:21–34
21. Yamano Y (1986) Comminuted fractures of the proximal humerus treated with hook plate. Arch Orthop Trauma Surg 105:359–363
22. Young TB, Wallace A (1985) Conservative treatment of fractures and fracture-dislocation of the upper end of the humerus. J Bone Joint Surg Br 77:373–377

Shoulder Arthroplasty for Proximal Humeral Fractures: Problems and Solutions

P. Boileau and G. Walch

Summary

Shoulder prosthesis positioning and tuberosity reconstruction in fractures have until now been very approximate. Because of the "eye-balling" involved in prosthesis positioning, tuberosity reconstruction was inaccurate. Not surprisingly, clinical results were poor and unpredictable, with a high rate of greater tuberosity migration. Anatomical reconstruction of the tuberosities is possible only if the prosthesis is positioned precisely for length and retroversion. The Aequalis fracture jig is a new device designed to help surgeons position the humeral implant correctly in both height and retroversion. The principle is simple: a ruler restores the length and a protractor restores the retroversion. This extramedullary guide helps to stabilize the prosthesis and minimizes the subjective assessment of the surgeon (whose experience is often limited) allowing better positioning of the prosthesis and therefore better reconstruction of the tuberosities. As no surgeon would now consider implanting a knee prosthesis without the appropriate jig, so we believe the same course should be followed when using a prosthesis for shoulder fractures.

Introduction

Depending on the patient's age, a shoulder prosthesis may be indicated in displaced or dislocated three- or four-part fractures of the proximal humerus. Neer was the first to emphasize the frequency of humeral head necrosis in displaced fractures and to propose in 1951 a replacement of the humeral head by a nonconstrained prosthesis associated with a reconstruction of the tuberosities [26]. However, apart from Neer, who obtained 80 %–90 % excellent or good results with shoulder prosthesis for fractures [27, 28], most authors achieved rather inferior results [10–15, 18, 19, 22, 25, 30, 31, 34, 36, 39]. Considering these ambiguous results, some surgeons have even opted for conservative treatment (or even no treatment at all) rather than surgical treatment for these complexe upper extremity fractures [40, 42].

Two questions are therefore raised: (a) Can the approximate anatomical reconstruction explain the inconsistent or misleading results? (b) What can we do to obtain a more reproducible anatomical reconstruction and thus be able to improve the functional results?

Since a preliminary clinical study highlighted the insufficiencies of anatomical reconstruction [2], we developed a new instrumentation to allow more precise positioning of the humeral prosthesis when used for displaced or dislocated proximal humeral fractures: the Aequalis fracture jig.

Poor Quality of Anatomical Reconstruction After Humeral Head Replacement for Proximal Fractures

With the exception of the two series published by Neer [27, 28], all others in the literature have shown poor functional results associated with shoulder prosthesis used in fractures. Table 1 summarizes these results and shows that active anterior elevation is low, averaging only the horizontal plane, and that shoulder replacement does not always produce a painless shoulder. Other studies report the high rate of complications of humeral head replacement for proximal humeral fractures and insist on the fact that most of the failure factors are technical errors of surgery [1, 8, 9, 24, 29, 41].

In 1990, because we were suspicious of the effect of approximate positioning of the prosthesis in four-part fractures, we performed measured X-rays of both humeri of patients who had undergone shoulder replacement with a Neer prosthesis [2]. We ascertained a poor quality of anatomical reconstruction with regards to length and width after shoulder replacement for fractures. Furthermore, we observed a *correlation between the quality of the anatomical reconstruction and the functional result.* In 1995, we participated in a multicenter retrospective study carried out by the French Orthopedic Society and performed the same measurements on a larger series of 188 patients reviewed at a mean follow-up of 52 months [19]. Our hypothesis that poor functional results are related to poor positioning of the prosthesis in fractures was confirmed by this larger series. These studies reflected what a surgeon might have experienced with the Neer pros-

Table 1. Results of shoulder arthroplasty in proximal humeral fractures according to the literature (na: non available)

Series, years	Number of cases	Mean age (years)	Follow-up (months)	Active Ant. elevation	External rotation	Internal rotation	Painful shoulder (%)
Neer (1970)	43	55	56	5>140° 34:90°–135° 4<90°	na	na	4 (9 %)
Kraulis (1976)	11	65	36	2>140° 9<90°	na	na	9 (81 %)
Tanner (1982)	16	69	38	101°	32°	na	12 (75 %)
Demarchais (1983)	18	59	36	3>140° 4:90°–135° 11<90°	na	na	11 (61 %)
Stableforth (1984)	16	67	60	11>90° 1<45°	8>25° 2<5°	15=T12	2 (12.5 %)
Huten (1986)	34	66	36	90°	10°	na	9 (26 %)
Neer (1988)	61	56	84	51>140° 9:90°–135° 1<90°	na	na	10 (16 %)
Pidhorz (1988)	10	63	18	80°	30°	L4	5 (50 %)
Frich (1991)	15	72	23	77°	17°	na	na
Moekel (1992)	22	70	36	119°	40°	T12	5 (23 %)
Pietu (1992)	21	65	49	109°	44°	L1	14 (66 %)
Green (1993)	20	65	37	110°	31°	L1	7 (35 %)
Hawkins (1993)	19	64	40	72°	16°	L1	11 (58 %)
Compito (1994)	64	62	33	127°	31>50° 22>30°	na	17 (26 %)
Huten et al. (1995)	188	67	52	80°	21°	L1	56 (30 %)

thesis implanted for fractures: the average Constant score, adjusted for gender and age, reached only 65.9 % partly due to fair results for mobility, with a mean anterior active elevation of less than 80°, an external rotation limited to 20° and internal rotation allowing only reaching the sacrum.

Three major technical errors need to be scrutinized because of their frequency and their biomechanical consequences on the glenohumeral joint: (a) tendency to diminution in the epiphyseal width, (b) tendency to shorten or lengthen the humerus, (c) tendency to excessive retroversion.

Tendency To Medialize with a Diminution in the Epiphyseal Width

Rietveld et al. [33] were the first authors to demonstrate a direct relationship between functional results and humeral width: the distance between the geometric center of the humeral head and the lateral border of the greater tuberosity is correlated to glenohumeral abduction. Our studies [2, 19], as others' [17, 21], confirm that there is a tendency to diminish the epiphyseal width, and that the poor active elevation after an hemiarthroplasty for fracture can be partly explained by the decreased lever arm of the deltoid and supraspinatus (Fig. 1). An average diminution of 5 mm (i.e., 10 %) of the humeral width was found in one study [19]. This diminution of humeral width can be explained by insufficient prosthetic head sizes and a tendency to position the prosthesis in valgus which leads to potential poor reconstruction of the greater tuberosity [2, 19].

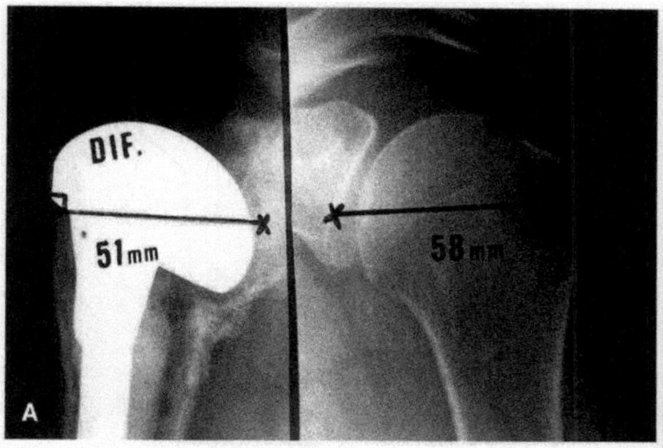

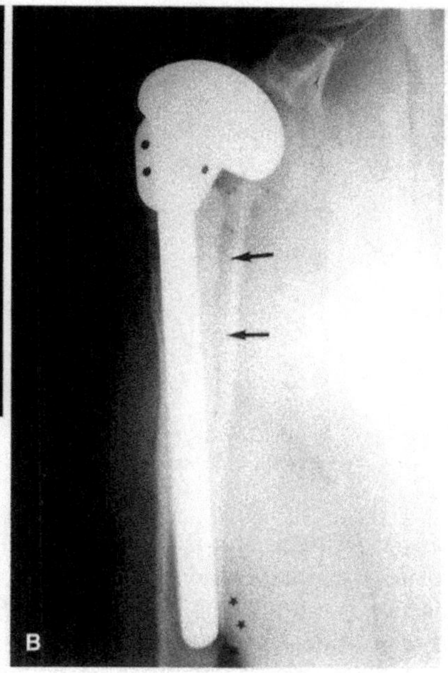

Fig. 1. Tendency to decrease the mediolateral offset of the humerus (**A**) and to implant the prosthesis in valgus (**B**). Notice that the greater tuberosity is not visible and probably migrated behind the prothesis in both cases

Tendency To Shorten or Lengthen the Humerus

Neer emphasized the importance of positioning the shoulder prosthesis with regard to height [26–29]. This positioning is particularly difficult in four-part fractures because the displacement of the tuberosities leads to loss of the proximal bony landmarks. Our studies [2, 19] show that there is a tendency to either shorten or lengthen the humerus (Fig. 2). Unless it is cemented, there is no way to hold and maintain the prosthesis at the correct height: either the prosthetic diameter is too large and the prosthesis has a tendency to be too proud, or it is too small and the prosthesis has a tendency to subside and be too low. Some surgeons have developed "home-made" tips to temporarily block the stem in the medullary canal using a surgical swab wrapped around the implant [41]. This may be helpful, but is not very accurate or reproducible.

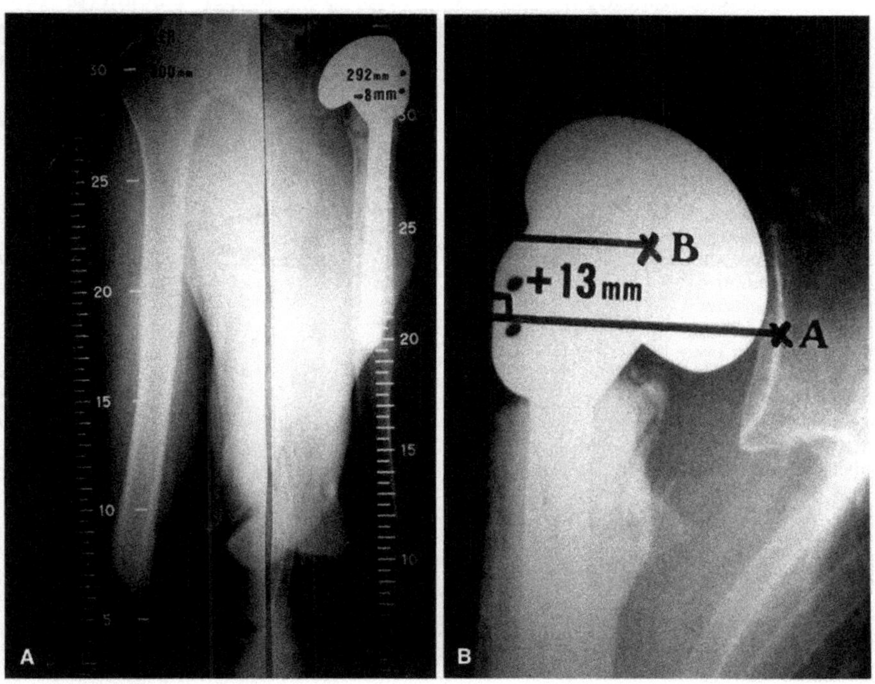

Fig. 2. Incorrect restration of humeral length can only be demonstrated with bilateral scaled X-rays.
A Example of shorten humerus with a low prosthesis (−8 mm).
B Example of lengthen humerus (+13 mm) with a proud prosthesis. Notice again that the greater tuberosity has disapeared because of the executive tensioning on the rotator cuff

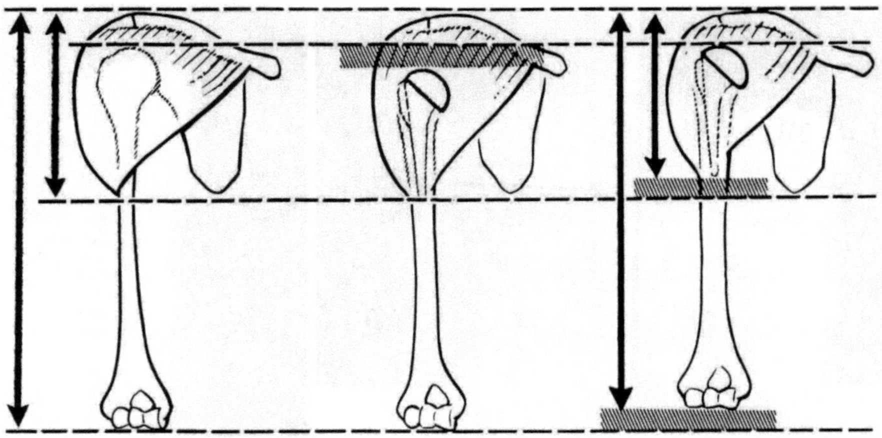

Fig. 3. Shortening of the humerus leads to shortening of the muscular fibers of the deltoid (to pull up the prosthetic head in front of the glenoid), thus decreasing the lever arm for active elevation

Humeral shortening is frequent and is usually due to the tendency to place the prosthesis on the medial part of the diaphysis as a result of the bone loss and the metaphyseal comminution. In an earlier study, 32 % of the prostheses displayed a humeral shortening greater than 10 mm [19]. As a result the muscular fibers of the deltoid are shortened, pulling up the humerus to make the prosthetic head face the glenoid. This permanent contracture of the deltoid and associated muscles can compromise anterior active elevation of the shoulder and explains why the true AP views may look normal, and why measured X-rays of the full humerus are necessary to detect this shortening (Fig. 2 and 3).

Humeral lengthening is also frequent and has even worse consequences, such as pain and limited mobility. The poor functional result is due to the superior humeral migration, leading to anterosuperior impingement (the supraspinatus being squeezed between the prosthetic head and the acromial arch) and nonunion between the greater tuberosity and the diaphysis (Fig. 4).

Tendency to Excessive Retroversion

Surgical publications recommend selecting 30°–40° of retroversion [8, 9, 27, 41]. However, the tendency is to insert the humeral prostheses in even greater retroversion, often over the recommended 40° (Fig. 5A). Prosthetic retroversion selection in four-part fractures can only be approximated and therefore is very often excessive. This is of particular concern as anatomical studies have shown that humeral retroversion is low with an average value of 20° in relation to the transepicondylar axis (Fig. 5B) [3, 7, 23, 32, 38]. Neer himself in one of his first papers on shoulder replacement published in 1955 [26] recommended a lower prosthetic retroversion and wrote: "The surgeon must remember that the normal humeral head faces posteriorly about 20°. The proper amount of retroversion can be reselected daily if the two epicondyles are palpated at the elbow and the head is turned about 20° from their plane."

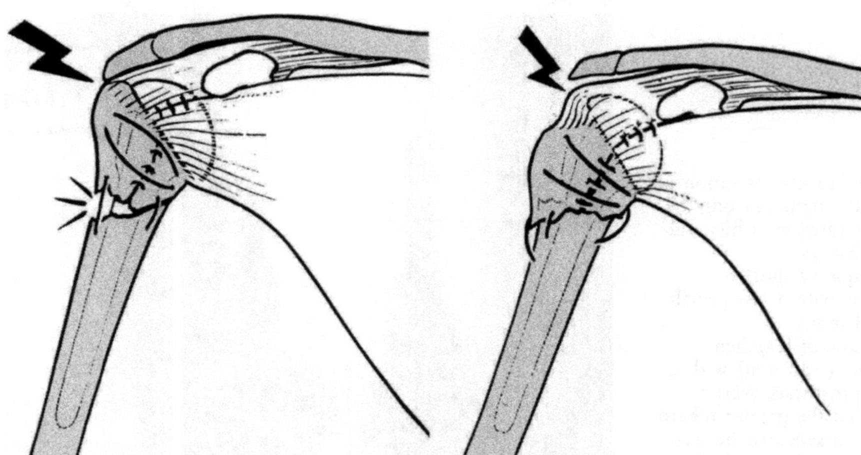

Fig. 4. Lengthening of the humerus because of a too proud prosthesis leads to nonunion between the greater tuberosity and the diaphysis (**A**) or to overtensioning and squeezing the supraspinatus against the coraco acromial arch with anterosuperior impingement (**B**)

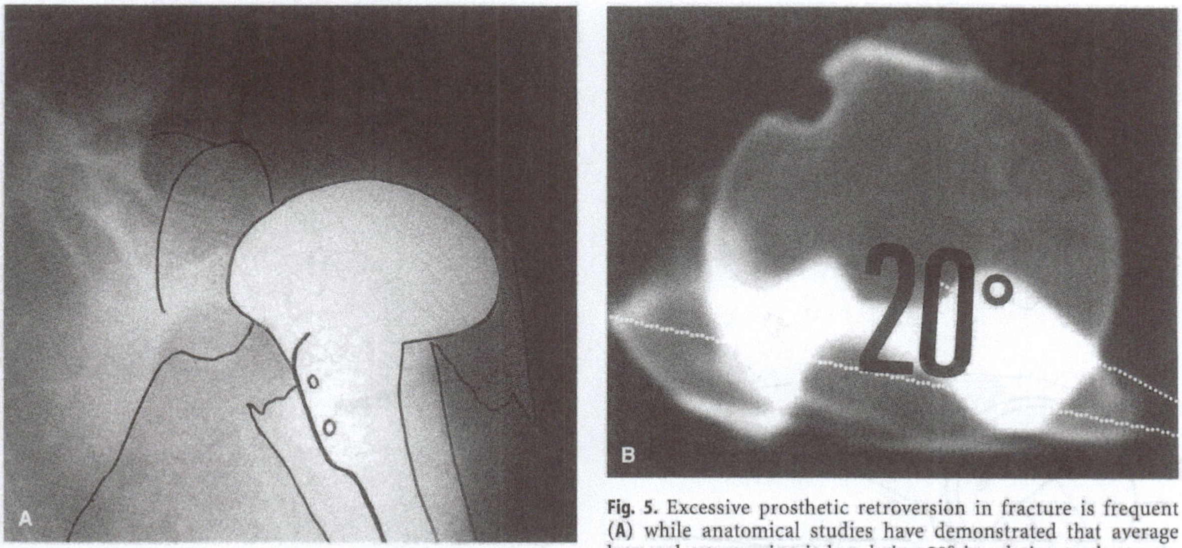

Fig. 5. Excessive prosthetic retroversion in fracture is frequent (**A**) while anatomical studies have demonstrated that average humeral retroversion is low, being 20° in relation to the trans-epicondylar line (**B**)

This excessive prosthetic retroversion is explainable by three independent and sometimes cumulative factors: (a) the fear of anterior dislocation due to the frequent anterior fracture-dislocations, (b) the use of imprecise distal landmarks such as the forearm whose valgus is variable because of a variable carrying angle of about 10° of the forearm [35], and (c) the use of an imprecise proximal landmark: *the bicipital groove.* Placing the prosthetic fin at a distance estimated at 5–10 mm behind the bicipital groove landmark has been proposed to help position the prosthesis and reconstruct the tuberosities [3, 37]. However, the bicipital groove is *not* an accurate landmark in four-part fractures because of the bone loss and the necessity to take into account the lower part of the groove as a surgical landmark. The direction of the bicipital groove is more axial than frontal at the level of the surgical neck. Placing the fin of the prosthesis in relation to the lower part of the bicipital groove (at the level of the surgical neck) leads to increase retroversion (Fig. 6). When the surgeon thinks he is implanting a prosthesis

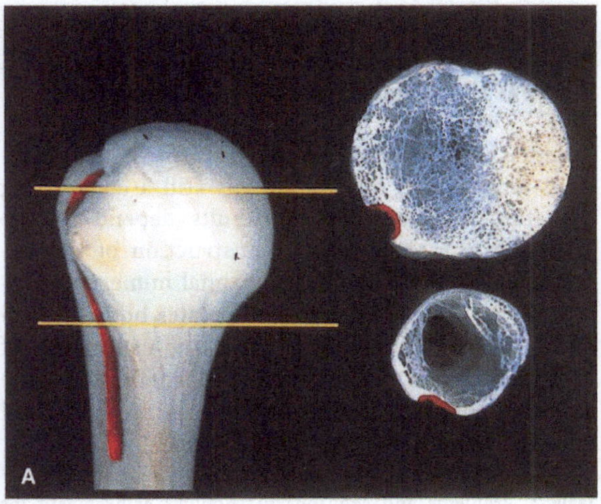

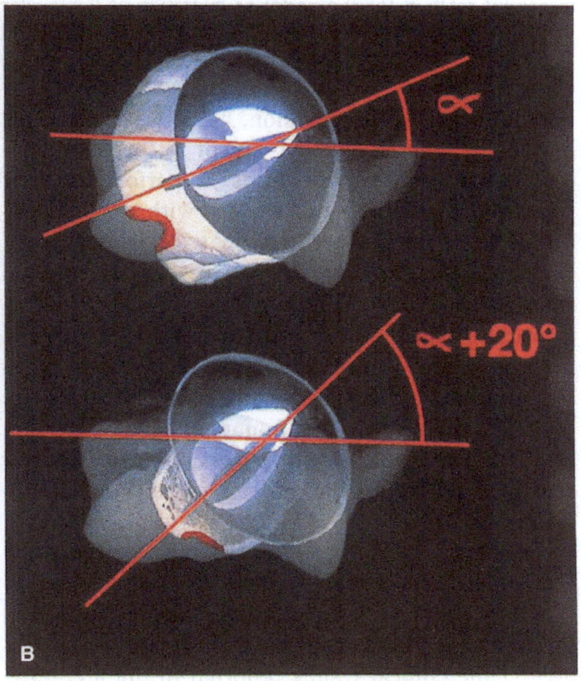

Fig. 6. The bicipital groove is S shaped and is axially oriented in its lower part (**A**). Orienting a shoulder prosthesis in relation to the lower part of the groove increases retroversion about 20° (**B**). Therefore, the bicipital groove is not an acurate landmark for implanting a shoulder prosthesis in fracture, because of the tendency to increase retroversion in this situation

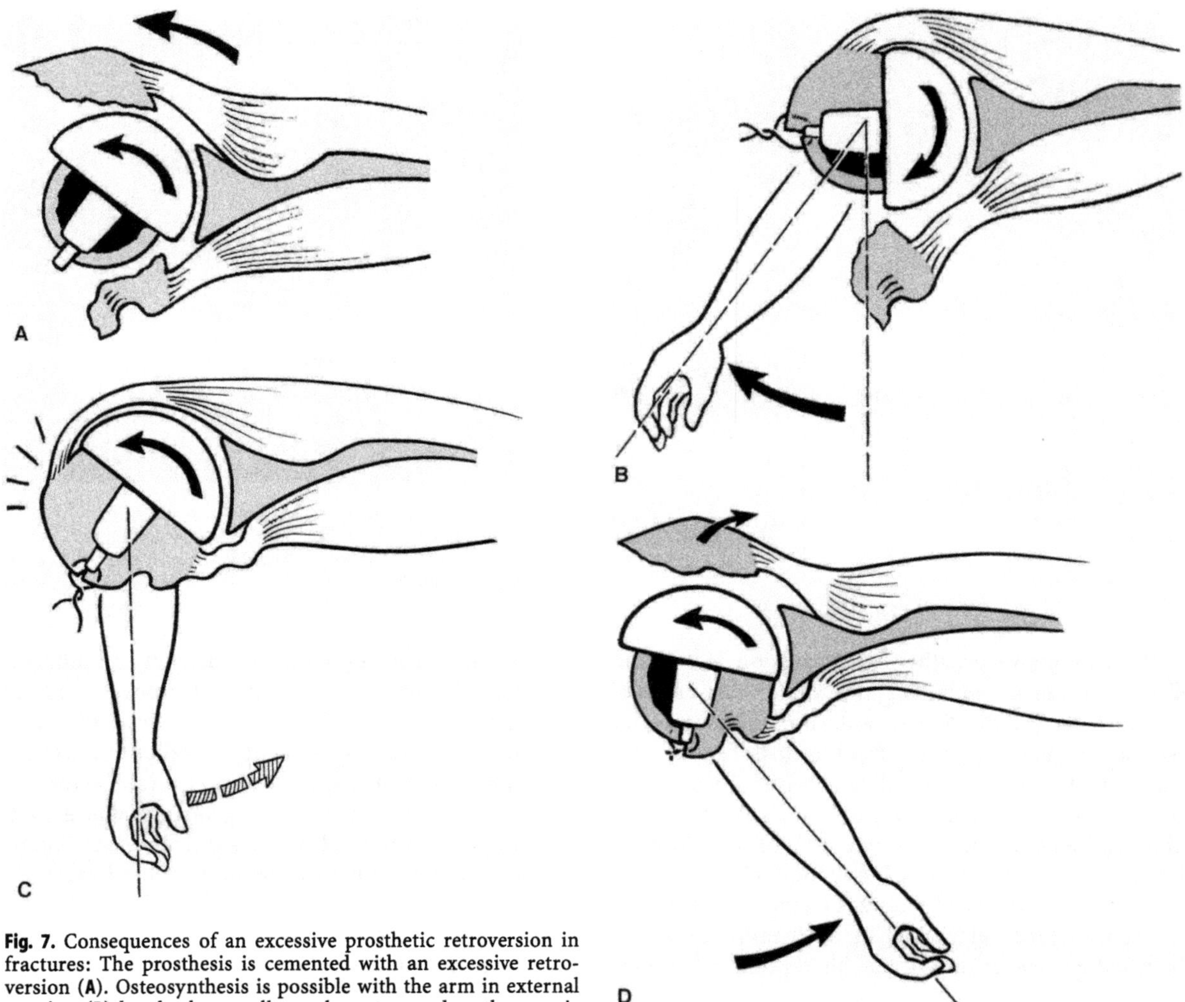

Fig. 7. Consequences of an excessive prosthetic retroversion in fractures: The prosthesis is cemented with an excessive retroversion (**A**). Osteosynthesis is possible with the arm in external rotation (**B**) but leads to pull-out the sutures when the arm is in neutral rotation (**C**) and posterior migration of the greater tuberosity when the arm is placed in internal rotation (arm in a sling at the end of the procedure) (**D**)

with 30 or 40° of retroversion, he is in fact implanting the prosthesis with 50°–60° of retroversion!

Excessive retroversion leads to perform a poor reconstruction of the tuberosities with overtensioning of the posterosuperior cuff. Excessive retroversion makes it necessary to put the arm in external rotation to reconstruct the greater tuberosity. Postoperatively the patients' arm is placed in internal rotation (hand on stomach), which leads to pull-out of the sutures and posterior migration of the greater tuberosity with nonunion and malunion (Fig. 7). This explains why excessive prosthetic retroversion is inadvisable and produces poor clinical results.

In summary, "eye-ball" positioning of the prosthesis explains the poor quality of anatomical reconstruction after humeral head replacement for proximal fractures and therefore the poor and somewhat unpredictable clinical results reported in the literature.

Restoration of the Anatomy Is Possible After Humeral Head Replacement for Proximal Fractures

Recent series in the literature confirm that humeral head replacement for fractures is still a challenging operation and that clinical results depend on the quality of the anatomical reconstruction of the humerus [1, 6–11, 13, 22, 28]. Proximal humeral reconstruction of displaced fractures creates both surgical and technical difficulties because the experience of each surgeon is limited. Table 2 summarizes the authors belief that technical problems can be solved with the help of the innovative surgical solutions:

Table 2. Problems and solutions in shoulder arthroplasty for fracture

Problems	Solutions
Humeral length Humeral retroversion	Aequalis fracture jig
Humeral width	Modular prosthesis

Restoration of Proper Humeral Width

Because of its modularity the Aequalis prosthesis allows the surgeon to preserve the humeral width or mediolateral offset [4–6, 16, 38]. A selection of head sizes allows the surgeon to address any variations in the dimensions of humeral head diameter and thickness that he may encounter. Selection of head size is based on caliper measurement of the fractured head (Fig. 8). Since diameter and thickness are related, the selected head size allows the surgeon to match the original head width. The Aequalis prosthesis also allows the surgeon to restore the average posterior offset of the articular surface by two preselected left and right positions marked on the eccentric dial head. Although the Aequalis prosthesis features several possible head/shaft angles (125°, 130°, 135°, and 140°), in fracture cases the 130° inclination is selected as this corresponds to the average value found in our anatomical work [6, 38]. Finally, the humeral stem must fill the medullary canal by selecting the appropriate diameter (6, 9, 12, or 15 mm).

Restoration of Proper Humeral Length and Retroversion

The Aequalis fracture jig is a new, patented system designed to help surgeons position the humeral implant correctly in both height and retroversion. The principle is simple: a ruler restores the length and a protractor restores the retroversion (Fig. 9). Since proximal anatomical landmarks are rare after a four-part fracture, the epicondyles must be used as they are the only reliable landmarks. Using an intramedullary guide is not a good option because of the "S" shape of the humerus, and because the medullary canal is closed at the level of the elbow.

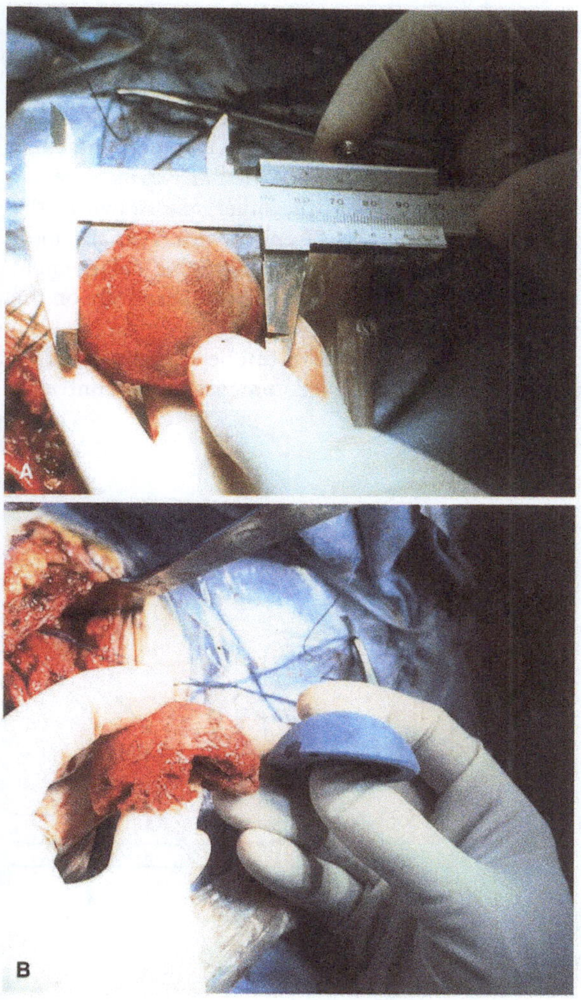

Fig. 8 A,B. Choice of the prosthetic head after measuring the head diameter with a caliper. There is a tendency to chose a prosthetic head which is too large in shoulder arthroplasty for fracture

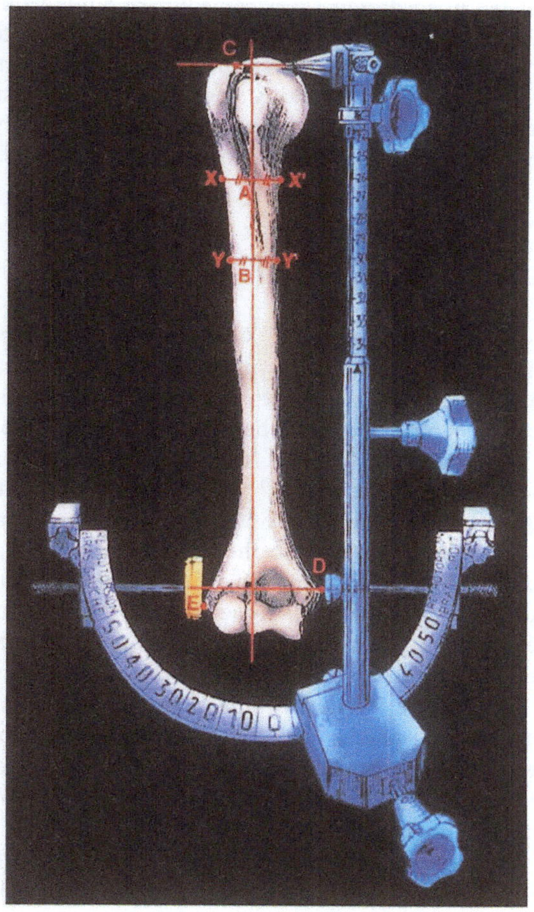

Fig. 9. The Aequalis fracture jig: a sliding ruler restores humeral length and a protractor restores humeral retroversion

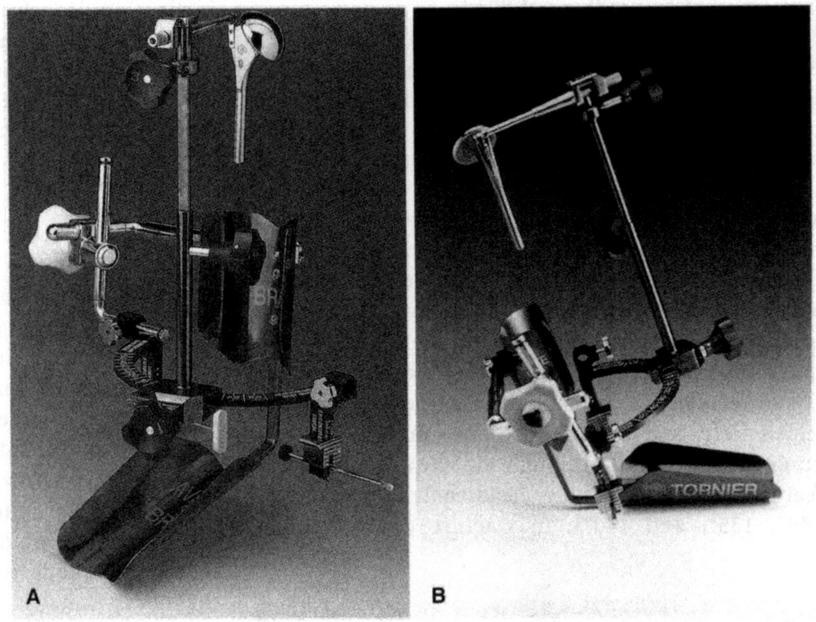

Fig. 10. The arm support of the fracture jig keeps the elbow flexed to avoid sliding of the skin on the bony landmarks (i.e., the two epicondyles) and is connected to the ruler and protractor with two squared linking roads (**A**). The prosthesis is fixed by its fin with the prosthesis holder (**B**)

This led us to design an extramedullary guide using an arm support to hold the elbow in flexion and to avoid the skin slipping over the elbow tuberosities. Two square, angled linking rods connect the arm support to the ruler/protractor assembly. Finally, the prosthesis is connected to the jig by a holder (Fig. 10).

Preoperative Planning

A preoperative calibrated X-ray of the unaffected humerus is essential to determine the humeral length. This X-ray can be taken with the patient erect or supine and must be performed in addition to the standard X-ray of the fractured humerus. The arm is abducted by 45° and the forearm cassette angle must also be 45°. A 100-mm-long magnification marker is taped onto the patient's arm so that radiographic enlargement can be taken into account. The patient must be positioned at 45° in order for the arm to lie flat on the cassette and minimize the risk of error. The preoperative planning must be carefully supervised by the surgeon: a humerus not lying flat on the cassette or a marker taped on the cassette (instead of the patient's arm) can modify the measurement by up to 2–3 cm for a 30-cm-long humerus (Fig. 11).

The humeral length is calculated as follows: The first step is to identify the prosthetic axis by marking the center of the medullary canal at the level of the surgical neck and approximately 10 cm lower. This prosthetic axis corresponds to the stem axis, which is different from the diaphyseal axis. This prosthetic axis is drawn down to the elbow level and up to the humeral head level. Length L' corresponds to the distance between two perpendicular lines: one drawn at the articular surface/greater tuberosity junction and the other one drawn at the most medial extremity of epitrochlea. Actual length (L) takes into account the radiographic enlargement (L=(L'×100/l') and is selected intraoperatively on the fracture jig ruler.

The humeral retroversion can be selected either by measuring on a computed tomogram the contralat-

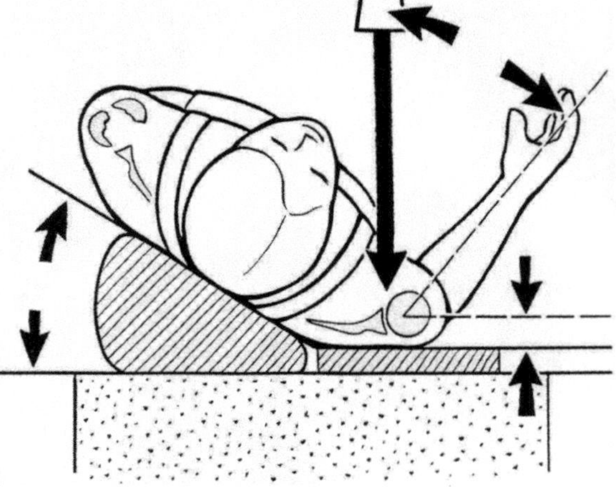

A

Fig. 11. Preoperative planning: humerus should be flat on the cassette (**A**) and markers should be parallel to the humerus (**B**) to allow exact calculation of true humeral length in relation with the prosthetic axis, the greater tuberosity and the medial (**C**)

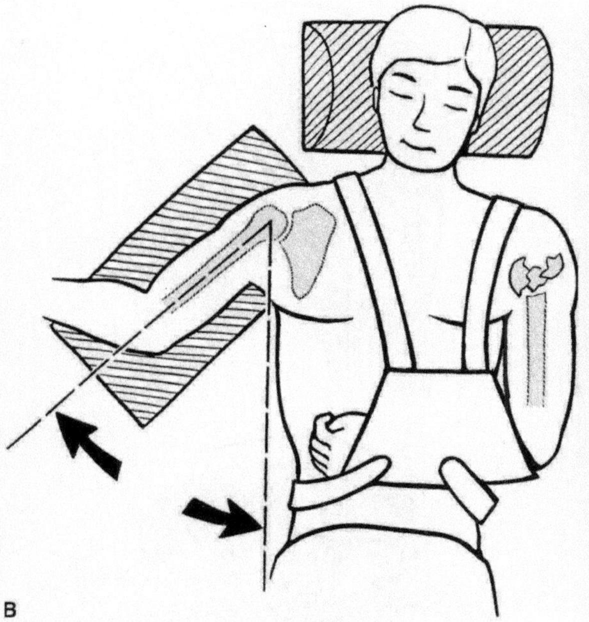

B

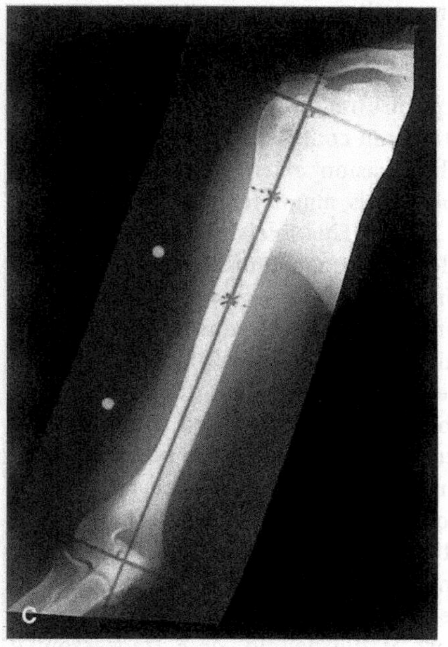

Fig. 11. (continued)

eral humeral retroversion or by choosing 20° as an average value. Our anatomical research demonstrates that retroversion between the left and right arms of the same individual can differ significantly, and that taking the average value of 20° may be a better choice [2, 3, 26].

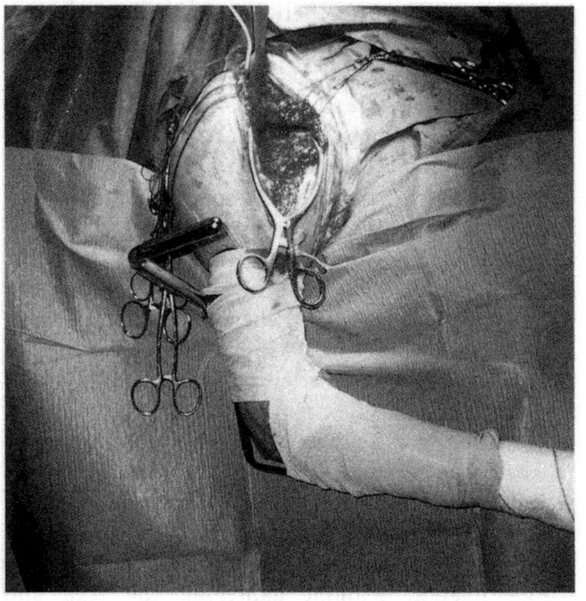

Surgical Technique Using the Aequalis Fracture Jig

The patient is placed in a beach-chair position with the shoulder clear of the table allowing the surgeon to place the arm in full extension so that the medullary canal can be reamed vertically without the coracoacromial arch getting in the way. The arm is positioned into the arm support with the larger linking rod already attached to it (Fig. 12).

Fig. 12. Shoulder is clear of the table to allow full extension and the arm is positioned into the arm support, leaving the elbow free

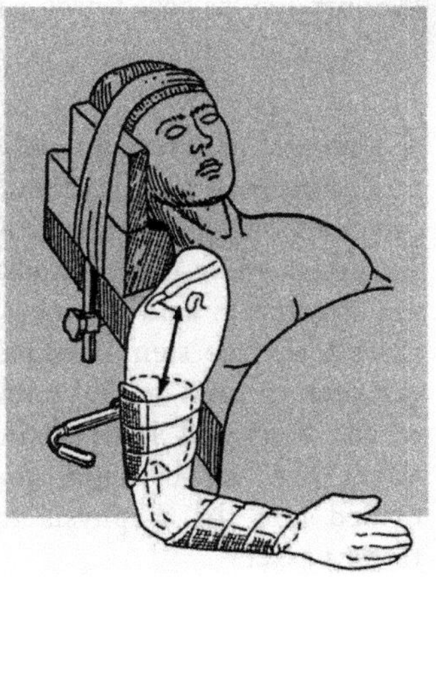

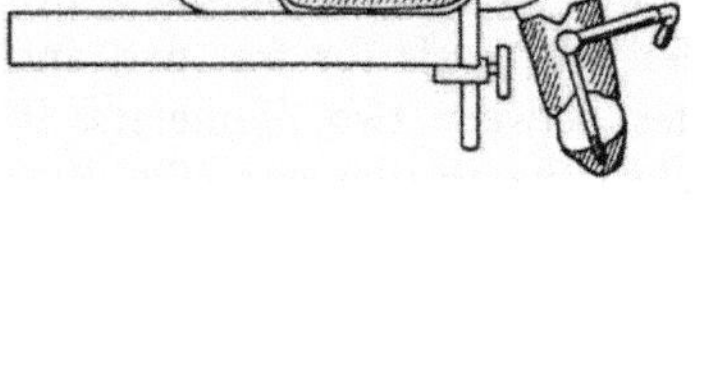

Approach and Preparation

An elongated deltopectoral approach is preferred, and proper exposure requires time and patience so that the operation can continue under optimum conditions [4]. The incision extends from the clavicle down to the pectoralis major tendon, which can be cut for 1 or 2 cm. This incision offers excellent access and allows adequate movement of the arm in abduction/internal rotation or adduction/external rotation, depending on the circumstances. Optimal exposure requires the use of a self-retaining retractor holding the deltoid laterally and the coracobiceps medially. A Homman retractor placed above the coracoid and a curved retractor on the acromion provide optimal retraction of the anterior part of the deltoid. The coracoacromial ligament should be preserved since it can be used as a landmark for length and avoids anterosuperior instability. Alternatively, an anterosuperior approach, through the anterior and medial part of the deltoid, or a transacromial approach are also possible ("cuff approaches").

Manipulation of the tuberosities should be minimized (Fig. 13). Once the biceps tendon has been found, the fracture site between tuberosities is identified and is usually posterior to the bicipital groove. If the two tuberosities are still attached to the diaphysis, this periosteal bridge must be preserved. The joint can be opened either by cutting longitudinally the rotator interval anteriorly or by dividing longitudinally the fibers of the supraspinatus posteriorly. The greater or lesser tuberosity is then retracted and the rotator interval opened up to the coracoid process. The long head of the biceps can be preserved, particularly when the bicipital groove is intact; however, it is sometimes necessary to carry out a tenodesis after resection of the intra-articular portion.

Horizontal sutures are inserted around the greater tuberosity at the bone-tendon junction, with the arm placed in abduction-internal rotation. A temporary suture is inserted around the lesser tuberosity, again at the bone-tendon junction, to obtain a strong fixation without damaging the frail and osteoporotic bone. The tuberosities are then gently retracted, "opening the book," and the humeral head is removed after resection of the capsular attachments. The glenoid is examined for defects or erosion. Verification of the capsule is carried out: any capsular tear or "Bankart lesion" should be sutured to avoid further instability. The diameter of the humeral head is measured with a caliper. There is a tendency to choose too big a prosthetic head in shoulder prosthesis for fracture, and if the surgeon hesitates between two diameters, it seems preferable to select the smaller one (Fig. 8).

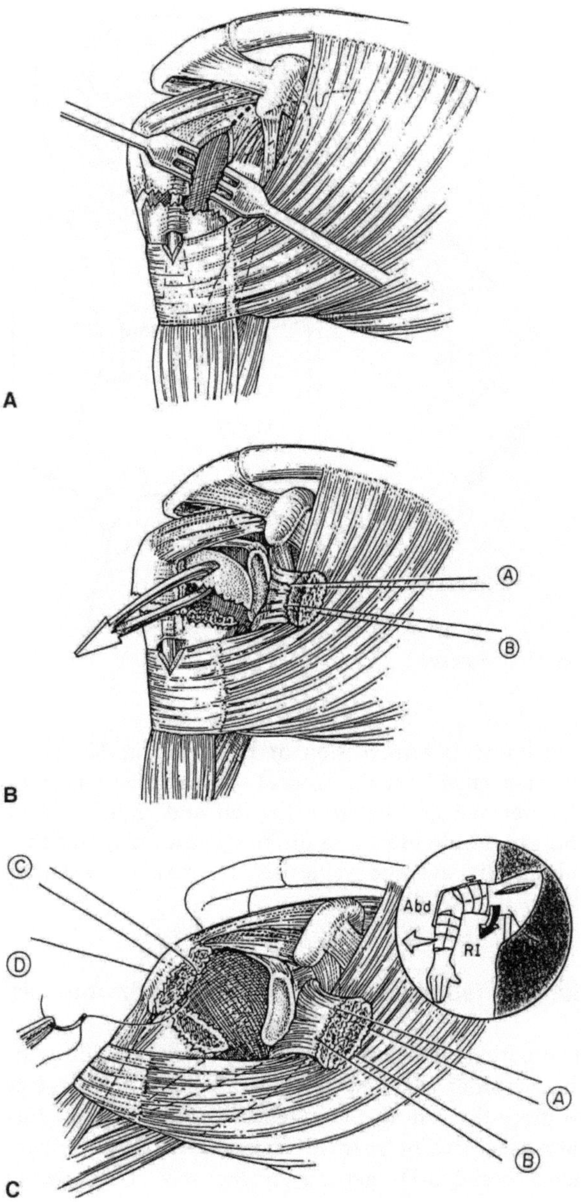

Fig. 13. Mobilization of the tuberosities: opening the rotator interval (**A**), removing the humeral head (**B**), and inserting the sutures at the bone-tendon junction (**C**)

Humeral preparation can begin, which allows the trial prosthesis to be chosen. The medullary canal is prepared using a cylindrical reamer of increasing diameters while the tuberosities are gently retracted, and the arm is held in extension. The trial implant is assembled: the stem diameter corresponding to the last reamer used, a 130° neck, a head corresponding to the fractured head diameter and assembled in either the left or right position. Four holes are drilled into the diaphysis to allow vertical sutures to be passed.

Insertion of the Trial Prosthesis with the Fracture Jig

The precise positioning of the humeral prosthesis for length and retroversion is performed with the help of the Aequalis jig. An average retroversion of 20° is selected by using *handle number one* while *handle number two* selects the preoperatively determined height (Fig. 14 A,B). The trial implant is attached to the prosthesis holder (left or right) and to the jig using *handle number three* (Fig. 14 C,D). The trial implant attached to the jig is gently inserted into the humeral shaft with the arm placed in extension and external rotation while still gently retracting the tuberosities. By placing the arm in flexion the prosthesis, with the jig in place, is reduced into the glenohumeral joint before attempting any positioning (Fig. 15).

Once the prosthesis is reduced into the joint cavity, the epicondylar guides can be positioned by the surgeon. The small round blue guide is the height landmark and must be placed over the epitrochlea. The rectangular yellow guide is the retroversion landmark and is placed over the lateral epicondyle (Fig. 16). This step is essential and determines the correct position of the prosthesis. In the case of a fat elbow or difficulty in palpating the bony landmarks, fluoroscopic control should be used to verify the position of the epicondylar guides. Once this position is acceptable, the assistant can assemble and tighten the two yellow linking rods, using *handle number four* (Fig. 17).

Fig. 14. After selecting humeral retroversion with handle (no. 1 (**A**) and humeral length with handle no. 2 (**B**), the prosthesis is fixed on the prosthesis holder to the jig with handle no. 3 (**C,D**)

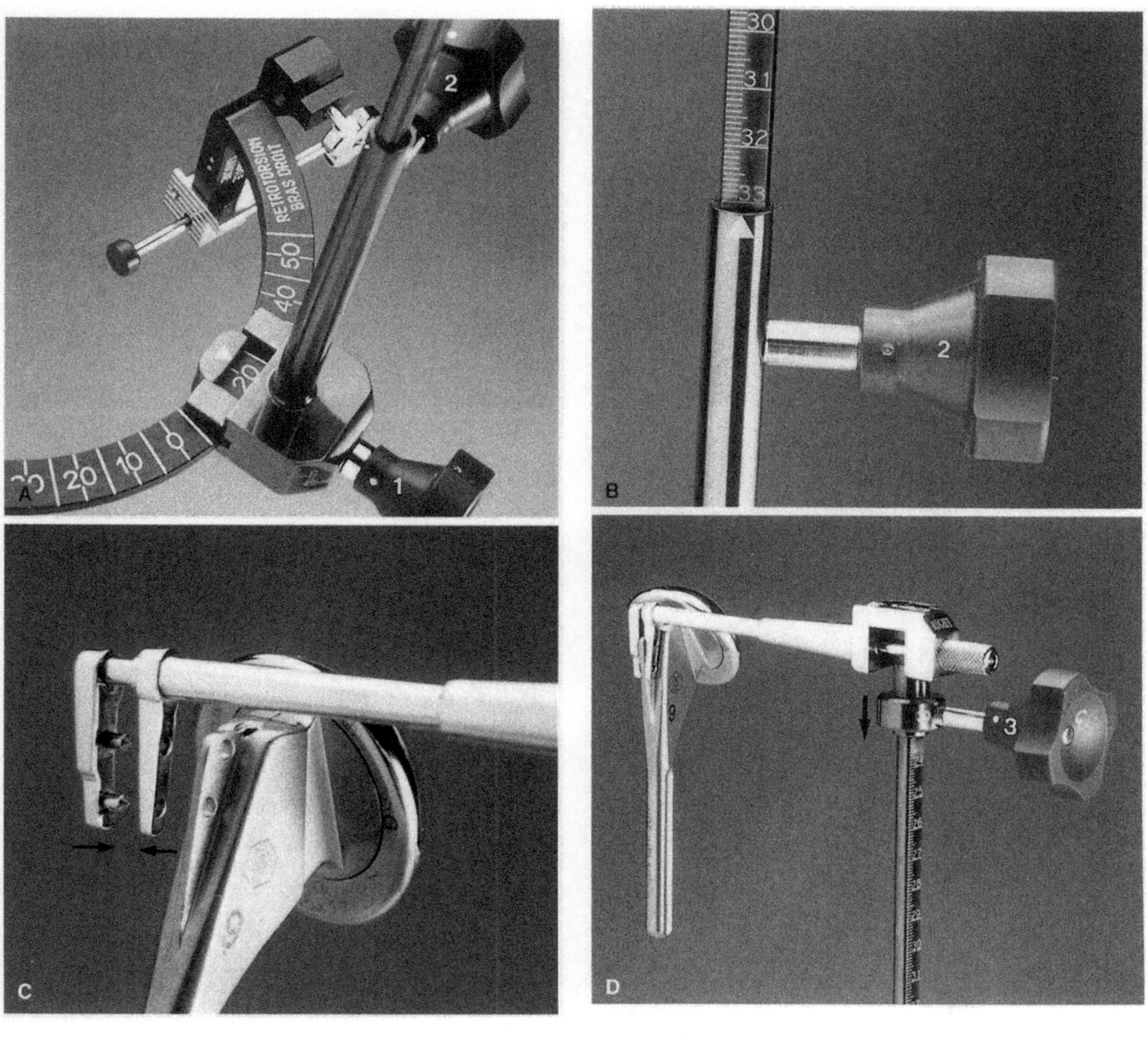

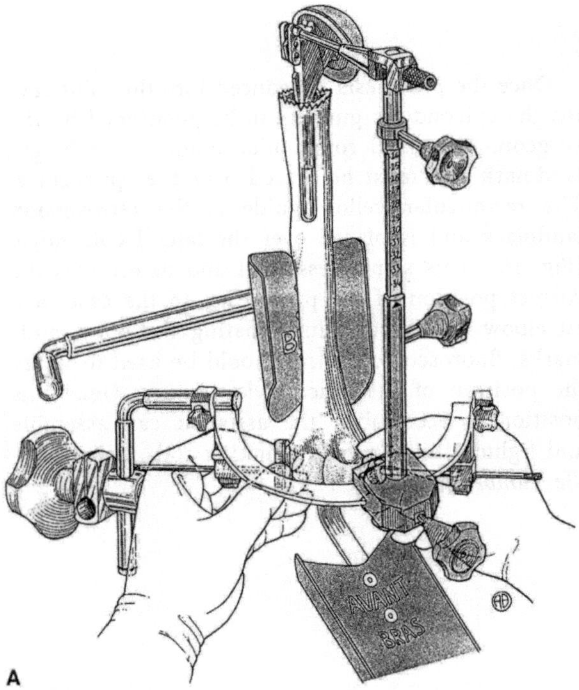

A

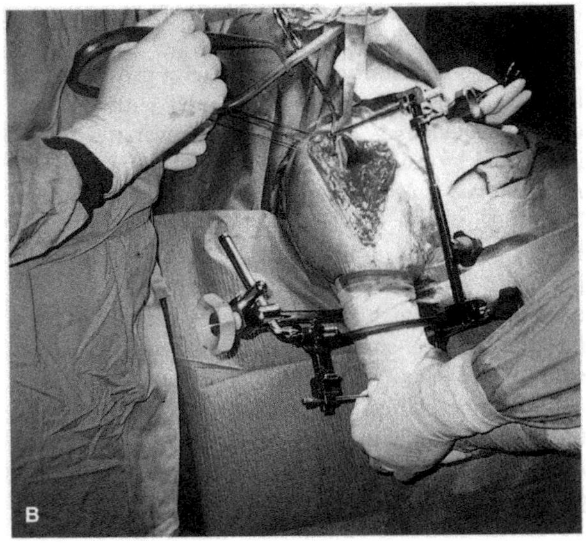

B

Fig. 15. The prosthesis is inserted in the medullary canal and reduced into the joint cavity (**A**) before looking for the bony landmarks of the elbow and connecting the two linking roads (**B**)

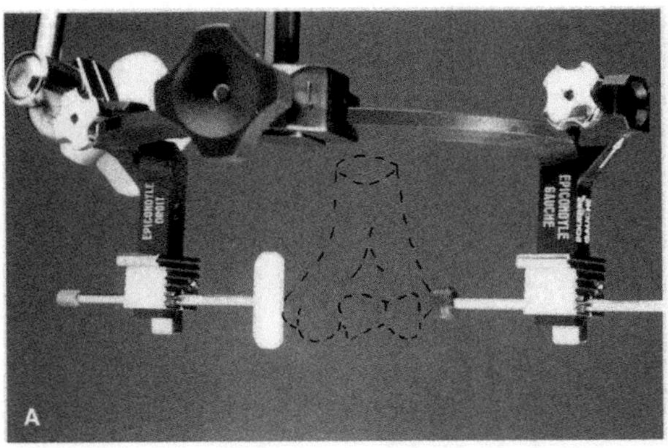

A

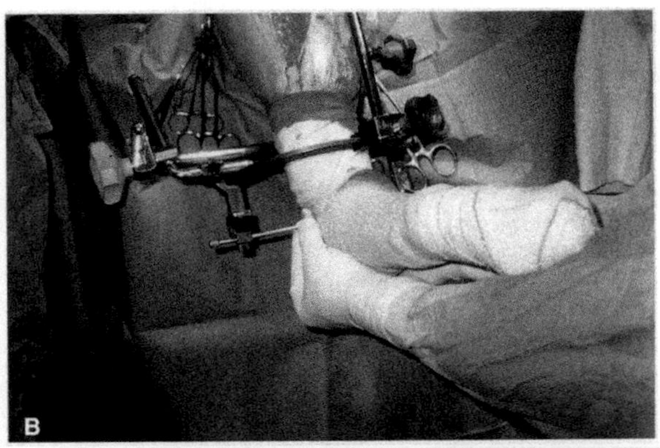

B

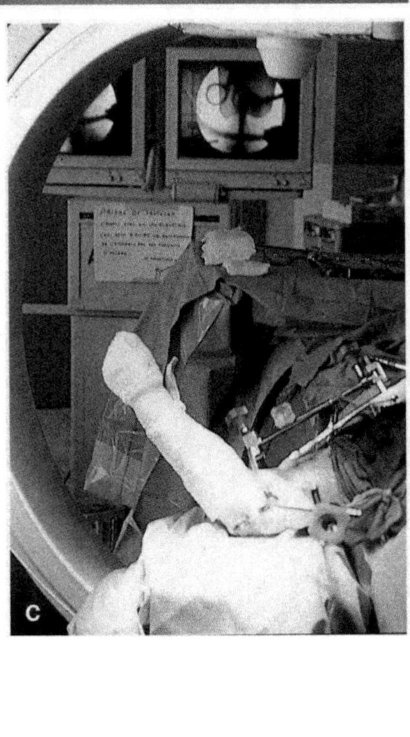

C

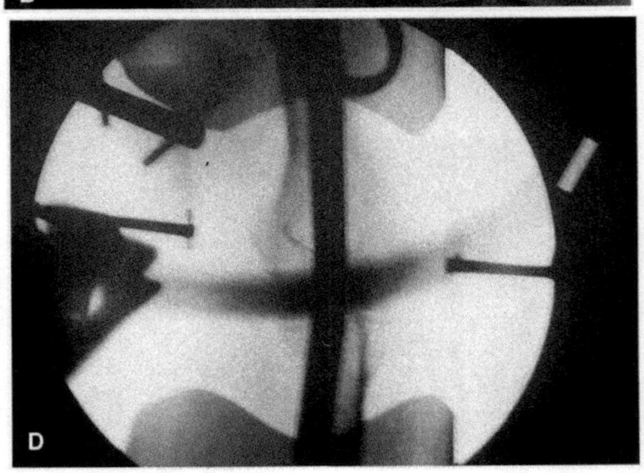

D

Fig. 16. Accurate positioning of the epicondylar guides (note that the two epicondyles are at different levels) is made by palpation (**A,B**) and under fluoroscopic control if needed (**C,D**)

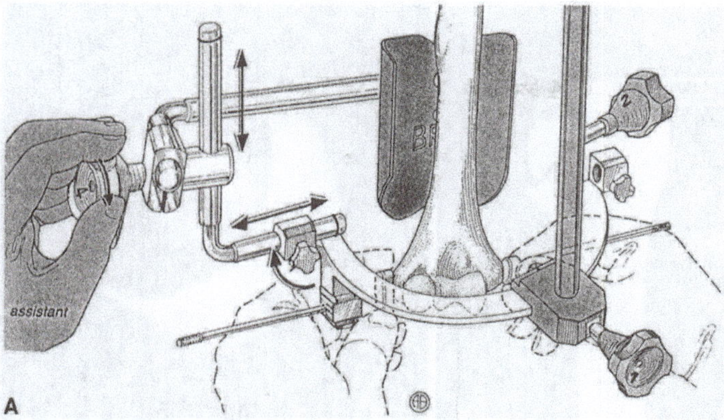

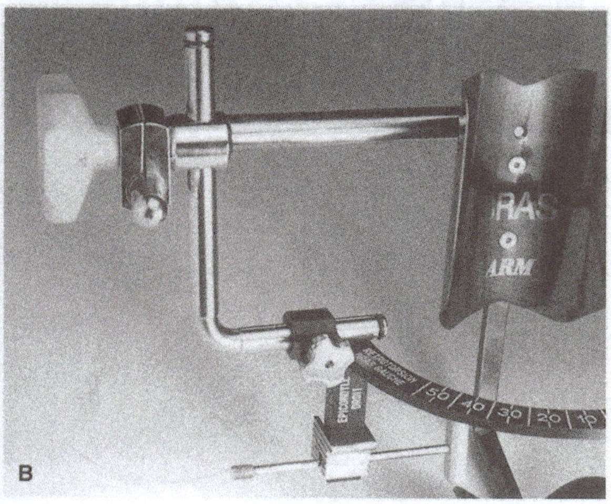

Fig. 17. The two linking roads are connected together with handle no. 4, giving a very stable device

Verification of the Proper Prosthesis Position

The prosthesis position can then be verified more easily as the prosthesis is stable and is, theoretically, maintained at the correct height and retroversion (Fig. 18). Once the prosthesis has been reduced into the joint, the greater and lesser tuberosities are placed alternatively under the prosthetic head to check their positioning (Fig. 19).

Proper humeral head width is usually not a problem as long as the head size has been correctly selected and stem retroversion is correct without valgus placement. The stem is usually well centered in the shaft when the neck-stem is in contact with the medial cortical diaphysis.

Evaluation of proper humeral length is carried out using the following five criteria:

- There must be no gap or overlapping between the greater tuberosity and the diaphysis (sometimes remnants of periosteal tissue help to asses the accuracy of the reduction).

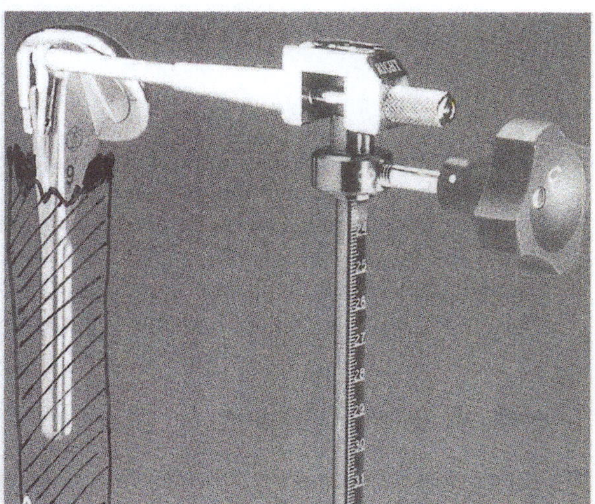

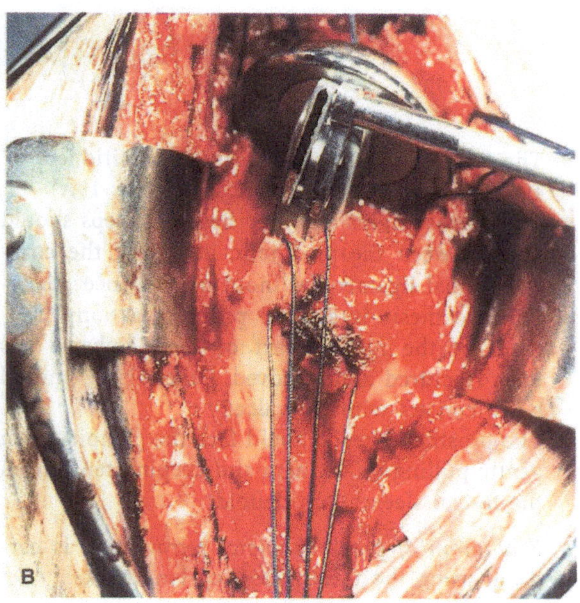

Fig. 18. Accurate positioning of the prosthesis for length and retroversion (A) together with stabilization of the prosthesis in proper position allows accurate reconstruction of the tuberosities (B)

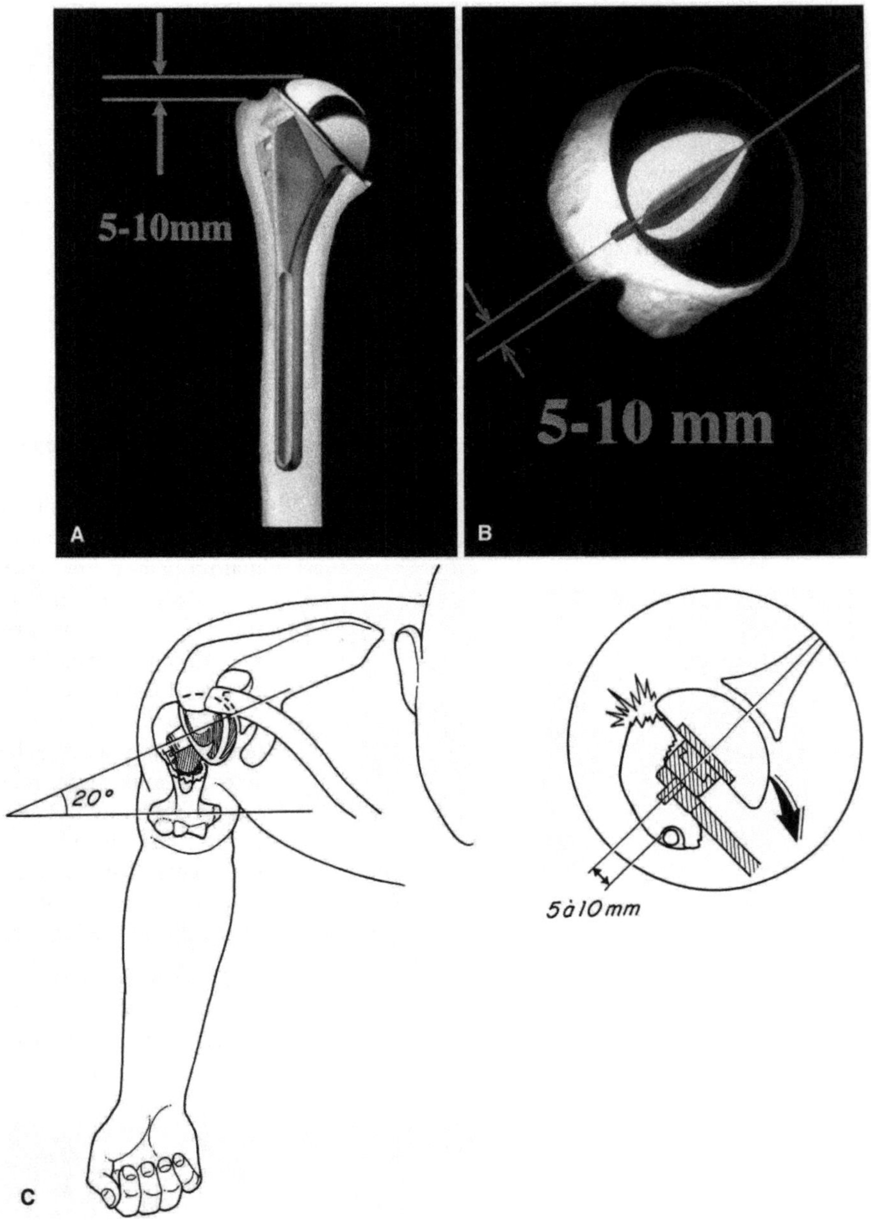

Fig. 19. Checking for anatomical restoration of the proximal humerus: the prosthetic head should be positioned 5–10 mm higher than the greater tuberosity (**A**) and the prosthetic fin must be positioned 5–10 mm behind the upper part of the bicipital groove (**B**). This corresponds to an aproximate retroversion of 20° related to the transepicondilar axis and 30° related to the fore-arm (**C**)

- The greater tuberosity must be positioned 5–10 mm below the prosthetic head (Fig. 19A).
- The supraspinatus and long head of biceps should pass between the prosthetic head and the coracoacromial ligament, without being squeezed.
- The prosthesis is slightly proud if a bony fragment of the medial part of the diaphysis has been fractured and removed. Otherwise it should be in contact with the calcar.
- The prosthetic head should face the glenoid when gently pulling on the arm and keeping tension on the fascial sleeves and deltoid.

Evaluation of proper humeral retroversion is carried out using the three following landmarks:

- When the arm is placed in neutral rotation, the prosthetic head must face the glenoid.
- The prosthetic fin must be positioned 5–10 mm behind the bicipital groove (Fig. 19B).
- The metaphyseal and diaphyseal parts of the bicipital groove must be aligned without "zig-zag."

Cementing the Definitive Prosthesis

If all the parameters are acceptable, the final implant can be cemented while the jig is kept in place attached to the arm. After having put the arm in extension to keep the prosthesis outside the wound, the trial implant is replaced by the final implant, using *handle number three.* The implant is cemented after the diaphysis has been plugged distally by a cement restrictor. While the implant is inserted into the medullary canal, the prosthesis holder is inserted in the ruler. Again, the prosthesis is reduced into the joint with the jig in place. The sutures must be inserted into the diaphysis before cementing to allow vertical reattachment of the tuberosities.

For the following reasons the authors recommend cementing the prosthesis in fracture cases: (a) The patients are often very elderly and osteoporotic with a large medullary canal with little or no cancellous bone and very thin cortical bone. (b) The prosthesis cannot be held by the tuberosities since they are fractured. (c) A "press-fit" prosthesis limits the ability to place the prosthesis at the correct height, with the tendency to position it too high.

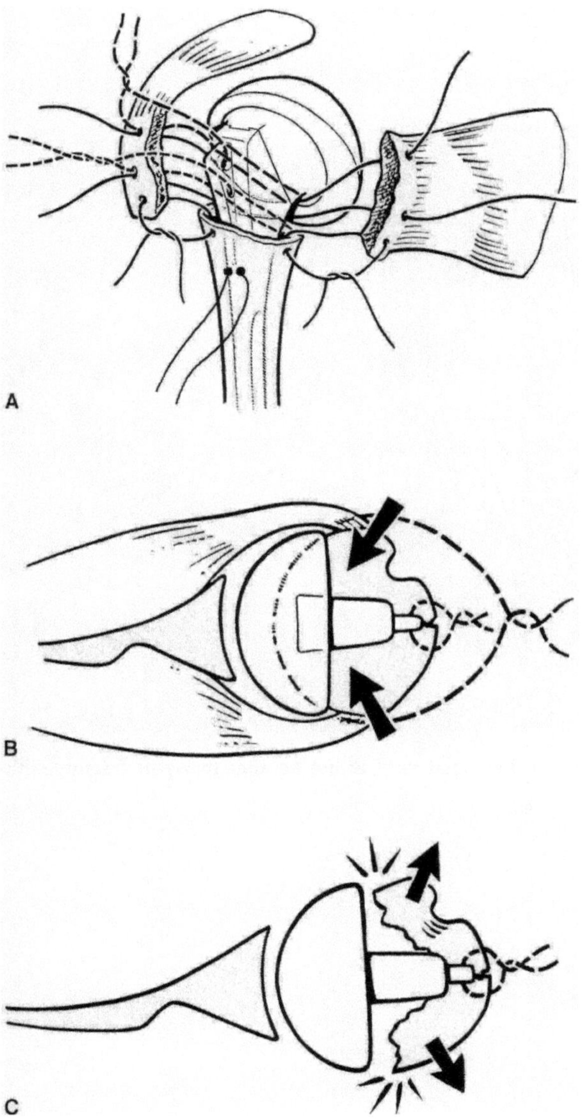

Fig. 20. The tuberosities should be secured with both horizontal and vertical sutures starting with the greater tuberosity (**A**). The horizontal sutures should not only be placed in the prosthetic fin but around the prosthetic neck to allow better stabilization and healing of the bone fragments (**B**). Passing the sutures in the fin of the prosthesis does not provide enough stability for healing of the bony fragments (**C**)

Reconstruction of the Tuberosities

This critical step of reconstruction of the tuberosities must be carefully performed (Fig. 20). The reconstruction is in two steps, attaching the greater tuberosity first, using anatomical landmarks (top of the greater tuberosity 5–10 mm below the prosthetic head, bicipital groove 5–10 mm in front of the prosthetic fin) to optimally reconstruct the upper part of the humerus.

Reconstruction of the tuberosities begins with the greater tuberosity using two horizontal sutures and one vertical suture. Placing the horizontal sutures in the prosthetic fin does not provide enough stability for the synthesis of the tuberosities. This is the reason why we recommend that the horizontal sutures be placed around the prosthetic neck to position the greater tuberosity correctly under the prosthetic head and to provide a more stable synthesis. The vertical suture between the greater tuberosity and the diaphysis is inserted in a "figure 8" manner into the fracture line to adjust the reduction to the optimal position and avoid any sliding and overlapping of the pieces of bone.

The next step is reconstruction of the lesser tuberosity, again using two horizontal sutures and one vertical suture. The two remaining sutures, initially tightened around the greater tuberosity, are inserted into the subscapularis tendon from inside to outside, allowing the lesser tuberosity to be drawn back under the prosthetic head. A vertical suture is also inserted between the lesser tuberosity and the diaphysis using the same "figure 8" technique.

A final vertical tightening is performed utilizing the two remaining sutures in the diaphysis using a tension band technique (Fig. 21). Passive elevation and external rotation is then checked to verify the stability of the reconstruction which allows early postoperative rehabilitation. Postoperative X-rays and the functional result demonstrates the quality of the humeral reconstruction (Fig. 22 and 23).

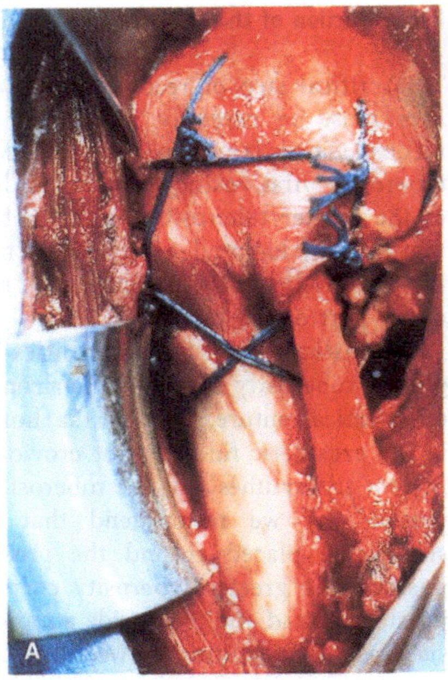

Fig. 21. Intraoperative view showing the vertical sutures in the diaphysis using a tension band technique and the correct alignement of the biceps and the bicipital groove (**A**). Incorrect alignement of the long head of the biceps and the groove is a witness of incorrect reduction of the tuberosities and/or incorrect retroversion of the prosthesis

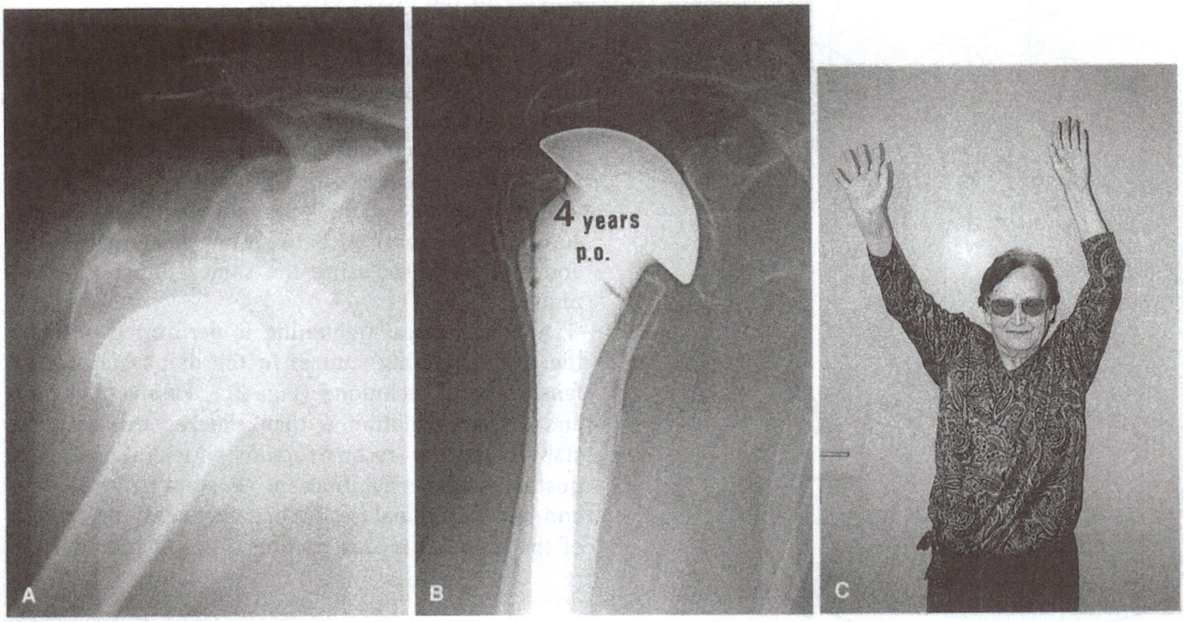

Fig. 22 A–C. Example of humeral reconstruction using the Aequalis prosthesis and the fracture jig after four-part fracture with anterior dislocation
A Preop-X-Ray: 4 part dislocated fracture
B Anatomical reconstruction and healing of the tuberosities
C Functional result

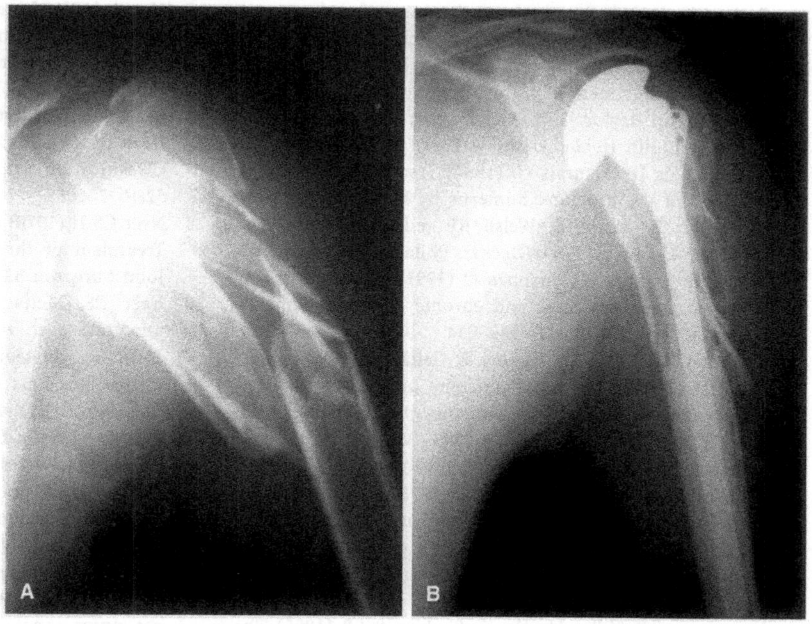

Fig. 23 A,B. Another example of reconstruction of the proximal humerus using the fracture jig. **(A)** Preop-X-Ray demonstrates a complexe metaphyso-diaphysal fracture. **(B)** Post-op X-Ray demonstrates the accuracy of the surgical reconstruction with restoration of humeral height and correct positioning of the greater tuberosity

Conclusion

The authors' philosophy of prosthetic shoulder reconstruction in fracture cases is based upon the following consideration: inaccurate articular reconstructions yield poor results. This is especially true in the shoulder joint. Because of the "eye-balling" of shoulder prosthesis positioning in fractures tuberosity reconstruction until now has been very approximate. Not surprisingly, clinical results were often poor and unpredictable. Shoulder prosthesis for a fracture should be considered as an "augmented osteosynthesis." This means that priority should be given to precise positioning of the prosthesis with regard to width, height, and retroversion, which allows anatomical reconstruction of the tuberosities.

The modularity of the Aequalis shoulder prosthesis allows the surgeon to restore the mediolateral offset (humeral width) by optimized filling of the medullary canal and by accurate selection of the articular surface diameter and thickness. The Aequalis fracture jig, which consists simply of a ruler and a protractor, allows the surgeon to correctly preserve the two other major parameters required for exact reconstruction of the proximal humeral anatomy: humeral height and retroversion. The Aequalis fracture jig minimizes the subjective assessment of the surgeon, whose experience may be often limited, allowing better positioning of the prosthesis and therefore better reconstruction of the tuberosities. By offering an instrument which is sufficiently simple and reliable, a reproducible technique for fracture reconstruction has been created. As no surgeon would now consider implanting a knee prosthesis without the appropriate jig, we believe the same course should be followed when using a prosthesis for shoulder fractures.

References

1. Bigliani LU, Flatow EL, McCluskey, Fischer RA (1991) Failed prosthetic replacement for displaced proximal humeral fractures. Orthop Trans 15:747–748
2. Boileau P, Chau E, Perraud M, Arcamone H, Argenson C (1993) Restoration of humeral length and humeral offset after shoulder prosthesis for fractures. Rev Chir Orthop 73:150
3. Boileau P, Walch G, Mazzoleni N, Urien JP (1993) In vitro measurement of humeral head retroversion. J Shoulder Elbow Surg 2(2):S12
4. Boileau P, Huten D (1995) Technique chirurgicale des prothèses de Neer pour fractures céphalo-tubérositaires. Rev Chir Orthop 81 [Suppl II]:85–88
5. Boileau P, Walch G (1996) Prothèses d'épaule pour fractures: problèmes et solutions. Maîtrise Orthopédique 6:18–23
6. Boileau P, Walch G (1997) Three dimensional geometry of the proximal humerus: implications for the surgical technique and prosthetic design. J Bone Joint Surg Br 79B:857–865
7. Broca P (1881) La torsion de l'humérus et le tropomètre, instrument destiné à mesurer la torsion des os (rédigée par L Mamouvier). Rev Anthrop 2(4):193–210, 385–423, 1577–1592
8. Compito CA, Self EB, Bigliani LU (1994) Arthoplasty and acute shoulder trauma, reasons for success and failure. Clin Orthop 307:27–36

9. Craig EV (1989) Prosthetic replacement for four part fractures of the proximal humerus. Tech Orthop 3:70–80
10. De Anquin CE, De Anquin CA (1982) Prosthetic replacement in the treatment of serious fractures of the proximal humerus. In: Bayley JL, Kessel L (eds) Shoulder Surgery. Springer, Berlin Heidelberg New York, pp 207–217
11. DesMarchais JE, Maurais G, (1984) Treatment of complex fractures of the proximal humerus by Neer's hemiarthroplasty. In: Bateman JE, Welsh RP (eds) Surgery of the shoulder. Mosby, St Louis/Decker, Philadelphia, pp 60–63
12. Frich LH, Sojberg JO, Sneppen O (1991) Shoulder arthroplasty in complexe acute and chronic proximal humerus fractures. Orthopaedics 14:949–954
13. Goldman RT, Koval KJ, Cuomo F, Gallagher MA, Zuckerman JD (1995) Functional outcome after humeral head replacement for acute three-and four-part proximal fractures. J Shoulder Elbow Surg 4(2):81–86
14. Green A, Barnard WL, Imbird RS, Providence RI (1993) Humeral head replacement for acute four-part proximal humerus fractures. J Soulder Elbow Surg 2:249–254
15. Hawkins RJ, Switlyk P (1993) Acute prosthetic replacement for severe fractures of the proximal humerus. Clin Orthop 289:156–160
16. Harryman DT, Sidles JA, Harris SI, Lippitt SB (1995) The effect of articular conformity and the size of the humeral head component on laxity and motion after glenohumeral arthroplasty: a study in cadavera. J Bone Joint Surg Am 77:555–563
17. Hsu HC, Wu JJ, Chen TH, Lo WH, Yang DJ (1993) The influence of a abductor lever-arm changes after shoulder arthroplasty. J Shoulder Elbow Surg 2:134–140
18. Huten D, Duparc J (1986) L'arthroplastie prothétique dans les traumatismes complexes récents et anciens de l'épaule. Rev Chir Orthop 72:517–529
19. Huten D, Boileau P, Bonnevialle P, Maynou C, Renault E, Vogt F, Postel JM, Candelier G, Fleure P (1996) Résultats et indications de l'arthroplastie prothétique dans les fractures récentes complexes de l'extrémité supérieure de l'humérus. Conférences d'Enseignement de la SOFCOT Expansion Scientifique Française, Paris, pp 125–140
20. Ianotti JP, Gabriel JP, Schneck SL, Evans BG, Miras S (1992) The normal glenohumeral relationships. An anatomical study of one hundred and forty shoulders. J Bone Joint Surg Am 74:491–500
21. Jacobson SR, Mallon WJ (1993) The glenohumeral offset ratio: a radiographic study. J Shoulder Elbow Surg 2, 3:141–146
22. Kraulis J, Hunter G (1977) The results of prosthetics replacement in fractures dislocations of the upper end of the humerus. Injury 8:129–131
23. Khral VE, Evans FG (1945) Humeral torsion in man. Am J Phys Anthrop 3:229–253
24. Muldoon MP, Cofield RH (1997) Complications of humeral head replacement for proximal humeral fractures. Instruct Course Lect 46:15–24
25. Moeckel BH, Dines DM, Warren RF, Altchek DW (1992) Modular hemiarthroplasty for fractures of the proximal part of the humerus. J Bone Joint Surg Am 74:884–889
26. Neer CS III (1955) Articular replacement of the humeral head. J Bone Joint Surg Am 37:215–228
27. Neer CS (1970) Displaced proximal humeral fractures. I. Classification and evaluation. J Bone Joint Surg Am 52:1077–1089
28. Neer CS II (1970) Displaced proximal humeral fractures. II Treatment of three and four part displacement. J Bone Joint Surg Am 52:1090–1103
29. Neer CS, McIlven SJ (1988) Remplacement de la tete humérale avec reconstruction des tubérosités et de la coiffe des rotateurs dans les fractures déplacées à 4-fragments. Résultats actuels et technique. Rev Chir Orthop 74 [Suppl II]:32–40
30. Pidhorz G, Saint-Cast Y, Grobost J, Boscher Y (1988) Traumatismes sévères récents de l'extrémité supérieure de l'humérus. Apport de la prothèse humérale (9 observations). Ann Orthop Ouest 20:31–37
31. Pietu G, Deluzarches P, Goin F, Letenneur J (1992) Traumatismes complexes de l'extrémité supérieure de l'humérus traités par prothèse céphalique: à propos de 21 cas revus avec un recul moyen de 4 ans. Acta Orthop Belg 58:159–169
32. Roberts SNJ, Foley APJ, Swallow HM, Wallace WA, Coughlan DP (1991) The geometry of the humeral head and the design of protheses. J Bone Joint Surg Br 73:647–650
33. Rietveld ABM, Dannen HAM, Rozing PM, Oberman WR (1988) The lever arm in gleno humeral abduction after hemi arthroplasty. J Bone Joint Surg Br 70:561–565
34. Stableforth PG (1984) Four part fractures of the neck of the humerus. J Bone Joint Surg Br 66:104–108
35. Steel FLD, Tomlinson JDW (1989) The carrying angle in man. J Anat 92:315–317
36. Tanner MW, Cofield RH (1983) Prosthetic arthroplasty for fractures and fracture dislocations of the proximal humerus. Clin Orthop 179:116–128
37. Tillett E, Smith M, Fulcher M, Shanklin J (1993) Anatomic determination of humeral head retroversion: the relationship of the central axis of the humeral head to the bicipital groove. J Shoulder Elbow Surg 2:255–256
38. Walch G, Boileau P (1991) Morphological study of the proximal humerus. J Bone Joint Surg Br 74 [Suppl I]:14
39. Willems WJ, Lim TEA (1985) Neer arthroplasty for humeral fractures. Acta Orthop Scand 56:394–395
40. Young TB, Wallace A (1985) Conservative treatment of fractures and fracture-dislocation of the upper-end of the humerus. J Bone Joint Surg Br 77:373–377
41. Zuckerman JD, Cuomo F, Koval KJ (1997) Proximal humeral replacement for complex fractures: indications and surgical technique. Instruct Course Lect 46:7–14
42. Zyto K, Kronberg M, Brostrom LA (1995) Shoulder function after displaced fractures of the proximal humerus. J Shoulder Elbow Surg 4:331–336

Preoperative Planning and the Use of the Fracture Jig

P. Boileau and G. Walch

Summary

The mistakes in positioning humeral components in height and retroversion have immediate or secondary consequences on the synthesis and union of the tuberosities. Our studies have demonstrated that tuberosity migrations are the main reason for failures in shoulder arthroplasty for 4-part fractures and that these tuberosity migrations are the consequence of poor prosthesis positioning leading to tuberosity malunion, nonunion and bone resorption. In order to decrease the mistakes in prosthesis positioning, we have designed a fracture instrumentation, i.e., the Aequalis fracture jig which allows to control humeral height and retroversion. This paper describes the preoperative planing and summarizes the use of the Aequalis fracture jig.

Introduction

Preliminary clinical studies had convinced us that our anatomical reconstructions using a shoulder replacement were insufficient in four-part displaced fractures of the proximal humerus [2, 4, 5] Because of this, we have designed and developed a fracture instrumentation which allows precise positioning of the humeral component with regard to height and retroversion: the Aequalis fracture jig (Tornier).

The Aequalis Fracture Jig

The Aequalis fracture jig is a totally original and patented system which is provided to assist the surgeon in inserting a shoulder prosthesis and to allow a precise match *of humeral height* and *humeral retroversion* (Fig. 1).

The principles are very simple: a *ruler* is needed to restore the humeral height and a *protractor* is needed to restore the humeral retroversion. The absence of landmarks at the proximal level, because of the fracture, had orientated us to choose the landmarks of the elbow.

Fig. 1. a The Aequalis fracture jig. **b** Details of the Aequalis fracture jig

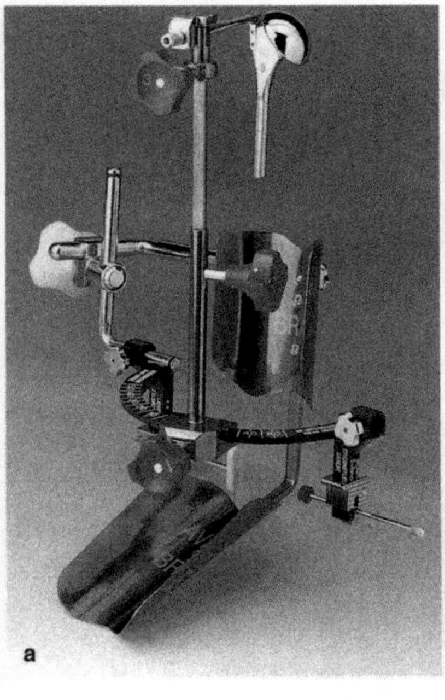

a

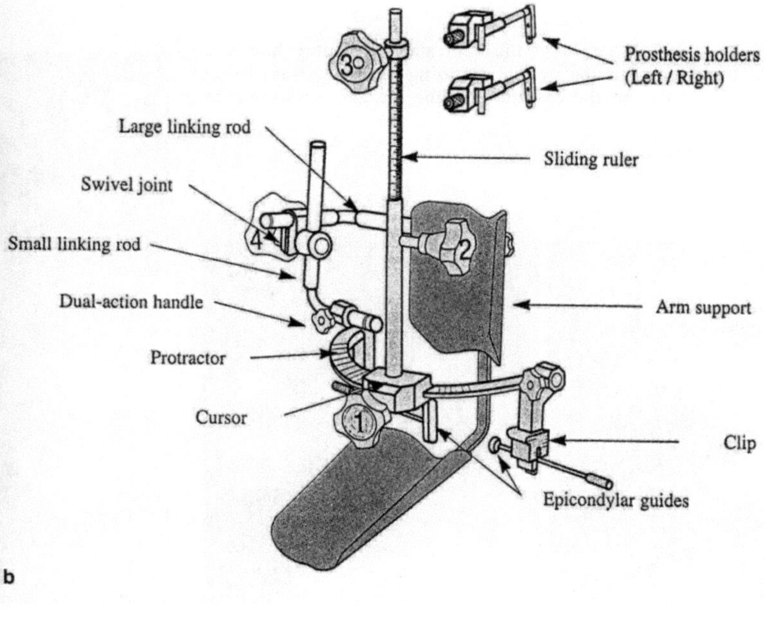

b

The other three parts of the fracture jig are:

- *The arm support* which keeps the elbow flexed and enables the prominence of the lateral and medial epicondyle to be identified, while preventing the skin from sliding over these prominence and giving false landmarks.
- *A prosthesis holder*, attached to the prosthetic fin.
- *Two squares* which allow to connect the arm-support with the ruler and protractor.

Preoperative Planning

In addition to an AP view, a lateral view and an axillary view of the injured shoulder (the trauma series of Neer), a scaled X-ray of the healthy contralateral humerus is needed.

The humeral height is predetermined using this scaled X-ray of the contra-lateral *healthy* humerus. A true anteroposterior radiograph of the humerus is needed. The humerus is positioned in neutral rotation with respect to the thorax and abducted 45°. The anteroposterior radiograph in the plane of the scapula is obtained by positioning the scapula flat on the cassette and aiming the beam at the joint. The beam makes a 45° angle with the cassette. A centimeter marker adjacent to the lateral humerus helps correct for radiographic magnification. The X-ray can be taken with the patient standing or lying (Fig. 2).

Measurement of the humeral height is determined by plotting the *prosthetic axis* (center of the proximal medullary canal) followed by the two perpendiculars to this axis: above, the tangent at the top of the greater tuberosity and below, the middle of the medial epicondyle (Fig. 3).

Details of the radiograph should be controlled by the surgeon himself to avoid false measurements: this is why we usually perform this scaled X-ray in the operating room just before starting the surgery. Many mistakes can be done: a humerus not positioned flat on the cassette (Fig. 4a) and/or a centimeter marker not adjacent to the humerus can give a false measurement by increasing humeral length (Fig. 4b).

The humeral retroversion is fixed at 20° from the mean value measured in our anatomical studies [3, 5, 6]. Intraoperative determination of prosthetic retroversion is impossible because of the disappearance of the usual landmarks: the humeral anatomical neck and/or the bicipital groove. Until now the totally approximate choice of retroversion depended on the experience of the surgeon. The usual tendency was to overretrovert the prosthesis, altering the centers of rotation and resulting in abnormal biomechanical situations.

Furthermore, the surgical literature usually recommended 35°–40° of retroversion for the humeral component. Our anatomical studies have shown that humeral retrotorsion is variable and certainly very much less: it seems reasonable to con-

Fig. 2 a,b. Scaled X-rays of the contralateral healthy humerus can be taken with the patient standing or lying. Notice that the arm is flat on the cassette and the marker is adjacent to the humerus

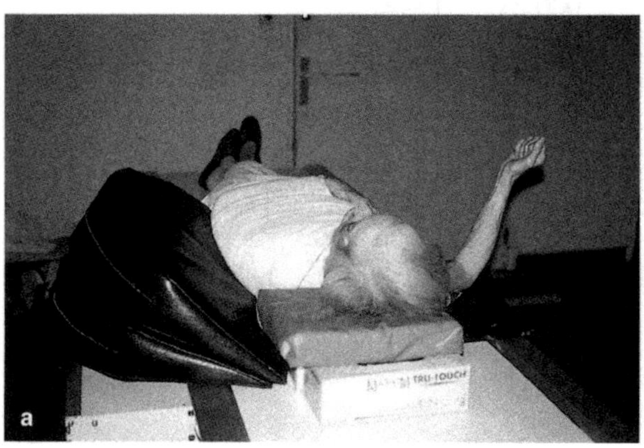

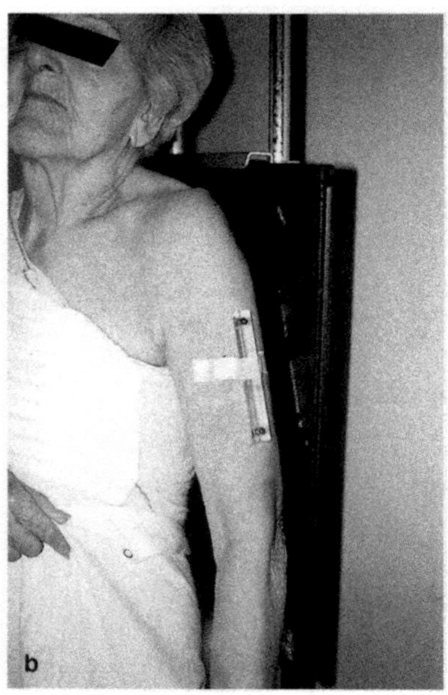

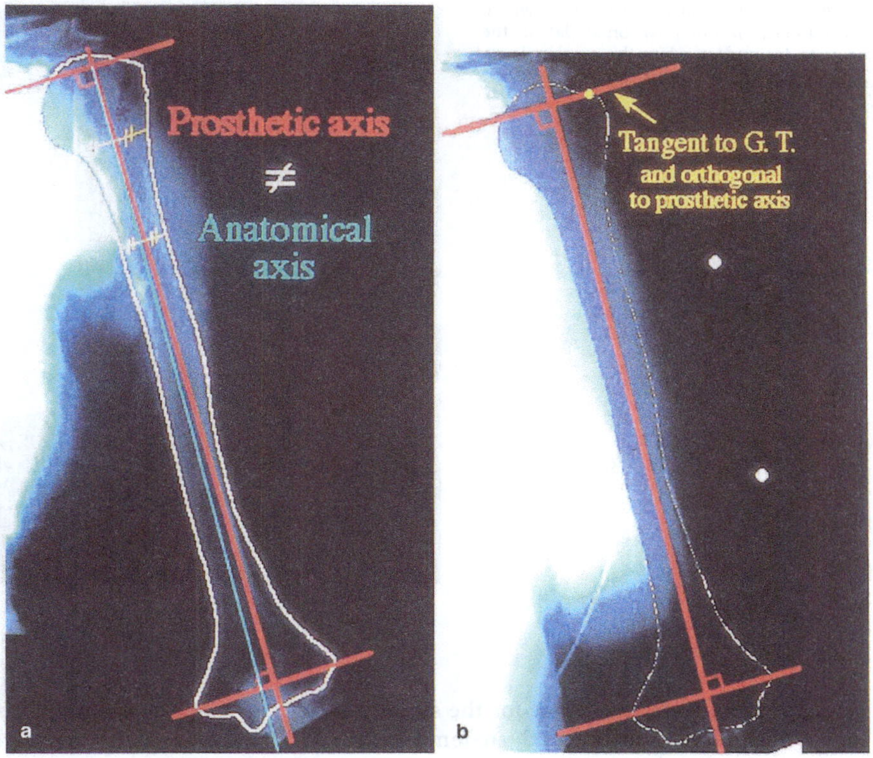

Fig. 3 a–d. Calculation of humeral length by taking into account the radiological magnification: The prosthetic axis (which is different from the anatomical axis) is plotted. **a** Two lines orthogonal to the prosthetic axis and tangent to greater tuberosity (**b**) and to medial epicondyle (**c**) are plotted. The X-ray magnification is taken into account with the metal markers

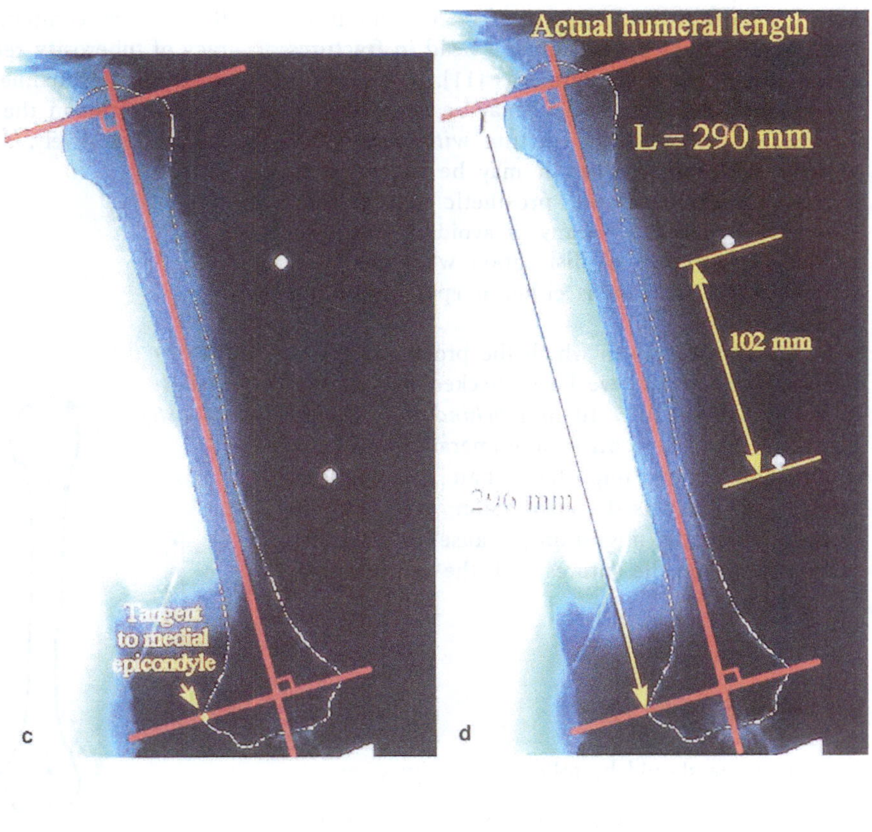

Fig. 3 c–d. (continued)

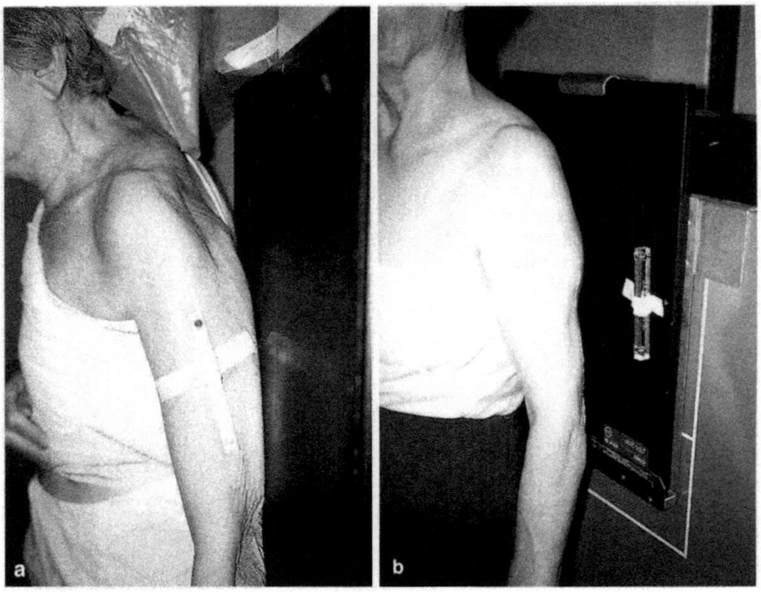

Fig. 4. False humeral measurements when the humerus is not positioned flat on the cassette (**a**) and/or when the marker is not adjacent to the humerus (**b**)

sider 20° as the reference value for the surgeon seeking to restore normal humeral anatomy [3, 6, 12]. This low retroversion had already been shown by older anatomical studies (Broca 1881; Khral 1944) and corresponds to the value recommended by Neer in its original publication of 1955 on the prosthetic replacement of the humeral head in fractures of the upper end of the humerus [11].

Obviously, this value of 20° may be modulated in the presence of a 4-part fracture *with anterior or posterior dislocation*, when it may be necessary to increase or decrease the prosthetic retroversion. This may represent a means of avoiding the postoperative recurrence of dislocation when the joint detachment or fracture is either irreparable or not repaired.

In the usual cases in which the prosthetic retroversion is set at 20°, we have checked that the fin of the prosthesis in 5–10 mm *behind the bicipital groove* [4, 5]. The control of humeral retroversion is probably more important than the humeral height: any increased retroversion will lead to greater tuberosity migration because of excessive pulling forces on the sutures with the arm in internal rotation.

Use of the Fracture Jig

The technique should be followed step by step:

- **Step 1: Preoperative planing:** As mentioned previously, a scaled X-ray of the healthy contralateral humerus should be taken with a ruler, taking into account the radiographic magnification. If the scaled X-ray has not been performed preoperatively, we still use the fracture instrumentation at least to control the retroversion and to stabilize the humeral component while checking the accuracy of tuberosity reconstruction. In this case, we make an approximate measurement of the humeral height on the healthy humerus and adapt it intraoperatively.

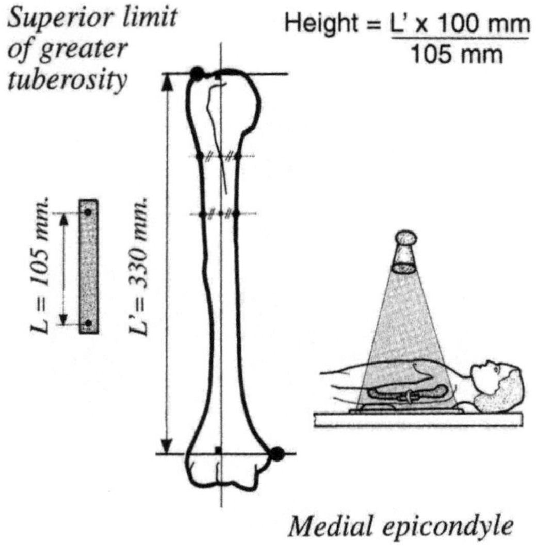

- **Step 2: Patient positioning:** The patient is in the beach-chair position, with the arm placed into its support and the whole shoulder free of the table to allow complete arm extension.

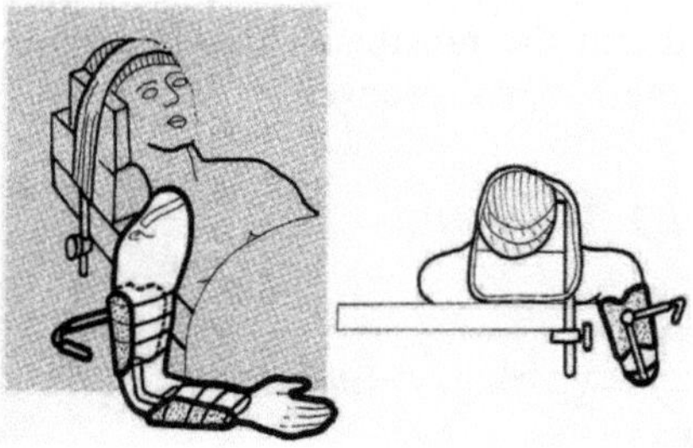

- **Step 3: Adjusting the retroversion and the height:** The retroversion usually chosen is 20° while the humeral length is predetermined using the preoperative measurements.

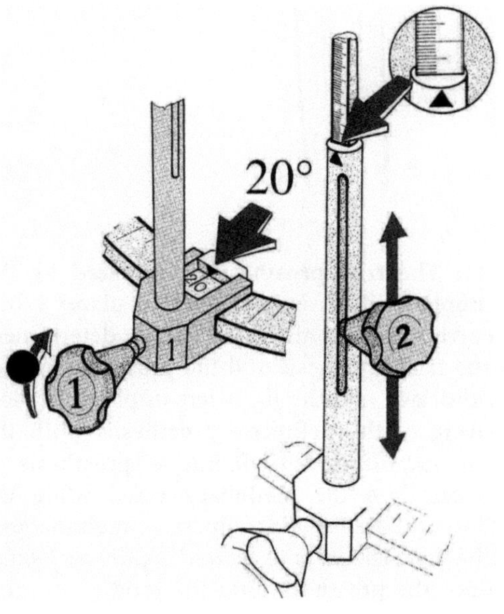

- **Step 4: Passing sutures through the tendon:** Stitches are passed through the subscapularis tendon and infraspinatus tendon.

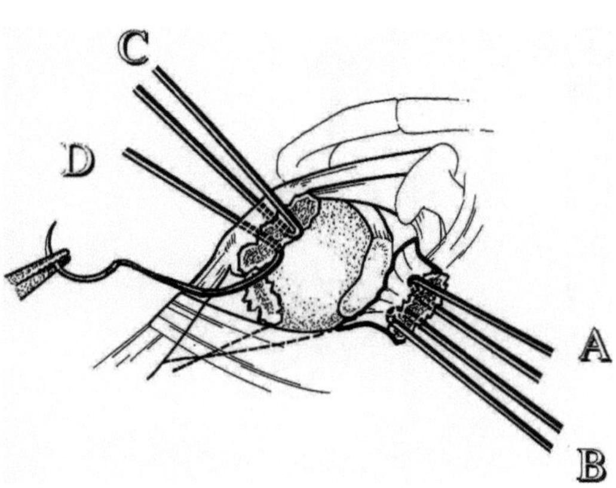

- **Step 5: Humeral reaming:** Cylindrical reamers of increasing sizes (6, 9, 12 mm) are advanced with the *arm in extension.*

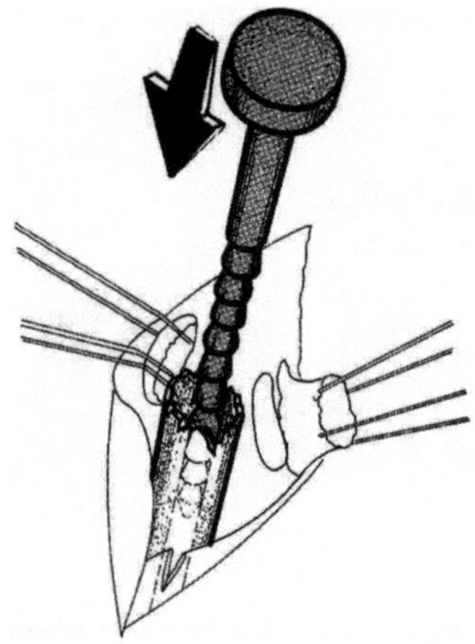

- **Step 6: Attachment of the trial implant to the jig:** The trial prosthesis is secured by its fin to the prosthesis holder which is fully inserted into the ruler.

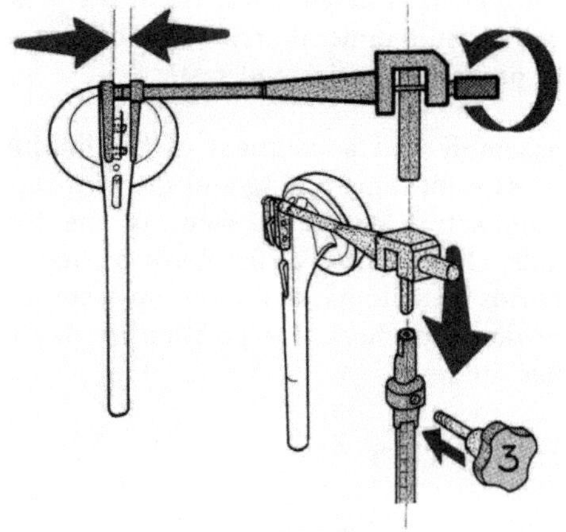

- **Step 7: Insertion of the trial implant into the humerus and intra-articular reduction:** With the *arm in extension*, the trial prosthesis, mounted in the ruler-protractor unit is slided gently into the medullary canal. The arm is then put *in flexion* to reduce the prosthesis into the joint.

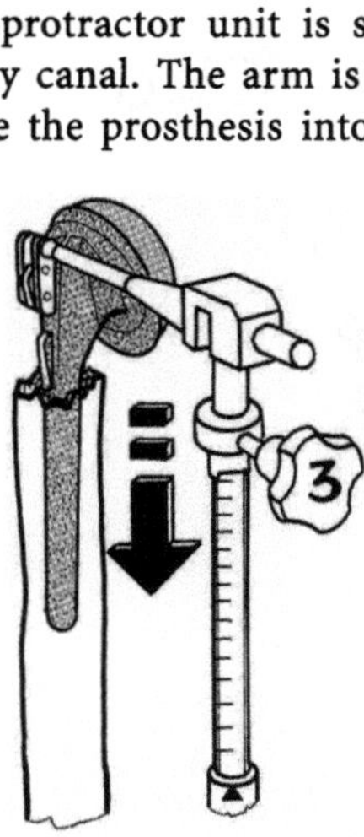

- **Step 8: Positioning the epicondylar guides:** With the *arm in flexion* and the prosthesis reduced into the joint, the surgeon identifies the prominence of the medial and lateral epicondyles.

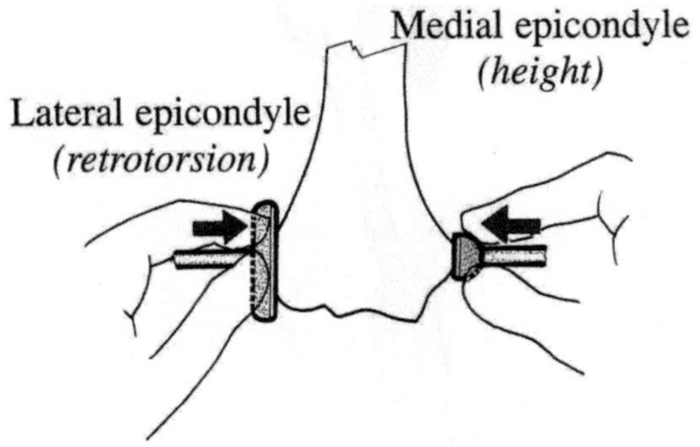

(NB: Identification of the bony landmarks of the elbow should not be performed with the prosthesis outside the joint. Positioning the epicondylar guides with the prosthesis inside the joint avoids mistakes of increased height (because of the presence of the acromiohumeral arch superiorly) and makes the procedure easier and faster.)

- **Step 9: Assembly and adjustment of the linking rods:** The assistant joins the jig and the arm support by connecting and then securing the two linking rods. (NB: In case of fat elbow or important edema or hematoma, a fluoroscopic control should be done to check the positioning of the epicondylar guides.)

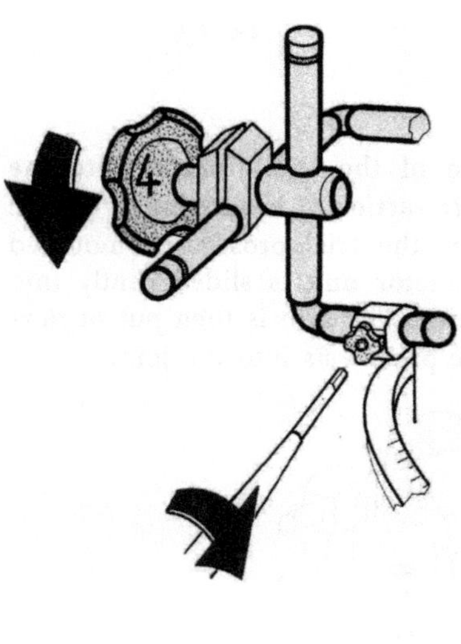

- **Step 10: Verification of the height and the retroversion:** While the tuberosities are replaced on the diaphysis and the prosthesis, the height and the retroversion are verified. The top of the greater tuberosity should be 5 mm below the prosthetic head and the prosthetic fin should be 5 mm behind the bicipital groove.

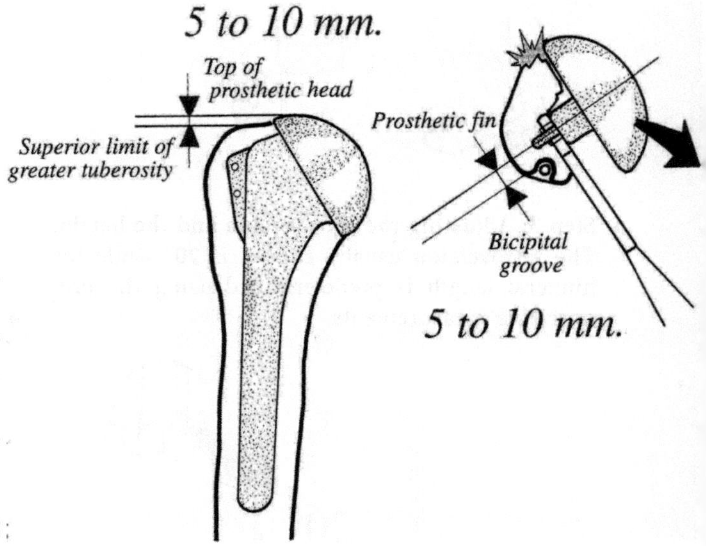

- **Step 11: The trial prosthesis is replaced by the final implant which is cemented in place:** When the correct positioning has been determined, only the trial prosthesis and the prosthesis holder are withdrawn and the jig is left in place to allow cementing of the definitive prosthesis. With the *arm in extension*, the definitive prosthesis is introduced into the medullary canal while the prosthesis holder is introduced simultaneously into the jig. The *arm is placed again in flexion* to reduce the prosthesis into the joint.

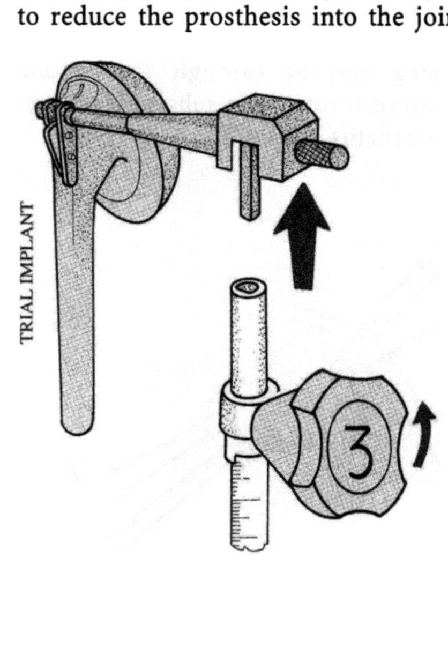

- **Step 12: Reattachment of the tuberosities:** The horizontal sutures are passed around the neck of the prosthesis (and not in the fin of the prosthesis) while the vertical sutures are tighten using the tension-band technique.

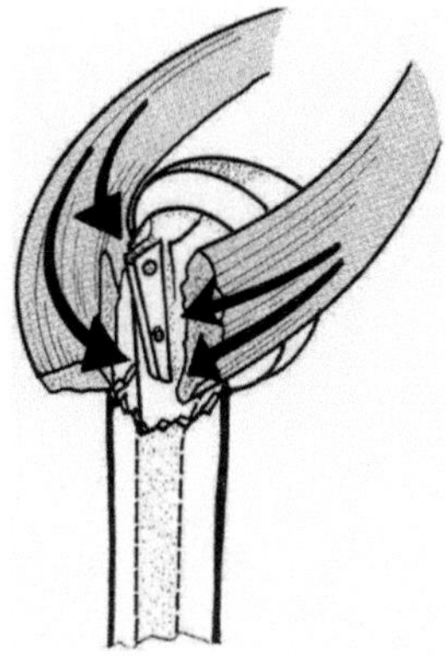

Conclusion

Shoulder prosthesis in 4-part fractures should be considered as an "improved osteosynthesis." This means that reconstruction of the tuberosities should be a priority and that the humeral component should allow to replace the articular head surface and help stabilizing and attaching the tuberosities. The Aequalis fracture jig, by decreasing the subjective part of the procedure, avoids the "eye ball operation" and provides a better positioning of the prosthesis and so a better quality of the humeral reconstruction.

References

1. Bigliani LU, Flatow EL, McCluskey, Fischer RA (1991) Failed prosthetic replacement for displaced proximal humeral fractures. Orthop Trans 15:747–748
2. Boileau P, Chau E, Perraud M, Arcamone H, Argenson C (1993) Restoration of humeral length and humeral offset after shoulder prosthesis for fractures. Rev Chir Orthop 73:150
3. Boileau P, Walch G, Mazzoleni N, Urien JP (1993) In vitro measurement of humeral head retroversion. J Shoulder Elbow Surg 2 (2):12
4. Boileau P, Huten D (1995) Technique chirurgicale des prothèses de Neer pour fractures céphalo-tubérositaires. Rev Chir Orthop 81 [Suppl II]:85–88
5. Boileau P, Walch G (1996) Prothèses d'épaule pour fractures: Problèmes et solutions. Maitrise Orthop 6:18–23
6. Boileau P, Walch G (1997) The three dimensional geometry of the proximal humerus: Implications for the surgical technique and prosthetic design. J Bone Joint Surg Br 79:857–865
7. Boileau P, Walch G (1995) The Aequalis Fracture Jig. Surgical Technique Overview. Tornier Inc, France (Booklet)
8. Compito CA, Self EB, Bigliani LU (1994) Arthoplasty and acute shoulder trauma, reasons for success and failure. Clin Orthop 307:27–36
9. Ianotti JP, Gabriel JP, Schneck SL, Evans BG, Miras S (1992) The normal glenohumeral relationships. An anatomical study of one hundred and forty shoulders. J Bone Joint Surg Am 74:491–500
10. Khral VE, Evans FG (1945) Humeral torsion in man. Am J Phys. Anthrop 3:229–253
11. Neer CS (1955) Articular replacement of the humeral head. J Bone Joint Surg Am 37:215–228
12. Walch G, Boileau P (1991) Morphological study of the proximal humerus J Bone Joint Surg Br 74 [Suppl I]:14

Tuberosity Osteosynthesis in Shoulder Arthroplasty

J. C. Le Huec, P. Boileau, R. Sinnerton, and I. Hovorka

Summary

Tuberosity osteosynthesis in shoulder arthroplasty remains a challenging problem: there is a high rate of nonunion or malunion and the number of failures is underdiagnosed. Proper synthesis of the tuberosities is closely linked to good positioning of the prosthesis with regard to length and retroversion. Nonunion of the tuberosities may be due to early or secondary bone migration because of malpositioning of the prosthesis and/or poor technique with tuberosity osteosynthesis. Migration of the tuberosities occurs either because there is excessive horizontal tension, if the prosthesis has been positioned in too much retroversion; excessive vertical tension, if the prosthesis has been cemented too high or by excessive oblique tension, if the stem has been cemented in valgus which shifts the upper part laterally, prevents intertuberosity contact, and causes over-tensioning.

Introduction

Osteosynthesis of the tuberosities is the final stage in the insertion of a shoulder hemiarthroplasty in fracture cases. However, despite whichever approach is used reinsertion of the tuberosities should be thought about from the onset because the final result depends to a great extent on the quality of this fixation. The bone quality is often poor in the older patients, and care must be taken not to damage these fragile fragments which provide an essential landmark in correctly positioning the prosthesis with regards to length and rotation. By systematically cementing the humeral stem at the correct anatomical length and retroversion by using the Aequalis fracture instrumentation, the tuberosities can be reconstructed onto the prosthesis. The proper positioning in length and retroversion of the prosthesis afforded by the jig is an important point and is detailed elsewhere. Nonunion between the tuberosities and with the diaphysis is not well recorded in the literature, with failure of the fixation often poorly diagnosed, and this is the cause of poor and unpredictable results.

Methods and Materials

Surgical Technique

Whenever possible the periosteal attachments between the tuberosities and with the diaphysis should be preserved. An approach via the avascular rotator interval or via the tendon of the supraspinatus (after incising the tendon in 1–2 cm) is preferred [3, 6, 7, 20]. A pragmatic approach should be taken to the biceps tendon: if it is undamaged in an unfractured groove, it should be preserved, but if it demonstrates tendinopathy, or if the tuberosity reconstruction is impaired by its presence, it should be divided and tenodesed.

An average 20° of retroversion related to the transepicondylar line should be selected [1]. The ease of osteosynthesizing the tuberosities depends on the site of the intertuberosity fracture line. The main fracture line is posterior to the bicipital groove in 80 % of cases (Fig. 1). The arm should then be

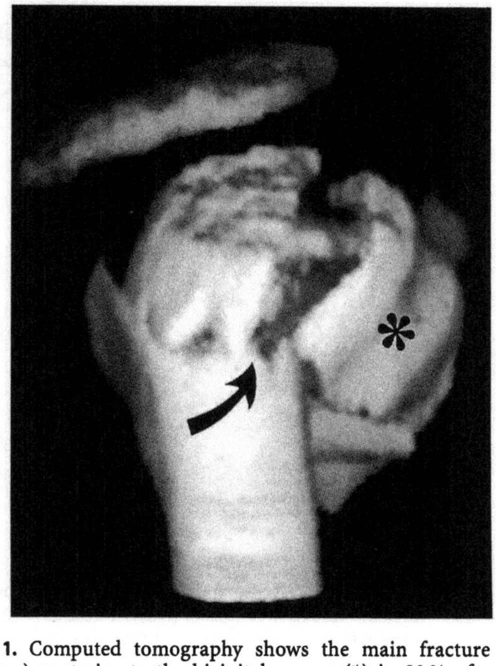

Fig. 1. Computed tomography shows the main fracture line (arrow) posterior to the bicipital groove (*) in 80 % of cases

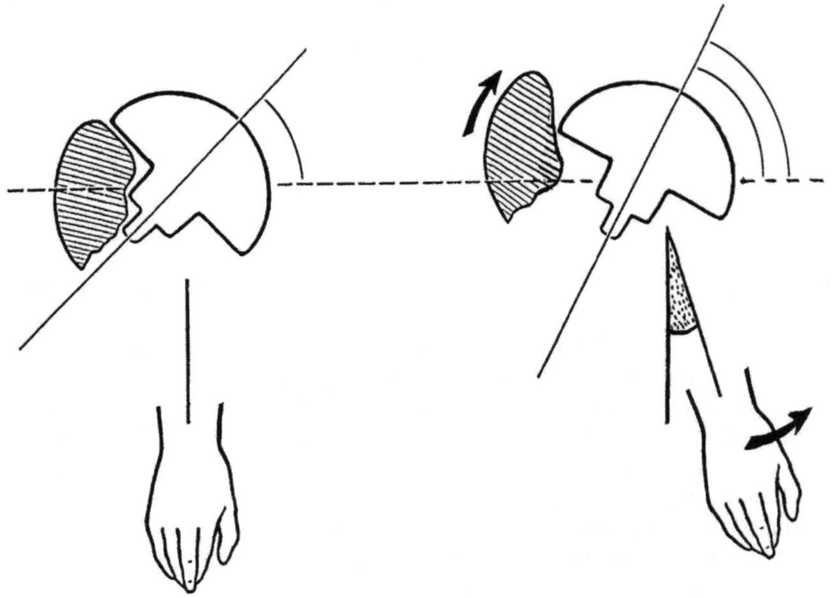

Fig. 2. If the prosthesis is overretroverted, the tuberosity fragment detaches when the arm is placed in internal rotation in a sling postoperatively (even if the fracture passes well behind the bicipital groove)

placed in neutral rotation to allow the greater tuberosity to seat onto the stem of the prosthesis without excessive tension. If the retroversion of the prosthesis is exaggerated, there is a source of tension on the horizontal sutures which may be the origin of an early failure especially as the patients are immobilized in internal rotation in a sling postoperatively (Fig. 2). The tuberosities need to be positioned flat onto the stem and not splayed out as can occur when, for the purpose of achieving intertuberosity contact, the tuberosities are tipped on the prosthetic fin (Fig. 3). Nonabsorbable sutures are passed

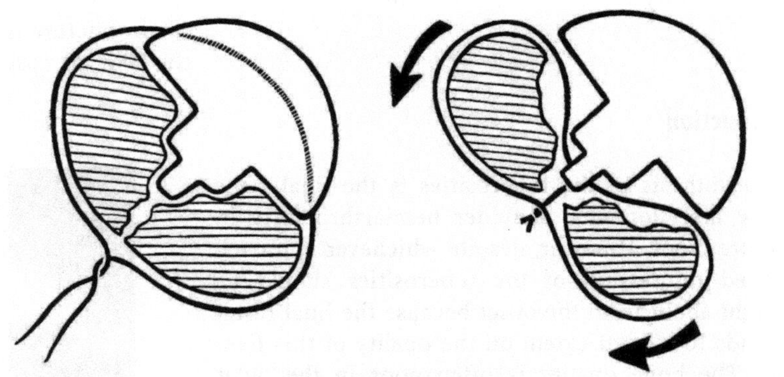

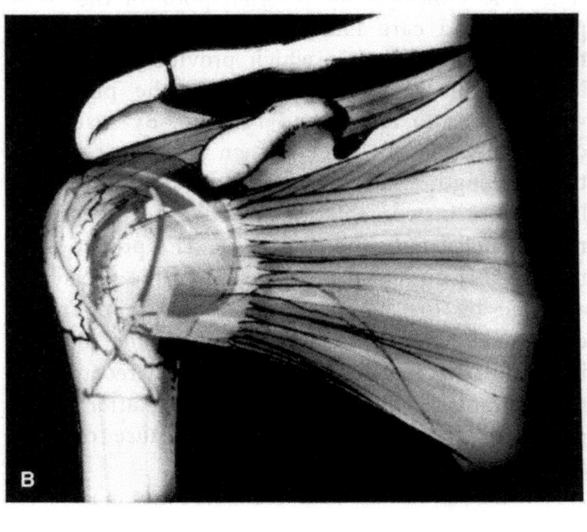

Fig. 3 A,B. The tuberosities should be secured with both horizontal and vertical sutures. **A** Passing the fixation sutures around the prosthetic neck allows the tuberosities to be perfectly seated and avoid their splaying out as occurs with the classical technique. **B** The vertical sutures are box-shaped or "figure-of-8" shaped

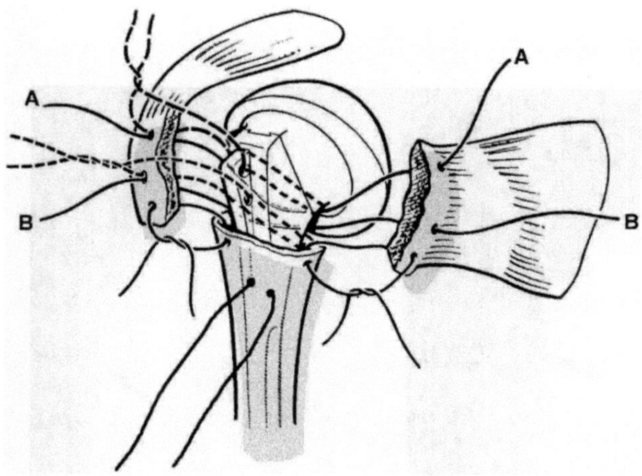

Fig. 4. Technique for passing the tuberosity fixation sutures. The sutures are passed through the bone-tendon junction, and those for fixation to the diaphysis should be passed before the stem is cemented

through the bone tendon junction so as to prevent damaging the often porotic bone. These sutures need to be flexible, as opposed to metal sutures, which are too rigid and saw through the bone.

By reattaching the tuberosities separately (Fig. 4) the anatomy can be matched better by controlling the positioning of the bicipital groove in relation to the prosthetic fin. This should be positioned 5–10 mm on average behind the bicipital groove at its upper part (Fig. 5). In fact, as it descends towards the diaphysis, the groove turns anteriorly and thus becomes a less reliable landmark. The greater tuberosity is always fixed first, both to the prosthesis and to the diaphysis. It is advisable to pass the sutures to be used for the vertical fixation through the diaphysis just prior to cementing the stem to avoid difficulties later. The holes in the fin can be used too. A corticocancellous bone graft taken from the humeral head is used to improve intertuberosity and diaphysis consolidation. While attaching the greater tuberosity it should be positioned so that its upper pole is about 5 mm lower than the upper margin of the prosthetic head and parallel to the diaphysis (Fig. 5). The lesser tuberosity attachment is then carried out, as a second step, and applied well onto the stem. The horizontal sutures passed around the neck of the prosthesis give optimal seating of the tuberosities onto the prosthesis.

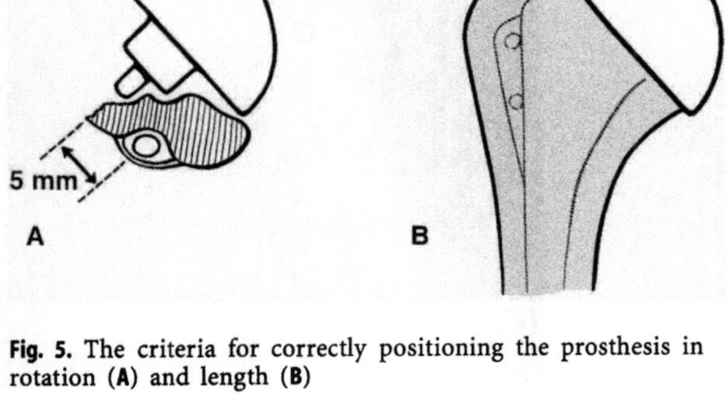

Fig. 5. The criteria for correctly positioning the prosthesis in rotation (**A**) and length (**B**)

Materials

A total of 73 patients underwent insertion of a prosthesis for head-tuberosity fractures, and whom 66 were available for review with a minimum follow-up of 12 months. There were 7 three-part fractures and 62 four-part, of which 21 were type II, 38 type III, and 3 type IV (see the classification in Le Huec et al. "Anatomical and Pathological Classification of Proximal Humeral Fractures," this volume). All the stems were cemented. The tuberosity synthesis was carried out using wire sutures in one case, nonabsorbable sutures in 58, and nonabsorbable sutures plus a Dacron tape in ten cases. Twenty-eight patients, including the ten with the Dacron tape underwent synthesis with the horizontal sutures passing around the neck of the prosthesis while the others underwent the classic approach [3, 6, 15–17]. All patients were immobilized with the elbow at the side and the hand on the abdomen in a sling and underwent early rehabilitation. The Constant score was evaluated at the last follow-up visit. All the patients had a radiographic examination consisting of an AP view in neutral rotation and a lateral outlet view profile. Computed tomography was performed on 23 patients at their last visit, and 39 had a measurement X-ray of the contralateral humerus.

Results

Thirty-five patients achieved an anatomical synthesis (Fig. 6A) which remained stable over time. Thirteen had a synthesis which was originally imperfect, associated with an error in positioning the prosthesis (too long in seven cases and excessive retroversion in six). Sixteen presented with secondary failure of the fixation; in seven cases this followed an imperfect initial synthesis and nine after a satisfactory initial appearance. A greater tuberosity visible on the radiograph in internal rotation but not visible in external rotation demonstrated at its posterior migration (Fig. 6B). Four patients showed bone resorption of the greater tuberosity confirmed

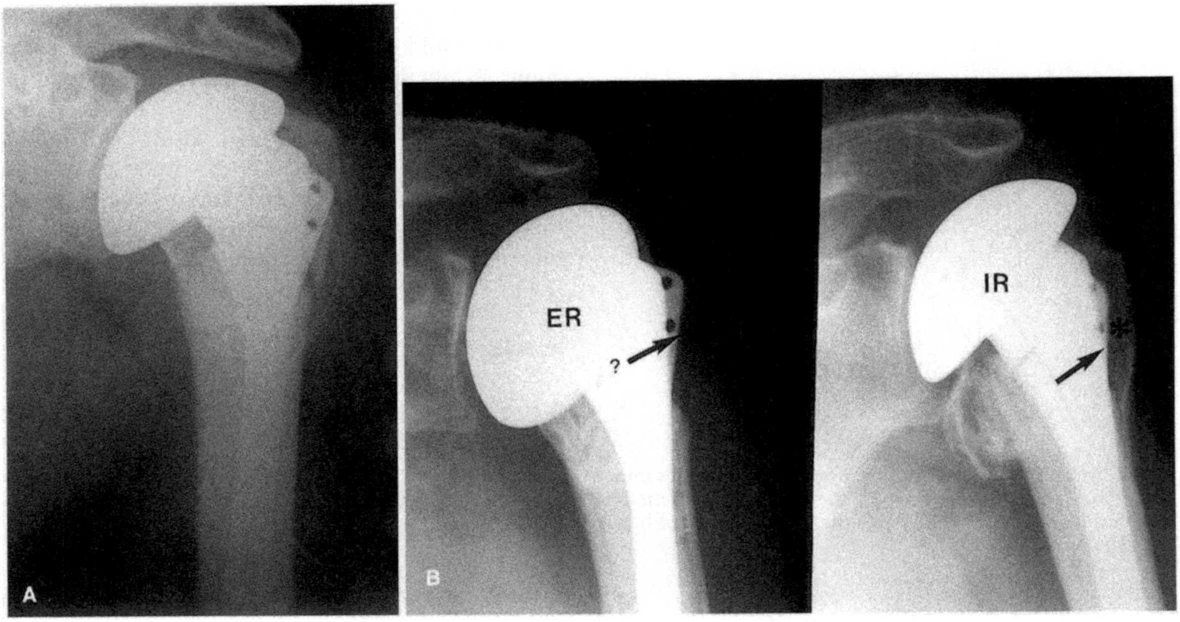

Fig. 6. A Proper fixation of the tuberosities which remains stable with time. The greater tuberosity is clearly seen on the AP radiograph in neutral rotation with the prosthesis at the correct height. **B** Improper fixation of the tuberosities: greater tuberosity is visible in internal rotation but is not visible in external rotation (the bone fragment is hidden by the prosthesis)

by computed tomography. One prosthesis dislocated anteriorly after a heavy fall downstairs in an 80-year old patient who presented only 6 months later but without pain and did not want to undergo revision.

Overall, the average absolute Constant score at review was 56 points. There were 47 % whose result was judged to be good or excellent, 33 % with an average result, and 20 % with a poor result.

When the prosthesis was correctly positioned with regard to length (less than 8 mm difference to the contralateral humerus) as occurred in 15 patients, the average Constant score was higher than 90 points. Errors in rotation were more difficult to analyze radiographically and were analyzed by computed tomography. An initially poor passive external rotation which increased sharply between two successive visits was often evidence of secondary failure of the fixation. In this series the average external rotation was 17.5° and internal rotation reached the L3 level. Failure of fixation was seen in 16 of the 66 cases, of which 7 where in patients who had an imperfect initial synthesis and 9 who had a prosthesis posi-

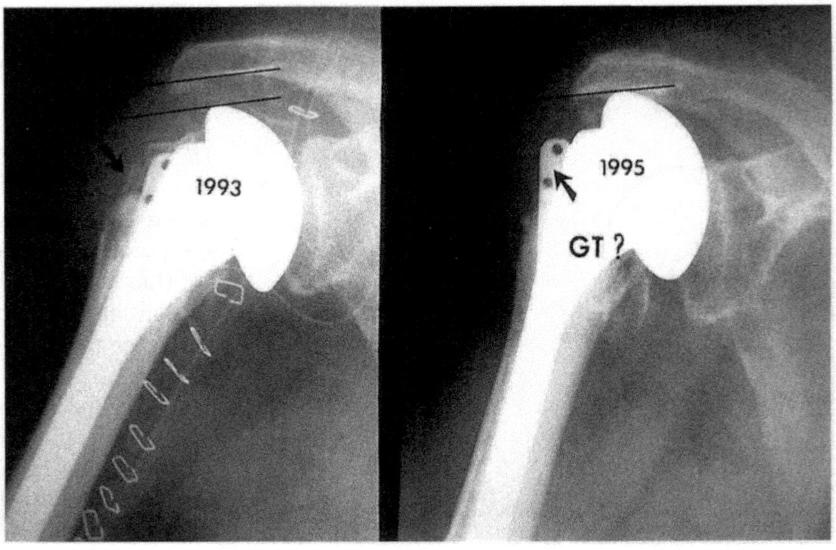

Fig. 7. Secondary posterior migration of the greater and lesser tuberosities leads to secondary proximal humeral migration

tioned too high (greater than 8 mm difference in comparison to the other shoulder) and/or with exaggerated retroversion (limitation of passive external rotation; Fig. 7). The prosthetic stems had been cemented in valgus with an angle superior to 10° in six cases, and this was correlated to a poor functional result with migration of the greater tuberosity (Fig. 8).

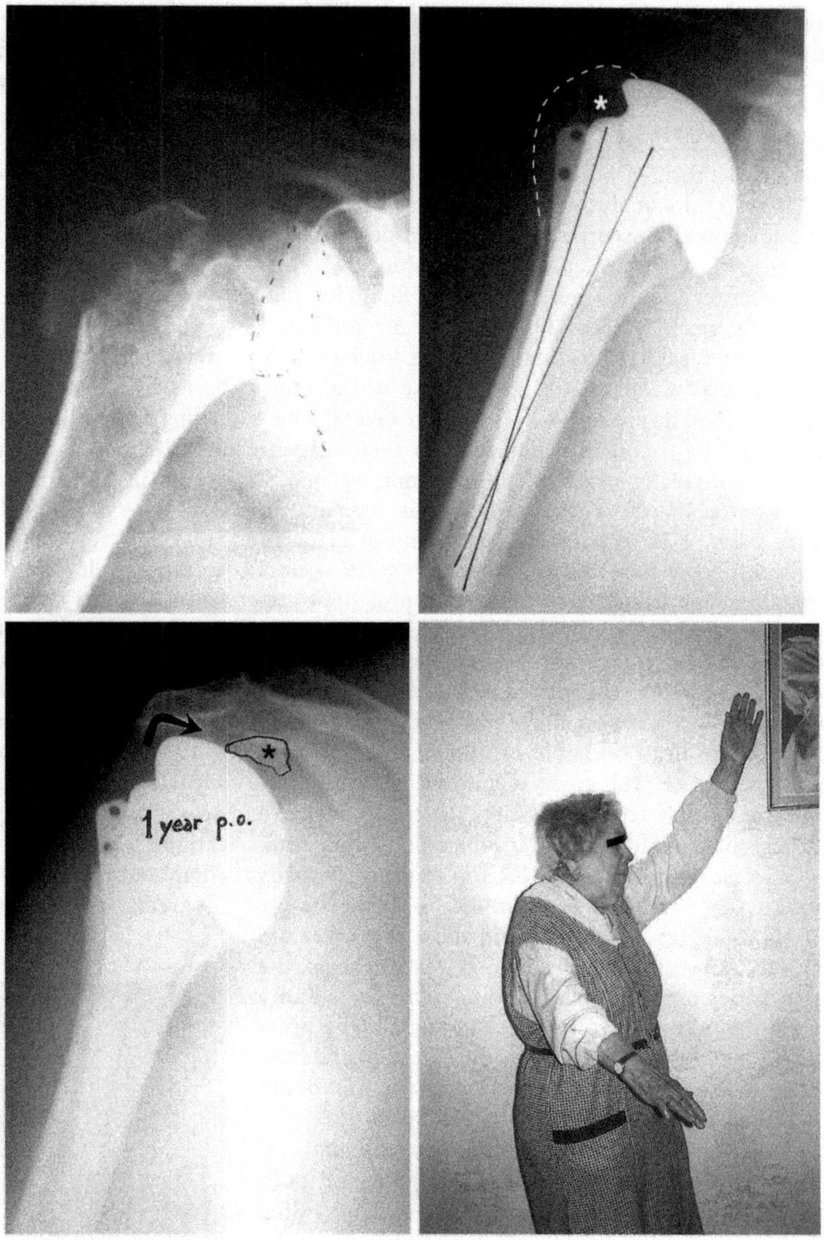

Fig. 8. Prosthetic valgus leads to oblique overtensioning of the rotator cuff with posterio-medial migration of the greater tuberosity (*) and poor functional result

Discussion

In this series proper synthesis of the tuberosities was closely linked with correct positioning of the prosthesis in length and retroversion. This idea of prosthetic length and retroversion had not been analyzed previously in the literature [3, 4, 6, 9, 13, 17, 18], and none has made use of a jig specifically designed to correctly position the prosthesis [1].

The results judged on the absence of pain and the recovery of a functional range of movement were similar to those of other series [3, 4, 9, 11, 14, 18, 19]. The results analyzed by the criteria of the Hospital for Special Surgery showed 81 % good results in a series of 22 patients reported by Moeckel [14]. Using the criteria of the "American Shoulder and Elbow Surgeors", Neer [17] reported 60 good and very good results in 61 patients. The level of very good results in these series reflects the use of scoring systems that are not very stringent (average elevation of 110°), and in which force is seldom mentioned in direct contrast to the Constant system.

Malunion between the tuberosities appears to cause pain. It is usually due to an initial error in positioning the tuberosities either by excessive horizontal tension because of exaggerated prosthetic retroversion (Fig. 2) or by increased vertical tension because the prosthesis is cemented too high or in valgus. We have also reported that when the greater tuberosity is visible on the AP radiograph in internal rotation and no visible on that in neutral rotation, the greater tuberosity synthesis is insufficient and the result often disappointing. To achieve proper, solid synthesis of the tuberosities it is advisable to place at least two horizontal sutures passing around the neck of the prosthesis and not simply through the fin as recommended in the literature [11, 13, 16–19]. This horizontal suture pulls the tuberosities onto the stem and augments the solidity of the fixation. The volume of the neck of the prosthesis is probably a factor in nonconsolidation between the tuberosities. This idea will no doubt be reanalyzed in the light of recent works [5].

Nonunion between the tuberosities and the diaphysis is also a source of persistent pain and poor results. This may be due either to a poor initial synthesis onto the diaphysis, which emphasizes the technical point of how important the vertical reinsertion of the tuberosities by sutures through the diaphysis is [3, 6], or to incorrect height positioning of the prosthesis, which leads to nonunion and painful subacromial impingement.

Failure of greater tuberosity fixation was high (23.5 %) and seems to have been increased in this series when the prosthesis was cemented too high and/or excessively retroverted. Failure of lesser tuberosity synthesis, which occurred less frequently, is a source of instability, with a risk of dislocation as occurred in one case in our series after a heavy fall. Secondary failures of fixation have been recorded in the literature: Green [9] reported 3 failures in 23 patients (13 %) and Moeckel [14] recorded one nonunion of the greater tuberosity in his series of 22 patients (4.5 %). Compito [4] reported 4 tuberosity fixation failures in 64 patients (6.2 %). Such a difference can only be due to a different analysis of the radiographs (Figs. 7–9), because our functional results were equal to those in the other series. It seems important to record an increased number of heterotopic ossification in those series, 10 % for Neer [17], 15 % for Cofield [3, 19] and 40 % for Moeckel [14]. Green [9] did not record this event.

It is probable that some of these ossifications are in fact undiagnosed secondary failures of fixation because the authors only had available one AP radiograph, which is clearly insufficient to make the diagnosis. In fact, failure of fixation, which occurs in our opinion very quickly after the operation, does not impede the obtention of a satisfactory functional result such as reported by Green [9] with an average elevation of 110°, external rotation of 31°, and the ability to carry out the activities of daily living, which in patients aged over 60 are often unnecessary as long as they can feed, wash, and dress themselves without assistance. None of these series analyzed the height of the prosthesis in comparison to the contralateral one. Moeckel [14] reported three superior subluxations in his series but did not suggest a diagnostic hypothesis. The heterotopic ossifications when analyzed with precision and the aid of computed tomography are often shown to be failure of greater tuberosity fixation, as demonstrated in

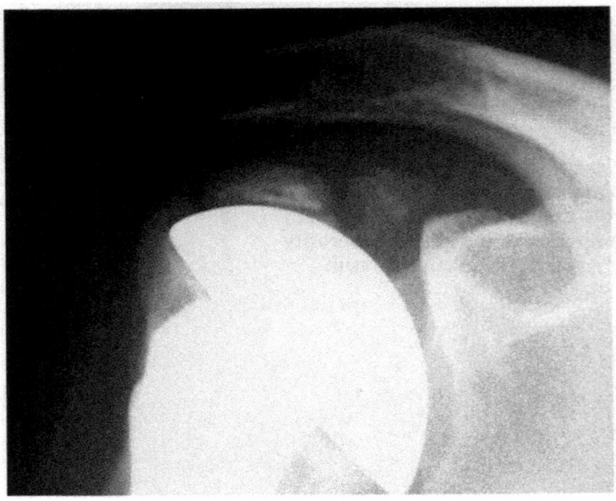

Fig. 9. «Heterotopic ossifications» which are in fact detachments of the tuberosities with posterosuperior migration of the greater tuberosity

Fig. 9. Thus the different series previously mentioned have a percentage of fixation failures equivalent to ours if this analysis of the ossifications is taken into account and explains why their functional results where equivalent to ours.

Conclusion

Overall, the results of humeral hemiarthroplasties in fractures of the proximal humerus are closely correlated with the quality of osteosynthesis of the tuberosities. This fixation which must be carefully carried out following exact rules and can be performed only when the prosthesis has been positioned at the correct height and retroversion and without any valgus. We underline again the importance of a jig to control these parameters while cementing the prosthesis. Carefully controlling the different technical steps of the procedure should help to obtain more predictable results in the elderly patients who wish an independent pain-free life.

References

1. Boileau P, Walch G (1995) Adaptabilité et modularité au cours des prothéses d'épaule. Acta Orthop Belg 61 [Suppl II]:50–61
2. Castagno AA, Shuman WP, Kilcoyne RF, Haynor DR, Morris ME, Matsen FA (1987) Complex fractures of the proximal humerus: role of CT in treatment. Radiology 165:759–752
3. Cofield RH (1988) Comminuted fractures of the proximal humerus. Clin Orthop 230:49–57
4. Compito CA, Self EB, Bigliani LU (1994) Arthoplasty and acute shoulder trauma, reasons for success and failure. Clin Orthop 307:27–36
5. Cook SD, Barrack RL, Salkeld SL, Prewett AB, Edmunds JO (1993) Bone ingrowth into a porous coated total shoulder component retrieved postmortem. J Arthropl 8:189–194
6. Craig EV (1989) Prosthetic replacement for four part fractures of the proximal humerus. Tech Orthop 3:70–80
7. Duparc J, Lagier A (1976) Les luxations-fractures de l'extrémité supérieure de l'humérus. Rev Chir Orthop 62:91–110
8. Gerber C, Schneeberger AG, Vinh T (1990) The arterial vascular.sation of the humeral head. An anatomical study. J Bone Joint Surg Am 72:1486–1494
9. Green A, Barnard WL, Imbird RS, Providence RI (1993) Humeral head replacement for acute four-part proximal humerus fractures. J Shoulder Elbow Surg 2:249–254
10. Hawkins RJ, Bell RH, Gurr K (1986) The three part fracture of the proximal part of the humerus: operative treatment. J Bone Joint Surg Am 68:1410–1414
11. Huten D, Duparc J (1986) L'arthroplastie prothétique dans les traumatismes complexes récents et anciens de l'épaule. Rev Chir Orthop 72:517–529
12. Jakob RP, Kristiansen T, Mayo K, Ganz R, Mulle ME (1984) Classification and aspects of treatment of fractures of the proximal humerus. In: Bateman JE, Welsh RP (eds) Surgery of the shoulder. Mosby, St Louis/Decker, Toronto, pp 330–343
13. Jakob RP, Miniaci A, Anson PS et al (1991) Four part valgus impacted fractures of the proximal humerus. J Bone Joint Surg Br 73:295–298
14. Moeckel BH, Dines DM, Warren RF, Altchek DW (1992) Modular hemiarthroplasty for fractures of the proximal part of the humerus. J Bone Joint Surg Am 74:884–889
15. Neer CS (1970) Displaced proximal humeral fractures. Part 2. J Bone Joint Surg Am 52:1077–1089
16. Neer CS, Brown TH, Mac Laughlin HL (1953) Fracture of the head of the humerus with dislocation of the head fragment. Am J Surg 85:252–258
17. Neer CS, Mac Ilveen SJ (1988) Replacement de la tête humérale avec reconstruction des tubérosités et de la coiffe dans les fractures déplacées à 4 fragments. Rev Chir Orthop 74 [Suppl II]:31–40
18. Nicholson GP, Flatow EL, Bigliani LU (1995) Shoulder arthroplasty for proximal humeral fractures. In: Friedman (ed) Arthroplasty of the shoulder. Thieme, Stuttgart, pp 183–193
19. Tanner MW, Cofield RH (1983) Prosthetic arthroplasty for fractures and fractures dislocations of the proximal humerus. Clin Orthop 179:116–128
20. Vichard P (1988) Luxations-fractures de l'épaule. Conférence d'énseignement de la SOFCOT. Expansion Scientifique Française, Paris

Results of Shoulder Arthroplasty in Acute Fractures of the Proximal Humerus

P. Boileau, L. Tinsi, J. C. Le Huec, D. Molé, R. Sinnerton, and G. Walch

Summary

Sixty-six patients with acute three and four-part proximal humeral fractures treated with humeral head replacement were reviewed and radiographed with an average follow-up of 19 months (12–57 months). At review, computed tomographic scans were available in 23 patients and scaled radiographs of both humeri were available in 39 patients. The most significant factors associated with a poor functional result were: (a) ***Migration of the greater tuberosity*** *either posterior (29 %) or superior (17 %), leading to nonunion, malunion and late bone resorption. (b)* ***Malposition of the prosthesis*** *because of inappropriate length, the prosthesis being too proud (15 %) or too low (29 %) and/or excessive retroversion (14 %).* ***There was a clear correlation between prosthesis positioning and greater tuberosity migration (p=0.001):*** *greater tuberosity migration was the consequence of malpositioning of the humeral prosthesis, particularly when the prosthesis was too proud, too retroverted. Multiple technical errors of prosthesis positioning may be associated and increase the risk of greater tuberosity detachment despite meticulous tuberosity reconstruction with associated bone graft and secure fixation with heavy nonabsorbable sutures. Prosthesis positioning is the key to greater tuberosity healing to the shaft and should be more accurate but is difficult because of the absence of proximal anatomical landmarks in three- and four-part fractures. The Aequalis fracture jig, a new device allowing for more accurate positioning of the prosthesis because of control of the humeral length and retroversion, has been designed because "eyeball" positioning of the prosthesis is insufficient. Its early use seems to be promissing.*

Introduction

In 1970 Neer reported the results of prosthetic replacement in three- and four-part fractures and fractures dislocations of the proximal humerus: excellent or satisfactory results were obtained in 90 % of the patients [29–31]. Other authors have reported less satisfactory or even disappointing results with stiff painful shoulders, demonstrating that shoulder replacement itself is no guarantee of a successful results [11–13, 15, 20, 24, 33, 39, 41, 43, 45]. Many authors have reported the difficulties of achieving correct prosthetic positioning in the absence of accurate anatomical landmarks and the incidence of tuberosity malunion, nonunion or bone resorption [1, 20, 27, 33, 41]. Technical considerations are clearly implicated in poor results and lack of experience of the orthopedic surgeons because of the relative infrequency of these fractures may be the cause of poor technique leading to poor and unpredictable functional results [2, 4, 44].

In 1990 in an earlier study we reviewed a series of three- and four-part fractures operated on with a Neer prosthesis and we looked specifically at humeral length by taking measured X-rays of both humeri [2]. We observed that poor results were clearly related to malpositioning of the prosthesis with regard to length. In another previous study we measured humeral retroversion on anatomical specimens [3] and observed that humeral retroversion is variable and that the average retroversion is low, being 20° when related to the transepicondylar axis. In an attempt to improve the prosthesis positioning in four-part fractures we developed a new extramedullary device, the Aequalis fracture jig (Tornier) which consists of a ruler and a protractor that are designed to allow more accurate placement of the prosthesis regarding length and retroversion.

Our hypothesis was that poor and unpredictable functional results observed with prosthesis for fractures are directly related to poor positioning of the humeral component for length and retroversion. Here we present our results with and without the use of this fracture jig for positioning of the prosthesis in the treatment of fractures of the proximal humerus.

Methods and Materials

Patients

Between January 1991 and April 1995, 73 acute proximal humeral fractures were operated on using the Aequalis shoulder arthroplasty in eight different orthopedic centers. All patients were operated on by or under supervision of senior shoulder surgeons. All the fractures were classified using the Neer [30, 32] and AO [23] systems (Table 1). The classification was established on the preoperative radiographs and on the intraoperative findings to minimize the intra- and interobserver lack of reproducibility of the different classifications [26, 36, 37]. Of the 66 fractures available at review there were 7 three-part fractures and 59 four-part fractures. Preoperatively, computed tomography (CT) was carried out in 38 cases which demonstrated the fracture lines between the tuberosities: the fracture line passed behind the bicipital groove in 26 cases (69%), through the groove in 2 (5%), and behind and through in 10 (26%). The fracture line did not pass in front of the groove in any of the cases. In two cases, an osteosynthesis had been attempted either in the days preceding the arthroplasty (one case) or at the same time as the arthroplasty (one case). In three cases an unsuccessful attempt at reduction under general anesthesia had been made. All the fractures underwent surgery within 3 weeks and, on average by the 5th day.

The average age of the patients at the time of the trauma was 66 years (range, 31–85). There was a clear predominance of women, with (68%) against only (32%) males. The right side was affected in 40% and the left in 60%. The dominant arm was involved in 46%. The cause of the fracture was a simple fall in 63%, a street accident in 30%, and a seizure leading to a fall in 7%. In eight cases there were associated injuries: four on the upper limb (one olecranon fracture, two distal radial fractures, one metacarpal fracture) and four on the lower limb (one pubic ramus fracture, one femoral fracture, one tibial fracture and one medial malleolar fracture).

Table 1. Anatomopathology of the fractures according to Neer and AO classification

Type of fracture	Number
• 4-part displaced or dislocated (C3)	30
Anterior	14
Posterior	3
Lateral	8
Inferior	5
• 4-part valgus impacted (C2)	21
• 4-part varus impacted (C2)	8
• 3-part with displaced greater tuberosity (B2)	4
• 3-part dislocation with surgical neck and greater tuberosity displaced (B3)	3
Total	66

Surgical Technique

The technique followed the principles detailed by Neer [4, 10, 31, 32, 44]. The patient was placed in the beach-chair position and was moved to the side of the table so that the upper extremity can be placed into maximum extension without obstruction by the operating table. The entire upper extremity was prepared and draped to allow full mobility during the procedure and great care was taken to keep the elbow free. The arm was draped into an arm support, which is part of the Aequalis fracture Jig, to maintain the elbow flexed. An extended deltopectoral approach without disinsertion of the anterior deltoid was used in all cases. Exposure was maximized by extending the incision upwards to just above the coracoid and distally to the tendon of pectoralis major, which was divided for 1–2 cm when necessary. The coracoacromial ligament, which acts as a guide to humeral length, was preserved in 48 cases. After excising the hematoma filled subacromial bursa, the tuberosities were identified. As noted above, the fracture line passed behind the bicipital groove in about 80% of the cases. The intra-articular approach was made either by incising the rotator interval longitudinally or by dividing the interval between supraspinatus and infraspinatus while gently retracting the tuberosities. In 40% there were comminuted fractures of the tuberosities and the bicipital groove was involved in the fracture in 31%.

After retracting the tendon of the long head of biceps, the humeral head fragment, stripped of any capsular attachments, was extracted. In the three-part fractures the lesser tuberosity still attached to the humeral head was osteotomized and the joint then approached in the same way. The subscapularis was never divided. There was a longitudinal cuff tear involving the supraspinatus in four cases of antero-inferior fracture-dislocation and this was repaired by side to side suture. Whenever possible the periosteal attachments between the tuberosities and the diaphysis were preserved. There were glenoid fractures in five cases which always occurred at the anteroinferior border of the articular surface and which were small enough to be ignored. After placing sutures through the tendon-bone junction of both the lesser and greater tuberosity fragments, the humerus was prepared using cylindrical rasps.

The arthroplasty used was the Aequalis prosthesis (Tornier) whose design is based on anatomical studies [6, 42]. The humeral component is both modular and adaptable and consists of three parts: a stem, a neck offering a choice of humeral inclination angle and a head available in a range of diameters and depths. The head has an eccentric dial system on its under surface which allows its position to be translated to match the posterior offset of the articular surface. There are eight available positions but two (one for left sided and one for right sided fractures) are preferred in fracture cases as these match the average posterior offset calculated statistically in previous studies [6, 42]. The inclination angle selected was 130° in 75 % of the cases, corresponding to the average value found in our anatomical studies. A 6-mm stem was used in 15 %, a 9-mm diameter stem in 68 %, and a 12-mm diameter stem in 17 % of the cases. The normal length stem was used in all but two cases where an extra-long stem was required due to extension of the fracture into the diaphysis.

The Aequalis fracture instrumentation jig (Tornier) is a new and original system consisting of an extramedullary sliding ruler and protractor which allows the prosthesis to be positioned to correctly match the normal humeral length and retroversion [5]. This device was used in 38 cases allowing its evaluation by the different surgeons. The length was selected based on measured radiographs of the unaffected humerus taken preoperatively with the arm in 45° of abduction, 45° of external rotation and with the upper arm actually flat on the X-ray plate. A radio-opaque ruler with metal markers was attached to the upper arm to allow true length to be calculated taking into account the radiographic enlargement [5]. Following our anatomical measurements and those from others [3, 7, 25, 34], an average humeral retroversion of 20° in relation to the transepicondylar axis was selected. The difference between surgical and anatomical retroversion is related to the carrying angle of the forearm [40]. The precision of the jig has been determined to be ±5 mm for length and 3° for retroversion [5].

The trial prosthesis was secured by its fin to the ruler and protractor. Once the prosthesis was introduced into the medullary canal and reduced into the joint cavity, the correct positioning for length and retroversion was determined by the surgeon who identified the prominences of the elbow and positioned the epicondylar guides on the medial and lateral epicondyles. The connection between the jig and the arm support was made by the assistant who assembled and tightened two linking rods. The greater and lesser tuberosities were then placed alternatively under the prosthetic head by pulling on the sutures to check the prosthesis and tuberosities positioning. When the correct positioning has been determined, the jig was left in place, the trial prosthesis was removed and replaced with the definitive prosthesis.

The humeral prosthesis was cemented and a cement restrictor was used in all cases. Heavy, non-absorbable sutures (no. 5 or 7) were used to attach the tuberosity fragments to the humeral shaft, to each other and to the prosthesis. The tuberosities were secured with both horizontal and vertical suturing [4, 31, 44]. Cancellous bone graft taken from the humeral head was put between the tuberosities and the diaphysis to improve bony union. The biceps tendon was tenodesed in 26 cases (43 %). Nine fractures which had metaphyso-diaphyseal extensions required complimentary osteosynthesis with cerclage using either sutures (eight cases) or wire (one case). The rotator cuff was repaired when necessary (four cases). No glenoid components were used. The goal of the procedure was to restore a normal offset for the glenohumeral joint [22, 35].

Rehabilitation was started on the first postoperative day with pendular exercises and was following the principles of early passive motion emphasized by Neer [18]. Forty-seven patients (78 %) were transferred to a rehabilitation center for an average stay of 6 weeks (3–12 weeks). This was done because of the importance of the rehabilitation and also because some elderly patients were not able to live alone and need assistance with their physical therapy. The initial rehabilitation period lasted about 6–8 weeks and consisted of only passive pendular exercises, passive external rotation and passive anterior elevation. Once consolidation had been achieved (after 6–8 weeks) then active rehabilitation was started. All patients participated in a supervised therapy program for at least 1 year. Unsatisfactory cooperation with the rehabilitation occurred with 20 patients (33 %) who were either very elderly, more than 80 years old (15 cases) or alcoholic (5 cases).

Follow-Up

Three patients who died and four patients who had not been followed-up for a minimum of 12 months were excluded, leaving 66 patients for evaluation. All the patients were reviewed clinically and with radiographs of the operated shoulder. The average follow-up was 19 months (12–57). The functional result was calculated using the Constant score, as adopted by the European Society for Shoulder and

Elbow Surgery [9]. This score covers pain (15 points), mobility (40 points), function (20 points) and force (25 points). A detailed questionnaire concerning ten tasks of daily living was used to evaluate patient's functional ability.

The radiographic examination at a minimum of one year follow up included anteroposterior radiographs in neutral, internal and external rotation, a lateral view and an axillary view when possible. The radiographs were analyzed to look at the quality of the humeral reconstruction. We specifically studied *the prosthetic positioning* by measuring the comparative humeral length and the acromiohumeral distance. Measured radiographs of both humeri taken at follow-up were performed in 39 cases to *measure and compare humeral length on both sides.* The humeral length was determined by plotting the prosthetic axis (middle of the proximal medullary canal) and by measuring the distance between two perpendiculars: one to the greater tuberosity and the other to the middle of the medial epicondyle. The *acromiohumeral distance* is the distance between the summit of the prosthetic head and the line of sclerosis of the acromion measured on AP view in neutral rotation. A distance inferior to 7 mm was synonymous of proximal migration of the humerus. We also specifically studied *the positioning and status of the tuberosities* by looking for posterosuperior migration and for malunion, nonunion or bone resorption. The greater tuberosity was considered as being correctly positioned when it was visible on an AP radiograph in neutral rotation and its summit being between 5 and 10 mm below the summit of the prosthetic head [21]. CT of the operated shoulder was carried out in 23 cases where the greater tuberosity could not be clearly seen on the standard radiographs. This also allowed prosthetic retroversion to be measured.

Finally, any periarticular *ectopic bone formation* as classified by Sneppen [38] and the *quality of the humeral cementing* were also evaluated. Radiolucent lines of 2 mm or more at the bone-cement interface or subsidence were considered as prosthetic loosening.

All the results were subjected to statistical analysis using Statview software (Abacus Concept, USA) and Student' *t* test, correlation, and regression tests were used. The value of $p<0.05$ was considered to be significant.

Results

Clinical Results

At review the average absolute *Constant score* was 56 points (20–95). Figure 1 summarizes the values of the absolute Constant score. The average Constant score, normalized for age and sex, was 74 % (31–116). We recorded excellent results in 15 cases (22.5 %), good in 16 (24.5 %), fair in 22 (33 %), and poor in 13 (20 %).

Table 2 summarizes the results for *pain.* On average this was 11.5 points out of a possible 15. The shoulder was totally or almost pain-free in 58 cases (87.%). Although there are many causes for persistent postoperative pain it would appear that it was mainly due to humeral lengthening (10 cases) or posterior migration of the greater tuberosity (19 cases).

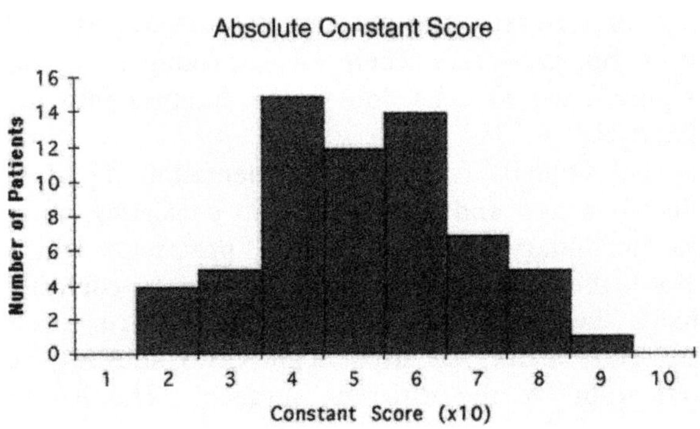

Fig. 1. Absolute Constant Score (mean score=56 points)

Table 2. Pain at review (average score: 11.5 points/15; n = 66)

Pain (Constant)	n	Purcentage
Severe (0–4)	1	1.5 %
Moderate (5–9)	7	11 %
Slight (10–14)	38	57.5 %
None (15)	20	30 %

Table 3. Active anterior elevation at review (average elevation: 101°; n = 66)

Active anterior elevation (Constant)	n	Purcentage
0–30° (0 points)	0	0 %
30–60° (2 points)	5	7.5 %
60–90° (4 points)	12	18 %
90–120° (6 points)	30	45.5 %
120–150° (8 points)	15	22.5 %
150–180° (10 points)	4	6.5 %

Table 4. Activity at review (average score: 12.5/20; n = 66)

Activity (Constant)	n	Purcentage
0–4 points	0	0 %
5–9 points	10	15 %
10–14 points	35	53 %
15–19 points	17	25.5 %
20 points	4	6.5 %

Table 3 summarizes the results for *mobility*. An average score of 22.1 points out of 40 was recorded. Anterior active elevation averaged 101° and ranged from 30°–175°. The average external rotation was 17.5° (0°–42) and internal rotation reached the L3 level on average and ranged from greater trochanter to T8. Suprisingly, supine passive elevation was much better than active elevation and averaged 135° (from 90°–175°).

Table 4 summarizes the results for *Activity:* 12.5 points out of 20 was the average score. The functional evaluation for activities of daily living is summarized in Table 5. Slipping on the affected side, carrying a weight, combing hair and using the hand above shoulder level were the most common limitations. The average *force* in elevation was 3.7 kg, ranging from 0–9 kg.

Patient satisfaction was also evaluated: 29 patients (45 %) were very satisfied with the results, 9 (13.5 %) were satisfied, 27 (41 %) were disappointed, and one was unhappy. The results from the constant score were in agreement with the patients' own opinion (p=0.001).

Several *clinical* parameters were correlated with a poor outcome: age greater than 60 years (p=0.05), operative delay longer than 10 days (p=0.001), the severity of the fracture and in particular fractures-dislocations (p=0.05). Other parameters were correlated with a good functional result: rehabilitation in a specialist center (p=0.03) and patient cooperation with the rehabilitation (p=0.03).

Table 5. Functional evaluation

Function (normal or with mild compromise)	Rating
Use back pocket	92 %
Wash opposite axilla	76 %
Comb hair	38 %
Carry 4–6 g with arm at side	56 %
Use hand with arm at shoulder level	65 %
Use hand with arm above the head	47 %
Care for perineum	87 %
Eat with ustensils	76 %
Sleep on affected side	56 %
Dress self	70 %

Radiological Results

Malposition of the prosthesis in length and retroversion was frequent and was correlated with a poor functional result. Table 6 shows that elongation greater than 10 mm (n=10), shortening greater than 15 mm (n=5), and retroversion superior to 40° (n=9) were detrimental for the functional result. The acromiohumeral distance was less than 7 mm in 15 cases (27 %), which indicates upward migration of the humeral head and is indirect evidence of a rotator cuff rupture or a nonfunctioning cuff. Narrowing of the acromiohumeral distance was correlated with both humeral lengthening (p=0.001) and excessive retroversion (p=0.003). Anterior active elevation was only 78° in average and external rotation was only 5.5° in case of excessive retroversion.

Migration of the greater tuberosity was also correlated with a poor functional result (Table 7). This migration was superior in 11 cases (17 %) and posterior in 19 cases (29 %). Initially we thought that when the tuberosity was not visible on the AP view, it must have undergone lysis. However, other radiographs, such as axillary views, and CT showed that the greater tuberosity was present but had migrated behind the prosthetic neck (Fig. 2). Migration of the lesser tuberosity occurred in only three

Table 6. Malposition of the prosthesis and correlation with a poor functional result

Malposition of the prosthesis	n	%	Correlation with a poor functional result (Constant score)
• Superior placement ≥ 10 mm	10	15	P = 0.02
• Inferior placement ≤ 10 mm (n = 14) ≤ 15 mm (n = 5)		29	≤ 10 mm, n.s. ≤ 15 mm, P = 0.05
• Excessive retroversion > 40°	9	14	P = 0.006

Table 7. Malposition of the greater tuberosity and correlation with a poor functional result

Migration of the greater tuberosity	n	%	Correlation with a poor functional result (Constant score)
• Superior migration (nonunion with the diaphysis)	11	17	P = 0.01
• Posterior migration (nonunion with lesser tuberosity)	19	29	P = 0.007

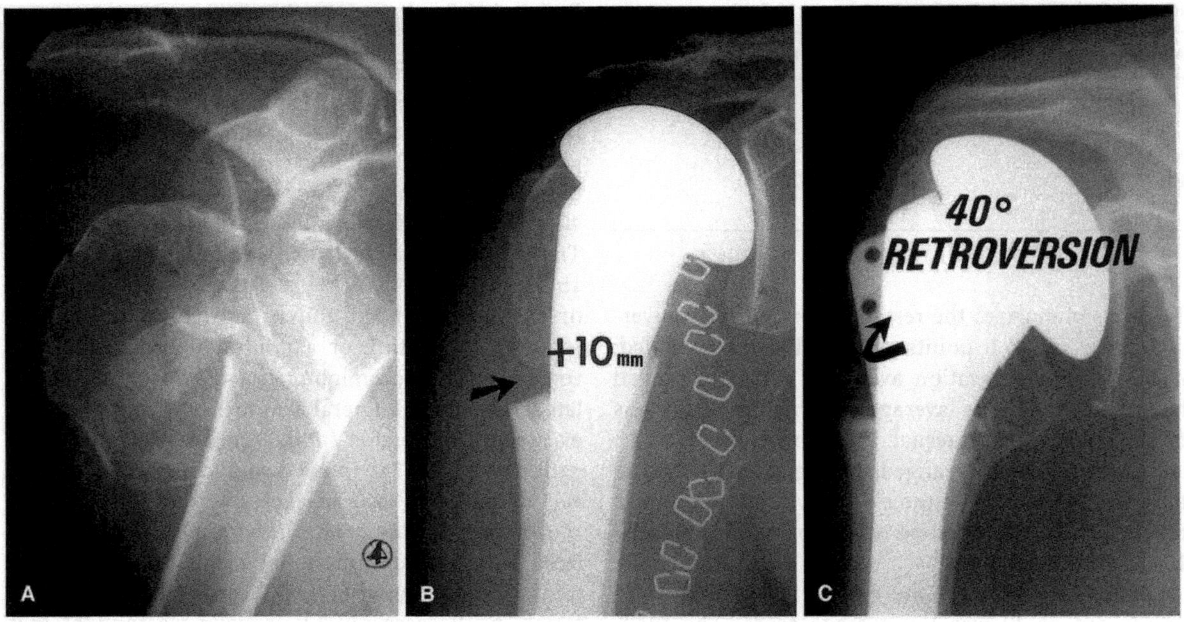

Fig. 2 A–F. Greater tuberosity migration related to poor prosthesis positioning for length and retroversion. **A** Four-part displaced fracture. **B** Postoperative X-rays: proud prosthesis (10 mm increased humeral length) with a gap between the greater tuberosity and the diaphysis. **C** Posterior migration of the greater tuberosity and proximal humeral migration at 2 years. **D** CT (2 years postoperatively): posterior migration of the greater tuberosity due to increased retroversion (>40° with nonunion between the tuberosities). **E,F** Poor functional result with poor abduction and poor external rotation

cases (5%), in association with greater tuberosity migration and was related to insufficient technique for suturing the tuberosities.

Migration of the greater tuberosity was correlated with malposition of the prosthesis. A proud prosthesis was more often associated with a superior migration of the greater tuberosity, leading to a *nonunion with the diaphysis* (p=0.04) while a prosthesis implanted with too much retroversion was more often associated with a posterior migration of the greater tuberosity, leading to a *nonunion with the lesser tuberosity* (p=0.001).

Technical errors may be combined, increasing the risk of migration of the greater tuberosity and of poor functional results. For instance, a proud and too retroverted prosthesis ("unhappy association") led always to migration of the greater tuberosity and poor functional result (Fig. 3).

We looked to the "anatomical profile" of the patients with excellent results and those with poor results (Table 8). We compared a group of 15 patients with excellent results (Constant score >90, active anterior elevation 147°, external rotation 31°, and internal rotation T12 level) with a group of

Table 8. Prosthesis positioning and final status of the greater tuberosity in two groups of patients with excellent and poor results

	Excellent Results (n = 15) Constant score > 90 Ant. Active Elev. = 147° Active Ext. Rot. = 31° Active Int. Rot. = T12	Poor Results (n = 13) Constant score < 60 Ant. Active Elev. = 70° Active Ext. Rot. = 10° Active Int. Rot. = L5	p
Prosthesis positioning			
High prosthesis (humeral lenghtening ≥ +10 mm)	0	7	0.02
Low prosthesis (humeral shortening ≥ −15 mm)	1	5	0.05
Prosthesis retroversion ≥ 40°	0	6	0.006
Migration of greater tuberosity			
Posterior migration	0	6	0.007
Superior migration	0	6	0.01

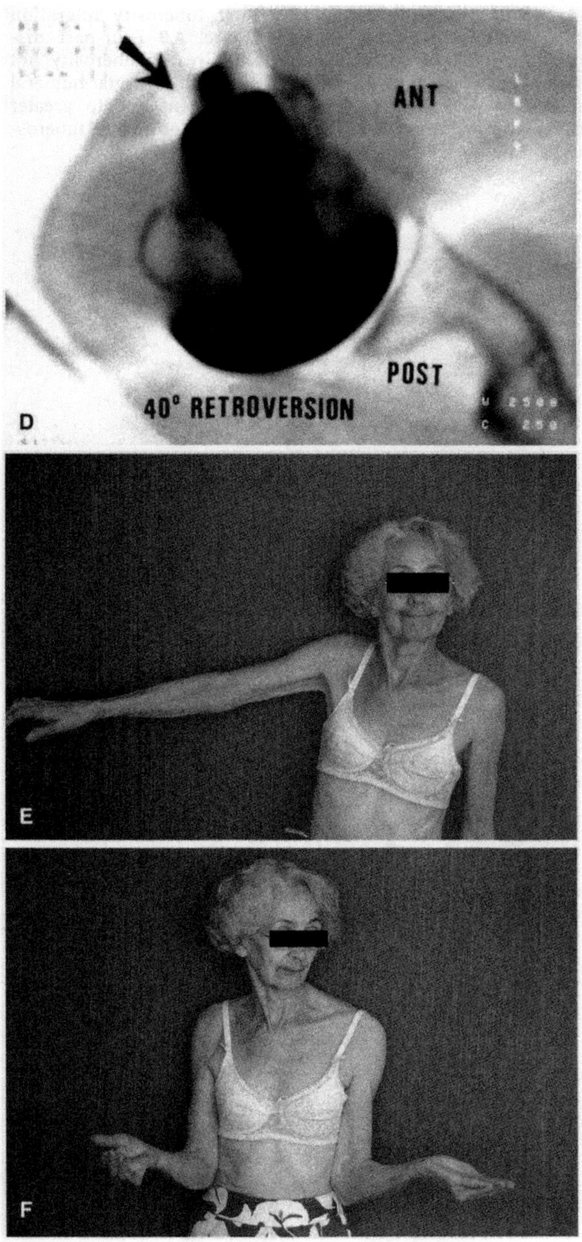

Fig. 2 A–F. (continued)

13 patients with poor results (Constant score <60, active anterior elevation 70°, external rotation 10°, and internal rotation L5 level). The most significant factor associated with a poor functional result was migration of the greater tuberosity leading to non-union, malunion and partial or total bone resorption. There was a clear correlation between prosthesis positioning and greater tuberosity migration: migrations of the greater tuberosity were the consequence of malposition of the humeral prosthesis in length (too proud) and/or excessive retroversion. Table 8 clearly shows the influence of the position of the prosthesis and the final status of the greater tuberosity on the functional results in the two groups of patients.

Finally, we looked at whether the *use of the Aequalis fracture jig* improved the positioning of the prosthesis for length and retroversion. Figure 4 confirms the effect on positioning of the prosthesis with regard to humeral length. Using the jig allows a positioning of the prosthesis within a precision of +5 to –5 mm while "eye-ball" positioning allows less precision (p=0.025). The prosthesis implanted with excessive retroversion were all inserted without the fracture jig. The fracture jig has been used in all but two of the excellent results of the present series, suggesting that "eye ball" positioning of the prosthesis may be insufficient. However, the use of the jig is not a guarantee for an accurate placement of the prosthesis in length: five patients had a proud positioning of the prosthesis despite the use of the jig. The reasons for this malposition was a mistake in the preoperative planning because of poor measured radiographs in three cases and a mistake in the identification of the bony landmarks of the elbow in two patients with fatty elbows.

Other Complications

Apart from the numerous tuberosity problems (non-unions and malunions) detailed above, we found three types of postoperative problem: nerve lesions, anterior instability and ectopic bone formation.

Nerve lesions were observed in three patients (4.5 %). In two cases the lesion involved the brachial plexus and in one case there was a axillary nerve injury which predated the surgery and was due to the initial trauma. The three lesions only partially recovered and affected the postoperative shoulder function.

Anterior instability was observed in one patient who sustained an anterior dislocation when she fell 18 months after surgery. The anterior dislocation was reduced under general anesthesia and the post-reduction radiographs showed the greater tuberosity to have been pulled off. The patient has not undergone revision surgery and currently has a chronic anterior dislocation. Although the functional result is poor, with active anterior elevation of only 45°, the patient is pain-free and does not wish to have further surgery.

Ectopic bone formation was observed in seven shoulders (11 %). There were grade II ossifications (occupying more than 50 % of the glenohumeral joint-line) in five cases (7.5 %) and grade III (a true scapulohumeral bridge) in two cases (3 %).

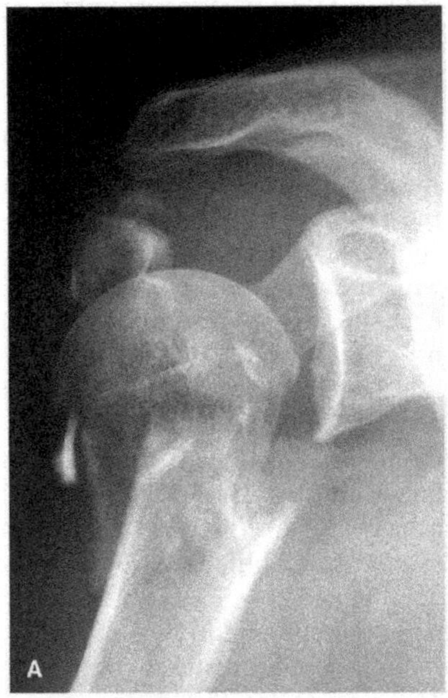

Fig. 3 A–G. Another example of greater tuberosity migration after shoulder replacement for fracture. **A,B** Four-part displaced fracture. **C** Proud prosthesis. **D** Greater tuberosity not visible on AP view in external rotation with proximal humeral migration. **E** Posterior glenoid impingement due to greater tuberosity malunion. **F** Posterior migration of greater tuberosity visible on CT-scan

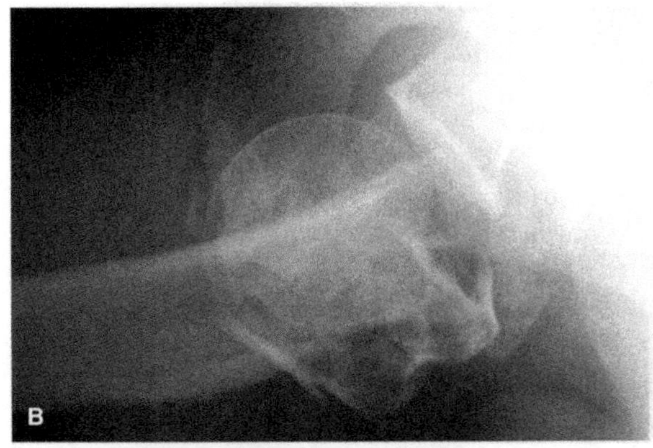

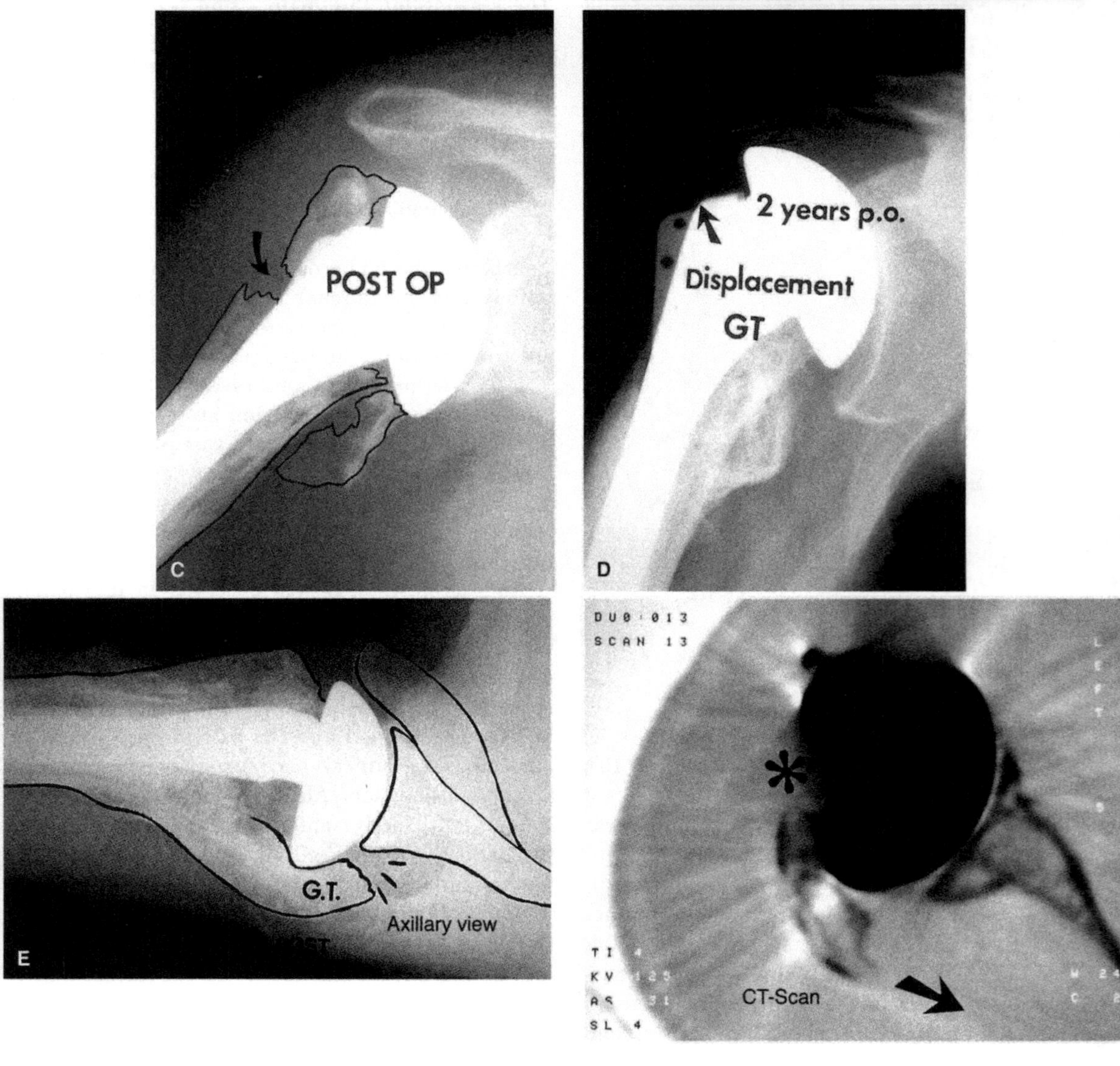

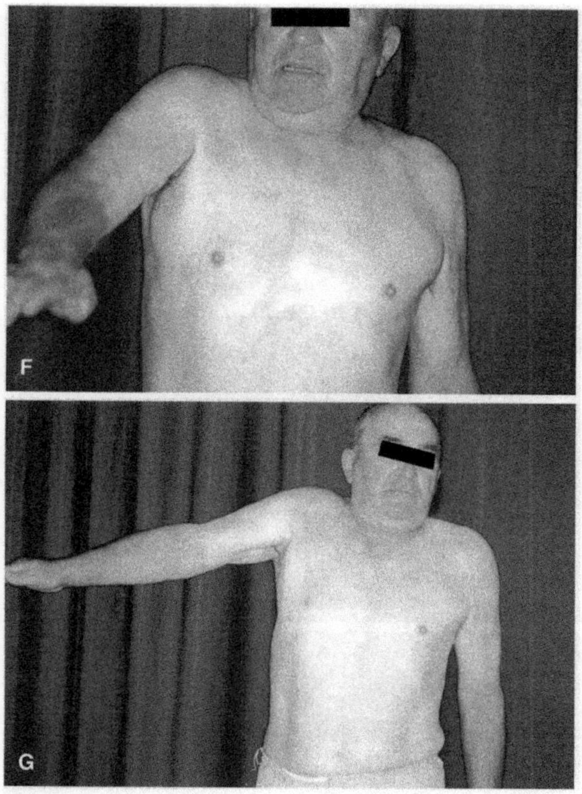

Fig. 3 A–G. (continued) G Poor active abduction and elevation

Although ossifications can be considered as complications, they did not effect the functional result in this series.

No humeral loosening was observed at follow up. However, 4 (16%) humeral components have a complete lucent line inferior to 2 mm at the bone-cement interface and 16 (24%) have an incomplete lucent line less than 1-mm in width.

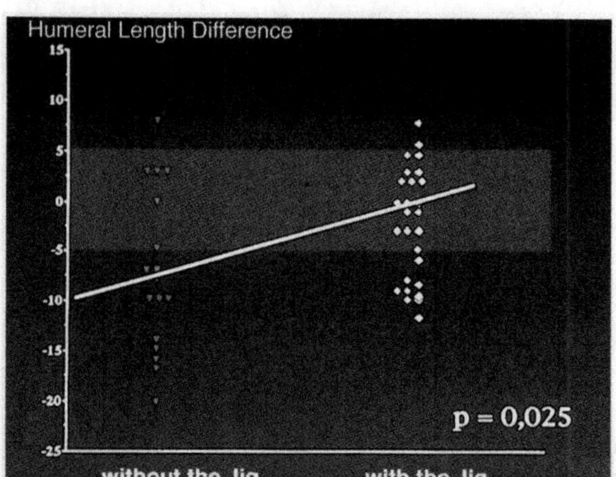

Fig. 4. Difference in humeral length after shoulder replacement with and without the Aequalis fracture jig. The jig allows a restoration of humeral length with a precision being between +5 and -5 mm

Discussion

Arthroplasty for fracture has a reputation for being a risky operation with uncertain results regarding mobility and function [11–13, 16, 20, 24, 27, 28, 39, 41, 43, 45]. Different factors related to poor outcomes have already been described in previous series [13, 15, 17, 41, 45] and were also identified in this study: age greater than 60 years with operative delay greater than 10 days; a fracture-dislocation and the absence of cooperation in the rehabilitation program. However, we were able to identify that the most significant factor associated with an unsatisfactory result was migration of the greater tuberosity. Moreover, we were able to demonstrate that greater tuberosity migration was related to malposition of the prosthesis for length and retroversion.

Poor positioning of the prosthesis for length leads to poor functional result and appears to be especially prejudicial. The present study confirms some of our previous works [2, 20]. Correctly setting the length of the humeral prosthesis is difficult in fracture cases because, except in rare cases, the proximal anatomical landmarks have disappeared due to bone loss and it is difficult to maintain the prosthesis in proper position: either the diameter of the stem is oversized and fills the canal placing the prosthesis in a proud position or it is undersized placing the prosthesis in a low position. Some shoulder surgeons have found helpful to use a surgical sponge wrapped around the implant to maintain the prosthesis in a proper position [44]. Although this may help, this may not be reproducible and enough accurate for less experienced surgeons.

In the present series any elongation greater than 10 mm was particularly detrimental with regard to active anterior elevation and pain. Lengthening of the humerus, because of a proud prosthesis, has two potential consequences: firstly, a possible non-union between the greater tuberosity and the diaphysis because the prosthesis protrudes from the shaft (p=0.04); secondly, a proximal migration of the humerus (p=0.001) leading to a possible cuff rupture because of excessive tension and squeezing of the supraspinatus between the prosthetic head and the coracoacromial arch (Figs. 2, 3). This is demonstrated indirectly at review by reduction in the acromiohumeral distance (less than 7 mm) with proximal humeral migration in the 15 patients with lengthening of the humerus. On the other hand, shortening of the humerus is better tolerated but becomes prejudicial when greater than 15 mm. A conclusion of this finding would be that: if in doubt, it is better to be short rather than long when implanting the humeral component. Our findings are in agreement with Neer who stated that loss

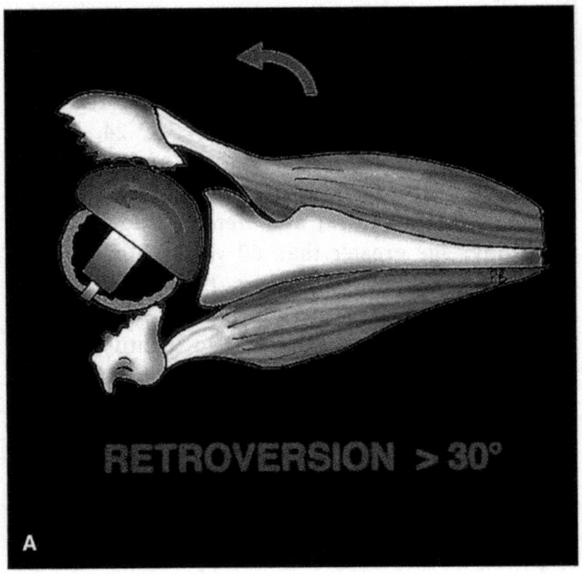

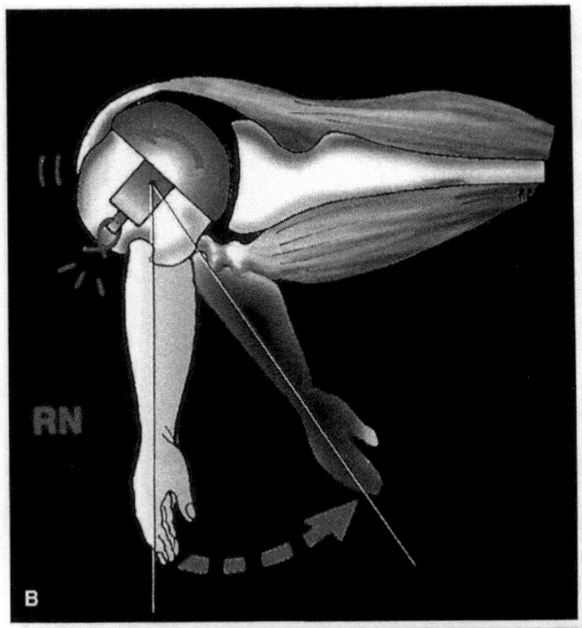

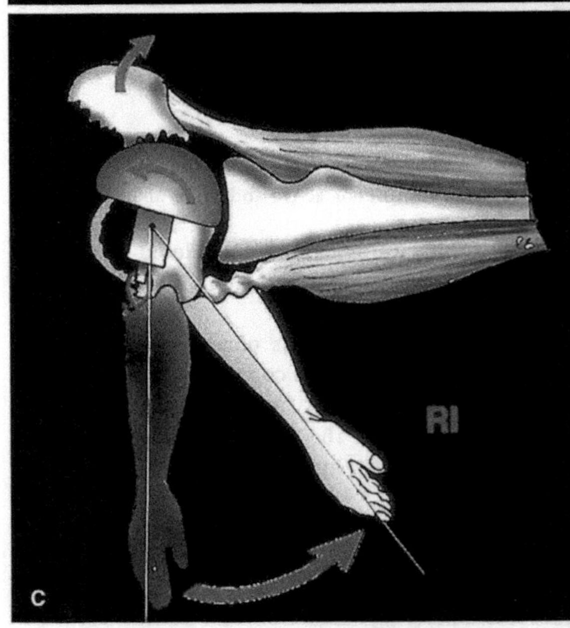

Fig. 5 A–C. Relationship between increased retroversion and posterior migration of the greater tuberosity. **A** Cementing the shoulder prosthesis with too much retroversion. **B** Synthesis of the greater tuberosity with the arm in neutral rotation is still possible. **C** However, once the arm is placed in internal rotation (in a sling at the end of the operation) there are too much pull-off strengths on the bone fragment which leads to posterior migration of the greater tuberosity

of humeral length is extremely common in prosthesis for fractures and that a loss of 2 cm or more leads to inadequate deltoid power [32].

Poor positioning of the prosthesis in retroversion, especially increased retroversion (>40°), is also a source of a poor functional result. Again, maintaining the prosthesis in the desired position of retroversion is difficult because of the possible rotation of the humeral component in the canal while reducing the tuberosities. Moreover, the bicipital groove is not an accurate landmark in four-part because it is often fractured (31 % of the cases) and only the lower portion of the groove could help for orientation in rotation of the prosthesis. Unfortunately, this lower portion of the groove is more axially oriented and leads to artificially increase the prosthetic retroversion as we have demonstrated in a previous study [5].

The consequences of increased retroversion of the prosthesis in fractures has been underestimated until now: the nine cases of our study with an increased retroversion of the prosthesis were all associated with a posterior migration of the greater tuberosity visible on axillary radiographs and CT at follow-up (Figs. 3, 4). Positioning the prosthesis with too much retroversion has the effect of inducing a pull-off of the greater tuberosity due to the excess tension on it when the arm is in internal rotation (the postoperative position in a sling). Intraoperatively, the tuberosity seems to be securely attached with the arm in neutral or external rotation but once internal rotation is applied, then the forces acting on the synthesis are too strong and the tuberosity migrates posteriorly (Fig. 5). This posterior migration of the greater tuberosity probably happens in the hours or in the days following the operation. When the tuberosity is not seen on the anteroposterior radiograph, then many authors have interpreted this as being due to "bone lysis" or "bone resorption" [8, 13, 27, 45]. Our study shows that the greater tuberosity is in fact present but hidden behind the metal neck of the prosthesis.

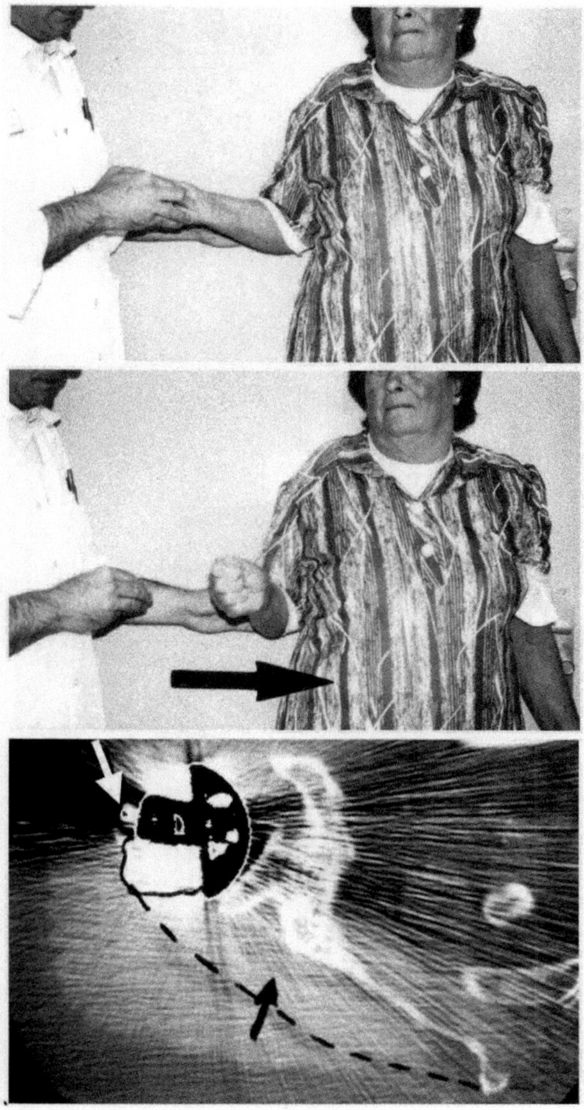

Fig. 6. Dropping sign in a patient with greater tuberosity nonunion (white arrow) and fatty degeneration of the infraspinatus (black arrow)

This posterior migration of the greater tuberosity equates to a massive tear of the rotator cuff involving supraspinatus, infraspinatus and teres minor as evidenced by the clinical loss of force in external rotation with a dropping sign and the fatty degeneration of the muscle belly visible on CT (Fig. 6). The weakness in external rotation as well as posterior glenoid impingement explain the poor active external rotation (5.5° in average) and poor anterior active elevation (78° in average) in cases where there is posterior migration of the tuberosity. Again, our findings are in agreement with Neer, who stated that the infraspinatus and teres minor supply more than 90% of the power for external rotation of the shoulder and that the deltoid alone is not capable of supplying the power for external rotation necessary for overhead use [32]. The dissociation between active anterior elevation (deficient) and passive anterior elevation (preserved) observed in this study demonstrate that this is not the stiffness or the scarring of the subacromial space and around the rotator cuff but rather the muscular weakness which is responsible for the poor functional results. Excessive retroversion leads also to proximal humeral migration with narrowing of the acromiohumeral distance.

Greater tuberosity displacement has been identified by Tanner and Cofield as being the most common complication after shoulder prosthesis for fracture [41]. Bigliani et al. recently examined the causes of failure after prosthetic replacement for proximal humeral fractures and found that although almost all failed cases had multiple causes, the most common single identifiable reason was greater tuberosity displacement [1]. In the present study, greater tuberosity migration was clearly associated with poor positioning of the prosthesis for length and/or retroversion. All the authors since Neer have stressed the necessity of meticulous and strong fixation of the greater tuberosity with nonabsorbable sutures [4, 8, 13, 31, 32]. We used very large diameter (#5 or 7) nonabsorbable sutures and secured the tuberosities with both horizontal and vertical suturing to assure better stability and enhance bony consolidation with the diaphysis. However, fixation of the tuberosities, regardless of their quality, cannot resist the excessive forces engendered when the prosthesis is positioned too high or too retroverted. Exact positioning of the prosthesis with regard to length and retroversion seems to be an essential step before embarking on any fixation. Our study has shown that poor positioning of the prosthesis has a direct influence on the position and final status of the greater tuberosity leading to nonunion and malunion. Separate fixation of the two tuberosities, starting with the greater, as recommended in the literature, allows the position of the greater tuberosity to be controlled in relation to the prosthetic head and the diaphysis [4, 8]. Rather than pass the sutures through the fin of the prosthesis, we now recommend to pass the sutures around the neck of the prosthesis in order to improve the approximation of the tuberosities.

The Aequalis fracture jig offers several advantages by standardizing the technique for positioning the humeral component for length and retroversion (Fig. 7). Most of the errors in restoring humeral length and retroversion occur because of "eye balled" positioning of the prosthesis in fractures and explain probably the inconsistent and somewhat unpredictable results observed in the literature [1, 2, 8, 13, 15, 19, 20, 33, 41, 43]. The fracture jig allows the trial prosthesis as well as the definitive prosthe-

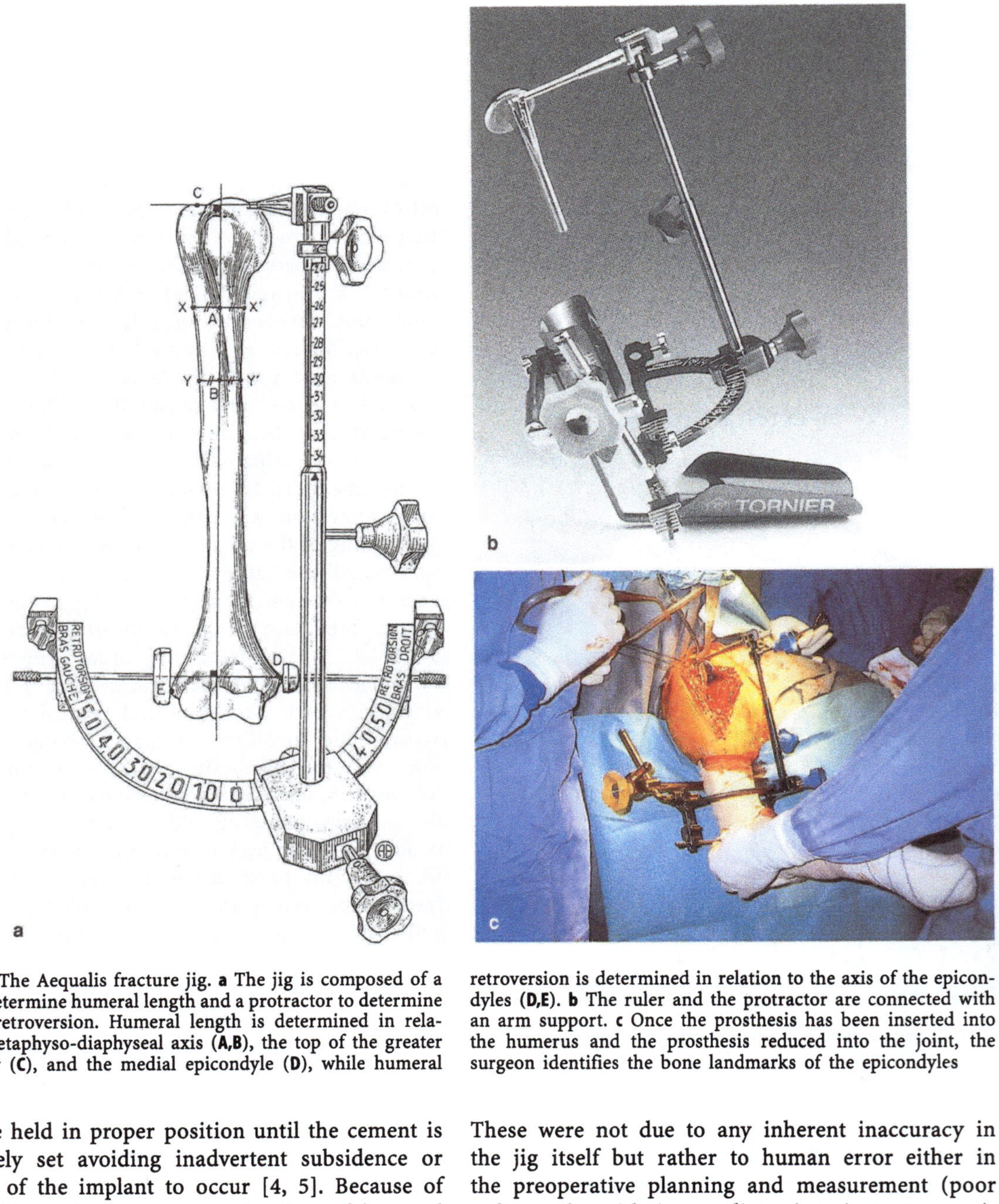

Fig. 7a–c. The Aequalis fracture jig. **a** The jig is composed of a ruler to determine humeral length and a protractor to determine humeral retroversion. Humeral length is determined in relation to metaphyso-diaphyseal axis (**A,B**), the top of the greater tuberosity (**C**), and the medial epicondyle (**D**), while humeral retroversion is determined in relation to the axis of the epicondyles (**D,E**). **b** The ruler and the protractor are connected with an arm support. **c** Once the prosthesis has been inserted into the humerus and the prosthesis reduced into the joint, the surgeon identifies the bone landmarks of the epicondyles

sis to be held in proper position until the cement is completely set avoiding inadvertent subsidence or rotation of the implant to occur [4, 5]. Because of the reliable and appropriate restoration of humeral length and retroversion offered by the jig, the surgeon can concentrate on the anatomical positioning and fixation of the tuberosities. More precise tensioning of the soft tissues in the vertical and horizontal planes allowed by properly positioned prosthesis minimizes stress on the bone sutures. This should aid in achieving union of the tuberosities to the shaft and proper functioning of the rotator cuff, essential in obtaining good functional results (Fig. 8).

However, even with the jig, mistakes in prosthesis positioning can be made as observed in five cases. These were not due to any inherent inaccuracy in the jig itself but rather to human error either in the preoperative planning and measurement (poor radiographs with image distorsion, improper positioning of the metal markers leading to mistakes in the calculation of the radiological magnification) or to difficulties in locating the intraoperative landmarks at the elbow in obese patients. This has led us to define more clearly the two most important steps in the use of the fracture jig [5] and these are repeated here: (a) the need to have a radiograph of the entire contralateral humerus avoiding two of the main causes for error in calculating radiographic enlargement: the humerus not flat on the cassette and the metal markers not parallel to the humerus; (b) the need to carry out a intraoperative radio-

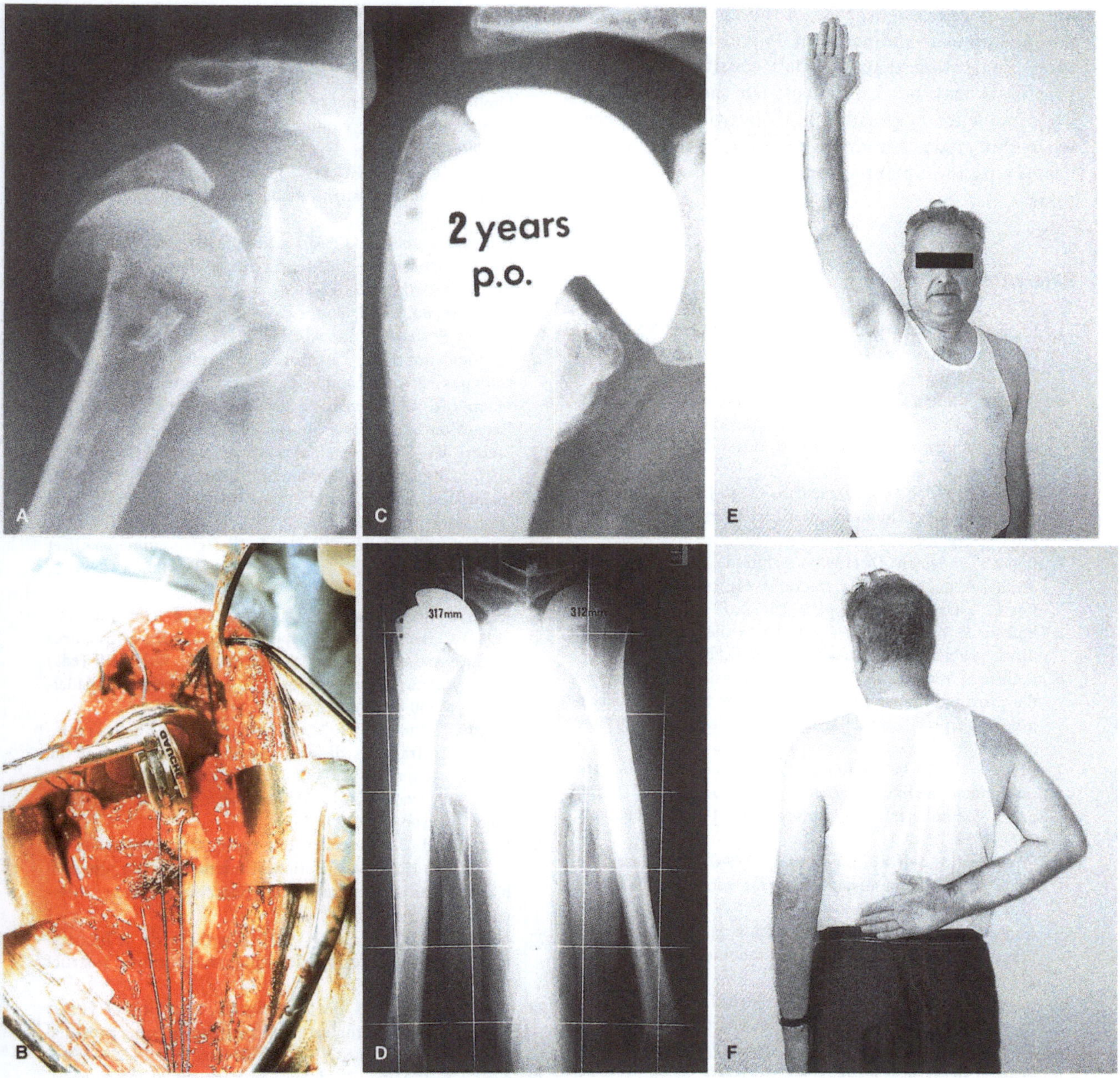

Fig. 8 A–F. Example of accurate reconstruction of the proximal humerus with a good functional result after a shoulder replacement for a four-part fracture. **A** Four-part fracture. **B** The fracture jig holds the prosthesis at proper length and retroversion. **C** Anatomical reconstruction of the greater tuberosity. **D** Restoration of humeral length (±5 mm). **E,F** Restoration of complete active mobility

graphic check of the position of the jig in relation to the elbow landmarks using an image-intensifier. In the next future CT should provide more accurate preoperative measurement of humeral length and should even allow to calculate true length and retroversion after tridimensional reconstruction of the fractured humerus [17].

Conclusion

There is a clear correlation between prosthesis positioning and greater tuberosity migration: posterosuperior migration of the greater tuberosity is the consequence of malpositioning the humeral prosthesis in height (too proud) and/or excessive retroversion. Prosthesis positioning is the key to greater tuberosity union to the shaft and should be more accurate but this is difficult because of the absence of proximal anatomical landmarks in 3- and four-part fractures, suggesting that "eye-ball" positioning of the prosthesis may be insufficient. On the basis of the high incidence of prosthetic malpositioning observed in this study, it may be relevant to consider the use of a jig to implant a humeral component in fractures.

References

1. Bigliani LU, Flatow EL, Mc Cluskey, Fischer RA (1991) Failed prosthetic replacement for displaced proximal humeral fractures. Orthop Trans 15:747–748
2. Boileau P, Chau E, Perraud M, Arcamone H, Argenson C (1993) Restoration of humeral length and humeral offset after shoulder prosthesis for fractures. Rev Chir Orthop 73:150
3. Boileau P, Walch G, Mazzoleni N, Urien JP (1993) In vitro measurement of humeral head retroversion. J Shoulder Elbow Surg 2(2):S12
4. Boileau P, Huten D (1995) Technique chirurgicale des prothèses de Neer pour fractures céphalo-tubérositaires. Rev Chir Orthop 81 [Suppl II]:85–88
5. Boileau P, Walch G (1996) Prothèses d'épaule pour fractures: problèmes et solutions. Maitr Orthop 6:18–23
6. Boileau P, Walch G (1997) Three dimensional geometry of the proximal humerus: implications for the surgical technique and prosthetic design. J Bone Joint Surg [Br] 79Br, 5:857–865
7. Broca P (1881) La torsion de l'humérus et le tropomètre, instrument destiné à mesurer la torsion des os (rédigé par L Mamouvier). Rev Anthrop 2(4):193–210, 385–423, 1577–1592
8. Compito CA, Self EB, Bigliani LU (1994) Arthoplasty and acute shoulder trauma, reasons for success and failure. Clin Orthop 307:27–36
9. Constant CR, Murley AHG (1987) A clinical method of functional assessment of the shoulder. Clin Orthop 214:160–164
10. Craig EV (1989) Prosthetic replacement for four part fractures of the proximal humerus. Tech Orthop 3:70–80
11. De Anquin CE, De Anquin CA (1982) Prosthetic replacement in the treatment of serious fractures of the proximal humerus. In: Bayley JL, Kessel L (eds): Shoulder Surgery. Springer, Berlin Heidelberg New York, pp 207–217
12. DesMarchais JE, Maurais G (1984) Treatment of complex fractures of the proximal humerus by Neer's hemiarthroplasty. In: Bateman JE, Welsh RP (eds) Surgery of the shoulder. Mosby, St Louis/Decker, Philadelphia, pp 60–63
13. Frich LH, Sojberg JO, Sneppen O (1991) Shoulder arthroplasty in complexe acute and chronic proximal humerus fractures. Orthopaedics 14:949–954
14. Goldman RT, Koval KJ, Cuomo F, Gallagher MA, Zuckerman JD (1995) Functional outcome after humeral head replacement for acute three-and four-part proximal fractures. J Shoulder Elbow Surg 4(2):81–86
15. Green A, Barnard WL, Imbird RS, Providence RI (1993) Humeral head replacement for acute four-part proximal humerus fractures. J Soulder Elbow Surg 2, 5:249–254
16. Hawkins RJ, Switlyk P (1993) Acute prosthetic replacement for severe fractures of the proximal humerus. Clin Orthop 289:156–160
17. Hurman WW, Jacobsen FS, AndersonJC, Chu WK (1987) Limb-length discrepency measured with computerised axial tomographic equipment. J Bone Joint Surg Am 69:699–705
18. Hughes M, Neer CS II (1975) Glenohumeral joint replacement and postoperative rehabilitation. Phys Ther 55:850–858
19. Huten D, Duparc J (1986) L'arthroplastie prothétique dans les traumatismes complexes récents et anciens de l'épaule. Rev Chir Orthop 72:517–529
20. Huten D, Boileau P, Bonnevialle P, Maynou C, Renault E, Vogt F, Postel JM, Candelier G, Fleure P (1996) Résultats et indications de l'arthroplastie prothétique dans les fractures récentes complexes de l'extrémité supérieure de l'humérus. Conférences d'Enseignement de la SOFCOT. Expansion Scientifique Française, Paris, pp 125–140
21. Ianotti JP, Gabriel JP, Schneck SL, Evans BG, Miras S (1992) The normal glenohumeral relationships. An anatomical study of one hundred and forty shoulders. J Bone Joint Surg Am 74:491–500
22. Jacobson SR, Mallon WJ (1993) The glenohumeral offset ratio: a radiographic study. J Shoulder Elbow Surg 2, 3:141–146
23. Jakob RP, Kristiansen T, Mayo K, Ganz R, Muller ME (1984) Classification and aspects of treatment of fractures of the proximal humeri. In: Bateman JE, Welsh RP (eds) Surgery of the shoulder. Mosby, St Louis/Decker, Philadelphia, pp 330–343
24. Kraulis J, Hunter G (1977) The results of prosthetics replacement in fractures dislocations of the upper end of the humerus. Injury 8:129–131
25. Khral VE, Evans FG (1945) Humeral torsion in man. Am J Phys Anthrop 3:229–253
26. Kristiansen B, Andersen LS, Olsen CA, Vasmarken JE (1988) The Neer classification of fractures of the proximal humerus: an assessment of interobserver variation. Skeletal Radiol 17:420–422
27. Muldon MP, Cofield RH (1997) Complications of humeral head replacement for proximal humeral fractures. Instruct Course Lect 46:15–24
28. Moeckel BH, Dines DM, Warren RF, Altchek DW (1992) Modular hemiarthroplasty for fractures of the proximal part of the humerus. J Bone Joint Surg Am 74:884–889
29. Neer CS III (1955) Articular replacement of the humeral head. J Bone Joint Surg Am 37:215–228
30. Neer CS (1970) Displaced proximal humeral fractures. I. Classification and evaluation. J Bone Joint Surg Am 52:1077–1089
31. Neer CS II (1970) Displaced proximal humeral fractures. II. Treatment of three and four part displacement. J Bone Joint Surg Am 52:1090–1103
32. Neer CS, Kirby RM (1982) Revision of humeral head and total shoulder arthroplasties. Clin Orthop 100:189–195
33. Pietu G, Deluzarches P, Goin F, Letenneur J (1992) Traumatismes complexes de l'extrémité supérieure de l'humérus traités par prothèse céphalique: à propos de 21 cas revus avec un recul moyen de 4 ans. Acta Orthop Belg 58:159–169

34. Roberts SNJ, Foley APJ, Swallow HM, Wallace WA, Coughlan DP (1991) The geometry of the humeral head and the design of protheses. J Bone Joint Surg Br 73:647–650
35. Rietveld ABM, Dannen HAM, Rozing PM, Oberman WR (1988) The lever arm in gleno humeral abduction after hemi arthroplasty. J Bone Joint Surg Br 70:561–565
36. Sidor ML, Zuckerman JD, Lyon T, Cuomo F, Shoenberg N (1992) The Neer calssification for proximal humeral fractures. J Bone Joint Surg Am 75:1745–1750
37. Siebenrock KA, Gerber C (1992) The reproductibility of classification of fractures of the proximal end of the humerus. J Bone Joint Surg Am 75:1751–1755
38. Sneppen O, Kjaersgaard-Andersen P, Frich LH (1990) Ectopic ossification after total shoulder arthroplasty. A study on 75 Neer total shoulder replacements. In: Post M, Morrey BF, Hawkins RT (eds) Surgery of the shoulder. Mosby-Year Book, St. Louis, pp 298–301
39. Stableforth PG (1984) Four-part fractures of the neck of the humerus. J Bone Joint Surg Br 66:104–108
40. Steel FLD, Tomlinson JDW (1989) The carrying angle in man. J Anat 92:315–317
41. Tanner MW, Cofield RH (1983) Prosthetic arthroplasty for fractures and fracture dislocations of the proximal humerus. Clin Orthop 179:116–128
42. Walch G, Boileau P (1991) Morphological study of the proximal humerus. J Bone Joint Surg Br 74 [Suppl I]:14
43. Willems WJ, Lim TEA (1985) Neer arthroplasty for humeral fractures. Acta Orthop Scand 56:394–395
44. Zuckerman JD, Cuomo F, Koval KJ (1997) Proximal humeral replacement for complex fractures: indications and surgical technique. Instruct Course Lect 46:7–14
45. Zyto K, Kronberg M, Bröstrom LA (1995) Shoulder function after displaced fractures of the proximal humerus. J Shoulder Elbow Surg 4:331–336

Section XII:

Sequelae of Proximal Humeral Fractures

Sequelae of Fractures of the Proximal Humerus: Surgical Classification and Limits of Shoulder Arthroplasty

P. Boileau, G. Walch, C. Trojani, R. Sinnerton, A.A. Romeo, and B. Veneau

Summary

This prospective multicenter study of 71 sequelae of fractures of the proximal humerus treated using a nonconstrained shoulder prosthesis demonstrates that osteotomy of the greater tuberosity is the most important factor for the functional result (p=0.05) because of persistent nonunion and/or bone resorption. This allows two types of fracture sequelae to be distinguished, whose functional results are completely different: (a) ***Intracapsular, impacted fracture sequelae*** *in which osteotomy of the greater tuberosity is* ***not*** *required. This type of sequelae, in which the greater tuberosity heals to the shaft with a slight malunion, includes cephalic collapse and necrosis (40 cases) and chronic, locked dislocations and fracture-dislocations (9 cases). (b)* ***Extracapsular, disimpacted fracture sequelae*** *in which an implant cannot be inserted without osteotomizing and repositioning the greater tuberosity. This type of sequelae, in which the greater tuberosity is not healed or heals away from the shaft, includes surgical neck nonunions (6 cases) and severe tuberosity malunions (16 cases). The necessity of performing a greater tuberosity osteotomy with the shoulder replacement in a fracture sequelae to reconstruct the proximal humerus should lead the surgeons to anticipate a "limited goal result" with a limited active anterior elevation, below the horizontal, and with residual pain.*

Introduction

Displaced proximal humeral fractures which have received either no treatment or inappropriate treatment may result in pain and disability of the shoulder. Some of these fracture sequelae may be indications for the insertion of a shoulder prosthesis. For example, some cases of avascular necrosis with subchondral bone collapse, certain locked dislocations and fracture dislocations, some nonunions of the surgical neck with a small osteoporotic head fragment, and some malunions of the tuberosities with incongruity of the humeral articular surface [5, 29]. However, treatment of the sequelae of proximal humeral fractures remains controversial because the possible benefit of arthroplasty in chronic problems has not yet been clearly established, and the prognosis remains unpredictable [11, 13, 29, 31, 40].

Neer was the first author to describe the technical difficulties, the high complication rate, and the poor and inconsistent functional results of shoulder arthroplasty in "old trauma" [28, 29]. However, there is disappointingly little in the literature on the subject because the number of cases in each series is limited [11, 13, 29, 31, 40]. Moreover, there is some confusion within heterogeneous groups of sequelae of the proximal humerus and the therapeutic results achieved by shoulder replacement within each group.

The lack of an updated classification of the sequelae of proximal humeral fractures may be instrumental in preventing communication and comparison of treatments between different centers. Furthermore, these posttraumatic sequelae usually occur in relatively young and active patients, making it even more crucial to know the preoperative prognosis when deciding on shoulder joint arthroplasty.

The purpose of this prospective multicenter study was to classify the sequelae of fracture of the proximal humerus, to evaluate the results achieved using a nonconstrained shoulder prosthesis, and to gather any information that would help establish guidelines for their treatment. A new surgical classification and a new biomechanical concept of fracture sequelae of the proximal humerus are proposed.

Methods and Materials

Patients

A prospective, multicenter study was undertaken on 71 sequelae of fractures of the proximal humerus operated on between 1991 and 1995 with a nonconstrained shoulder prosthesis. Thirteen orthopedic centers were involved in the study (Table 1). The charts, operation notes, initial and late radiographs, and computed tomograms, when available, were reviewed. There were 70 patients (40 men and 30 women). One patient had been operated on

Table 1. Origin of the 71 fractures sequelae

Center	Surgeon	*n*
Giens	Basso M	2
Nice	Boileau P	11
Tours	Favard L	2
Marseille	Franceschi JP	4
Paris	Gouttallier D, Scheffer JC	2
Stuttgart	Habermeyer P	17
Strasbourg	Kempf JF	2
Bordeaux	Le Huec JC	4
Lyon	Lévigne C	5
Lille	Mestdagh H	2
Nancy	Molé D	3
Lyon	Walch G	17

both shoulders. The average age of the patients at the time of the operation was 59 years (between 30 and 87). The right side was involved in 44 cases (62 %) and the dominant side in 42 cases (59 %). The cause of the initial fracture was a simple fall in 31 cases, a car accident in 12, a seizure in 4, and unknown in 24. Preoperatively there were no vascular lesions, but two transient axillary nerve lesions were observed. There was one associated glenoid fracture in a patient with a posterior fracture dislocation.

The Neer [24] and the AO classification of fractures [19, 20] of the proximal humerus was used to classify the initial fracture. The initial lesions and initial treatment are summarized in Table 2. Forty-three patients had had nonoperative treatment and 22 had undergone a previous operative procedure. Of these, 3 had had two revisions. The average delay between the initial fracture and the insertion of the prosthesis was 5 years and 5 months, but this varied greatly between the different fracture sequelae (Table 2).

A clinical and radiological review of all the patients was carried out with a mean follow-up of

Table 2. The four groups of sequelae of fractures of the proximal humerus according to the initial fracture, initial treatment, and delay before shoulder prosthesis

Fracture sequelae	Initial fracture	*n*	Initial treatment		Delay before prosthesis
			Orthopedic	Surgical	
Cephalic collapse or necrosis (n=40)	Four-part valgus impacted	20	35	5	8 years, 2 months
	Four-part varus impacted	12			
	Four-part displaced	1			
	Two-part anatomical neck	3			
	Two-part surgical neck	4			
Chronic dislocation and fracture-dislocation (n=9)	Posterior locked dislocation	7		None	1 year, 7 months
	Posterior fracture-dislocation	1			
	Anterior fracture-dislocation	1			
Nonunion of surgical neck (n=6)	Two-part surgical neck displaced	2	2	5 (one reoperation)	3 years
	Three-part geater tuberosity	2			
	Four-part, already operated on	2			
Severe tuberosity malunion (n=16)	Four-part displaced or dislocated fractures	16	6	12 (two reoperations)	2 years
Entire series (n=71)		71	43	22	5 years, 5 months

Table 3. Type of prosthesis (total or hemi-), associated bone procedures and status of the rotator cuff in the four groups of sequelae of fractures of the proximal humerus

Fracture sequelae	Prosthesis type		Associated bone procedure		Status of the rotator cuff		
	Humeral	Total	GT osteotomy	LT osteotomy	Normal	Thin	Torn
Cephalic collapse of necrosis (n=40)	19	21	0	2	19	17	4
Locked dislocation (n=9)	8	1	0	1	2	5	2
Nonunion of surgical neck (n=6)	6	0	6	2	4	0	2
Severe tuberosity malunion (n=16)	13	3	11	6	4	7	5
Entire series (n=71)	46	25	17	11	29	29	13

GT, Greater tuberosity; LT, lesser tuberosity.

19 months (12–48 months). The clinical evaluation was made using the Constant scoring system which covers pain, activity, mobility, and force and can be adjusted for age and sex [8, 9]. Radiographic examination consisted of anteroposterior views of the shoulder in neutral, internal, and external rotation, a scapular profile view (58 cases), and an axillary view (50 cases).

The radiological review was made separately and then together by two observers (P.B. and C.T.). Difficult or controversial cases were definitively classified by the two observers after discussion to reduce misinterpretation. Statistical analysis were carried out using Student's *t* test on Stateview software (Abacus Concept, USA).

Surgical Technique

All the patients were operated on by a senior surgeon using the same technique and a single implant. An extended deltopectoral incision was used in all the cases in this series except one in which a superior transacromial approach was used. Table 3 shows the type of prosthesis (hemi- or total), the associated tuberosities osteotomy, and the status of the rotator cuff. On 8 occasions the joint was approached via an osteotomy of the lesser tuberosity with subscapularis attached to improve mobilization. Where the displacement was moderate, the greater tuberosity was not osteotomized. However, in 20 cases there was severe displacement of the greater tuberosity, and an osteotomy was required. Tuberosity osteotomies were performed with an osteotome or a saw. Great care was taken to leave enough bone attached to the rotator cuff to allow solid fixation of the tuberosities to the diaphysis. After the osteotomy had been performed, the rotator cuff was released medially on its deep and superficial surfaces. Any capsular retraction was released at the glenoid edge to allow the tendon to be advanced laterally. At the end of the procedure the tuberosities were fixed to the implant and to the humeral shaft using heavy nonabsorbable sutures. An autologous bone graft taken either from the residual humeral head or from the iliac crest was performed in eight cases.

A rotator cuff tear was reported and repaired in 13 cases (Table 3): in seven of these, the rupture involved two tendons (supra- and infraspinatus), and in six, there was a single tendon rupture (four supra- and two infraspinatus tears. The biceps tendon was tenodesed nine times (13 %). Fifteen acromioplasties were performed with the goal of improving the space for the tuberosities under the coracoacromial vault or to protect a cuff repair. The head was carefully dislocated in adduction, external rotation, and retropulsion to minimize the risk of a shaft fracture. Despite this attention there were four diaphyseal and one metaphyseal fractures in the series. The humeral head cut was usually minimal and was not even required in some cases of collapse and necrosis after impacted fractures. Because of the bony distortion reaming the medullary canal was difficult. All the stems were cemented in place after inserting a cement restrictor.

The implant used was the Aequalis prostheses (Tornier). This shoulder prostheses is a new, unconstrained prosthesis whose conception was based on anatomical studies which demonstrated changes in the dimension and especially the shape of the proximal humerus [2, 3]. Forty-six were hemiarthroplasties (65 %) and 25 total shoulder replacements (35 %). In the 25 total shoulders, a polyethylene glenoid component was used in 23 cases, and this was always cemented. In two cases, a metal-backed component was used whose primary bony fixation comes from two expansion screws.

Postoperatively, passive mobility was started the day after surgery as per Neer's recommendations [28]. No active muscular activity was started until a complete range of passive movement had been achieved, and there was bony consolidation of the tuberosity osteotomies (6–8 weeks). The patients had home physiotherapy but 45 patients benefited from a stay in a specialist rehabilitation center for an average of 35 days.

Anatomopathological Classification

Faced with the enormous variability of the lesions seen and their many possible combinations, we were initially confronted with a problem of terminology and classification of the different sequelae of fractures of the proximal humerus. Originally, the fracture sequelae were presented as a heterogeneous series within which various different lesions may coexist, for example, malunion with avascular necrosis of the humeral head, nonunion, or a locked fracture-dislocation. A review of the published series showed the same confusion making any comparison of the results impossible [11, 13, 20, 29, 31, 40]. Most authors studied limited, heterogeneous groups of old fractures and combined the results obtained for avascular necrosis with moderate tuberosity malunions with those for major fracture sequelae. Some authors included nonunions of the surgical neck and locked fracture-dislocations in their series [29, 31, 40] while others either excluded them or studied them separately [11, 13, 31].

It therefore seemed to us that the inconsistent results achieved using shoulder prostheses to treat fracture sequelae are probably due in part to this enormous variability in the anatomical lesions. Starting from this basis it seemed logical to try first of all to categorize the sequelae of fracture of the proximal humerus. A study of the natural history of the different fractures and how they developed into their sequelae allowed us to start to understand the lesions which presented later. By studying the initial radiographs and those at later stages and by reading the operation notes we were able to describe four basic lesions which, when present, dominated the clinical picture and allowed the fracture sequelae to be classified into one of the following groups:

Group 1: Humeral Head Collapse and Necrosis with Moderate Tuberosity Malunion (n=40). Necrosis was classified as stage IV in 21 cases and stage III in 19. The initial fractures in this group were dominated by four-part fractures impacted either in valgus (20 cases) or varus (12 cases). The initial treatment had been nonoperative in 35 cases (simple immobilization) and operative in only five. Overall the time between the initial fracture and the prosthetic replacement was very long, averaging 8 years and 2 months, and six of the patients underwent surgery more than 20 years after their fracture.

Group 2: Locked Dislocations and Fracture-Dislocations (n=9). This group consisted of seven locked posterior dislocations with greater than 50% head collapse; one locked, two-part, posterior fracture-dislocation and one locked, impacted, anterior fracture-dislocation. In the latter two cases the tuberosity malunion was moderate, and partial osteotomy of the greater tuberosity was required only in the anterior dislocation case. In all the cases the lesion had gone unrecognized and received no treatment. The time between the initial trauma and prosthetic replacement was 1 year and 7 months on average.

Group 3: Nonunion of the Surgical Neck (n=6). This group was always combined with a severe malunion of the tuberosities to the shaft. All the nonunions of the surgical neck followed nonoperated three-part fractures with rotation of the humeral head fragment and significant displacement of the greater tuberosity or two- and four-part fractures which had undergone primary surgery. The time between the initial fracture and the prosthesis was on average 3 years.

Group 4: Severe Malunion of the Tuberosities (n=16). The initial fracture was a displaced or dislocated four-part fracture with disimpaction of the head. In 6 cases the initial treatment had been nonoperative, and the other 10 had undergone 12 interventions (2 revisions). The operations were one attempted surgical reduction combined with a posterior bone block, one surgical reduction revised after 2 years to clear the joint of para-articular ossifications and eight open reduction and internal fixations with various materials (screws, plates, staples, intramedullary nails). The average delay between the initial trauma and shoulder replacement was 2 years.

A New Surgical Classification of Sequelae of the Proximal Humeral Fractures

Although useful, this anatomopathological classification is not reliable in predicting the results expected with a shoulder arthroplasty. From a surgical point of view, two types of fracture sequelae can be distinguished whose natural history, functional outcome, and prognosis are very different: *Intracapsular, impacted fracture sequelae,* in which an osteotomy of the greater tuberosity is *not* required, and *Extracapsular, disimpacted fracture sequelae* in which a humeral implant cannot be inserted without osteotomy and repositioning of the greater tuberosity. Cephalic collapse and necrosis and chronic fracture dislocation or fracture-dislocation are usually associated with *impacted intracapsular fracture sequelae,* while nonunions of the surgical neck and severe malunions of the tuberosities are associated with *disimpacted extracapsular fracture sequelae* (Fig. 1).

We observed that it is major displacement of the humeral head, above all, which causes significant and intolerable displacement of the tuberosities. The sequelae of proximal humeral fractures can be divided into moderate and major, depending on the *impaction/disimpaction* of the humeral head and the *connection/disconnection* of the tuberosities, especially of the greater tuberosity (Fig. 2). The disimpaction of the humeral head and the disconnection of the greater tuberosity from the shaft are more frequent in case of extracapsular fractures of the proximal humerus, i.e., very displaced or dislocated fractures.

Most of the complex fracture sequelae in our series were found when there was a *disimpaction* (two- and four-part displaced or dislocated fractures) *and/or a rotation* of the head fragment (three-part fractures). This disimpaction of the head is a reflection of high-energy trauma leading

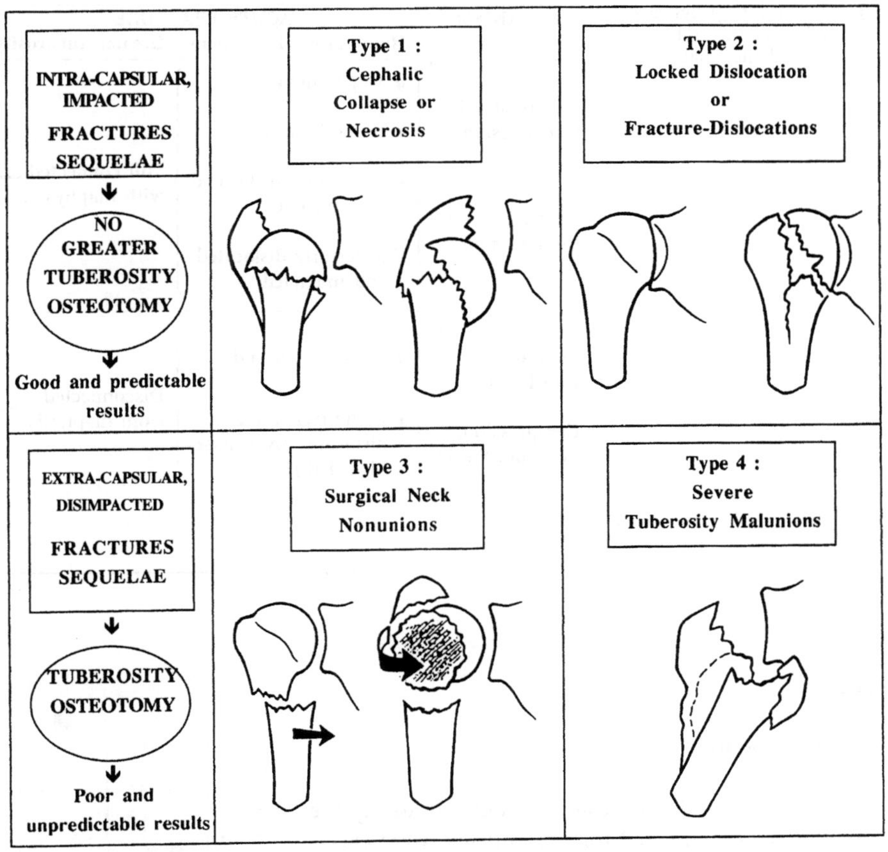

Fig. 1. A new surgical classification of sequelae of the proximal humerus fractures

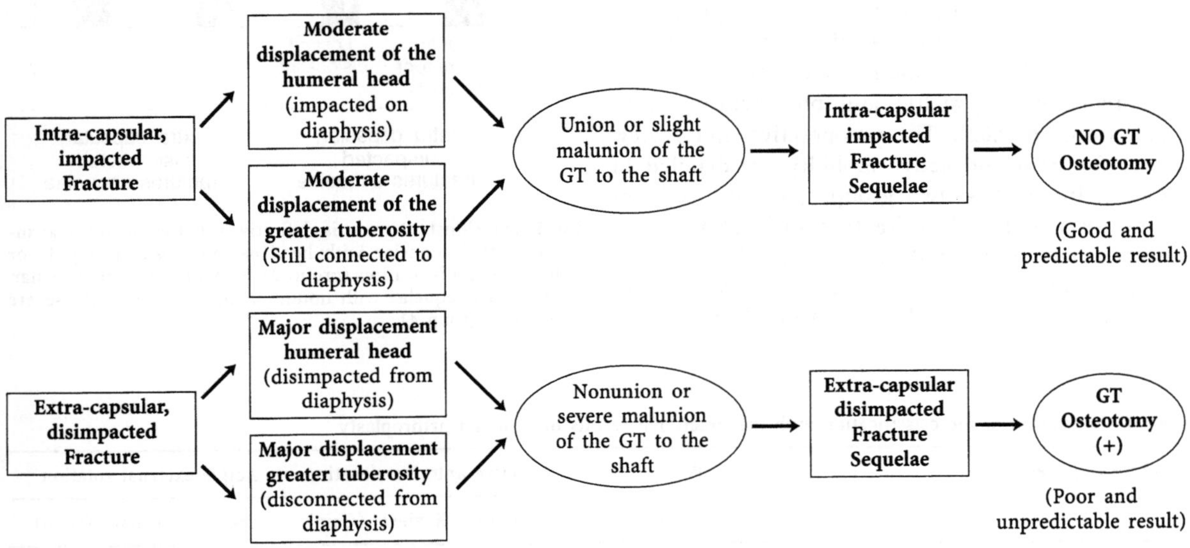

Fig. 2. Relationship between the necessity of tuberosity osteotomy and the pathophysiological mechanism (GT: Greater Tuberosity)

to permanent dislocation of the head fragment anteriorly, posteriorly, laterally, or inferiorly. Conversely, *impaction of the humeral head* (three- and four-part valgus impacted in fractures and varus) usually lead to simple and tolerable malunions of the tuberosities, although it is associated with late head collapse and necrosis and/or chronic (locked) dislocation (Fig. 1 and 2).

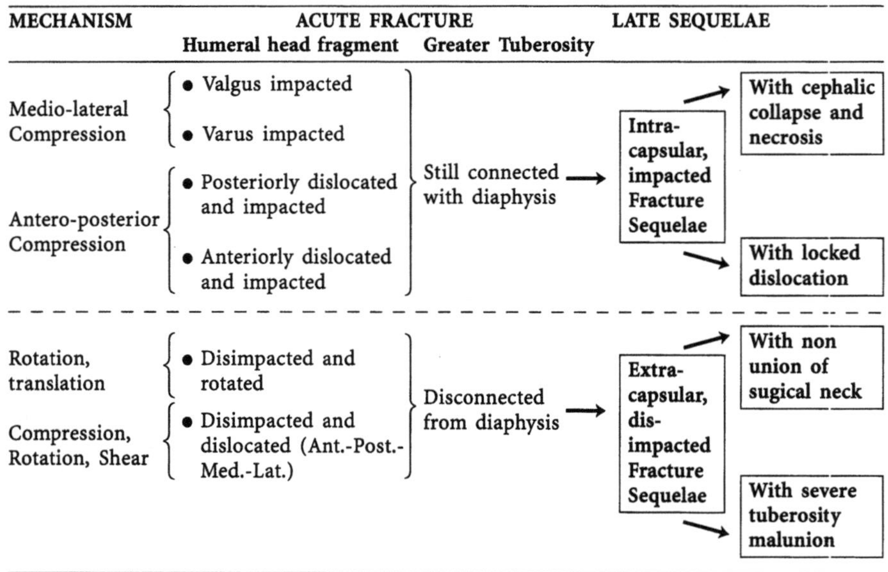

Fig. 3. Relationship between mechanism of the initial fracture and the final sequelae

Results

Functional Results

The overall functional results calculated using the Constant score, adjusted for age and sex, were excellent in 11 cases (16 %), good in 19 (26 %), average in 18 (25 %), and poor in 23 (33 %). The results differed significantly depending on the type of the lesion. Figure 4 shows that the type of fracture sequelae *(moderate or major)* was correlated with the preoperative (p=0.01) and postoperative Constant score (p=0.02). The preoperative and review scores for pain and active mobility are detailed in Table 4. In the first two groups (cephalic collapse or necrosis and locked fracture dislocations), the results where both good and predictable, resulting in significant pain reduction and recovery of active anterior elevation beyond the horizontal. In the sec-

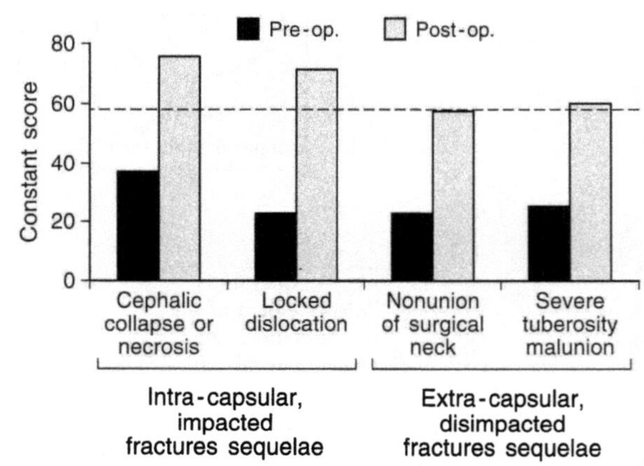

Fig. 4. The Constant score is definitively better in intra-capsular, impacted sequelae with head osteonecrosis (group 1) or with chronic dislocation (group 2) than in the extra-capsular, disimpacted sequelae with nonunion (group 3) or with severe malunion (group 4)

Table 4. Correlation of the classification with the functional results of shoulder arthroplasty

Fracture sequelae	Pain	Active anterior elevation			Active external rotation		
	(Constant score)	Preop.	Review	(Gain)	Preop	Review	(Gain)
Intracapsular, impacted fractures sequelae							
Cephalic collapse or necrosis (n=40)	12/15	87° →	133°	(+46°)	0° →	40°	(+40°)
Locked dislocation or fracture-dislocation (n=9)	11.5/15	57° →	114°	(+57°)	-2° →	42°	(+44°)
Extracapsular, disimpacted fractures sequelae							
Surgical neck nonunion (n=6)	7/15	50° →	63°	(+13°)	10° →	26°	(+16°)
Tuberosity malunion (n=16)	9.5/15	58° →	91°	(+32°)	-5° →	20°	(+25°)
Entire series (n=71)	10.7	74° →	102°	(+28°)	0° →	34°	(+34°)

ond two groups (nonunion of the surgical neck and severe tuberosity malunion), the results were both poor and unpredictable, with slight reduction in pain and no recovery of anterior elevation beyond the horizontal.

Of the 71 patients in the series 59 (81%) reported themselves as being satisfied or very satisfied with the result, although they did all have some degree of limitation in the operated shoulder. The ten patients who were disappointed with the operation and the two who were unhappy all belonged to groups 3 and 4.

Table 5. Complications following shoulder arthroplasty for fracture sequelae

Complications	*n*
Intraoperative fractures (4 diaphysis, 1 metaphysis)	5
Greater tuberosity early loss of fixation	1
Greater tuberosity nonunion	4
Greater tuberosity osteolysis	4
Anterior dislocation	1
Transitory neurological lesions (radial nerve)	1
Late infection	2
Total	18

Greater Tuberosity Osteotomy: The Reason for Poor Results

Greater tuberosity osteotomy was necessary in all cases of nonunion by remaining fibrous tissue and by bone cutting in tuberosity malformations. Osteotomy of the greater tuberosity either in isolation (12 cases) or in combination with lesser tuberosity osteotomy (8 cases), was the most prejudicial intervention, and allowed no recovery of movement beyond the horizontal and limited active anterior elevation to only 82° (p=0.05). On the other hand, isolated lesser tuberosity osteotomy was not prejudicial as active anterior elevation on the five cases in our series reached on average 132° at the time of review.

Intracapsular, impacted fracture sequelae did not necessitate a greater tuberosity osteotomy while in most of the *Extracapsular, disimpacted fracture sequelae,* a humeral prosthesis could not be implanted without performing a greater tuberosity osteotomy. This GT osteotomy was necessary in the surgical neck nonunions in severe tuberosity malunion following displaced or dislocated four-part fractures.

Complications and Reoperations

There were 18 recorded complications, of which 6 occurred during operation. These complications demonstrate the technical difficulties of this surgery and are summarized in Table 5. They were more frequent in *Extracapsular, disimpacted fracture sequelae with greater tuberosity osteotomy* and were correlated with a poor functional result (p=0.0001). All the complications concerning the greater tuberosity (nonunion, bone resorption) occurred following greater tuberosity osteotomy and resulted in a worsening of the functional results in the Constant score (p=0.0001).

Four patients required revision surgery, and of these three had an *extra-capsular, disimpacted fracture sequelae.* In two cases, this was to remove the prosthesis in late-presenting infection. These two patients had had previous attempts to reduce and fix the initial fracture. One patient underwent an acromioplasty 9 months postoperatively for signs of anterosuperior impingement and with radiographs that showed the greater tuberosity to be higher than the level of the head by 6 mm. Finally, one patient who presented with failure of the fixation of the greater tuberosity underwent revision 3 weeks postoperatively when, having achieved complete passive elevation, she complained of pain and a sudden loss of function. The radiographs showed posterior and upward migration of the greater tuberosity, and this was reattached using metal sutures. The functional result was mediocre, with elevation of 90° and episodic pain.

Discussion

The sequelae of fracture of the proximal humeral fractures is one of the more difficult categories to deal with when considering shoulder replacement surgery. An anticipated functional result is usually difficult to establish because of the complexity of the bone loss and deformity. For these reasons shoulder arthroplasty is considered by many authors to be an unpredictable treatment for fracture sequelae of the proximal humerus [5, 9, 11, 13, 14, 17, 21, 28, 31, 33, 35, 39, 42]. However, because the patients tend to be younger and more active than those operated on for osteoarthritis or rheumatoid arthritis, a preoperative prognosis is even more crucial when deciding on shoulder joint replacement. In the present study important differences were seen between the fracture sequelae where a *greater tuberosity osteotomy* was performed and those where this procedure was not required.

A New Surgical Classification

The analysis and categorizing of the different lesions in our series leads us to propose a new surgical classification by showing a number of specific correlations within each group. Two types of fracture sequelae can be distinguished: (a) *Intracapsular, impacted fracture sequelae following cephalic collapse or necrosis and chronic dislocation or fracture-dislocation* in which an osteotomy of the greater tuberosity is *not* required; (b) *Extracapsular, disimpacted fracture sequelae following surgical neck nonunion and severe tuberosity malunion* in which an implant usually cannot be inserted without osteotomy and repositioning of the greater tuberosity (Fig. 1). A posttraumatic sequelae of fractures of the proximal humerus is considered to be major when it is the end-result of an extracapsular (displaced or dislocated) fracture. In this case there is a disimpaction and/or a rotation of the humeral head. This major displacement of the humeral head, which remains outside the capsule, leads to a major and nontolerable displacement of the tuberosities (Figs. 2, 3). The initial fractures, the functional outcomes, the delay between the trauma and the insertion of a prosthesis, the technical difficulties, the complications, and the functional results are different for the two types of fracture sequelae. This classification gives a coherent pathophysiological basis for the sequelae of shoulder fractures and allows the operative indications to be clearly defined as well as anticipating any technical problems.

The simplification necessarily brought by this classification should not obscure the fact that other factors may affect the bony lesions, both initially and later, making their interpretation and classification more difficult if not impossible. At least three factors must be mentioned which, in addition to making the classification difficult, also change the prognosis for operations on fracture sequelae: (a) There may be neurological lesions (brachial plexus, circumflex nerve, suprascapular nerve) or soft-tissue lesions (cuff-tears, deltoid retraction oreitrophy) concomitant with the bone and joint damage [6, 29]. These should be considered in the preoperative investigations, and if there is any doubt EMG, arthrography, or GT scan better than magnetic resonance imaging should be requested. (b) The length of time between the initial trauma and the insertion of the prosthesis allow the lesions to deteriorate, with severe soft-tissue retraction which becomes less elastic and leads to progressive degradation of the glenoid cartilage. (c) Previous surgery to internally fix fractures often prejudices the outcome as it increases the risk of tuberosity devascularization, infection, and ossification [9, 31].

Intracapsular, impacted fracture sequelae do not require a greater tuberosity osteotomy and give good and predictable results. These include humeral head collapse or necrosis and chronic unreduced dislocations or fracture-dislocation. *Collapse and necrosis of the humeral head* associated with slight tuberosity malunion makes up the largest group of fracture sequelae of the proximal humerus (40 cases in our series). Many authors have stressed the great functional tolerance for head necrosis when it is combined with moderate malunion of the tuberosities. This was confirmed in our series where we noted that there was usually a very long delay between the initial fracture and the implantation of a prosthesis: 8 years and 2 months on average with 6 patients operated on after 20 years. Shoulder replacement for intracapsular fracture sequelae with humeral head collapse or necrosis gave the best functional results among the sequelae of fractures with an average normalized Constant score of 75 % (Fig. 4, Table 4). *The chronic, locked dislocation or fracture-dislocation* (9 cases) all presented with an impacted fracture with complete devascularization of the head fragment. In all the cases the long delay between the initial trauma and the insertion of the prosthesis (1 year and 7 months, on average) demonstrates a failure in making the initial diagnosis. Shoulder arthroplasty also gave good functional results (Fig. 4, Table 4). The normalized Constant score was 71 % and in four cases was greater than 80 % which indicates a good or excellent outcome. The improvement in mobility was significant in elevation (average 57°) as well as in external rotation (average 44°).

We believe that the good results observed in these intracapsular fracture sequelae are due to the fact that we did not have to perform an osteotomy of the greater tuberosity. There is usually a false impression of upward migration of the greater tuberosity because of impaction of the humeral head. Measurement of the greater tuberosity-acromion distance demonstrates only slight displacement. Because the greater tuberosity is only slightly displaced, it is often possible to remove enough bone from the deep surface of the greater tuberosity to allow implantation of the humeral component and still maintain continuity of the tuberosity and the rotator cuff, as recommend by Neer [28]. Moreover, we had at our disposal a third-generation shoulder prosthesis (the Aequalis prosthesis) adaptable to the distorted anatomy, which can reapproximate the anatomy of the proximal humerus by changing the inclination or the offset of the prosthetic articular surface.

Extracapsular, disimpacted fracture sequelae do require a greater tuberosity osteotomy in most of the cases and give poor and unpredictable results. These include nonunion of the surgical neck and severe major tuberosity malunion. *Nonunion of the surgical neck* (6 cases of the present series) are found in two different etiologies. Firstly, in displaced fractures which have undergone surgery with poor fracture fixation and, secondly, in three-part fractures with rotation of the head fragment which were mistakenly not operated on (leading to a persistent rotation of the head fragment). The functional result achieved with shoulder arthroplasty where the worst in our series with a Constant score of only 57% (Fig. 4). None of the patients had elevation above the horizontal, and three still had annoying pain (mean pain score of 7). The only real benefit of the surgery was the recovery of a satisfactory range of external rotation (Table 4). These poor results were the consequence of persistent nonunion with bone resorption (2 cases) despite bone grafting in four cases. Bridging the nonunion with the stem of the prosthesis plus a cancellous bone graft was not enough to achieve healing. *Severe tuberosity malunions* includes 16 cases where union of the greater tuberosity to the shaft was obtained but with a major displacement secondary to an extracapsular fracture with disimpaction of the humeral head. This disimpaction of the head causes major displacement and retraction of the tuberosities and explains why such sequelae always occur in four-part displaced or dislocated fractures (Fig. 1). This criteria, which can be seen on the preoperative radiographs, demonstrates the significance of the malunion in that 11 of our 16 cases required a greater tuberosity osteotomy (Table 3). Previous internal fixation makes the implantation of a humeral prosthesis more difficult due to secondary ossification and severe adhesions between the tuberosities and the deltoid [9, 31].

The poor results with shoulder arthroplasty in nonunions and severe malunions are also found in other series in the literature [9, 11, 15, 17, 28, 30, 33, 42]. These poor results are related to a persistent nonunion of the greater tuberosity (4 cases) or bone resorption (4 cases) because of bone devascularization. As emphasized by Neer, greater tuberosity nonunion is responsible for weakness of the infraspinatus which is one of the key muscle in depressing the humeral head.

Conclusion

The results of shoulder arthroplasty in sequelae of fractures of the proximal humerus appear to depend on the original fracture pattern: intracapsular, impacted fractures lead to moderate nonunions without the necessity of performing a greater tuberosity osteotomy while extracapsular, disimpacted fractures lead to major malunions and nonunions in which a humeral component cannot be inserted without performing a greater tuberosity osteotomy.

The requirement to perform a greater tuberosity osteotomy in the treatment of fracture sequelae should lead the surgeon to anticipate a "limited result" and should help him in the decision making process. However, using a shoulder prosthesis which can be adapted to the distorted anatomy, because of its variable inclination and translocation of the articular surface, is of particular use in the treatment of fracture sequelae, because the need to perform a greater tuberosity osteotomy may be avoided.

References

1. Boileau P, Chau E, Perraud M, Arcamone H, Argenson C (1993) Restoration of humeral offset and humeral length after hemiarthroplasty for displaced 4-part fractures of the proximal humerus. Rev Chir Orthop 79 [Suppl I]:150
2. Boileau P, Walch G (1995) Adaptability and modularity in shoulder arthroplasty. Acta Orthop Belg 61 [Suppl I]:49–61
3. Boileau P, Walch G (1997) Three dimensional geometry of the proximal humerus: implications on the technique and the prosthetic design. J Bone Joint Surg Br 79 Br, 5:857–865
4. Brooks CH, Revell WJ, Heatley FW (1993) Vascularity of the humeral head after proximal humeral fractures an anatomical cadaver study. J Bone Joint Surg Br 75:132–136
5. Cofield RH (1987) Shoulder replacement: prognosis related to diagnosis. In: Kölbel R, Helbig B, Blauth W (eds) Shoulder replacement. Springer, Berlin Heidelberg New York, pp 157–161
6. Compito CA, Self EB, Bigliani LU (1994) Arthroplasty and acute shoulder trauma: reasons for success and failure. Clin Orthop 307:27–36
7. Constant CR, Murley AHG (1987) A clinical method of functional assessment of the shoulder. Clin Orthop 214:160–164
8. Dines DM, Klarren RF, Altcheck DW, Moeckel B (1993) Posttraumatic changes of the proximal humerus: malunion, nonunion, and osteonecrosis. Treatment with modular hemiarthroplasty or total shoulder arthroplasty. J Shoulder Elbow Surg 2(1):11–21
9. Duralde XA, Flatow EL, Pollock RG, Nicholson GP, Self EB, Bigliani LO (1996) Operature treatment of the surgical neck of the humerus. J Shoulder Elbow Surg 5(3):169–180
10. Flatow EL, Neer CS II (1993) Chronic anterior dislocation of the shoulder. J Shoulder Elbow Surg 2(1):2–10

11. Frich LH, Sjoberg JO, Sneppen O (1991) Shoulder arthroplasty in complex acute and chronic proximal humerus fractures. Orthopaedics 14:949–954
12. Gerber C, Schneeberger AG, Vinh TS (1990) The arterial vascularisation of the humeral head, an anatomic study. J Bone Joint Surg Am 72 10:1486–1494
13. Hawkins RJ, Neer CS II (1987) Locked posterior dislocation of the shoulder. J Bone Joint Surg Am 69:9–18
14. Healy WL, Jupiter JB, Kristiansen TK, White RR (1990) Nonunion of the proximal humerus. In: Post M, Morrey BF, Hawkins RJ (eds) Surgery of the soulder. Mosby Year Book, St Louis, p 59
15. Huten D, Duparc J (1986) L'arthroplastie prothétique dans les traumatismes complexes récents et anciens de l'épaule. Rev Chir Orthop 72:517–529
16. Ianotti JP, Gabriel JP, Schneck SL, Evans BG, Misra S (1992) The normal glenohumeral relationships. An anatomical study of one hundred and forty shoulders. J Bone Joint Surg Am 74:491–500
17. Ianotti JP, Sidor ML (1997) Malunions of the proximal humerus. In: Warren JP, Ianotti JP, Gerber C (eds) Complex and revision problems in shoulder surgery. Lippincott-Raven, Philadelphia, pp 245–264
18. Jakob RP, Kristiansen T, Mayo K, Ganz R, Muller ME (1984) Classification and aspects of treatment of fractures of the proximal humerus. In: Bateman JE, Welsh RP (eds) Surgery of the shoulder. Decker, Philadelphia, pp 330–334
19. Jakob RP, Miniani A, Anson PS (1991) Four part valgus impacted fractures of the proximal humerus. J Bone Joint Surg Br 73:295–298
20. Keene JS, Huizenga RE, Engber WD, Rogers SC (1983) Proximal humeral fractures: a correlation of residual deformity whith long term function. Orthopedics 6:173
21. Kyle RF, Conner TN (1981) Post-traumatic avascular necrosis of the humeral head in displaced proximal humeral fractures. J Trauma 21:788–791
22. Laing PG (1956) The arterial supply of the adult humerus. J Bone Joint Surg Am 38:1105–1116
23. Lee CK, Hansen HR (1981) Post traumatic avascular necrosis of the humeral head in displaced proximal humeral fractures. J Trauma 21:788–791
24. Neer CS II (1970) Displaced proximal humeral fractures. I. Classification and evaluation. J Bone Joint Surg Am 52:1077–1089
25. Neer CS II (1970) Displaced proximal humeral fractures. II. Treatment of three and four part displacement. J Bone Joint Surg Am 52:1090–1103
26. Neer CS II, Watson KC, Stanton FJ (1982) Recent experience in total Shoulder replacement. J Bone Joint Surg Am 64:319–337
27. Neer CS (1983) Nonunion of the surgical neck of the humerus. Orthop Trans 3:389
28. Neer CS (1990) Old trauma in glenohumeral arthroplasty. In: Shoulder reconstruction, vol 3. Saunders, Philadelphia, pp 222–234
29. Nicholson GP, Flatow EL, Bigliani LU (1994) Soulder arthroplasty for proximal humeral fractures. In: Friedman RJ (ed) Arthroplasty of the shoulder. Thieme, New York, pp 183–193
30. Norris TR, Turner JA, Bovill D (1990) Nonunion of the upper humerus: an analysis of the aetiology and treatment in 28 cases. In: Post M, Morrey BF, Hawkins RJ (eds) Surgery of the soulder. Mosby Year Book, St Louis, p 63
31. Norris TR, Tuner JA (1995) Late prosthetic shoulder arthroplasty for displaced proximal humerus fractures. J Shoulder Elbow Surg 4:271–280
32. Pritchett JW (1987) Prosthetic replacement for chronic unreduced dislocations of the shoulder. Clin Orthop 216:89–93
33. Razemon JP, Baux S (1969) Les séquelles des fractures de l'extrémité supérieure de l'humérus. Rev Chir Orthop 55:479–490
34. Resch H, Beck E, Bayley I (1995) Reconstruction of the valgus impacted humeral head fracture. J Shoulder Elbow Surg 4:74–80
35. Rowe CR, Zarins B (1982) Chronic unreduced dislocations of the shoulder. J Bone Joint Surg Am 64:494–505
36. Scheck M (1982) Surgical treatment of nonunions of the surgical neck of the humerus. Clin Orthop 167:255–259
37. Siebenrock, Gerber C (1993) The reproducibility of classification fractures of the proximal end of the humerus. J Bone Joint Surg Am 75:1751–1755
38. Sidor ML, Zuckerman JD (1993) The Neer classification system for proximal humerus fractures. J Bone Joint Surg Am 75:1745–1750
39. Tanner MW, Cofield RH (1983) Prothetic arthroplasty for fractures and fractures dislocations of the proximal humerus. Clin Orthop 179:116–128
40. Walch G, Boileau P, Martin B, Dejour H (1990) Unreduced posterior dislocations and fracture-dislocations of the shoulder. A review of 30 cases. Rev Chir Orthop 76:546–558
41. Walch G, Badet R, Nove-Josserand L, Levigne C (1996) Nonunions of the surgical neck of the humerus: surgical treatment with an intramedullary bone peg, internal fixation and cancellous bone grafting. J Shoulder Elbow Surg 5:161–168
42. Watson KC (1987) Indications and considerations of shoulder replacement in post-traumatic conditions. In: Kölbel R, Helbig B, Blauth W (eds) Shoulder replacement. Springer, Berlin, Heidelberg New York, pp 129–133
43. Wirth MA (1994) Complications of shoulder arthroplasty. Clin Orthop 307:47–69

Sequelae of Fractures of the Proximal Humerus: Results of Shoulder Arthroplasty without Greater Tuberosity Osteotomy

P. Boileau, G. Walch, C. Trojani, B. Veneau, and R. Sinnerton

Summary

We isolated two types of fractures sequelae of the proximal humerus that can be treated with a shoulder arthroplasty without having to perform a greater tuberosity osteotomy: humeral head collapse or necrosis (40 cases) and chronic dislocation or fracture dislocation (9 cases). These old traumas feature tolerable displacement of the greater tuberosity, which makes an implantation of a humeral component possible while still maintaining continuity of the tuberosity and rotator cuff to the shaft. The Aequalis shoulder prosthesis was used in all cases and was particularly indicated in these challenging post traumatic conditions since it offers the possibility to be adapted to this distorted anatomy. Adjustment of inclination and/or translation of articular prosthetic surface allows some tuberosity osteotomies to be avoided. The risk of nonunion of the greater tuberosity after osteotomy should lead surgeons to abandon the idea to reconstruct a normal anatomy of the proximal humerus at any costs. In these two specific etiologies, the surgeon can accept some deformity of the proximal humerus but with good functional results.

Introduction

Fractures sequelae of the proximal humerus are rare but serious: their treatment using a shoulder prosthesis is complex and their prognosis remains unpredictable [5, 10, 12, 13, 16, 18, 27, 29, 31, 34, 36–38]. Because of previous disappointing experiences with shoulder replacement in fractures sequelae of the proximal humerus, we hypothesized that poor results could be related to the necessity to perform a greater tuberosity osteotomy [2]. We decided to accept some anatomical deformities of the proximal humerus and to try to implant a shoulder prosthesis without performing a greater tuberosity osteotomy. We observed that intra-capsular fractures, with impaction of the humeral head on the diaphysis, usually lead to tolerable malunion of the tuberosities and allow implantation of a humeral component while maintaining a continuity of the tuberosity and rotator cuff to the shaft. This group of fracture sequelae includes cephalic collapse or necrosis and chronic unreduced dislocation and fracture dislocations.

Since 1991 we have been using a new shoulder prosthesis to treat these difficult pathologies the Aequalis shoulder prosthesis (Tornier, France) which allows any variations of the shape of the proximal humerus to be matched, thanks to its adaptability [1–3]. The ability to alter the inclination angle of the neck and to translate the position of the prosthetic articular surface in all planes of movement means that the humeral implant can be adapted to fit the distorsed anatomy which is often found in intra-capsular fracture sequelae.

This chapter presents the results achieved in post-traumatic collapse or necrosis and chronic unreduced dislocations or fracture dislocations of the proximal humerus using the Aequalis prosthesis without performing greater tuberosity osteotomy. Details concerning the surgical technique and the prosthesis positioning are described.

Material and Methods

Patients

Between 1991 and 1995, 49 shoulders in 48 patients have been operated on with a shoulder prosthesis, for a cephalic collapse or necrosis (40 cases) and a chronic locked dislocation or fracture dislocations (9 cases). There were 20 males and 29 females. The average age of the patients at the time of the operation was 58 years (between 34 and 87). The right side was involved in 30 cases (61 %) and the dominant side in 29 cases (59 %). The initial fracture was a four-part fracture in 33 cases, a two-part fracture in 7 cases, a posterior fracture dislocation (with impression fracture of the head greater than 50 %) in 7 cases, a posterior dislocation in one case and an anterior fracture dislocation in one case (Table 1). There was one associated glenoid fracture in a patient with a posterior fracture dislocation.

A clinical and radiological review of the 49 patients was carried out at a mean follow-up of 19 months (12–48 months). The clinical evaluation was made using the Constant scoring system which evaluates pain, activity, mobility and force and can be adjusted to allow for age and sex [8, 9]. All the patients were reviewed in clinic with a radiographic examination consisting of AP views of the shoulder in neutral, internal and external rotation, a scapular profile view (42 cases) and an axillary view (38 cases). Measured radiographs of both humeri were available in 3 cases and CT scans in 3 cases.

Anatomopathology

Two types of lesion can give an intra-capsular, impacted sequelae after a proximal humeral fracture *without* requiring to perform a greater tuberosity osteotomy: a cephalic collapse or necrosis with tolerable tuberosity malunion and a chronic locked dislocation or fracture-dislocation (Table 1).

Humeral head collapse or necrosis with tolerable tuberosity malunion was found in 40 cases. Necrosis was classified as stage IV in 21 cases and stage III in 19. This group involved four part fractures impacted, either in valgus (20 cases) or varus (12 cases). The initial treatment had been conservative in 35 cases (simple immobilisation) and surgical in 5 cases. One oblique surgical neck fracture had been reduced and fixed by screws and had developed a necrosis two years later. One four-part displaced fracture had been fixed with multiple intramedullary nails with a necrosis after four years. One fracture of the upper third of the diaphysis had been treated by closed reduction which resulted in gleno-humeral osteoarthritis after twenty years due to consolidation of the fracture in about 40° of internal rotation at the epiphysis. One four-part fracture impacted in varus had been treated by closed reduction and resulted in cephalic collapse and necrosis after four years and one four-part fracture impacted in varus had been fixed with screws resulting in necrosis after three years. Overall, the time between the initial fracture and the prosthetic replacement was very long averaging eight years and two months and 6 of the patients had surgery more than twenty years after their fracture.

Chronic, locked dislocations and fracture-dislocations were found in 9 cases. This group consisted of seven locked posterior dislocations with greater than 50 % head collapse, one locked, two part, posterior fracture-dislocation and one locked anterior fracture-dislocation. In all cases the lesion had not been identified and thus received no treatment. The time between the initial trauma and prosthetic replacement was one year and seven months on average.

Table 1. Characteristics of the intra-capsular, impacted sequelae of fractures of the proximal humerus

	Cephalic collapse and necrosis with moderate tuberosity malunion (n=40)	Chronic dislocation and fracture-dislocations (n=9)
Initial fracture		
4-part valgus impacted	20	–
4-part varus impacted	12	–
4-part displaced	1	–
2-part anatomical neck	3	–
2-part surgical neck	4	–
Posterior locked dislocation	–	7
Posterior fracture-dislocation	–	1
Anterior fracture-dislocation	–	1
Initial treatment		
Orthopadic	35	–
Surgical	5	–
Delay before shoulder arthroplasty	8 years, 2 months	1 year, 7 months
Type of shoulder prosthesis	19 Hemi, 21 Total	8 Hemi, one Total
Cuff tear	4	2

Surgical Technique

All the surgeons involved in this prospective study used the same surgical technique and the same prosthesis. The patient was placed in a beach-chair position with the shoulder free of the table edge. An elongated delto-pectoral incision was used in all cases in this series except one, where a superior trans-acromial approach was used. The dissection was always difficult because of soft-tissue retraction and bony distortion especially where there had been previous open surgery. The main landmark was the biceps tendon which acted as a guide for the surgeon towards the rotator interval and as a help to locate the subscapularis. Releasing the capsule beneath the subscapularis and dividing the coraco-humeral ligament were done routinely. On three occasions (6 %) the joint was approached by an osteotomy of the lesser tuberosity with subscapularis attached to improve mobilisation (two head necrosis and one locked posterior fracture-dislocation) and was fixed at the end of the procedure by using non-absorbable sutures. No greater tuberosity osteotomy was performed except on one occasion where a partial, uniplane, greater tuberosity osteotomy was carried out in one chronic unreduced anterior fracture-dislocation. A rotator cuff tear was reported and repaired in six cases. In two of these, the rupture was of two tendons (supra and infraspinatus) and in four it was a single tendon rupture (three supra and one infraspinatus). The cuff was considered to be thin in 22 cases (45 %) and normal in 21. The biceps tendon was tenodesed 9 times (18 %). Seven acromioplasties were performed with the goal of improving the space for the tuberosities under the coraco-acromial vault or to protect a cuff repair. The head was carefully dislocated in adduction, external rotation and retropulsion to minimise the risk of a shaft fracture. Despite the precautions, three diaphyseal and one metaphyseal fractures were reported in the series. The humeral head cut was usually minimal and was even not required in some head collapse or necrosis. Because of the bony distortion, reaming the medullary canal was often difficult and was carried out using cylindrical rasps of increasing diameters.

Forty-nine Aequalis prostheses were used of which 27 were hemiarthroplasties and 22 were total shoulder replacements. Within the range of humeral stem sizes, the nine mm stem was used 28 times (57 %), the six mm stem in 13 cases (26 %) and the twelve mm stem in 8 cases (16 %). All stems were cemented in after placing a cement restrictor. Out of the 22 total shoulders, a polyethylene glenoid component was used in 21 cases and was always cemented. In one case a metal-backed component was used whose primary bony fixation comes from two expanding screws. The conception of the humeral component is based on anatomical studies which demonstrated variations in the dimension and more specifically the shape, of the proximal humerus [1, 3]. Modularity is achieved by the availability of seven articular heads of increasing diameter and thickness. Variations in the inclination of the humeral neck and antero-posterior and medio-lateral translation of the articular surface have been found to be geometrical parameters of critical importance. Adaptability is possible due to the available variable inclination thanks to a choice of four neck angles of 125°, 130°, 135° and 140°. An inclination guide allows the angle to be measured intraoperatively and then the appropriate neck can be selected. Of the range available the 130° neck was used 12 times (24 %), the 135° on 16 occasions (32 %), the 125° on 11 patients (22 %) and the 140° was used in 10 cases (20 %). Adaptability is also possible due to the ability to translate the humeral head. An original eccentric dial system on the under surface of the head allows it to be translated into one of eight positions both supero-inferiorly and medio-laterally until the bony surface is best covered. The goal was to restore the lever arm for the cuff and deltoid muscles [17, 33].

Post-operatively the arm was immobilised in a sling with the elbow at the side. Passive mobility was started the day after surgery following Neer's recommendations [25, 26]. No active muscular activity was started until a complete passive range of movement had been achieved and there was bony consolidation of the tuberosity osteotomies (6–8 weeks). Thirty patients benefited from a stay in a specialized rehabilitation centre for an average of 35 days. Eight patients had home physiotherapy and in eleven cases the type of rehabilitation was not detailed.

Results

Clinical Results

Functional results are summarized in Table 2. The adjusted Constant score at review averaged 75 %. Using the Constant criteria [8, 9] we reported 9 excellent, 16 good, 12 average and 12 poor results, i.e. 51 % good or excellent. Evaluated using the Neer system [25, 26], the objective results were 11 excellent, 23 good, 11 fair and 4 poor, i.e. 69 % good or excellent. The pain score at review was 11 points out of 15 on average for the head necrosis and 11.7 points for the locked dislocations and fracture dislocations. The mean score for active mobility

Table 2. Detailed Constant score

Results	Cephalic collapse and necrosis with moderate tuberosity malunion (n=40)			Chronic dislocation and fracture-dislocation (n=9)		
	Preop	Postop	(Gain)	Preop	Postop	(Gain)
Pain (/15 points)	5.2 →	11	(+ 5.8)	3.6 →	11.7	(+ 8.1)
Activity (/20 points)	7.7 →	15.9	(+ 8.2)	5.7 →	13.8	(+ 8.1)
Mobility (/40 points)	13.7 →	28	(+14.3)	7.5 →	25.5	(+18)
Strength (/25 points)	2.8 →	5	(+ 2.2)	1.1 →	4	(+ 2.9)
Absolute Constant score	29.5 →	60	(+30.5)	17.6 →	56	(+38.4)
Normalised Constant score	37 % →	75 %	(+38 %)	22 % →	71 %	(+49 %)

at review was 27.6 out of 40, and increase from 12.2 preoperatively. Forty-seven out of the forty-nine patients in the series (95 %) declared themselves as being satisfied or very satisfied with the result. Two patients were disappointed with the operation because of persistent pain and reduced mobility.

Radiological Results

The greater tuberosity position was studied on a true AP view in neutral rotation. It should be recalled that the average distance between the top of the humeral head and the top of the greater tuberosity is 8 mm with a minimum of 5 mm and a maximum of 13 mm and that the greater tuberosity is never above the top of the humeral head [19]. In eight cases the top of the greater tuberosity was above the top of the prosthetic humeral head demonstrating non-optimal reconstruction of the proximal humerus anatomy. In seven cases the top of the greater tuberosity was at the level of the top of the head. Finally, in 34 cases (69 %) the greater tuberosity position was considered to be anatomical, below the summit of the head by 7.5 mm on average (28 head collapse and necrosis, and 6 chronic locked dislocations or fracture dislocations).

The humeral cement mantle was examined along the entire length of the stem and was normal in 41 cases (84 %). An incomplete lucent line was recorded in 5 cases (10 %), complete in 3 cases (6 %) but were considered non-progressive. There were no lucent lines greater than 2 mm. The glenoid fixation was studied in the 21 polyethylene components and seemed normal in 11 cases. There were ten cases with a lucent line of which 80 % (8 out of 10) were visible immediately post-operatively. The lucent line was complete in 7 cases and incomplete in 3 cases.

Ossifications were found in 5 cases (10 %). Using the Sneppen classification [40] we reported two ossifications grade I (ossification of less than half the joint line), two ossifications grade II (more than half the joint line), and one ossification grade III (ossifications forming a scapulo-humeral bridge). In the last two cases there were pre-existing ossifications and no correlation was found with the functional result.

Complications and Revision

The three intra-operative fractures of the diaphysis were the only complications recorded. They were minimally displaced and were treated nonoperatively. The functional result was not altered by these complications. No neurological damages and no infection were observed. Only one patient underwent revision surgery to perform an acromioplasty at nine months post-operation for clinical antero-superior impingement. The radiographs showed that the greater tuberosity was above the level of the head by 6 mm. After the revision surgery elevation reached 140° with an adjusted Constant score of 66 %. Although this did not increase the elevation, it did improve the pain status and the patient was satisfied with his shoulder.

Discussion

Shoulder arthroplasty in sequelae of fractures of the proximal humerus is considered a risky operation with poor and unpredictable functional results.

Post-traumatic Collapse and Necrosis of the Humeral Head

Collapse and necrosis of the humeral head associated with moderate tuberosity malunion, makes up the largest group of fracture sequelae of the proximal humerus being 40 cases in our series. These avascular necrosis are the consequence of fractures which interrupt the blood supply to the head which comes essentially from the antero-lateral ascending branches of the anterior circumflex vessels and the postero-medial branches of the posterior circumflex vessels [4, 14, 23]. The minor contribution from the muscle and capsular attachments plus the absence of a round ligament (cf. the femur) certainly partly explains the frequency of necrosis of the humeral head. Nor does necrosis seem to be just the domain of the elderly because the mean age of the patients in this group was 58 years.

Head collapse and necrosis occur in our series after four-part fractures impacted in valgus (20 cases) or in varus (12 cases). Initially, these fractures may be erroneously evaluated as minor condition. They are not included in Neer's classification since as they are considered as minimally displaced fractures [25, 26]. Jakob, in 1984, was the first to include fractures impacted in valgus or varus within the AO classification and to emphasize their frequency calculated as 14% of all proximal humeral fractures [20, 21]. Other fractures acting as the originator of head necrosis with tolerable malunion are much less uncommon: essentially these are displaced fractures of the anatomical (3 cases) or surgical neck (4 cases). Surgical treatment, which is a possible cause of devascularising the humeral head, can-

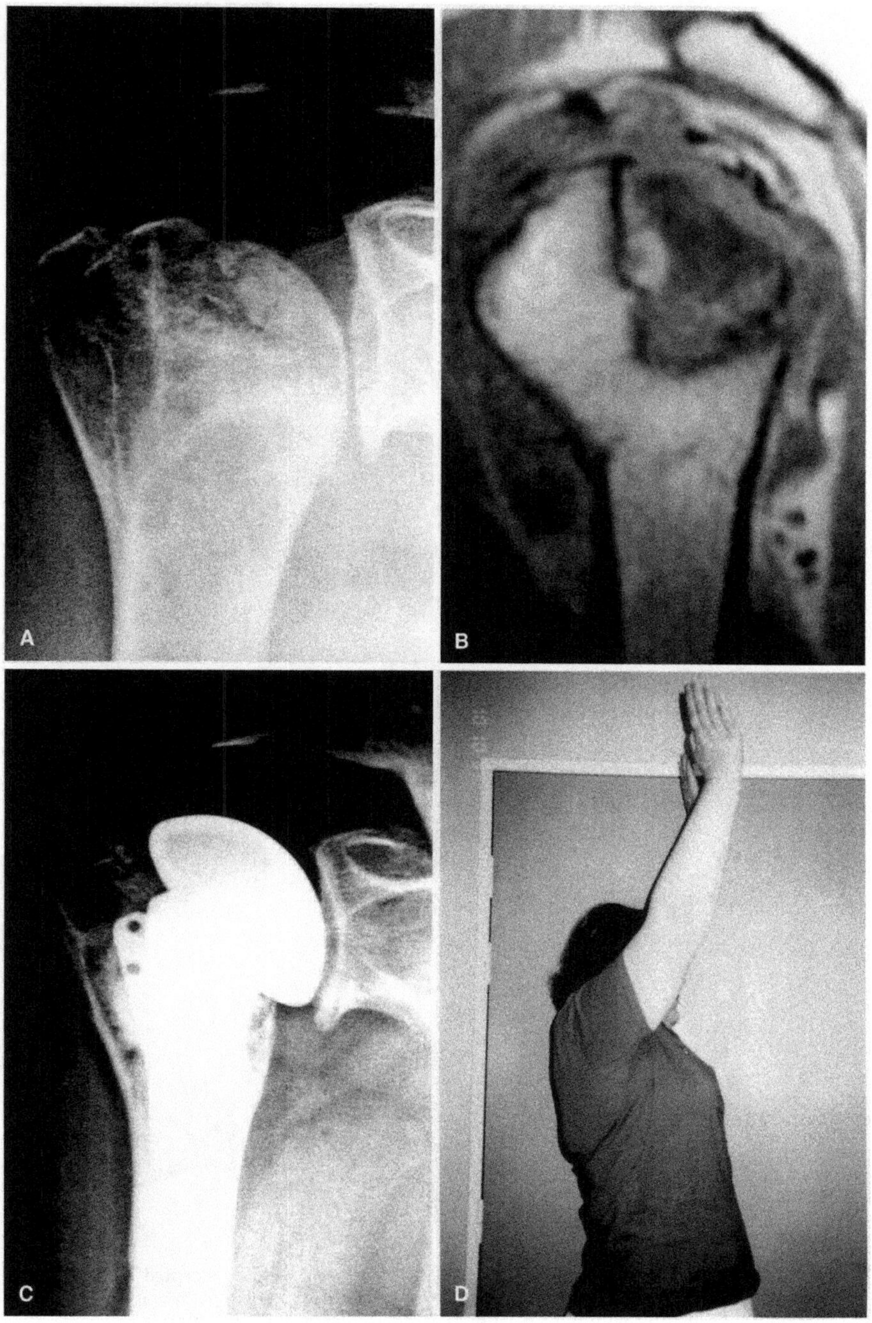

Fig. 1. Example of arthroplasty in a sequelae of a 4-part fracture impacted in valgus. **A** Stage III necrosis with pseudo-ascension of the greater tuberosity (note the normal acromio-humeral distance). **B** MRI showing the head necrosis and slight malunion of the greater tuberosity. **C** Adaptable shoulder prosthesis positioned with a superior offset avoiding the necessity to perform a greater tuberosity osteotomy. **D.** Three years postoperatively: almost normal active elevation

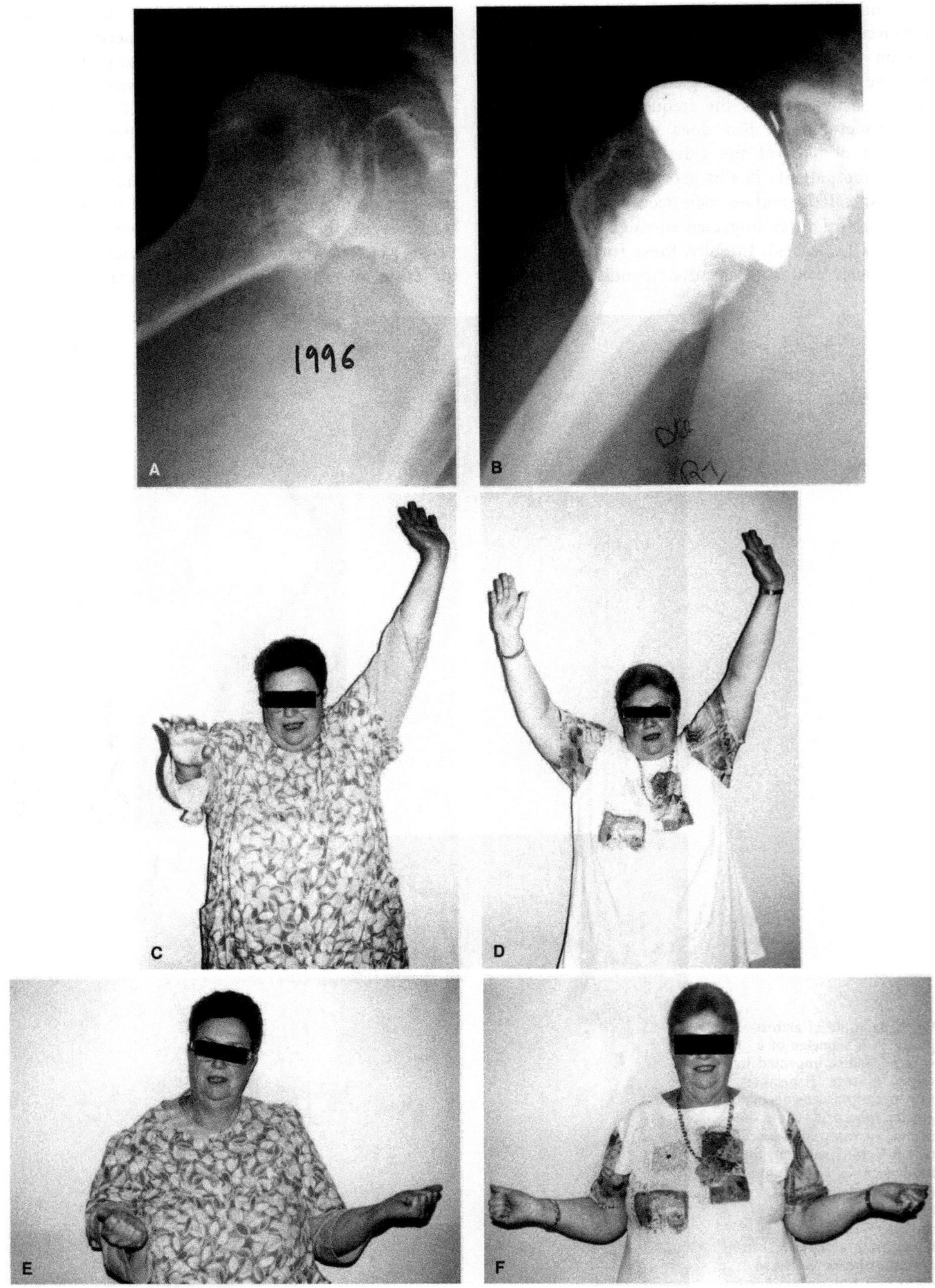

Fig. 2. Another example of cephalic collapse and necrosis after 4-part impacted fracture. **A.** Cephalic collapse and necrose with greater tuberosity malunion. **B** Shoulder arthroplasty with accepted deformity of the proximal humerus. **C,D** Pre and postoperative active elevation. **E,F** Pre- and postoperative active rotation

not be blamed for the necrosis because in 35 out of the 40 fractures which developed a necrosis the treatment had been non-operative. These findings agree with that of Razemon and Baux in 1969 [31].

Many authors have emphasized the great functional tolerance for head collapse and necrosis when it is combined with slight malunion of the tuberosities [14, 31, 32]. This was confirmed in our series where we noted that there was usually a very long time interval between the initial fracture and the implantation of a prosthesis: eight years and 2 months on average, six patients were operated on after twenty years. After a period during which the fracture consolidates, the initial satisfactory result deteriorates because of a progressing head necrosis (Fig. 1 and 2). In 19 cases in our series, the necrosis was classified as stage III confirming that it is the depression and deformation of the head which causes the pain and compromises mobility and function [26, 31]. The pain becomes then severe, particularly at night and then leads the patient to seek medical help. Twenty-one cases had stage IV necrosis with glenoid damage therefore justifying a total arthroplasty (Fig. 2). Malunions of the tuberosities following four-part impacted fractures are usually tolerable as evidenced by the retention of a relatively satisfactory range of preoperative movement in anterior elevation: 87° on average in this series.

Chronic, Locked Dislocations and Fracture Dislocations

The indications for shoulder arthroplasty in chronic locked posterior dislocations and fracture dislocations have been defined in the literature [16, 30, 34, 37]. The seven locked posterior dislocation, in our series all featured with an impacted fracture involving more than 50 % of the articular surface of the head. One case of locked posterior fracture dislocation was a sequela of a 2-part fracture with complete devascularisation of the head fragment. In all cases except one, where glenoid damage required a total arthroplasty, a hemi-arthroplasty was performed. Chronic, locked anterior dislocations usually occurs in the very elderly and are generally well tolerated, then rarely justifying any surgical intervention [12]. Even so we did have one case of a poorly tolerated anterior fracture dislocation which benefited from a hemiarthroplasty. In all

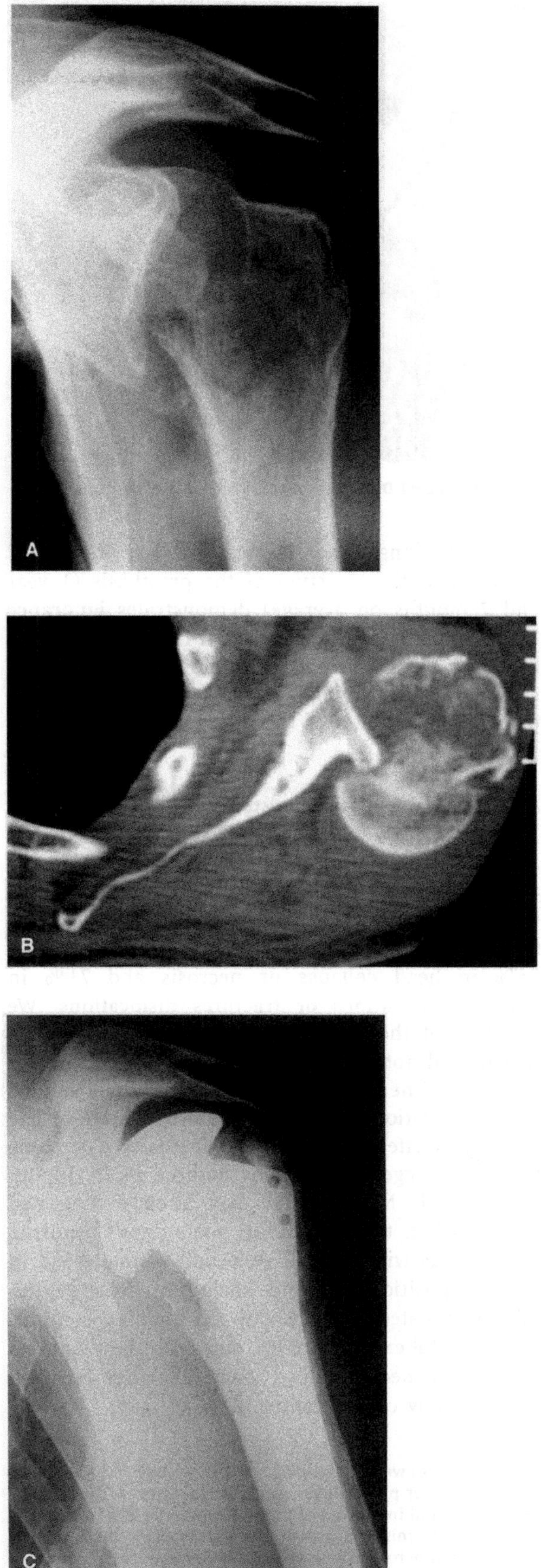

Fig. 3. Example of shoulder arthroplasty in a locked posterior fracture dislocation. **A** AP view of a locked posterior fracture dislocation diagnosed three months after trauma. **B** CT scan shows the head fragment hooked on the posterior edge of the glenoid. **C** Hemiarthroplasty was implanted without having to perform a greater tuberosity osteotomy

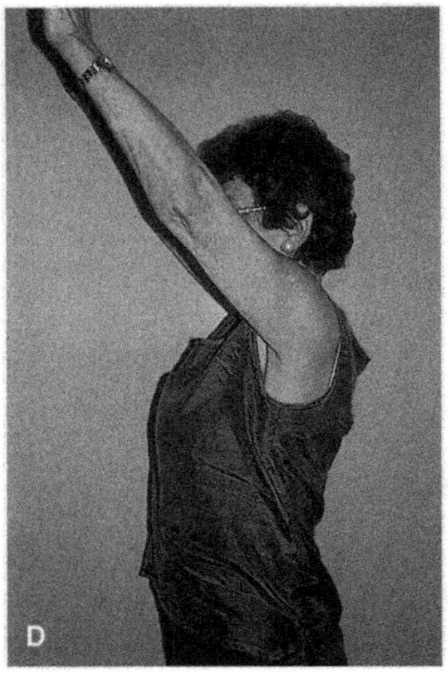

Fig. 3. (continued) D Active elevation above the horizontal level

cases, the long time interval between the initial trauma and the insertion of the prosthesis (1 year and 7 months on average) demonstrates ignorance in making the initial diagnosis. The delto-pectoral approach was sufficient in all the cases to allow to reduce the dislocation and to perform the arthroplasty after excision of the fibrous tissue (Fig. 3).

Avoiding Greater Tuberosity Osteotomy

Shoulder replacement for head collapse or necrosis and chronic unreduced dislocations or fractures dislocations gives good and predictable functional results: the average adjusted Constant score was 75% in head collapse or necrosis and 71% in chronic dislocations or fractures dislocations. We believe that these good results are due to the fact that we did not perform an osteotomy of the greater tuberosity. The improvement in mobility was significant in elevation as well as in external rotation. The prejudicial effect of a greater tuberosity osteotomy has been suggested by many authors [6, 7, 10, 13, 22, 28, 29]. Neer himself has already suggested "cheating" in the "borderline malunions" by using a prosthesis with a small stem and a small head in a varus position to avoid having to do a greater tuberosity osteotomy [28]. By maintaining continuity of the tuberosity and the cuff with the diaphysis there is no need to slow down rehabilitation until there is bony consolidation [2, 26].

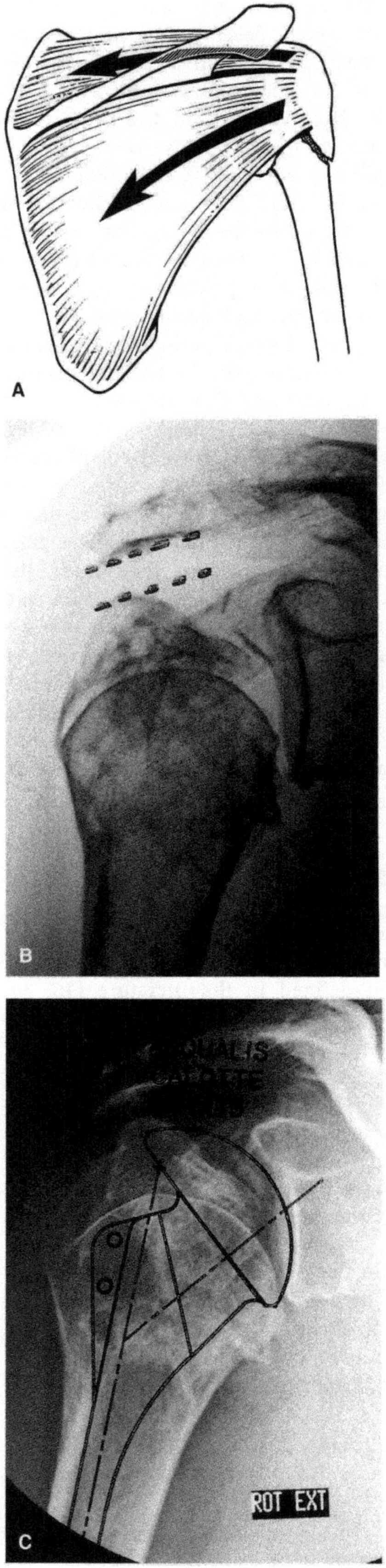

Fig. 4. False upward migration of the greater tuberosity in sequelae of four-part valgus impacted fractures. **A** The balance between the pulling forces of the supraspinatus and infraspinatus with teres minor avoids a marked superior retraction of the greater tuberosity. **B** Radiological example. **C** Preoperative planning anticipating supero-lateral offset

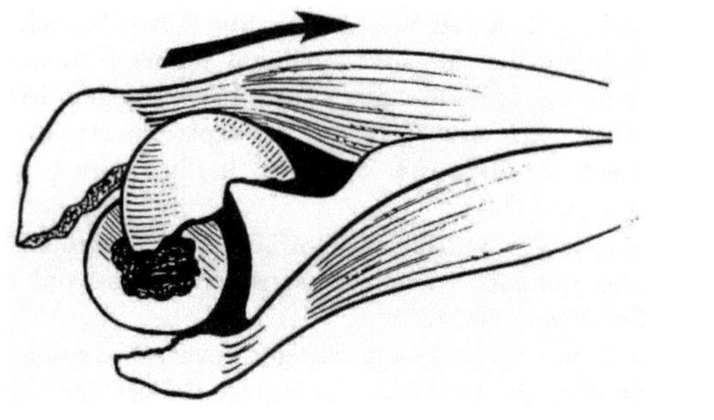

Fig. 5. Limited backward migration of the greater tuberosity in posterior chronic dislocation or fracture dislocation: the locked head fragment avoids a marked posterior retraction of the greater tuberosity

In post-traumatic sequelae of four-part varus impacted fractures, there is a *false upward migration of the greater tuberosity:* it is not the greater tuberosity which moves upward but rather the humeral head which falls downward by being impacted into the diaphysis, giving an "ice-cream cone" appearance to the humeral epiphysis. Measurement of the tuberosity-acromial distance on a AP view in neutral rotation shows that this distance is almost normal (Fig. 4). This led us to avoid performing greater tuberosity osteotomies despite the worrying appearance of a tuberosity 'door-stop' seen on the preoperative radiographs. In fact, the medial displacement of the greater tuberosity is minimal because of the balance between the supraspinatus, pulling upward and the infraspinatus et teres minor pulling downward. The bone fragment which is usually important remains hooked by the diaphysis because of this neutralising forces. Similarly, medial displacement of the greater tuberosity in posterior chronic fracture dislocation is also limited because of the presence of the head fragment, hooked on the posterior glenoid rim (Fig. 3 and 5).

By contrast, displacement of the lesser tuberosity can be marked with medial retraction of the bone fragment and contracture of the anterior capsule and subscapularis. In three cases we carried out an isolated osteotomy of the lesser tuberosity which did not prejudice the outcome and allowed active anterior elevation of 130° and external rotation of 40°. In one case, however, we did not perform a lesser tuberosity osteotomy and the poor functional result, in addiction to a radiographs in internal rotation showing a tuberosity doorstop, made us think this osteotomy probably would have been appropriate. The beneficial nature of an isolated lesser tuberosity osteotomy has already been pointed out by Neer who described the possibility of partially or totally excising the lesser tuberosity to reattach the subscapularis to the supraspinatus in order to recover full external rotation in these difficult post traumatic conditions [31].

Prosthetic Adaptability

The use of a modular and adaptable prosthesis offers several advantages and is particularly useful in intra-capsular, impacted fracture sequelae: the ability to adjust inclination and to translate the articular surface allows the humeral implant to be adapted to the encountered anatomical distortions without having to perform a greater tuberosity osteotomy (Fig. 6 and 7). Prosthetic adaptability is a new concept which effectively allows a customized prosthesis to be constructed intraoperatively [11]. Two techno-

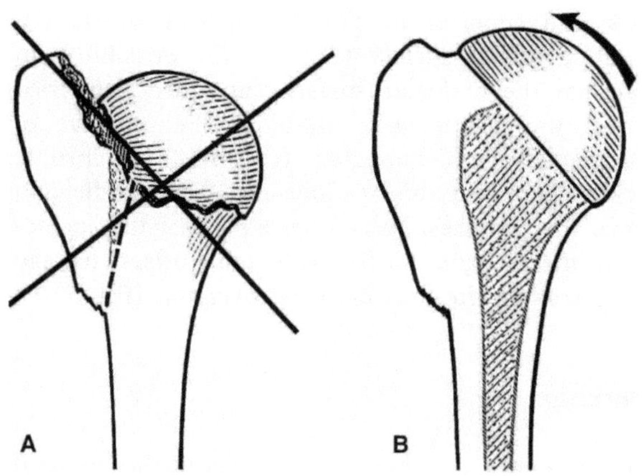

Fig. 6. A Greater tuberosity osteotomy should be avoided in sequelae of 4-part valgus impacted fracture because of the difficulties to achieve bone union. **B** This is possible when using an adaptable humeral prosthesis with a variable inclination and a variable supero-lateral offset

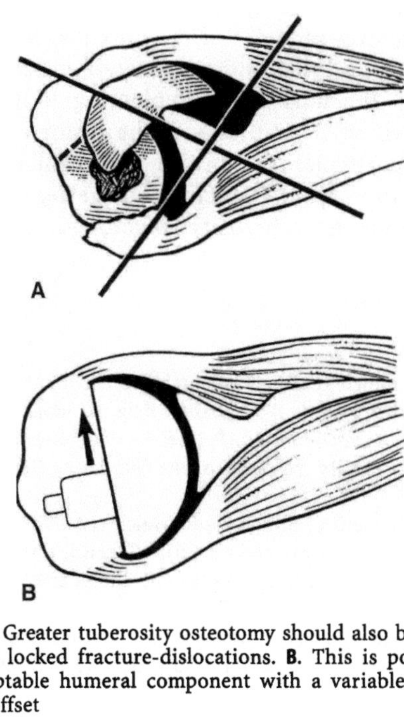

Fig. 7. A Greater tuberosity osteotomy should also be avoided in chronic locked fracture-dislocations. **B.** This is possible using an adaptable humeral component with a variable antero-posterior offset

logical innovations have allowed this implant's adaptability: a variable neck which allows the inclination to be adjusted from 125° to 140° and an eccentric dial system on the under surface of the head which anteroposterior and mediolateral offset to be respected.

Positioning the top of the articular surface 5–10 mm above the top of the greater tuberosity was achieved in 69% (28 cases out of the 40 cases) of cephalic collapse and necrosis with tuberosities malunions. The post-operative radiographs show that the prosthesis was most often positioned using a small stem in valgus (13 cases) or lateralised along the lateral cortex (10 cases) with a 130° or 135° neck and superior or postero-superior translation of the articular surface (Fig. 6). The possibility to translate the articular surface superiorly (superior offset) was particularly useful in the sequelae of four-part valgus impacted fractures. In chronic locked posterior dislocations or fracture-dislocations, the prosthesis was inserted translating posteriorly the articular surface (posterior offset) instead of decreasing the prosthetic retroversion (Fig. 7).

Conclusion

Post-traumatic collapse and necrosis of the humeral head and locked posterior dislocations and fracture dislocations can be treated by implantation of a shoulder prosthesis without having to perform a greater tuberosity osteotomy. The present study demonstrates that shoulder arthroplasty can give good and predictable functional results for these types of fractures sequelae of the proximal humerus, resulting in pain relief and recovery of active elevation beyond the horizontal. Implanting a shoulder prosthesis which is adaptable to the distorsed anatomy is of particular use in the treatment of such impacted, intra-capsular fractures sequelae, avoiding the need of greater tuberosity osteotomy.

References

1. Boileau P, Walch G (1994) Adaptability and modularity in shoulder arthroplasty. Acta Orthop Belg 61[Suppl. I]:69–61
2. Boileau P, Walch G, Liotard JP, Noel E (1994) Neer shoulder prosthesis: results related to the etiology. Rev Rhum 61:539–547
3. Boileau P, Trojani C, Sinnerton R, Walch G (1997) Sequelae of fractures of the proximal humerus. Surgical classification and limits of shoulder arthroplasty. J Shoulder 6(2):195
4. Boileau P, Walch G (1997) Three dimensional geometry of the proximal humerus: implications for technique and prosthetic design. J Bone Joint Surg Br 79(5):857–865
5. Brooks CH, Revell WJ, Heatley FW (1993) Vascularity of the humeral head after proximal humeral fractures an anatomical cadaver study. J Bone Joint Surg Br 75:132–136
6. Cofield RH (1987) Shoulder replacement: prognosis related to diagnosis. Springer, Berlin Heidelberg New York, pp 157–161
7. Compito CA, Self EB, Bigliani LU (1994) Arthroplasty and acute Shoulder trauma: reasons for success and failure. Clin Orthop 307:27–36
8. Constant CR (1986) Age related recovery of shoulder function after injury. Thesis, University College Cork, Ireland
9. Constant CR, Murley AHG (1987) A clinical method of functional assessment of the shoulder. Clin Orthop 214:160–164
10. Dines DM (1993) Posttraumatic changes of the proximal humerus: malunion, nonunion, and osteonecrosis. Treatment with modular hemiarthroplasty or total shoulder arthroplasty. J Shoulder Elbow Surg 2(1):11–21
11. Duralde XA, Flatow EL, Pollock RG, Nicholson GP, Self EB, Bigliani LU (1996) Operature treatment of the surgical neck of the humerus. J Shoulder Elbow Surg 5(3):169–180
12. Flatow EL, Neer CS II (1993) Chronic anterior dislocation of the shoulder. J Shoulder Elbow Surg 2(1):2–10
13. Frich LH, Sojberg JO, Sneppen O (1991) Shoulder arthroplasty in complexe acute and chronic proximal humeral fractures. Orthopaedics 14:949–954
14. Gerber C, Schneeberger AG, Vinh TS (1990) The arterial vascularisation of the humeral head, an anatomic study. J Bone Joint Surg Am 72(10):1486–1494
15. Green A, Lloyd B, Richard S, Limbird MD, Providence RI (1993) Humeral head replacement for acute, four-part proximal humerus fractures. J Shoulder Elbow Surg 2:249–254
16. Hawkins RJ, Neer CS II (1987) Locked posterior dislocation of the shoulder. J Bone Joint Surg Am 69:9–18
17. Hsu HC, Wu JJ, Chen TH, Lo WH, Yang DJ (1993) The influence of abductor lever-arm. Changes after shoulder arthroplasty. Shoulder Elbow Surg 2:134–140
18. Huten D, Duparc J (1986) L'arthroplastie prothétique dans les traumatismes complexes récents et anciens de l'épaule. Rev Chir Orthop 72:517–529
19. Ianotti JP, Sidor ML (1997) Malunions of the proximal humerus. In: Warren JP, Ianotti JP, Gerber C (eds) Complex ans revision problems in shoulder surgery. Lippincot-Raven, Philadelphia, pp 245–264
20. Jakob RP, Kristiansen T, Mayo K, Ganz R, Muller ME (1984) Classification and aspects of treatment of fractures of the proximal humerus. In: Bateman JE, Welsh RP (eds) Surgery of the shoulder. Decker, New York, pp 330–334
21. Jakob RP, Miniani A, Anson PS (1991) Four part valgus impacted fractures of the proximal humerus. J Bone Joint Surg Br 73:295–298
22. Knight RA, Mayne JA (1957) Comminuted fractures and fractures dislocation involving the articular surface of the humeral head. J Bone Joint Surg 39A:1343
23. Kraulis J, Hunter G (1977) The results of prosthetics replacement in fractures dislocations of the upper end of the humerus. Injury 8:129–131
24. Kyle RF, Conner TN (1981) Post-traumatic avascular necrosis of the humeral head in displaced proximal humeral fractures. J Trauma 21:788–791
25. Laing PG (1956) The arterial supply of the adult humerus. J Bone Joint Surg 38A:1105–1116

26. Lee CK, Hansen HR (1981) Post traumatic avascular necrosis of the humeral head in displaced proximal humeral fractures. J Trauma 21:788–791
27. Neer CS II (1970) Displaced proximal humeral fractures part 1: classification and evaluation. J Bone Joint Surg Am 52:1077–1089
28. Neer CS II (1970) Displaced proximal humeral fractures part 2: treatment of three and four part displacement. J Bone Joint Surg Am 52:1090–1103
29. Neer CS II (1970) Displaced proximal humeral fractures part 2: treatment of three and four part displacement. J Bone Joint Surg 52A(6):1090–1103
30. Neer CS II, Watson KC, Stanton FJ (1982) Recent experience in total Shoulder replacement. J Bone Joint Surg Am 64:319–337
31. Neer CS (1990) Old trauma in glenohumeral arthroplasty. In: Shoulder reconstruction, vol 3. Saunders, Philadelphia, pp 222–234
32. Norris TR (1995) Late prosthetic shoulder arthroplasty for displaced proximal humerus fractures. J Shoulder Elbow Surg 4:271–280
33. Pritchett JW (1987) Prosthetic replacement for chronic unreduced dislocations of the shoulder. Clin Orthop 216:89–93
34. Razemon JP, Baux S (1969) Les séquelles des fractures de l'extrémité supérieure de l'humérus. Rev Chir Orthop 55:479–490
35. Resch H, Beck E, Bayley I (1995) Reconstruction of the valgus impacted humeral head fracture. J Shoulder Elbow Surg 4:74–80
36. Rietveld ABM, Dannen HAM, RozingPM, Oberman WR (1988) The lever arm in gleno-humeral adduction after hemi arthroplasty. J Bone Joint Surg Br 70:561–565
37. Rowe CR, Zarins B (1982) Chronic unreduced dislocations of the shoulder. J Bone Joint Surg Am 64:494–505
38. Siebenrock, Gerber C (1993) The reproducibility of classification fractures of the proximal end of the humerus. J Bone Joint Surg Am 75:1751–1755
39. Sidor ML, Zuckerman JD (1993) The Neer classification system for proximal humerus fractures. J Bone Joint Surg Am 75:1745–1750
40. Sneppen O, Kjaersgaard-Andersen P, Frich LH (1990) Ectopic ossification after total shoulder arthroplasty. A study on 75 Neer total shoulder replacements. In: Post M, Morrey BF, Hawkins RJ (eds) Surgery of the shoulder. Mosby Year Book, St. Louis, pp 298–301
41. Tanner MW, Cofield RH (1983) Prothetic arthroplasty for fractures and fractures dislocations of the proximal humerus. Clin Orthop 179:116–128
42. Walch G, Boileau P, Martin B, Dejour H (1990) Luxations et fractures luxations postérieures invétérées de l'épaule. A propos de 30 cas. Rev Chir Orthop 76:546–558
43. Watson KC (1987) Indications and considerations of shoulder replacement in post-traumatic conditions. In: Kölbel R, Helbig B, Blauth W (eds) Shoulder replacement. Springer, Berlin Heidelberg New York, pp 129–133
44. Wirth MA (1994) Complications of shoulder arthroplasty. Clin Orthop 307:47–69

Sequelae of Fractures of the Proximal Humerus: Results of Shoulder Arthroplasty with Greater Tuberosity Osteotomy

P. Boileau, C. Trojani, G. Walch, R. Sinnerton, and P. Habermayer

Summary

We isolated two types of sequelae of fractures of the proximal humerus where a shoulder prosthesis could not be inserted without having to perform tuberosity osteotomy: surgical neck nonunions (6 cases) and severe tuberosities malunions (16 cases). Analysis of the clinical and radiological results demonstrates that greater tuberosity osteotomy is the most prejudicial factor ($p<0.05$) and does not allow active elevation beyond the horizontal (average active elevation: 85°). Performing a greater tuberosity osteotomy in these posttraumatic conditions leads to poor and unpredictable results for shoulder arthroplasty. For this reason, it is usually better to avoid tuberosity osteotomy when possible. In surgical neck nonunions, rather than a shoulder replacement, an isolated bone graft should be carried out, in order to obtain a bone union with the diaphysis. In severe malunions, where a shoulder arthroplasty with a greater tuberosity osteotomy has to be performed, the surgeon should anticipate a limited goal result and should inform the patient before the surgery.

Introduction

Nonunion of the surgical neck of the humerus or severe malunion of the tuberosities often results in painful shoulder with limited motion. These significant sequelae of proximal humerus fractures occur following extracapsular, disimpacted fractures, which have either been non treated or treated with a poor surgical technique.

Prosthetic replacement associated with anatomical reconstruction of the proximal humerus may be needed in these severe posttraumatic cases. However, the distorted anatomy means that a shoulder prosthesis cannot be inserted without performing a greater tuberosity osteotomy.

This chapter presents the results achieved with shoulder arthroplasty used in this group, i.e., extracapsular fracture sequelae where a greater tuberosity osteotomy was performed.

Material and Methods

Patients

Between 1991 and 1995, 22 shoulders in 22 patients where operated on using a shoulder prosthesis for either a surgical nonunion (6 cases) or a severe tuberosity malunion (16 cases). There were 12 males and 10 females. The mean age of the patients at the time of the operation was 62 years (37–82). Details of the initial fractures, initial treatment and time interval before shoulder arthroplasty are given in Table 1.

A clinical and radiological review of the 22 patients was carried out at a mean follow-up of 19 months (12–36 months). The clinical evaluation was made

Table 1. Characteristics of the extracapsular, disimpacted sequelae of fractures of the proximal humerus

	Surgical neck nonunions (n=6)	Major tuberosity malunion (n=16)
Initial fracture	Two-part surgical neck, (2); three-part greater tuberosity, (2); four-part displaced, (2)	displaced or dislocated Four-part fractures
Initial treatment	Orthopedic, (2); surgical, (5) (one reoperation)	Orthopedic, (6); surgical, (12) (two reoperations)
Delay before shoulder arthroplasty	3 years	2 years
Type of shoulder prosthesis	6 Hemi	13 Hemi, 3 Total
Cuff tear	2	5

using the Constant scoring system which covers pain, activity, mobility and force and can be adjusted to allow for age and sex [7, 8]. All the patients were reviewed in clinic with a radiographic examination consisting of AP views of the shoulder in neutral, internal and external rotation, a scapular profile view (16 cases) and an axillary view (12 cases). Measured radiographs of both humeri were available in 4 cases and CT scans in 3 cases.

The radiographic analysis looked at the quality of the humeral reconstruction (position of the stem, epiphyseal width, humeral length and status of the greater tuberosity); the glenohumeral relationship, i.e., superior or inferior subluxation of the head (by measuring the acromiohumeral distance on the AP radiograph in neutral rotation); the status of the prosthesis fixation (by examining the humeral and glenoid cement mantle); any periarticular ectopic ossifications, using Sneppen's classification [31].

Anatomopathology

Two types of lesions can result in an extracapsular disimpacted fracture of the proximal humerus with the need to perform a greater tuberosity osteotomy: nonunions of the surgical neck and major malunions of the tuberosities.

Nonunion of the surgical neck (6 cases) was often seen after previous open reduction and internal fixation. In two cases, there were displaced fractures of the surgical neck of the humerus which had undergone primary surgery and in which the head had then progressively collapsed and resorbed. These had been internally fixed using a plate in one case, and multiple intramedullary nails in the other. There were two cases of three-part fractures with rotation of the humeral head fragment and significant displacement of the greater tuberosity treated nonoperatively. The last two cases were four-part displaced fractures treated operatively with multiple intramedullary nails plus staples in one case and by a plate and screws in the other. The time interval between the primary surgery and the prosthesis was on average 3 years.

Severe malunion of the tuberosities (16 cases) occurred secondary to displaced or dislocated four-part fractures with disimpaction of the head. In 6 cases the initial treatment had been nonoperative, and the other 10 had undergone 12 interventions (two revisions). The operations were: one attempted surgical reduction combined with a posterior bone block; one surgical reduction revised after 2 years to clear the joint from some periarticular ossifications; and various osteosynthesis: intramedullary nail (three cases), screws (three cases), or plate (three cases). The average time interval between the initial trauma and shoulder replacement was 2 years.

Surgical Technique

The patient was placed in a beach-chair position with the shoulder free of the table edge. An elongated deltopectoral incision was used in all cases in this series. The dissection was always difficult because of soft-tissue retraction and anatomical distortion especially where there had been previous open surgery. The main landmark was the biceps tendon used as a guide for the rotator interval and to locate the subscapularis. On 12 occasions the joint was approached via an osteotomy of the lesser tuberosity with the subscapularis still attached in order to improve mobilization. A lesser tuberosity osteotomy was carried out two times in nonunions of the surgical neck and six times in major malunions of the tuberosities. A greater tuberosity osteotomy was carried out in all but five cases. The greater tuberosity osteotomy was large enough to allow solid fixation to the diaphysis. Fourteen patients had had previous open surgery. A rotator cuff tear was reported and repaired in seven cases. Five of these tears were a two tendons rupture (supra and infraspinatus) and two were a single tendon rupture (one supra- and one infraspinatus). The cuff was thin in seven cases and normal in eight. The biceps tendon was tenodesed six times and left free in its groove in three cases despite signs of damage (inflammation or erosion). Eight acromioplasties were performed in order to the space for the tuberosities under the acromiocoracoid vault or to protect a cuff repair. The head was carefully dislocated in adduction, external rotation and retropulsion to minimize the risk of a shaft fracture. Despite this precaution, only one diaphyseal peroperative fracture was reported in the series. The humeral head cut was usually minimal. Reaming the medullary canal was difficult due to the anatomical distortion.

Twenty-two Aequalis prostheses were used. Nineteen were hemiarthroplasties and three were total shoulder replacements (Table 1). The Aequalis shoulder is an unconstrained prosthesis whose conception is based on anatomical studies which demonstrated variations in the dimensions, and especially the shape, of the proximal humerus [2, 3]. Consisting of three sections (head, neck and stem), this implant allows the prosthesis to be adapted to the anatomy rather than having to adapt the anatomy to the prosthesis. Modularity is achieved by the availability of seven articular heads of increasing diameter and thickness. Adaptability is possible due to the variable inclination offered by a choice of four neck angles of 125°, 130°, 135°, and 140°. An inclination guide allows the angle to be measured intraoperatively and then the appropriate neck can be selected. Out of the available range the 130° neck was used 15 times (68 %) the 135 on 3 occasions (14 %) and the 125 on 4 patients (18 %). Adaptability is also possible due to the ability to translate the humeral head. An eccentric dial system on the under surface of the head allows it to be translated into one of eight positions both superoinferiorly and mediolaterally until the bony surface is best covered.

In seven cases (five malunions and two nonunions), the humeral prosthesis was inserted using the Aequalis fracture jig [1]. This jig allows humeral length to be restored based on measurements taken from a radiograph of the unaffected humerus. It also helps to select the appropriate retroversion. The landmarks used are the lateral and medial epicondyles. A cemented polyethylene glenoid component was used in the three cases of total shoulder arthroplasty. A cancellous bone graft was used in eight cases and was always taken from the humeral head.

Postoperatively the arm was immobilized in a sling with the elbow at the side. Passive mobility was started the day after surgery following Neer's recommendations [17–19]. No active muscular activity was started until full passive movement had been achieved and there was bony consolidation of the tuberosity osteotomies (6–8 weeks). Fifteen patients benefited from a stay in a specialized rehabilitation center for an average of 35 days. Two patients had home physiotherapy and in five cases the type of rehabilitation was not detailed.

Results

Clinical Results

The adjusted Constant score at review averaged 59 % (Table 2). Using the Constant criteria we recorded 2 excellent, 3 good, 6 fair, and 11 poor results, i.e., 23 % good or excellent. The objective results evaluated according to the Neer system were 3 excellent, 7 good, 5 fair, and 10 poor, i.e., 32 % good or excellent.

Pain. At review the mean pain score was 9.5 (out of a possible 15); an increased from 3.1 preoperatively. There were only 2 cases (9 %) where the shoulder was completely pain free (score of 15). There were 7 cases (32 %) where the shoulder was almost painfree (score between 1 and 14); there was pain limiting the use of the upper limb (score between 5 and 10) in 11 cases (11 %), and incapacitating pain (score between 0 and 1) in 2 cases (9 %). Although pain was due to multiple causes, we noticed greater tuberosity resorption or persistant nonunion.

Active Mobility. At review the mean score was 20.8 out of 40. Mobility was quite poor with active anterior elevation not passing the horizontal (63° in the nonunions and 90° in the malunions) and unsatisfactory external rotation (20°). Internal rotation which, overall, was zero preoperatively (hand to the level of the greater trochanter) reached the L5 level at follow-up.

Activity. This was recorded as 11.8 out of 20 at review as opposed to 5 preoperatively. All the patients where able to carry out the activities of daily living such as washing, dressing and putting their hand to their mouth, whereas two-thirds could not do so before their surgery.

Strength. The average strength in elevation was 3.3 points at review increased from 1.2 preoperatively. It was greater than 5 points in only 32 % of patients (7 cases).

Table 2. Detailed Constant score in extracapsular, disimpacted sequelae of fractures of the proximal humerus

	Surgical neck nonunion (n=6)			Major tuberosity malunion (n=16)		
Results	Preop	Postop	(Gain)	Preop	Postop	(Gain)
Pain (/15 points)	3.5 →	8.3	(+ 4.8)	2.8 →	9.8	(+ 7.0)
Activity (/20 points)	4.7 →	10.6	(+ 5.9)	5.1 →	12.3	(+ 7.2)
Mobility (/40 points)	8.3 →	19.5	(+11.2)	9.5 →	21.6	(+12.1)
Strength (/25 points)	1.1 →	3	(+ 1.9)	1.3 →	3.4	(+ 2.1)
Absolute Constant score	17.6 →	41.4	(+23.8)	18.7 →	47.1	(+28.4)
Normalized Constant score	22 →	57	(+35)	24 →	60	(+36)

Subjective Results. Of the 22 patients in the series 12 (54 %) declared themselves satisfied or very satisfied with the result, although they all had some degree of limitation in the operated shoulder. Eight patients were disappointed with the operation and two were unhappy. One of these was because of persistent pain and reduced mobility for no clear reason and the other had to have the prosthesis removed for infection.

Radiographic Results

Humeral Length

Calculating humeral length on comparative, measured radiographs was only possible in the 5 cases of major tuberosity malunions where the fracture jig was used. The length difference between the healthy and operated humeri was minimal (between +4 and -8 mm).

Epiphyseal Width

This is the sum of the medial offset of the humeral head (the distance between the metaphysodiaphyseal axis and the medial edge of the prosthesis) plus the lateral offset of the greater tuberosity (distance between this axis and the lateral border of the greater tuberosity). Measurement of restoration of the medial offset is the only significant value [14, 27]. The mean medial offset measured in 9 cases was 32.5 mm on the operated side against 31.9 mm on the healthy side. The mean lateral offset in the 9 cases was 18.1 mm on the operated side and 17.5 mm on the healthy side. The mean epiphyseal width was 50.6 mm on the operated side and 49.4 on the healthy side.

Greater Tuberosity Position

It should be recalled that the mean distance between the top of the humeral head and the top of the greater tuberosity was 8 mm (with a minimum of 5 mm and a maximum of 13 mm) and that the greater tuberosity is never above the top of the humeral head (13). In 3 cases the top of the greater tuberosity was above the top of the prosthetic humeral head demonstrating poor reconstruction of the proximal humeral anatomy. In 3 cases the top of the greater tuberosity was at the level of the top of the head and in 12 cases (55 %) it was below the top of the head by an average of 7.5 mm on average. This last situation occurred in 4 nonunions of the surgical neck and 8 major malunions of the tuberosities.

Acromiohumeral Distance

The acromiohumeral distance measured on the AP radiograph in neutral rotation had been altered in 7 cases (32 %) where the space had become less than 5 mm or where there was a superior migration. This reduction in the acromiohumeral distance may be explained by a cuff tear in two cases, by an increasingly thin cuff in three cases and by nonunion of the greater tuberosity in one case. The restoration of humeral length had not been achieved in these cases.

Prosthetic Fixation

The Humeral Cement Mantle. This was examined along the entire length of the stem and was normal in 16 cases (73 %). An incomplete lucent line was recorded in 4 cases (18 %). A complete lucent line was recorded in 2 cases (9 %) but was considered nonprogressive. There were no lucent lines greater than 2 mm. One infective loosening was reported.

The glenoid fixation was studied in the 3 polyethylene components and featured a lucent line. In 2 cases there was an incomplete lucent line and in 1 case a complete lucent line resulting in removal of the prosthesis because of deep infection.

Ossifications

These were found in three cases (14 %). According to Sneppen's classification we reported: one grade I (ossification of less than half the joint line); one grade II (more than half the joint line), which was present before the joint replacement; one grade III (ossifications forming a scapulohumeral bridge): in this case there was preexisting grade II ossification. The ossifications had increased from grade II to grade III after open surgery to clear the joint.

Complications and Revisions

Thirteen complications were reported among which one occurred intraoperatively, demonstrating the technical difficulties of this surgery.

Intraoperative Complication. The only was a diaphyseal fracture which was fixed by screws and cerclage wiring. This case was complicated by a radial nerve palsy following fixation using a plate and screws reinforced by injection of intramedullary cement. Two years after, the patient had no functional sequelae with 140° of elevation and an adjusted Constant score of 97 % and was very happy with the outcome.

Early Postoperative Complications (n=3). One patient presented with a diaphyseal fracture around the prosthesis following a fall one month postoperatively. He was treated nonoperatively and consolidated in 3 months. At the last follow-up, the had achieved only 60° of elevation and an adjusted Constant score of 34 %. Another patient presented with a failure of the greater tuberosity fixation at 3 weeks postoperatively and had to undergo revision surgery to reattach the fragment. One patient who had a nonunion of the surgical neck and had already had surgery, presented with an immediate postoperative anterior dislocation. This was due to insufficient retroversion plus deficient anterior musculo-capsular structures. Despite a closed reduction there was a persistent anterior subluxation. At the latest review, the patient had 50° of elevation and an adjusted Constant score of 34 % and was disappointed with the outcome.

Late Postoperative Complications (n=9). Four postoperative cases of *resorption of the greater tuberosity* were observed. A greater tuberosity osteotomy in all cases was the main reason. Three *nonunions of the greater tuberosity*, one of which existed preoperatively, were observed (one nonunion of the surgical neck and two severe tuberosity malunions). Again, an osteotomy of the greater tuberosity or a preexisting nonunion were the mean reasons for persistent nonunion. Finally, two late infections presented at 18 months and required prosthetic removal.

Revision Surgery

Three patients required revision surgery. The first case was the patient who presented a failure of the fixation of the greater tuberosity. Having achieved complete passive elevation, she complained of pain and a sudden loss of function 3 weeks postoperatively. The radiographs showed upward migration of the tuberosity and this was refixed using metal sutures. The functional result was mediocre with elevation of 90° and episodic pain. In the second case, the prosthesis was removed due to late infection. Hemiarthroplasty had been achieved in a patient who had already undergone two operations to fix a proximal humeral fracture. The infection manifested itself at 18 months with the appearance of a fistula. Two attempts were made to débride the tract but both failed and finally the humeral prosthesis, which was not loose, had to be removed. The patient was left with a hanging shoulder. The third case was a total arthroplasty which never achieved a good functional result (elevation of 90°, adjusted Constant score 50 %) and presented with radiological signs of humeral and glenoid loosening (complete humeral and glenoid lucent lines and cement fracture at the tip of the stem). This case required the removal of both components and all the cement.

Discussion

Our study demonstrates that it is almost impossible to obtain a functional shoulder in fracture sequelae where a greater tuberosity osteotomy has to be performed in the same time than a humeral prosthesis.

Nonunion of the Surgical Neck

Nonunion of the surgical neck occurred in two different groups. Firstly, in displaced fractures which had undergone previous surgery and where the fixation has contributed to both periosteal destruction and distraction of the fracture. This was the case for surgical neck fractures fixed using a plate or even with multiple intramedullary nails and for displaced four-part fractures with attempted fixation with plates. Secondly, they occurred in three-part displaced fractures which did not undergo surgery: the rotationally displaced humeral head, which still had part of the rotator cuff attached to it, is usually in contact with the diaphysis thus making bony union difficult if not impossible [15, 17, 18].

Most authors emphasize of the difficulties of operating on nonunions of the surgical neck [9, 20, 23, 24, 28]. The functional results achieved after shoulder arthroplasty for surgical nonunion were the poorest in our series with a Constant score of 57 % at review. None of the patients had elevation above the horizontal and three still had disabilitating pain. The only real benefit of the surgery was the recovery of a satisfactory range of active rotation of the upper arm. These poor results were the consequence of a persistent nonunion and/or tuberosity lysis. Bridging the nonunion with the stem of the prosthesis plus a cancellous bone graft was not enough to achieve consolidation (Fig. 1). Our experience highlighted that the insertion of a prosthesis should always be combined with a large cancellous auto graft plus additional fixation with nonabsorbable bone sutures. The bone graft should be taken from the humeral head and even this is often insufficient and may need additional graft from the iliac crest.

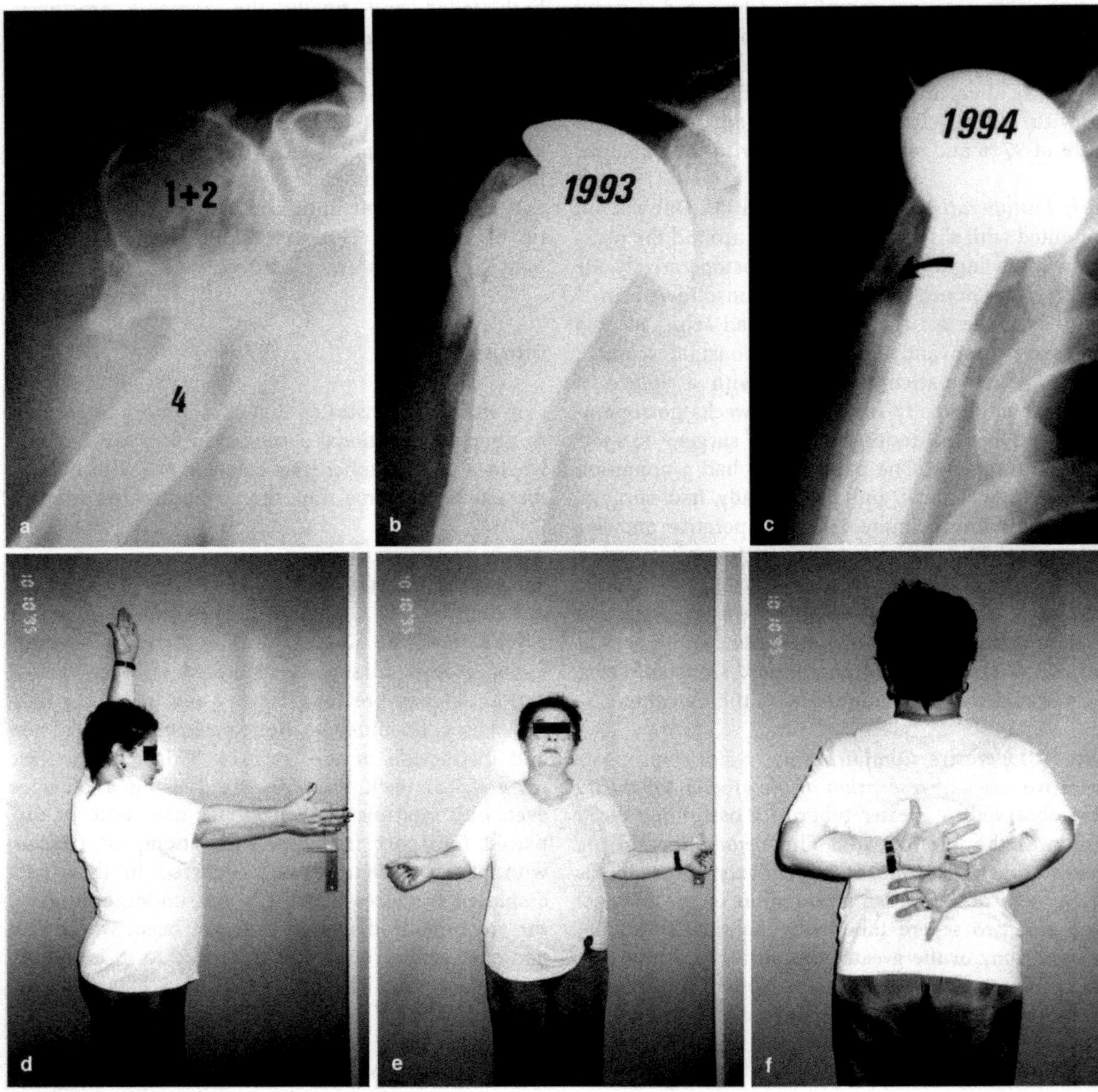

Fig. 1 a–f. Example of nonunion of the surgical neck after a three-part greater tuberosity fracture. **a** Radiograph of the fracture sequelae with preexisting nonunion. **b** Aequalis prosthesis (osteotomy and graft). **c** After 1 year: persistent greater tuberosity nonunion seen on the lateral view (arrow). **d,e,f** Poor active anterior elevation but satisfied external and internal rotation

Performing a shoulder replacement in nonunions of the surgical neck may even be questionable. Treatment of nonunion of the surgical neck is a difficult task, as illustrated by the fact that there were 35 failed repair attempts in the 50 nonunions in Neer's 1983 series [20]. Nicholson and Bigliani [22] are the only authors to report that humeral head replacement is comparable, if not superior, to open reduction and internal fixation, providing 60%–80% satisfactory results. Our own experience and that of others [9, 11, 12, 21, 25] runs contrary to this. Our impression is that filling of the medullary canal by the prosthesis prevents union of the tuberosities to the humeral shaft. For this reason, we think that union of the tuberosities to the shaft should be the primary goal and can be obtained by using a large intramedullary autogenous iliac graft: this should be the first and may be the only treatment resulting in satisfactory function and mobility of the shoulder [33]. Replacement arthroplasty should only be proposed in cases of longstanding nonunion where the humeral head has resorbed or collapsed [32]. Three out of the six cases in the present series could have been treated by using a bone graft alone without a shoulder replacement.

Severe Malunions of the Tuberosities

Consolidation of a proximal humeral fracture in a very malunited position is usually not well tolerated because of pain, even at rest, and a very limited range of movement. In these posttraumatic conditions it is usually impossible to implant a shoulder prosthesis without performing a greater tuberosity osteotomy. Within this group we included 16 cases where consolidation of the tuberosities with severe malunion was associated with disimpaction of the humeral head. It is this disimpaction of the head which led to major displacement and retraction of the tuberosities and explains why such outcomes always occur in four-part displaced or dislocated fractures (Fig. 2). This criterion, which can be assessed on the preoperative radiographs, demonstrates the seriousness of the malunion, and require a tuberosity osteotomy. The failure of the initial surgical treatment shows how very unstable these

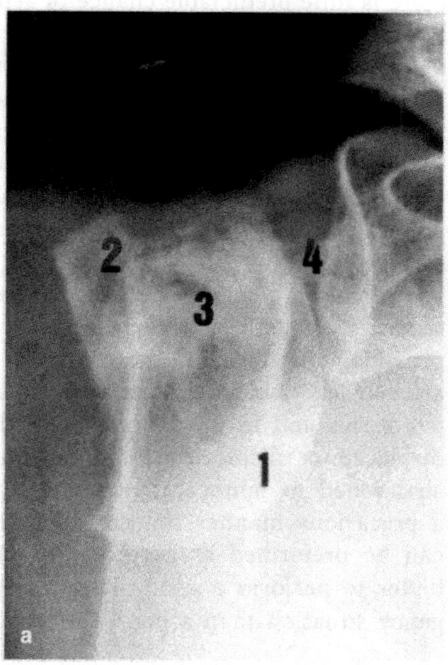

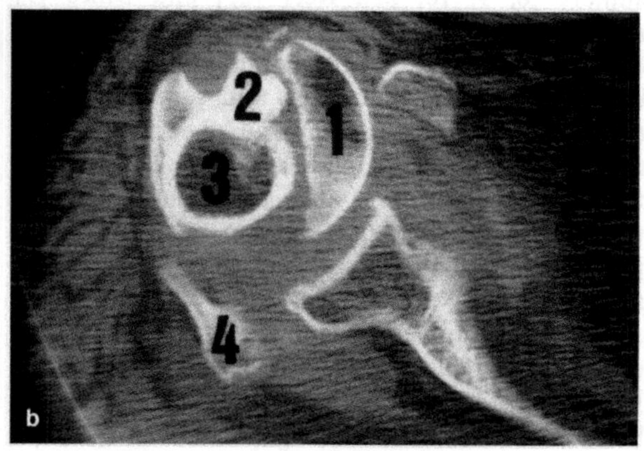

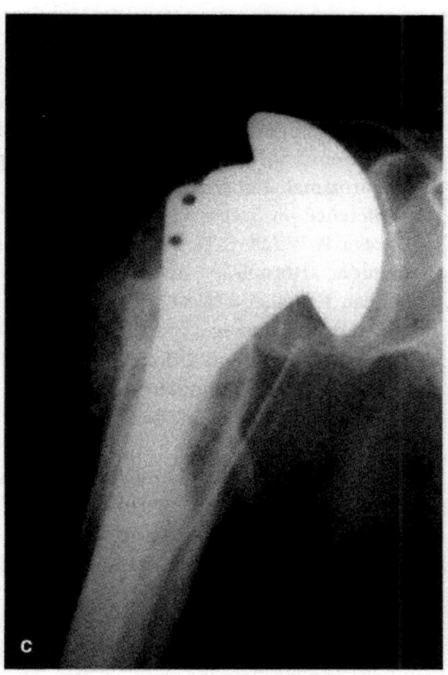

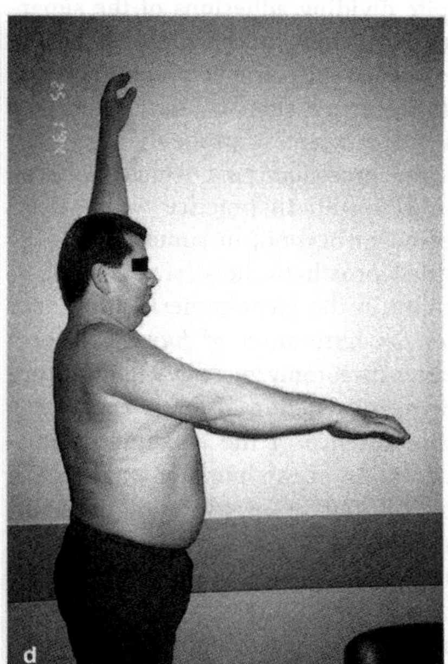

Fig. 2 a–d. Example of severe malunion of the tuberosities after a displaced four-part fracture initially treated nonoperatively. **a** Extra-capsular, disimpacted fracture sequela. **b** The four bone fragments shown on CT scan: *1*, head; *2*, lesser tuberosity; *3*, diaphysis; *4*, greater tuberosity. **c** reconstruction around a prosthesis after tuberosity osteotomy and graft from the humeral head. **d** Poor active anterior elevation lesions are, being difficult to fix internally. In ten cases attempted fixation, either closed or open, acted only to perpetuate already significant displacements. Two patients even underwent two surgeries. Moreover, previous internal fixation makes the implantation of a humeral prosthesis even more difficult due to secondary ossification and adhesions between the tuberosities and the deltoid [4, 9, 21, 24, 35].

Osteotomy of the Greater Tuberosity: the Main Reason for Poor Results

The poor results achieved with shoulder arthroplasty in tuberosity malunions are also found in other series in the literature [4, 13, 19, 20, 21, 32] and in our opinion are due, to *devascularization of the greater tuberosity* after osteotomy leading to tuberosity nonunion, migration and resorption. The complications have already been recorded by other authors [6, 9, 10, 21]. Neer [21] and Dines [9] recommend taking a fragment of the greater tuberosity which is sufficiently large to have enough bone still attached to the cuff and sufficiently long to favor bony contact between the repositioned tuberosity and the diaphysis. We always tried to favor revascularization and consolidation of the tuberosities by replacing the cement at the upper part of the diaphysis by cancellous graft taken from the head.

Two other problems should be solved at the time of shoulder replacement in tuberosity malunions. Firstly, *loss of elasticity in the soft tissues* which have been retracted for long periods of time [9, 10, 24, 32]. Despite dividing adhesions of the superficial layers and performing a capsulotomy of the deep layers, the rotator cuff usually remains inelastic. Although we were not able to check this with preoperative CT scans, there is probably also fatty degeneration in the muscular part which compromise the functional result. In practice we have no answer to this problem beyond, in some cases, suggesting that a small prosthetic head size is used to allow some mobility in the glenohumeral joint. Secondly, *difficulties for restoration of humeral length* [1, 21]. A tuberosity osteotomy recreates the fracture and should allow reconstruction of the normal anatomy. However, the absence of the anatomical landmarks makes restoration of the humeral length difficult. This is shown in our series where we observed some cases of superior migration of the prostheses. This problem has already been observed in fresh fractures [1, 6]. It is for this reason that we developed the Aequalis fracture jig designed to help the surgeon to accurately restore the humeral retroversion and length by using a preoperative measured radiograph of the healthy humerus. This jig was used in the last five cases of major tuberosity malunion and a prospective study is currently being carried out to evaluate the validity of the jig's design and use.

Conclusion

Our experience suggests that it is better to avoid performing an arthroplasty in cases of surgical neck nonunion and of severe tuberosity malunion requiring a greater tuberosity osteotomy, because there is little predictable chance of achieving a functional shoulder. In such cases, only incapacitating pain with significant functional impairment would make us consider inserting a prosthesis. The numerous technical problems (freeing retracted soft tissues, restoration of humeral length and retroversion, osteolysis and persistent greater tuberosity nonunion) have not yet been resolved and need further studies.

Prevention remains the best answer in trying to reduce the number of sequelae of fractures of the proximal humerus. The poor results after shoulder arthroplasty for nonunions and malunions both in our series and in the literature clearly show that a displaced or dislocated fracture should neither be abandoned to nonoperative treatment nor fixed in a precarious manner thinking that an arthroplasty can be preformed as a secondary procedure. It is better to perform a good arthroplasty in the emergency situation than a poor one later.

References

1. Boileau P, Chau E, Perraud M, Arcamone H, Argenson C (1992) Restoration of humeral offset and humeral length after hemiarthroplasty for displaced 4-part fractures of the proximal humerus. Presented at the 5th International Conference on Surgery of the Shoulder. Paris
2. Boileau P, Walch G (1994) Adaptability and modularity in shoulder arthroplasty. Acta Orthop Belg 61 [Suppl I]:49–61
3. Boileau P, Walch G (1997) Three dimensional geometry of the proximal humerus: implications on the technique and the prosthetic design J Bone Joint Surg Br 79 (5):857–865
4. Cofield RH (1987) Shoulder replacement: prognosis related to diagnosis: Springer, Berlin Heidelberg New York, pp 157–161
5. Cofield RH (1988) Comminuted fractures of the proximal humerus. Clin Orthop 230:49–57
6. Compito CA, Self EB, Bigliani LU (1994) Arthroplasty and acute shoulder trauma: reasons for success and failure. Clin Orthop 307:27–36
7. Constant CR (1986) Age related recovery of shoulder function after injury. Thesis, University College Cork

8. Constant CR, Murley AHG (1987) A Clinical Method of functional assessment of the Shoulder. Clin Orthop 214:160–164
9. Dines DM (1993) Posttraumatic changes of the proximal humerus: malunion, nonunion, and osteonecrosis. Treatment with modular hemiarthroplasty or total shoulder arthroplasty. J Shoulder Elbow Surg 2 (1):11–21
10. Duralde XA, Flatow EL, Pollock RG, Nicholson GP, Self EB, Bigliani LU (1996) Operature treatment of the surgical neck of the humerus. J Shoulder Elbow Surg 5(3):169–180
11. Healy VL, Jupiter JB, Kristiansen TK, White RR (1990) Nonunion of the proximal humerus. In: Post M, Morrey BF, Hawkins RJ (eds) Surgery of the shoulder. Mosby Year Book, Chicago, pp 59–62
12. Huten D, Duparc J (1986) L'arthroplastie prothétique dans les traumatismes complexes récents et anciens de l'épaule. Rev Chir Orthop 72:517–529
13. Ianotti JP, Sidor ML (1997) Malunions of the proximal humerus. In: Warren JP, Ianotti JP, Gerber C (eds) Complex and revision problems in shoulder surgery. Lippincot-Raven. Philadelphia, pp 245–264
14. Jacobson SR (1993) The glenohumeral offset ratio: a radiographic study. J Shoulder Elbow Surg 2, 3:141–146
15. Jakob RP, Kristiansen T, Mayo K, Ganz R, Muller ME (1984) Classification and aspects of treatment of fractures of the proximal humerus. In: Bateman JE, Welsh RP (ed) Surgery of the shoulder. Decker, pp 330–334
16. Jakob RP, Miniani A, Anson PS (1991) Four part valgus impacted fractures of the proximal humerus. J Bone Joint Surg Br 73:295–298
17. Neer CS (1970) Displaced proximal humeral fractures. I Classification and evaluation. J Bone Joint Surg Am 52:1077–1089
18. Neer CS (1970) Displaced proximal humeral fractures. II Treatment of three and four part displacement. J Bone Joint Surg Am 52:1090–1103
19. Neer CS, Watson KC, Stanton FJ (1982) Recent experience in total shoulder replacement. J Bone Joint Surg Am 64:319–337
20. Neer CS (1983) Nonunion of the surgical neck of the humerus. Orthop Trans 7:389
21. Neer CS (1990) Old trauma in glenohumeral arthroplasty, first edn. In: Shoulder reconstruction. Saunders, Philadelphia, pp 222–234
22. Nicholson GP, Flatow EL, Bigliani LU (1994) Shoulder arthroplasty for proximal humeral fractures. In: Friedman RJ (Ed) Arthroplasty of the shoulder. Thieme, Stuttgart, pp 183–193
23. Norris TR, Turner JA, Bovill D (1990) Nonunion of the upper humerus: an analysis of the etiology and treatment in 28 cases. In: Post M, Morrey BF, Hawkins RJ (eds) Surgery of the shoulder. Mosby-Year Book, Chicago, pp 63–67
24. Norris TR (1995) Late prosthetic shoulder arthroplasty for displaced proximal humerus fractures. J Shoulder and Elbow Surg 4:271–280
25. Razemon JP, Baux S (1969) Les séquelles des fractures de l'extrémité supérieure de l'humérus. Rev Chir Orthop 55:479–490
26. Resch H, Beck E, Bayley I (1995) Reconstruction of the valgus impacted humeral head fracture. J Shoulder Elbow Surg 4:74–80
27. Rietveld ABM, Dannen HAM, Rozing PM, Oberman WR (1988) The lever arm in gleno humeral adduction after hemi arthroplasty. J Bone Joint Surg Br 70:561–565
28. Scheck M (1982) Surgical treatment of nonunions of the surgical neck of the humerus. Clin Orthop 167:255–259
29. Siebenrock, Gerber C (1993) The reproducibility of classification fractures of the proximal end of the humerus. J Bone Joint Surg Am 75:1751–1755
30. Sidor ML, Zuckerman JD (1993) The Neer classification system for proximal humerus fractures. J Bone Joint Surg Am 75:1745–1750
31. Sneppen O, Kjaersgaard-Andersen P, Frich LH (1990) Ectopic ossification after total shoulder arthroplasty. A study on 75 Neer total shoulder replacements. In: Post M, Morrey BF, Hawkins RJ (eds) Surgery of the shoulder. Mosby-World Book, St. Louis, pp 298–301
32. Tanner MW, Cofield RH (1983) Prosthetic arthroplasty for fractures and fractures dislocations of the proximal humerus. Clin Orthop 179:116–128
33. Walch G, Boileau P, Martin B, Dejour H (1990) Unreduced posterior dislocations and fracture-dislocations of the shoulder. A review of 30 cases. Rev Chir Orthop 76:546–558
34. Walch G, Badet R, Nové-Josserand L, Lévigne C (1996) Nonunions of the surgical neck of the humerus: surgical treatment with an intramedullary bone peg, internal fixation and cancellous bone grafting. J Shoulder Elbow Surg 5:161–168
35. Watson KC (1987) Indications and considerations of shoulder replacement in post-traumatic conditions. In: Köbel R, Helbig B, Blauth W (eds) Shoulder replacement. Springer. Berlin Heidelberg New York, pp 129–133

Section XIII:
Rehabilitation

Rehabilitation Following Shoulder Arthroplasty: Experience at a Rehabilitation Centre

J.P. Liotard

Summary

We report our experience of rehabilitation in shoulder arthroplasty through a series of 130 patients operated on with an Aequalis prosthesis from 1991 to 1994. Because our Health Care System has provision for impatient rehabilitation, patients were rehabilitated in a specialised rehabilitation center with a swimming pool. The aetiologies were osteoarthritis in 58 cases, rheumatoid arthritis in 21, old fractures in 16 and 34 other causes: osteonecrosis (5 cases), revision surgery (12 cases), locked posterior dislocations (4 cases), cuff tear arthropathies (5 cases), complexes fractures (8 cases), arthritis after radiotherapy (1 case), necrosis after large cuff tear (1 case). Our rehabilitation was directly inspired by Neer's protocol. However, we added rehabilitation in a warm swimming pool which has simplified the programme. The immediate use of a pool heated to 35 °C and a suspensory system have allowed the patients to make breast-stroke movements without gravity, whether or not they know how to swim, and has quickly removed the early muscular shakes and postoperative inhibition with recovery of passive movement.

Introduction

In 1975 Hughes and Neer [3] presented their protocol for shoulder rehabilitation after arthroplasty. In 1982 [5] Neer described the results of shoulder arthroplasty depending on their aetiology and separated those shoulders in which rehabilitation could have only *limited goals* from those where a *full exercise programme* could be used. By 1987 [6] he had proposed the idea of *early recovery of passive movement* with the aim of achieving between 140° and 160° of passive anterior elevation by the end of the first postoperative week. By 1990 [7] Neer's protocol had become established and had created a common rehabilitation system for all shoulder operations with the progression through the exercise programme dependent on the operative findings, the procedure and scar healing. With unconstrained shoulder arthroplasties most authors, for example, Cofield, Rockwood and Matsen [1] have adopted the Neer protocol. We have also adopted the protocol, but, as we are able to follow the programme on in-patients at a rehabilitation centre, we have been able to add early rehabilitation in a warm swimming pool. Taking into account the functional anatomy of the shoulder, we visualise the recovery of the range of joint movement [4] as starting with elevation in the scapular plane, passing from the "zero position" to 150° of elevation (Saha) [8] and ending with exercising the shoulder to recover the last few degrees of movement. The 130 shoulders included in this study present the results achieved by the same medical, surgical and physiotherapy team.

Material and Methods

Between November 1991 and August 1994, 130 patients who had undergone the implantation of a non-constrained Aequalis shoulder arthroplasty were admitted to our specialist centre for postoperative rehabilitation. The aetiologies, age, postoperative day of entry and length of stay are detailed in Table 1. We can see that there was a predominance

Table 1. The 130 Aequalis prostheses in the series

Aetiology	OA (*n*=62)	Bilat. (*n*=38)	Unilat. (*n*=24)	RA (*n*=21)	PTA (*n*=13)	AF (*n*=6)	Rev. (*n*=12)	CTA (*n*=5)	Misc. (*n*=11)
Age at operation (years)	66	68	62	57	63	73	65	71	57
Admission (days postop.)	11	10	12	17	7	12	8	5	17
Length of stay (days)	30	29	30	31	38	55	30	36	28

OA, osteoathritis; RA, rheumatoid arthritis; PTA, posttraumatic arthritis; AF, acute fracture; Rev., operative revision; CTA, cuff tear arthritis; Miscellanous [chronic dislocation (4), atraumatic necrosis (3), complex fracture (2), postradiotherapy arthritis (1), necrosis with cuff tear (1)]

of osteoarthritis patients (62 cases) with a clear under-representation of recent fractures with only 6 cases (4.5 %) whereas in the multi-centre study they made up 16 %. The rehabilitation after fracture is dealt with by Caligaris-Cordero et al. ("Rehabilitation Following Shoulder Arthroplasty for Fracture", this volume).

Postoperative Rehabilitation in a Specialist Centre

We use a consistent rehabilitation protocol based on one objective which is the early postoperative recovery of the passive range of motion, carried out in a rehabilitation centre which specialises in the shoulder. The Service has 40 in-patient beds and the three physiotherapists involved have access to a pool and a gymnasium and did not deal with patients other than those who had undergone shoulder surgery. Between 1991 and 1994 there were 1425 other patients mixed with the 130 arthroplasty patients, and 462 of these had undergone rotator cuff repairs. The postoperative rehabilitation followed the same principles for all the operated shoulders.

The immediate postoperative rehabilitation programme used between 1991 and 1994 is as follows:

The patients arrive at the centre during the second postoperative week and have control radiographs taken which consist of AP views (double oblique) of both shoulders to rule out the presence of any problem with the prosthesis and allows the state of the opposite shoulder to be evaluated. The scar is checked by a doctor. Plans are made on admission, based on the operation details, for the way in which their rehabilitation will be carried out both while in the centre and, importantly after they have left.

The patient is then placed in the care of the physiotherapist and, depending on the medical and surgical indications, they begin passive elevation movements with the patient supine on a couch. The physiotherapist decides on the potential for rehabilitation for each individual by examining the opposite shoulder to assess their normal joint type, by gauging the physical and mental aptitude of the patient to relax, and then details the do's and don'ts to be respected during and between sessions. The patient starts auto-mobilisation in elevation while supine on the bed with the hands joined (Fig. 1).

By the end of the second postoperative week, and after the clips or stitches have been removed, the patient starts to exercise in the warm swimming pool (34°). Initially, the patient remains standing, lets the arms float and practices movements below the horizontal level. Firstly they swing their arms, with one coming forward just up to the surface while the other is swung backwards and then alternating them (Fig. 2). Secondly, they swing one arm across the body in horizontal adduction so that the hand reaches the opposite shoulder while the other arm swings behind the back in vertical adduction (Fig. 3). The patient can be made to feel weightless by being connected to a harness, whether they

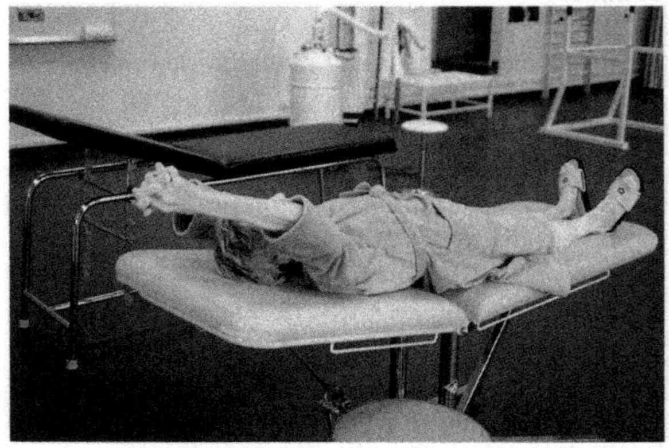

Fig. 1. Symetrical self-mobilisation used to passively elevate the arm in supine position (prier position)

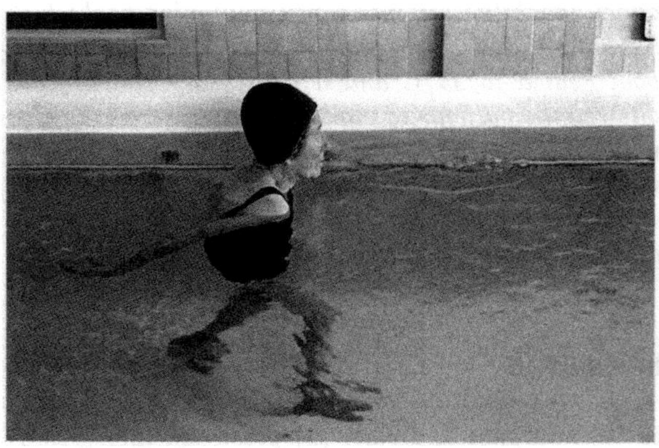

Fig. 2. Alternate mouvement combining flexion and extension (under horizontal level) in the warm swimming pool

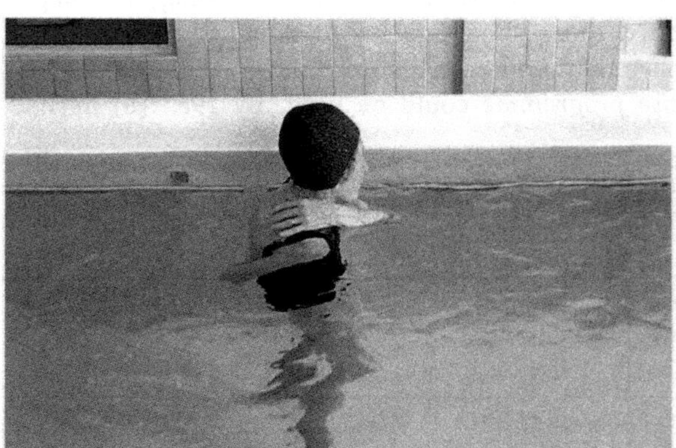

Fig. 3. Alternate mouvement combining horizontal adduction and internal rotation in the warm swimming pool

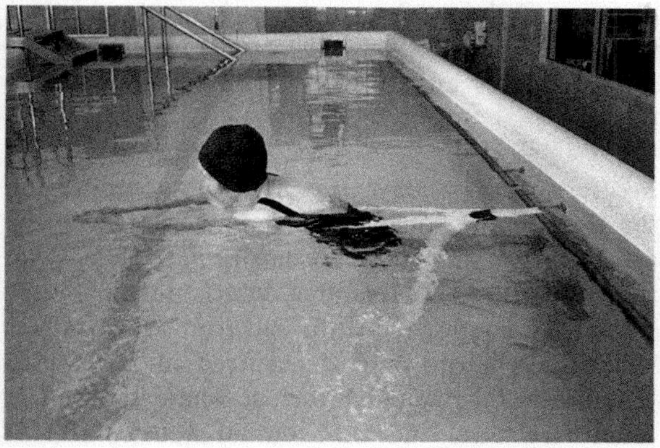

Fig. 4. Patient swimming brest-stroke while being attached: symetric elevation in. weightlessness

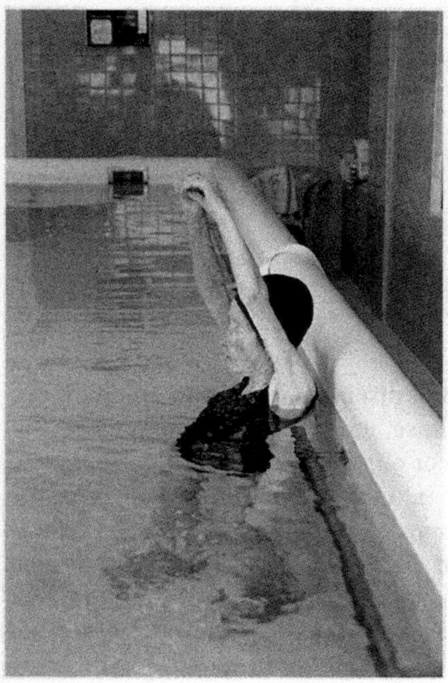

Fig. 5. Symetrical self mobilisation in passive elevation in standing position with the arm in the "zero position"

can swim or not, and does breast-stroke movements with the arms coming forward in at least 100° of elevation from the starting position (Fig. 4). Later they auto-mobilise with joined hands, standing in the water (Fig. 5) with their arms progressively leaving the water (100°) and finally reaching maximal elevation (150°). Thus, they are carrying out auto-passive movements against gravity but with the beginning of the range of movement, up to the horizontal, being protected by the water. When auto-passive elevation reaches about 150° then the arms can be placed behind the head with the fingers linked in the 'siesta' position and the elbows moved alternatively forwards and backwards (Figs. 6a and b).

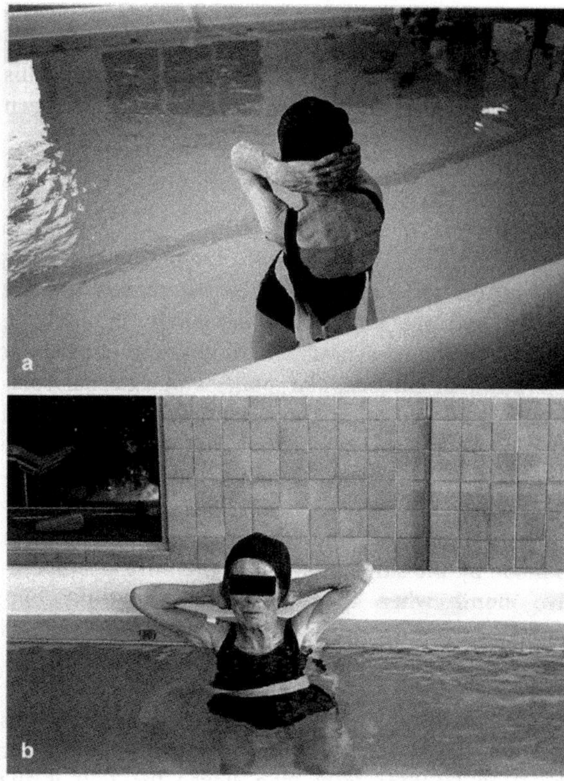

Fig. 6. a "Siesta position" with elbows forward: stretching of the posterior capsule and muscles. **b** "Siesta position" with elbows backward: stretching of the anterior capsule and muscles

Indications for Limited Goal or Complete Rehabilitation

The rehabilitation programme is not just based on the operative indications but also on the postoperative state and it is the surgeon who decides the limits. It should be remembered that osteoathritis patients should go for complete rehabilitation, if the cuff and tuberosities are intact, and this means there should be rapid recovery of passive elevation above the horizontal. Active mobility is not worked on as this comes spontaneously and is helped by simply removing the sling and leaving the patient free to perform movements within the limits of pain. In the case of a prosthesis inserted for a fresh fracture, where the tuberosities and tendinous insertions need time to consolidate and heal, rehabilitation is limited temporarily. Passive movements are unrestricted (except in specific cases) but a sling must be worn between physiotherapy sessions and, when spontaneous active mobility starts, then the patient must be told to remain very careful because bony and tendinous healing takes from 3–6 months. Finally, the rehabilitation is said to have a *limited goal* when the final result is clearly going to be limited to achieving a pain-free shoulder with mobility reduced to below the horizontal. This is typically the case where a prosthesis has been inserted for cuff-tear arthritis.

Results

The results were assessed when the patient left the Centre and are detailed by aetiology in Table 2. The elements measured where; passive movement (elevation in the scapular plane and external rotation with the elbow at the side), functional internal rotation (hand passing behind the back) and active elevation. At this stage usually about 6 weeks postoperatively it is not necessary to make a full functional examination, and the first overall assessment is made by the surgeon at about the third postoperative month when they also assess how the outpatient rehabilitation is coming along as well as the recovery after the initial in-patient period.

Length of Stay at the Centre. All the prostheses patients stayed for 1 month on average except for the fresh fracture cases who stayed for 2. It is the patient who decides when they are capable of leaving once they have recovered their independence and have a painfree shoulder. This delay varied within each aetiological group, sometimes directly related to the state of the shoulder and sometimes due to social conditions (elderly or living alone), but this does not alter the rehabilitation programme followed.

Recovery of Passive Movement. On leaving the Rehabilitation Centre, a satisfactory elevation would be greater than 140°, external rotation of at least 30° and internal rotation which allows the hand to reach behind the back. Oddly, in osteoarthritis, bilateral disease gave better results than unilateral disease and the results were even better in rheumatoid arthritis. By contrast, the results were worse for fresh fractures and, obviously, in the limited goal cases.

Recovery of Active Movement. This was dependent on the state of the rotator cuff and was judged to be satisfactory if it passed the horizontal. This is not the case with fresh fractures, which do not healed within 2 months or with cuff-tear arthropathies where there is no cuff. It occurred in 1 out of 3 cases with rheumatoid arthritis, where the cuff is often very thin, and in 2 out of 3 osteoarthritis cases: remembering that this measurement is made at about 6 weeks postoperation

Complications. One patient had an injection due to persistent stiffness. Two patients were treated with calcitonin for frozen shoulder. Two patients improved after manipulations for cervical arthritis which had been limiting their rehabilitation. Eight patients had a second stay and nine patients stayed for longer than 2 months.

Discussion

The purpose of the discussion is not to compare our methods with those used by others but rather to detail the basics of our system. We would emphasise the three steps in our programme related to the functional anatomy of the shoulder: passive elevation of the arm in the scapular plane up to the "zero position" of the shoulder, exercising the shoulder to recover the last few degrees of movement and rehabilitation in a warm swimming pool.

Table 2. Results at the end of the Rehabilitation Centre stay

Aetiology	OA (*n*=62)	Bilat. (*n*=38)	Unilat. (*n*=24)	RA (*n*=21)	PTA (*n*=13)	AF (*n*=6)	Rev. (*n*=12)	CTA (*n*=5)	Misc. (*n*=11)
Length of stay (days)	30	29	30	31	38	55	30	36	28
Admission (days postop.)	41	39	42	48	45	67	38	41	45
Passive ant. elev. >140° (%)	55	63	42	62	31	17	42	20	36
External rot. 1>30° (%)	52	55	46	81	54	17	50	40	55
Internal rot. (%)	73	63	88	86	54	50	83	40	64
Active ant. elev >90° (%)	69	68	71	33	46	0	42	0	36

OA, osteoathritis; RA, rheumatoid arthritis; PTA, posttraumatic arthritis; AF, acute fracture; Rev., operative revision; CTA, cuff tear arthritis; Misc., chronic dislocation (4), atraumatic necrosis (3), complex fracture (2), post radiotherapy arthritis (1), necrosis with cuff tear (1)

Passive Elevation in the Scapular Plane up to the "Zero Position"

Elevation in the Scapular Plane. Elevation in the scapular plane is the shoulders preferred movement. Neer presented the clinical evidence for forgetting pure abduction and pure flexion and sticking to elevation in the scapular plane which allows recovery of the maximum degree of movement with the most ease. The biomechanical evidence has been verified in the laboratory by Gagey [2] who described limitation in pure flexion due to tension in the coraco-humeral ligament and limitation of pure abduction by tension in the inferior gleno-humeral ligament whilst elevation in the scapular plane occurs with a balance in tensions in the two ligaments occurring later in the range. This idea of optimal elevation in the scapular plane demonstrates the fundamental role played by the capsulo-ligamentous apparatus in modifying the mutual positioning of the humerus and the scapula. During rehabilitation, mobilising the arm in the scapular plane places these guiding ligaments under their optimal tensions and moves the scapula over the thoracic cage to achieve total overall movement. This simple humeral movement has supplanted all the other techniques which control and limit scapular movement because limiting scapula movement while the humerus ascends inevitably leads to acromio-tuberosity impingement.

Passive Movement. During passive movement the deltoid is at rest, and initially this is the easiest way to avoid acromio-tuberosity impingement as the ascending action of the deltoid is not involved and the greater tuberosity can slide under the acromial vault. During passive movement, the rotator cuff is not under tension, either at the start or finish of elevation, because the supraspinatus tendon relaxes progressively from its long to its short status, while the biceps tendon is progressively swallowed up by and stabilised within the bicipital groove. Finally, in passive movement, the joint capsule, as well as the inferior gleno-humeral ligament and coraco-humeral ligament, are progressively extended throughout the movement. This is the simplest way to avoid persistent postoperative capsular stiffness.

Zero Position of the Shoulder. The "zero position" of the shoulder corresponds to elevation of 150° in the scapular plane with the hand at the zenith [8]. Having the hand at the zenith does not mean that the arm is vertical, as this is a separate result from the recovery of the final few degrees of elevation when the arm moves from 150° to 180°. The term "zero position" was suggested in 1950 by Saha [8] to characterise the position of optimal balance in the gleno-humeral joint with regards to the tensions imposed on the rotator cuff. The shoulder has a unique joint pattern from the point of view of the bones, capsule, ligaments, muscles and tendons which combine to provide a configuration which makes rehabilitation very interesting. Reaching the zero position is a major stage in the recovery of passive movement. *Any capsulitis can be avoided* (Fig. 7A) because achieving 150° implies that physiological capsular movement has been recovered, especially in the inferior gleno-humeral ligament. *All bony impingement is avoided* (Fig. 7B) as the greater tuberosity has already passed under the acromial vault because of the posterior tilt of the scapula and because ascending component of the deltoid is neutralised. The rotator cuff is protected (Fig. 7C) because the supraspinatus is relaxed, the biceps tendon passes into its groove and the infraspinatus and subscapularis are in reciprocal balanced tension.

Automatic and Associated Rotation. Elevation to 150° in the scapular plane involves automatic rotation: external moving up and internal moving down. At the limits of the zero position, the arm (humerus) remains in the scapular plane and the patient produces a spontaneous, associated, external rotation

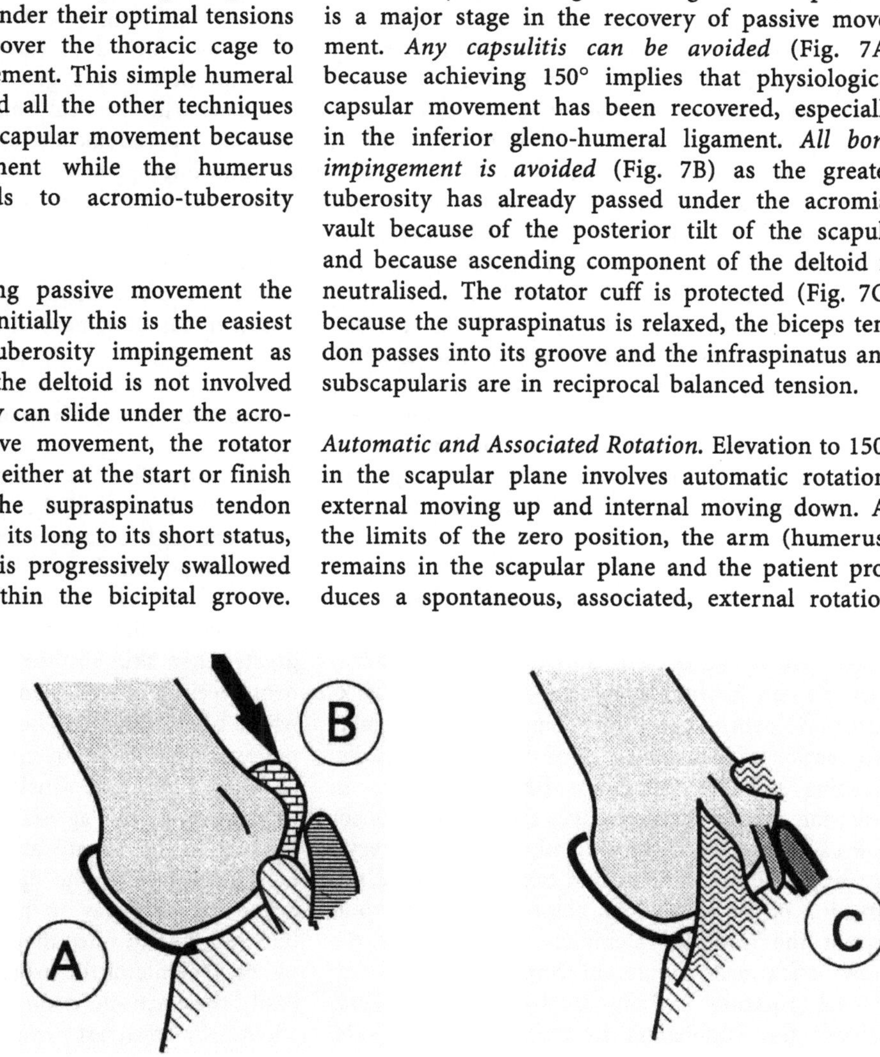

Fig. 7. The benefits of the "zero position" of the shoulder. **A,** No postoperative stiff shoulder; **B,** deltoid contraction does not lead to proximal humeral migration; **C,** optimal balancing between external and internal rotators

above 150° (hand behind the head) and, when descending, an associated internal rotation (hand behind the back). During rehabilitation, when patients recover passive elevation to 150°, they often also recovered functional rotation.

The Final Degrees of Movement and Exercising the Shoulder

Exercising the Shoulder. When the passive movements are judged to be satisfactory and the zero position having been reached, the next goal is to recover complete mobility in the shoulder by regaining the final degrees of elevation. We call this 'athletic' exercising of the shoulder because, in practice, the movements used to regain these last degrees go beyond simply repeating those movements used in daily life but involve stretching techniques as practised by athletes.

The Final Degrees of Movement. Completing elevation beyond 150° has the purpose of fully releasing the subacromial bursa which, at the end of elevation, is swept in and out by the greater tuberosity, beyond the acromio-coracoid vault as far as the acromio-clavicular joint. In complete external rotation (ER2), the goal is to recover the same subacromial freedom when the greater tuberosity above the horizontal plane sweeps from front to back under the acromion. These extreme positions in elevation and external rotation are not recovered spontaneously, especially in patients over 65-year-old. In practical terms, recovery of complete elevation and external rotation can be achieved by doing a very simple exercise: the fingers are linked and the hands positioned, with the palms up, behind the head in the 'siesta' position and the degree of movement gradually increased. This exercise is only started once passive elevation is about 150°.

The "Siesta Position." This is carried out with the patient standing, their chest straight and the fingers linked behind the occiput and the elbows alternatively pushed forward and back (Fig. 6). The backward movement of the elbow comes from the synergistic action of many muscles of the scapular girdle: trapezius and the rhomboids fix the scapulae in adduction on the thoracic cage; the spinal extensor muscles reduce the kyphosis and support the cervical spine; the posterior deltoid holds horizontal retropulsion of the arm which completes the retropulsion of the shoulder. Complete movement of the elbows backwards results in complete recovery of external rotation beyond horizontal (ER2) and achieves full suppleness in the anterior capsule. The elbows are pulled forwards by the combined action of the anterior deltoid and the pectoralis major, and the movement is complete when the elbows touch. This has the effect of stretching the posterior muscles and the posterior capsule. The exercise is bilateral and symmetrical and is facilitated by the muscles of the operated and healthy sides acting in synergy. This siesta movement is a protected exercise for the scapulo-humeral joint, done in the auto-passive mode because all the movements are carried out with the hands joined behind the occiput. In this position of auto-passive elevation with the arms beyond 100°, the greater tuberosity has already passed under the coraco-acromial vault, so there is no risk of acromio-tuberosity impingement: the "siesta-position" is a non-impingement position.

Completion of Stretching with the Hands at the Zenith. From the position where the fingers are crossed behind the head and with the hands remaining linked together, the patient stretches the arms up towards the ceiling with the palms upwards and the elbows locked in full extension at the end of the movement. This gives maximal elevation with the arms truly vertical both sagittally and frontally. It is also, paradoxically, an auto-passive movement without impingement which does not induce any damaging forces and this movement brings into play most of the peri-scapular musculature and has a noticeable effect on toning up these muscles which are often flabby in elderly patients whose shoulder has been painful and stiff for a long time.

Rehabilitation in a Warm Pool

Empirically. Year by year, as our experience has grown, we have used the warm pool at an ever earlier stage and for ever increasing periods. The first sensation which the patient experiences when they enter the water at 34°, is an immediate thermal comfort because the water temperature is just slightly greater than skin surface temperature and this cutaneous feeling of well-being leads to relaxation of the whole body which can be quite remarkable to see in patients who have so recently undergone surgery and, as such, are sensitive to pain. The second impression is the agreeable sensation of their arm floating in the warm water as opposed to the problems they face in the open air where they do not know the best way to hold the arm to prevent it hurting. Finally, once they start performing the simple movements in the protocol, they are amazed how easily these can be done and at the absence of pain where, by contrast, even the first stage in the movements had appeared almost impossible on dry land.

Connective Tissue, Collagen and Warm Water. The benefit of the warm water also has an effect by modifying the behaviour of the dense connective tissues. The soft-tissues surrounding the arthroplasty and acting to make it move, are made up of connective tissues and collagen: synovium, capsule, ligaments, tendons, muscular aponeuroses, fascia and bursae. At 34°, the water has a beneficial effect on collagen fibres which is manifest in many ways. The temperature increases the plasticity of connective tissue so improving its ability to stretch. The 34° temperature has this effect in comparison to the usual ambient air temperature of 20° rather than in comparison to the body temperature of 37°. The thermal comfort evoked at the skin interface does not have any risks, as has often been reported, and is safe, and indeed beneficial, for cardiac and rheumatoid patients.

Weightlessness. During movement, the connective tissues, which are ready to be stretched, undergo reduced tensions because of the weightless effect from the water. This effect acts in combination with the fact that movements, which had been limited and painful on dry land, are now easier to perform. When the patient exercises against the water, the weightlessness becomes a facilitating effect due to Archimedes principle. The muscle action required is minimal and, because of this, the intra-articular forces and the friction forces are diminished: always assuming that the patient carries out the movements slowly without fighting against the resistance imparted by the water.

Neuro-physio-Therapeutic Effect. The pool is an environment which is perfectly adapted to providing a total neuro-physio-therapueutic effect on the operated shoulder. The thermal comfort and the physical facilitation means that movements are recovered more easily and quickly than in the open air. We have abandoned decontracting massages and antalgic physiotherapy and replaced it with morning and afternoon sessions in the pool. At the end of each session the patient feels very relaxed and often likes to repose in their room before returning gently to the normal atmosphere of the centre: postoperative stress is literally left in the pool.

Conclusion

Since 1994 our protocol has evolved towards an increased use of the warm pool whose temperature has now risen to 35°. The use of a non-allergic, waterproof but air permeable dressing (Lumiderm) now allows us to start therapy in the pool as soon as the patient arrives at the centre rather than having to wait until the sutures had been removed and this means an extra week can be gained. A mask and snorkel are now the rule in order to relax the cervical spine when swimming the breaststroke in the fixed harness. More and more patients now use a weighted belt in order to do their exercises completely submerged and seem extremely happy. In the same way, movements in the siesta position can be done seated while wearing the weighted belt. It is only when the patient can comfortably carry out the movements in the water that they also do the same on dry land. This evolution, which may appear rather spectacular, is simply a development of Neer's early passive motion concept carried out in water. This development using the pool must be run in parallel with two ideas: (a) the results of rehabilitation should not, strictly speaking, be judged until after the first 3 months and not the first 3 weeks; and (b) an assessment of the cost, including all the different means of administering postoperative rehabilitation, is difficult, but it is clear that as the years have gone by, the Centre provides a short extension to the postoperative period after a standard arthroplasty but with a functional result when the patient leaves.

References

1. Cofield RH (1990) Degenerative and arthritic problems of the glenohumeral joint. In: Rockwood CA, Matsen FA (eds) The shoulder. Saunders, Philadelphia, pp 735–736
2. Gagey O, Bonfait H, Gillot C, Mazas F (1988) Anatomie fonctionnelle et mécanique de l'élévation du bras. Rev Chir Orthop 74:209–217
3. Hugues M, Neer CS (1975) Glenohumeral joint replacement and postoperative rehabilitation. Phys Ther 55:850–858
4. Liotard JP, Expert JM, Mercanton G, Padey A (1995) Rééducation de l'épaule. Encycl Med Chir Kinésithérapie-Rééducation fonctionnelle, 26210-A-10, Editions techniques, Paris, p 23
5. Neer CS, Watson KC, Stanton FJ (1982) Recent experience in total shoulder replacement. J Bone Joint Surg Am 64:319–337
6. Neer CS, McCann PD, McFarlane EA, Padilla N (1987) Earlier passive motion following shoulder arthroplasty and rotator cuff repair. A prospective study. Orthop Trans 11:231
7. Neer CS (1990) Shoulder rehabilitaion In: Shoulder reconstruction. Saunders. Philadelphia, pp 487–533
8. Saha AK (1950) Mechanism of shoulder movements and a plea for the recognition of "zero-position" of glenohumeral joint. Indian J Surg 12:153

Rehabilitation Following Shoulder Arthroplasty for Osteoarthritis with Massive Cuff-Tear

M. Mezzana, J.C. Scheffer, and D. Goutallier

Summary

Rehabilitation following shoulder arthroplasty for osteoarthritis associated with massive cuff-tears must be completely changed to adapt to this rare surgical indication: perfect gleno-humeral movement is not sought and active stability of the shoulder should be achieved. This rehabilitation should aim for function without pain and remain very modest in these ambitions.

Introduction

Despite a poor reputation, shoulder arthroplasty can give an improvement in pain more than function in patients with painful and pseudoparalysed shoulders secondary to osteoarthritis associated with massive cuff-tears.

Limited Goal Surgery and Rehabilitation

In osteoarthritis with massive cuff-tear, the prosthesis replaces a damaged glenohumeral joint which has lost all of its normal relationships and its ability for active and passive recentering. Repair of the ruined cuff cannot be envisaged and even the surgical approach itself can cause instability in the prosthesis. The goal therefore, is limited, and if the patient is not to be left in the same state, then the aim is to relieve pain. The rehabilitation programme must be totally altered to adapt to these rare surgical cases and the aim is not to try to achieve complete recovery of glenohumeral movement but to try and achieve active stability within the joint. Whatever function is recovered must occur without pain and only modest results can be expected. The rehabilitation must be adapted to the implant used and above all avoid excessive mechanical forces acting on the joint.

Recovery of Articular Mobility

The outcome should remain within reasonable limits in the knowledge that, in the osteoarthritic case with an associated cuff-tear, one would generally not expect to achieve active elevation greater than 70°. There is therefore no point in trying to achieve a very mobile gleno-humeral joint at all costs as this may worsen any instability.

Recovery of mobility in the scapulo-thoracic joint should, however, play a part in the rehabilitation of these shoulders as a large part of the result depends on the function achieved here. This joint is often used by the patients who have become used to a humeral head which has migrated superiorly, sometimes with a subacromial neo-articulation.

Active Shoulder Stabilisation

Due to the state of the rotator cuff, mobility and cooptation is carried out only by the deltoid (but strengthening it will only worsen the superior head migration!), the short head of biceps and triceps. By bringing all these muscles into play and by balancing their respective forces, a suitably trained subject can achieve a stable humeral prosthesis. Similarly, these elevating forces are balanced by strengthening the shoulder depressors (pectorals, latissimus dorsi). In aiming for a functional result, there is no point in wrestling against the compensatory actions of any compensatory movements, e.g. shoulder elevation by the trapezius.

Pain-Free Function

This is the primary aim of the shoulder arthroplasty. Any joint, regardless of how damaged, will have improved function when it is painfree. This means that the rehabilitation needs to be carefully and patiently carried out in a confident subject. Active movements after shoulder arthroplasty does not involve the use of any athletic exercising of the shoulder but rather depends on more gradual techniques placing minimal forces on the prosthesis.

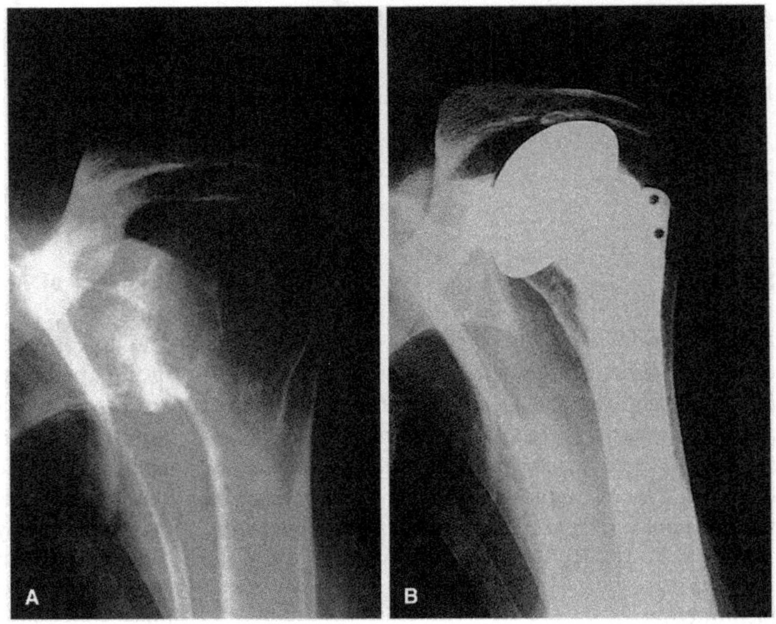

Fig. 1. Anatomical considerations. **A** Preoperatively: typical aspect of osteoarthritis with massive cuff-tear. **B** Postoperatively: the humeral component articulates with both the acromion and the glenoid and have a new fulcrum

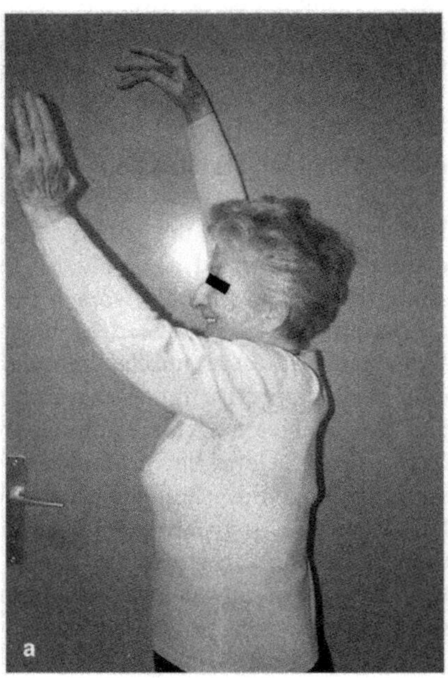

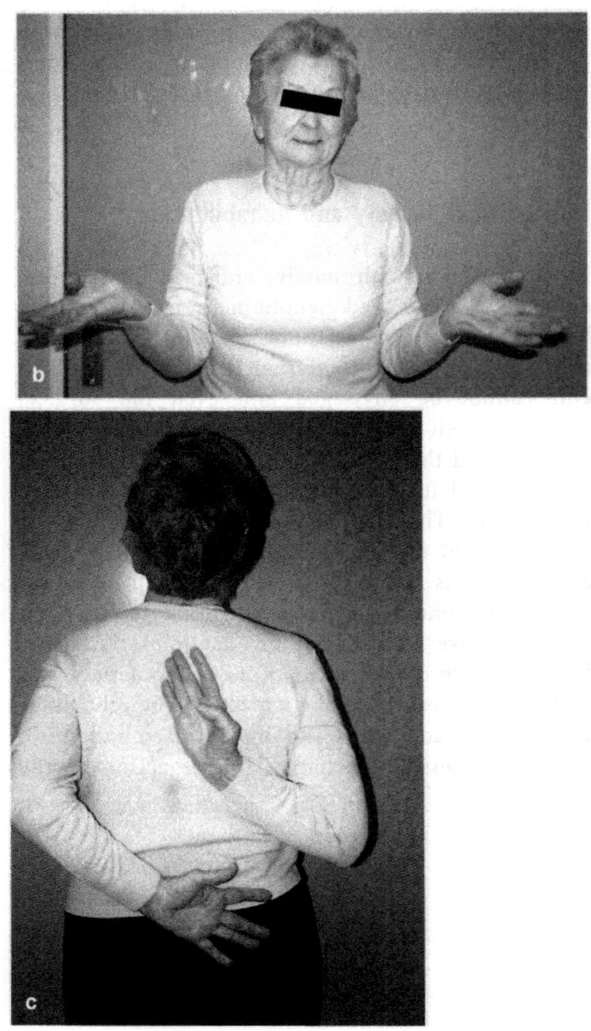

Fig. 2. Functional considerations. **a** Active painfree elevation above the horizontal. **b** Symetrical external rotation. **c** Internal rotation allows to reach the fifth lumbar vertebra (limited goal surgery and rehabilitation)

These techniques are oriented to 'reawaken' the muscles and to facilitate movement: repeated movements of the contra-lateral agonists, and eccentric rehabilitation. Different muscle strengthening exercises are also used: static isometric exercises, dynamic isotonic exercises, isokinetic muscle exercises at constant speed but with variable resistance.

This group of exercises should be carried out both concentrically (by bringing the two ends of the muscle towards each other) and eccentrically (lengthening the muscle) with the muscle tension less than the load. In daily practice, the progression is from concentric to eccentric exercise.

The functional rehabilitation should finally involve the simple movements of daily living (eating, washing and dressing), always ensuring maximal shoulder stability. They may be complemented by ergotherapy and psychotherapy.

Conclusion

Despite its poor reputation for this indication, shoulder arthroplasty can help improve pain relief and function in patients with osteoarthritis and massive cuff-tear. In some specific cases, where the humeral head has upward migrated but has find a new stability position, the functional result can be surprisingly good with active elevation above the horizontal and recovery of external and internal rotations (Fig. 1 and 2).

References

1. Brems JJ (1994) Rehabilitation following total shoulder arthoplasty. Clin Orthop 307:70–85
2. Cofield RH (1990) Degenerative and arthritic problems of the glenohumeral joint. In: Rockwood CA, Matsen FA (eds) The shoulder. Saunders, Philadelphia, pp 735–736
3. Craig EV (1986) Continuous passive motion in the rehabilitation of the surgically reconstructed shoulder: a preliminary report. Orthop Trans 10:219
4. Donatelli R (1987) Physical theraphy of the shoulder. Churchill Livingstone, New York
5. Hughes M, Neer CS II (1975) Gleno-humeral joint replacement and post-operative rehabilitation. Phys Ther 55:850–858
6. Kisner C, Colby LA (1990) Therapeutic exercise foundations and techniques, 2nd edn. Davis, Philadelphia, pp 241–270
7. Maybach A, Schlegel TF (1995) Shoulder rehabilitation for the arthritic glenohumeral joint: preoperative and postoperative considerations. Semin Arthroplasty 6:297–304
8. Neer CS (1990) Shoulder reconstruction. Saunders, Philadelphia, pp 487–530
9. Neer CS, McCann PD, Macfarlane EA, Padilla N (1987) Earlier passive motion following shoulder arthroplasty and rotator cuff repair: a prospective study. Orthop Trans 11:231
10. Mezzana M, Auvity J, Scheffer J (1992) Le centrage passif et actif du pivot huméral. L'Epaule et sa Rééducation, Expansion Scientifique Française, pp 40–48

Rehabilitation Following Shoulder Arthroplasty for Fracture

B. Caligaris-Cordero, F. Payeur, R. Sinnerton, and P. Boileau

Summary

Forty-three patients (46 shoulders) who underwent shoulder arthroplasty after fracture of the proximal humerus underwent rehabilitation and follow-up at a special reeducation center for an average of 3 months (1–6). The rehabilitation followed the protocol recommended by Neer (recovery of passive joint movements, muscular strengthening and stretching) to which were added hydrotherapy, physiotherapy and occupational therapy. The functional results, assessed after an average follow-up of 19 months, were disappointing with a normalised Constant score of only 60.2 %. There appeared to be two factors which explained these poor results. Firstly, the advanced age of the population (52 % older than 70) who was often poorly or non-motivated (22 %) and debilitated (21 % chronic alcoholics) and who had significant medical and neuro-psychiatric histories. Secondly, incompletely resolved anatomical and surgical problems: damage to the circumflex nerve (6.5 %), early migration of the greater tuberosity (6.5 %), secondary migration with malunion (15 %) and/or nonunion (11 %) of the greater tuberosity. These anatomical and surgical problems should be suspected clinically in patients who have an abnormally painful shoulder in the immediate postoperative period (16 cases in our series) and later if there is a dissociation between active anterior elevation (deficient) and passive anterior elevation (preserved) or if the range of active movement plateaus or regresses with time (24 % and 9 % of the patients in this series). The discrepancy between active and passive motion elevation suggests that limited motion is not caused by gleno-humeral scaring but instead by weakness of the deltoid (because of axillary lesion) and/or of the external rotators (because of greater tuberosity migration).

Introduction

Many authors, most of them surgeons, have reported their experience using arthroplasty to treat fresh fractures of the proximal humerus [6, 7, 10, 12–14, 16–18, 21, 23–25, 30, 32]. In the course of their work none of these authors have discussed the problems of rehabilitation after shoulder arthroplasty for fracture. Only Neer in his publications stresses the importance of rehabilitation and to the different stages this must involve in achieving a functional outcome [15, 22–24]. However, after shoulder arthroplasty, all the conditions combine to lead to shoulder stiffness: the anatomy of the proximal humerus has been completely altered; a haemarthrosis may be the start of intra-articular fibrosis, peri-articular haematoma may be the origin for adhesions at the level of the bursae; muscular bruising may be a source of contracture and finally capsular dehisences may be the onset of instability. The often disappointing clinical results bear witness to both the difficulties in surgical reconstruction around the prosthesis [1–3, 7, 9, 17, 26] and to the rehabilitation [4, 5, 10, 15, 19, 20].

Aware of the importance of shoulder rehabilitation after treatment for fracture, in obtaining a satisfactory functional result, we undertook a prospective study of 43 patients (46 shoulders) who had undergone this surgery and received rehabilitation at a specialist center. The goal of the study was to evaluate the importance, duration and problems posed by rehabilitation after arthroplasty for fracture using the stringent review available thanks to their receiving their treatment as inpatients.

Methods and Materials

Rehabilitation Principles

The functional rehabilitation used in our center (Centre Helio-Marin de Vallauris, France) follows the principles described by Neer to which we have added hydrotherapy, physiotherapy and occupational therapy [5, 10, 19, 20]. Neer's shoulder rehabilitation is a complete but flexible system based on a simple premise, which consists of three main phases [4, 15, 24].

Phase 1 is the essential, early recovery of the passive range of movements ("early passive motion"). This starts the day after surgery and continues once the patient is transferred to the center (1–2 weeks postoperative). A pain-free shoulder is achieved by immobilisation and physiotherapy. The shoulder is immobilised depending on the surgeons instructions and usually with the elbow at the side in internal or neutral rotation or, occasionally, in an abduction brace. The physiotherapy involves the application of heat at the start of each session, to loosen the muscles, and cold at the end of the session to reduce inflammatory reactions, as well as micro-wave treatments. We also carry out upper spinal massage. During this period antalgics, anti-inflammatories and muscle relaxants may be used. The recovery of joint movement comes only from the use of passive exercises which the patient must learn to do themselves and is encouraged to carry out many times a day. Passive mobilisation by the physiotherapist works on two essential movements: anterior elevation and external rotation. Anterior elevation of the arm is carried out with the patient lying on their back and aims to move the humeral head under the acromion with the palm of the hand towards the ceiling. External rotation is worked on in the same way but without going beyond 30°–40° – depending on the surgeons instructions. Internal rotation with the hand behind the back is not started in this first stage as there is a risk of damaging the fixation of the greater tuberosity. Auto-passive exercises are done using pendular movements with the patient lying on their front or leaning forward with the head on the opposite arm, and letting the operated arm fall. Anterior elevation of the operated arm can also be done using the healthy arm while lying on the back. The patient carries out a series of 10 successive movements repeating this up to 3 times in each session. Anterior elevation can also be worked at with the patient standing and sliding the hand horizontally across a smooth table-top. External rotation is worked on using a baton with the elbow held to the side with a strap or against a wall. Hydrotherapy is started once the scar has healed and using a float which allows passive exercises to be performed with the effects of gravity and pain eliminated. Occupational therapy using a pulley allows the patient to start practicing some of the functions of daily living.

Phase 2 consists of muscular recovery, initially isometrically. This stage starts once bony consolidation has been achieved which is at about 6 weeks. By this stage passive mobility should have been almost fully recovered. The recovery of muscular strength is achieved using three types of exercise:

- Stabilisation of the raised arm. The patient lies on their back stabilising the arm vertically; the physio applies multidirectional forces to the arm which the patient resists. This is a true proprioceptive exercise. The muscular reactivation is complete when the patient can fully control the descent of the operated arm.
- Eccentric exercises [19] consist of applying progressive tension to the rotator cuff. In practice, during passive mobilisation in anterior elevation, the supraspinatus is at rest. The patient stabilises the hand at the top of the movement and then controls the descent of the arm. This equates to applying an eccentric tension on the tendon and muscle of supraspinatus. Progressive increases in weight, speed and amplitude apply longitudinal tension on the tendon and thus have a trophic effect on the strength of muscular contraction. The same principles are used to work on internal and external rotation with the elbow at the side. Movements in pure abduction are not used as these increase subacromial impingement in the same way that antepulsion in internal rotation increases impingement with the coracoacromial ligament.
- Isometric exercises are carried out with the patient standing with their elbows at the side and against resistance for 5 seconds followed by a similar length rest period. This exercise is carried out using a baton or a towel for the rotators or against a hard surface for the deltoid and retropulsers. Dynamic exercises against resistance using elastic bands or a pulley, strengthen the shoulder depressors and the cuff muscles.

Hydrotherapy also allows work against the resistance from the water using a hand fin. Occupational therapy studies the patients professional movements and develops exercises to help recover these functions. When the patient has recovered sufficient strength, they start arm elevation in the scapular plane standing in front of a mirror and trying to avoid moving the shoulder before having lifted the hand and arm first.

Phase 3 consists of recovering the extremes of the passive range of movement by stretching. This starts once active work against resistance is allowed. Once the tuberosities have consolidated then passive stretching exercises become essential to recover the last few degrees of movement. They allow the tissues, and especially the joint capsule, to recover their elasticity. The patient caries out these exercises either alone or with the physio, for short periods repeated frequently (5 min, 5 times a day). Heat should always be applied before starting the exercises to prevent injury and ice at the end to limit inflammation. Passive stretching and muscular strengthening of infraspinatus allows the complete recovery of external rotation which is essential in gaining complete anterior elevation. This stage can also be started earlier in the swimming-pool. During the rehabilitation programme, we also work on proprioception of the operated shoulder using different diameters balls. Work on the deltoid can start from the 10th week, especially if their is damage to the circumflex nerve. The shoulder consists of 5 joints which, throughout this rehabilitation programme, are rehabilitated along with the gleno-humeral joint and with the same goal of obtaining near normal function.

The hydrostatic, muscle relaxing and sedative effects of water at 32° means that movements can be carried out in weightless conditions which limit the mechanical forces acting on the prosthesis. Water is used at all stages of the programme; as a support in carrying out passive movements (phase 1); as resistance in strengthening muscles of the cuff and deltoid (phase 2) and again as a support to help in stretching (phase 3). The physiotherapists use peripheral nerve stimulators for their antalgic effect, the motor stimulating effect of electricity helps to prevent amyotrophy and pulsed short-wave treatment for its antalgic and anti-inflammatory effects. Occupational therapy plays its part by analysing the exercises, coordinating the patients movements and allowing them to readapt to the activities of daily living. On leaving the center the patient must continue with rehabilitation for at least 6 months.

Patients

Between December 1990 and December 1994, 46 shoulder arthroplasties for fresh fractures of the proximal humerus underwent rehabilitation at the Centre Helio-Marin de Vallauris. This prospective series consisted of 43 patients (5 men and 38 women) with 3 having bilateral procedures. The dominant arm was fractured in 20 cases (43.5 %). At the time of surgery the average age was 68 (37–88). Figure 1 shows the significant percentage of patients aged greater than 70 years (52 %). There was a large female predominance at 88.4 % (ratio of 7.6 females to 1 male). The mechanism of injury was variable: 34 suffered an accidental fall, 4 were involved in street accidents, 3 had alcohol induced fits and 2 had direct blows. The average delay to surgery was 8 days: 34 were operated on in the first week, 4 between weeks one and two and 8 between the second and third weeks. The fracture type was determined from the radiographs and the operation note. They were classified using the Neer system [22, 23, 27, 28] resulting in 42 four-part fractures (of which 22 were fracture dislocations) and 4 three-part fractures. There were some associated injuries: 3 rib fractures, 2 pelvic fractures, 1 ipsilateral wrist fracture and 1 ankle fracture. Depending on their site and significance, these can slow up the rehabilitation programme.

The patients were referred from five different hospitals and were operated on by experienced surgeons. Three types of arthroplasty were used: the Global shoulder (Depuy) in 2 cases, the Modular shoulder (3 M) in 27 cases and the Aequalis (Tornier) in 17. The average period of functional rehabilitation was 3 months at the center (1–6). A majority of the patients presented with associated problems as detailed in Table 1. Of particular note are the number with psychiatric and/or chronic alcoholic problems. On their arrival at the center 27 patients (59 %) had large haematomas affecting the whole upper limb which in 10 cases extended onto the ipsilateral hemithorax. Sixteen patients (37 %) presented with abnormal and unusual pain in the operated shoulder which required analgesics and anti-inflammatories. These pains interfered with the smooth running of the programme and in 3 cases lead on to an algodystrophy. In 3 cases, circumflex nerve

Table 1. Medical problems associated

Medical problems	*n*	%
Cardiovascular	23	53
Diabetis (treated)	8	18
Phychiatric (treated)	13	30
Alcoholism	9	21
Neurological	5	11
Neoplasia	1	2

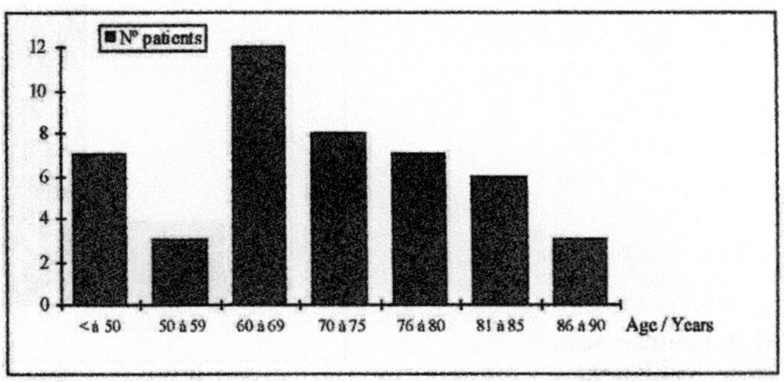

Fig. 1. Age of the patients at operation. Notice that about half of the patients were more than 70-year-old

damage was diagnosed and confirmed by postoperative EMG. This nerve injury resulted in a reduction in the range of anterior elevation of the upper limb due to damage to the control of deltoid. One superficial skin infection in the scar was reported and treated with the appropriate antibiotics. In this series there were no recorded deep infections of the joint or peri-articular tissues. One anterior dislocation occurred at 3 months postoperatively in a patient who had had bilateral surgery. There were no posterior dislocations.

During their stay at the center, 3 patients presented with early migration of the greater tuberosity. In one case, immobilisation was recommended which meant there was no rehabilitation during that period. In two cases, revision surgery was carried out, at 2 weeks and at 4 months, to reattach the tuberosity. Finally, several patients had medical complications during their stay which required transfer to Intensive Care Unit and thus their programmes were stopped: two cases of acute pulmonary oedema and one GI bleed.

We carried out a clinical and radiographic review of 40 patients. At follow-up we recorded 3 deaths (pancreatic cancer, neurological complications and acute alcohol poisoning). These 3 were included in the study because they had a minimum of 8 months follow-up. The average follow-up was 19 months (12–72). The clinical evaluation was made using the Constant score which covers pain, activity, mobility and strength [8]. This can be normalised for age and sex. All the patients were followed-up at the rehabilitation center and then seen in consultation for a clinical and radiographic evaluation. The radiographic study was made on AP views taken in neutral, internal and external rotation plus a scapular and an axillary view. These were mainly used to look for peri-articular ossifications using the Sneppen classification [28] and to assess the position and consolidation of the greater tuberosity. All the data underwent statistical analysis using Statview software (Abacacus Concept, USA).

Results

Constant Score. When evaluated using the Constant score, the functional result was excellent (a score greater than 100) in 4 cases (9.3 %), good (between 80 and 100) in 1 case (2.9 %), average (between 60 and 80) in 14 cases (32.6 %) and poor (greater than 60) in 24 cases (55.8 %). The normalised Constant score was 60.2 % on average (Fig. 2). Pain had a mean score at follow-up of 9.5 out of a possible 15.

In terms of *pain*, the shoulder was totally painfree (15/15) in 11 cases (26 %), almost painfree (10–14) in 17 cases (39 %). In 11 cases (26 %) pain limited the use of the upper limb (5–10) and the pain was incapacitating (<5) in 4 patients (9 %). We identified a group of 16 shoulders who, on arrival at the rehabilitation center, had immediate intense postoperative pain making rehabilitation difficult if not possible. The pain was present even at rest and responded poorly to analgesics and cryotherapy.

Active mobility had a mean score of 18.3 out of a potential 40. At the time of follow-up, active anterior elevation was 95°, although passively this reached 124°. Table 2 demonstrates this difference between active and passive mobility which was evident 3 months after shoulder arthroplasty.

Activity scored 12.7 points on average out of 20. Function was considered normal or good in 64 % of the patients, difficult in 16 % and possible only with help in 20 % (Table 3). Finally, the average force was 3.5 out of 25.

The subjective result was judged on the 40 patients questioned: 9 of these (22 %) were very satisfied, 15 (38 %) were satisfied and 16 patients (40 %) declared themselves disappointed with the intervention. The cooperation from the patients was arbitrarily judged as satisfactory, average or poor. For 25 shoulders (54 %) the patients cooperation was judged to be good, in 11 cases (24 %) it was average and in 10 cases (22 %) we were confronted with a poor level of cooperation often related to psychiatric or alcoholic problems.

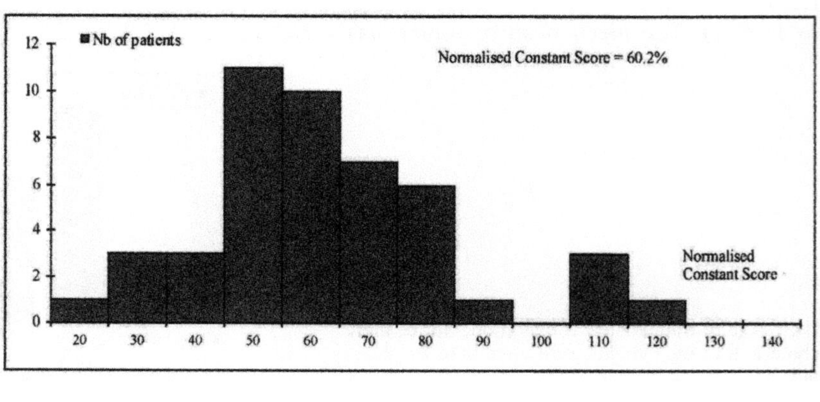

Fig. 2. Constant Score normalised for age and sex

Regarding the *progression of recovery,* we distinguished three groups of patients based on their results on leaving the Centre (30–90 days) and at follow-up (Fig. 3). In the first group of 8 shoulders the result remained stable (24 %), the second group of 23 shoulders showed an improvement in the functional state (67 %) and finally a third group of 3 shoulders had a functional regression (9 %).

The radiographic results were often disappointing with disappearance, malunion or nonunion of the greater tuberosity. In 7 cases the tuberosity was not seen on the standard AP radiographs (15 %) due to late migration. In 5 cases (11 %) there was nonunion of the greater tuberosity. Ossifications were looked for and classified using the Sneppen system [29]. In our series we only saw 5 cases with grade III (ossifications causing a true scapulo-humeral bridge). The patients who presented with these ossifications had suffered four-part fractures without dislocation and all came from the same hospital. We therefore believe that a technical operative problem was the origin of this complication. A failure of peri-operative lavage has been suggested as a possible cause [7].

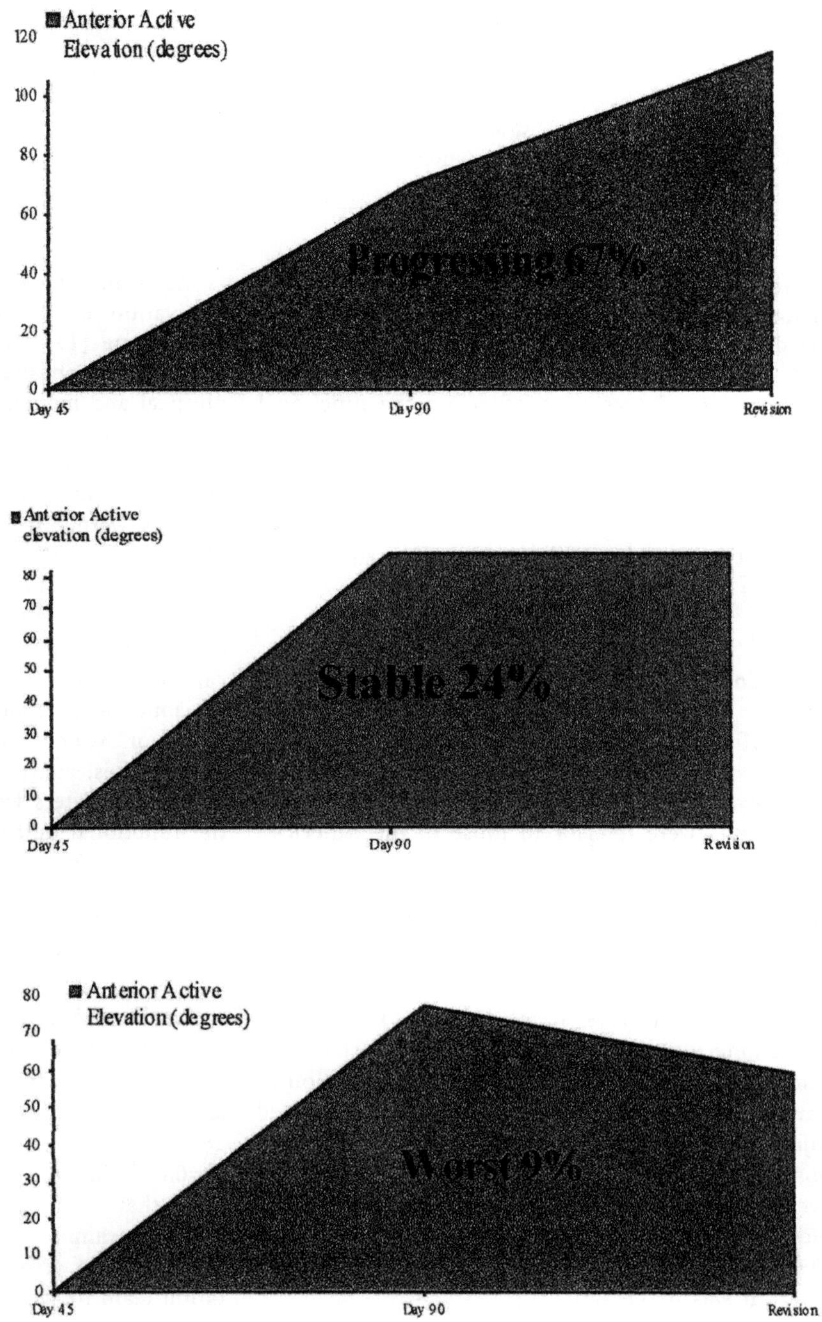

Fig. 3. Three groups of patients could be distinguished when considering evolution of anterior active elevation after 3 months

Table 2. Evolution of mobility (Na: Non available)

Mobility	Day 45	Day 90	Revision
Passive anterior elevation	108°±25° (40°–160°)	127°±32° (80°–180°)	123°±29° (60°–180°)
Active anterior elevation	Na	73°±30° (0°–150°)	96°±35° (10°–180°)
Passive external rotation	11.5°±9° (0°–40°)	19°±13° (0°–50°)	19.5°±12° (0°–50°)
Active external rotation	9°	Na	11°±10° (0°–30°)

Table 3. Functional results

Function	Normal or good	Difficult	Helped or impossible
Use the back pocket	43	0	0
Wash opposite underarm	38	4	1
Comb hair	14	11	18
Carry 4–6 kg arm at side	15	9	19
Use arm at the shoulder level	20	7	16
Use arm above shoulder level	9	8	26
Reach behind back, fasten brassiere	41	2	0
Eat with ustensil	40	3	0
Sleep on operate shoulder	26	8	8
Daily activities	26	13	4
Dress oneself	31	9	3

We looked for *correlations* between different parameters and the functional result as determined by the degree of anterior elevation at review. It seems that the following parameters have a deleterious effect, to one degree or another, on the functional outcome: a dislocation combined with the fracture ($p=0.05$), a preoperative delay of greater than 7 days ($p<0.01$), the presence of intense immediate postoperative pain ($p=0.05$), absence of the greater tuberosity on the follow-up AP radiographs ($p>0.01$) or tuberosity nonunion ($p<0.001$).

Discussion

It is difficult to make comparisons of our functional results with those in the literature because of the different evaluation methods used by different authors. Our results were inferior to those of the American series [7, 11, 13, 21, 23, 31] but comparable to those of the Europeans and Canadians [14, 16, 17, 25, 30]. The principle difference was in average active mobility, which, in our series, was 95° for active anterior elevation and 20° of external rotation whereas in Compito's series [7] for example, the active anterior elevation was 127° and external rotation greater than 30°. A stricter patient selection in particular with regard to the age and associated injuries, certainly explains, in part, the better results observed by Neer and his school [7, 22–24]. The average age in our series was 68 years (with 52% older than 70) and this was much lower with Neer [23] where the average was 56 years and for Compito where it was 62 [7].

Many authors have stressed the cooperation and motivation of the patient with the rehabilitation programme [13, 21, 23, 30, 31]. Hawkins [14] and Pietu [25] emphasised the importance of the general physical and mental state of the patients. The significant proportion of patients who had an on-going psychiatric problem often combined with chronic alcoholism must be noticed in our series. These patients were difficult to reeducate, depressed and often rebelled against all the rules and came into the poor result group. Similarly, there was often a significant history of medical problems (Table 1): several elderly patients in our series presented with cardiac pathologies, mental state deterioration, and, for some, a generally physically weak postoperative condition which slowed down and, in the most severe cases, contraindicated some of the exercises. Other parameters which had a deleterious effect on the functional outcome have already been reported and were seen in our series: an associated dislocation [21], a preoperative delay greater than 7 days [7, 17, 21, 23, 25] and, malunion or secondary displacement of the greater tuberosity [2, 7, 17, 21, 31].

We identified a group of 16 shoulders who, on their immediate postoperative arrival at the center, had abnormal, intense pain making the operated shoulder untouchable by the physiotherapist. These 16 shoulders came into the poor results in our series ($p=0.05$). This early clinical sign seems important to us in that it will delay or slow down the rehabilitation programme. The appearance of a hyperalgic shoulder after arthroplasty should alert the rehabilitation team to search for anatomical problems: mal-

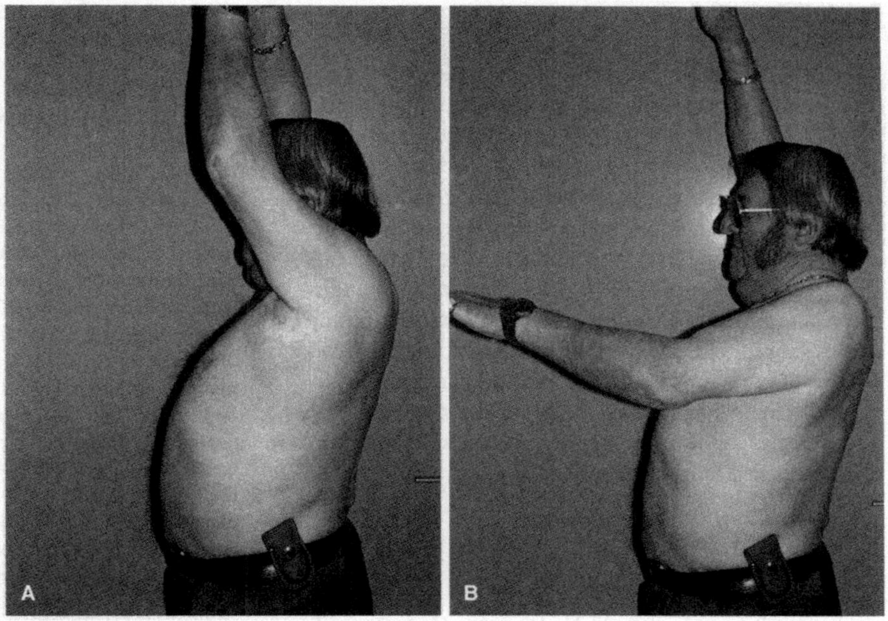

Fig. 4. Example of patients who has complete passive elevation (**A**) and limited active elevation (**B**) after shoulder arthroplasty for fracture. Complete passive motion is the proof that there is no scarring tissue. Limited active motion is related to muscular weakness (often because of GT migration)

union or migration of the tuberosities and, in particular, the greater tuberosity.

We were interested to find that in some patients there was a dissociation between passive and active anterior elevation. The regularly repeated daily exercises allowed the passive range of movement to recover quickly even when the active range remained difficult to achieve. This active/passive dissociation seems to be due to damage to the circumflex nerve (3 cases, 6.5 %) and to anatomical problems such as primary or secondary malunion of the tuberosities, especially the greater tuberosity (15 %). This damage was due either to direct trauma from displacement of the bony fragments, from attempts at reducing a dislocation or occurred during the procedure, as shown by Compito in his study [7]. Some authors state that the nerve always recovers [7, 17] while others suggest that recovery is only partial [13]. The three nerve injuries that we followed for at least 1 year did not recover and ended up in the poor outcome group in this series. Often unrecognised due to the difficulties of the initial examination in a trauma case, the frequency of neurological lesions and their effect on the functional outcome means that they must be systematically looked for as they are undoubtedly underestimated. [7, 13].

Several authors [7, 21, 23, 30] assessed their results after 2 years and stressed the importance of continuing rehabilitation for at least 1 year. This supposition was not found in our series where everything that was going to be recovered had been recovered by 6 months and often by 3 months (Table 2). Review at 6 months and 1 year seems to be long enough, as with Green [13] and Hawkins [14], to judge the functional result. Function can improve after 1 year, but not significantly as shown in our results, and for some the result can regress. In fact with regard to the progression we distinguished three groups of patients (Fig. 4); for 24 % the functional outcome achieved when they left the center remained static, for 67 % there was progression from 6 months to 1 year and finally for 9 % the outcome, already poor when they left the center, regressed between then and follow-up. This rule of *"all or nothing by 3 months"*, as well as the different progression profiles, are new concepts which have not previously been reported in the literature.

Again, a plateauing or regression in the range of movement with time, should alert the rehabilitation team or the surgeon to look for complications related to the greater tuberosity. Nonunion of the greater tuberosity (11 %) and/or primary or secondary malunion (15 %) were the most common cause of a poor functional result. All authors [13, 14, 16, 17, 25] have reported a significant percentage of secondary tuberosity migration, occurring particularly with early rehabilitation [7, 31]. We believe it is the surgeons who hold the answer by ensuring that they carry out a solid fixation of the tuberosities both to the prosthesis and to the humeral shaft. However, we [1–3] have stressed the difficulties in positioning of the prosthesis with regards to height and retroversion because of the loss of the normal humeral anatomical landmarks. We have shown in particular that a tuberosity fixation which appears to be perfect but carried out on an approximately positioned prosthesis, can lead to secondary migration of the greater tuberosity and a poor functional result.

Conclusion

Rehabilitation after shoulder arthroplasty for fracture remains difficult and disappointing. Despite rehabilitation following Neer's protocol with the addition of hydrotherapy and, in particular, despite strict supervision of the patients in a rehabilitation center for an average of 3 months, we did not achieve the same level of results as many American authors. There appear to be two factors to explain these disappointing results: a different patient population (more elderly and with significant medical and psychiatric problems) and anatomical and surgical problems which have not been fully resolved (the frequency of circumflex nerve injury and malunion, migration and nonunion of the greater tuberosity).

References

1. Boileau P, Chau E, Perraud M, Arcamone H, Argenson C (1992) Restoration of humeral offset and humeral length after hemiarthroplasty for displaced 4- part fractures of the proximal humerus. Presented at the 5th International Conference on Surgery of the Shoulder, Paris
2. Boileau P, Huten D (1995) Technique chirurgicale des prothèses de Neer pour fractures céphalo-tubérositaires. Rev Chir Orthop 81 [Suppl II]:85–88
3. Boileau P, Walch G (1996) La prothèse d'épaule dans les fractures à 4 fragments: problèmes et solutions. Maîtrise Orthopédique 6:18–23
4. Brems JJ (1994) Rehabilitation following total shoulder artroplasty. Clin Orthop 307:70–85
5. Caligaris-Cordero B, Boileau P (1993) Rééducation de l'épaule après prothèses pour fracture-luxation à 4 fragments: intérêt du séjour en centre de rééducation. In: Bonnel F, Blotman F, Mansat M (eds) L'Épaule. Springer, Berlin Heidelberg New York, pp 554–560
6. Cofield RH (1988) Comminuted fractures of the proximal humerus. Clin Orthop 230:49–57
7. Compito CA, Self EB, Bigliani LU (1994) Arthroplasty and acute Shoulder trauma: reasons for success and failure. Clin Orthop 307:27–36
8. Constant CR, Murley AHG (1987) A Clinical Method of functional assessment of the shoulder. Clin Orthop 214:160–164
9. Craig EV (1989) Prosthetic replacement for four-part fractures of the proximal humerus. Technique Orthop 3:70–80
10. Demblans-Deschans B, Heuleu JN (1988) Rééducation de l'épaule pré et post-chirurgicale. Cahier d'enseignement de la SOFCOT no. 33, Expansion Scientifique Française, Paris, p145
11. Dines DM, Waren RF (1994) Modular shoulder arthroplasty for acute fractures. Clin Orthop 307:18–26
12. Frich LH, Söjberg JO, Sneppen O (1991) Shoulder arthroplasty in complexe acute and chronic proximal humerus fractures. Orthopaedics 14:949–954
13. Green A, Lloyd B, Richard S, Limbird MD, Providence RI (1993) Humeral head replacement for acute, four-part proximal humerus fractures. J Shoulder Elbow Surg 2:249–254
14. Hawkins RJ Switlyk P (1993) Acute prosthetic replacement for severe fractures of the proximal humerus. Clin Orthop 289:156–160
15. Hughes M, Neer CS (1975) Gleno-humeral joint replacement and post-operative rehabilitation. Phys Ther 55:850–858
16. Huten D, Duparc J (1986) L'arthroplastie prothétique dans les traumatismes complexes récents et anciens de l'épaule. Rev Chir Orthop 72:517–529
17. Huten D, Candelier G, Fleure P (1995) La prothèse de Neer dans les fractures récentes complexes de l'extremité supérieure de l'humérus. Rev Chir Orthop 81 [Suppl II]:75–83
18. Kraulis J, Hunter G (1977) The results of prosthetics replacement in fractures dislocations of the upper end of the humerus. Injury 8:129–131
19. Liotard JP, Expert JM, Mercanton G, Padey A (1995) Rééducation de l'épaule. Enc. Med Chir., Kinésithérapie et Rééducation Fonctionnelle, 26210 A10. Editions Techniques, Paris, p 23
20. Mezzana M, Auvity J, Scheffer J (1992) Le centrage passif et actif du pivot huméral. L'Epaule et sa Rééducation, Expansion Scientifique Française, pp 40–48
21. Moeckel BH, Dines DM, Warren RF, Altchek DW (1992) Modular hemiarthroplasty for fractures of the proximal humerus. J Bone Joint Surg Am 74 884–889
22. Neer CS (1970) Displaced proximal humerus fractures. I. Classification and evaluation. J Bone Joint Surg Am 52:1077–1089
23. Neer CS (1970) Displaced proximal humerus fractures. II. Treatment of three-part and four-part displacement. J Bone Joint Surg Am 52:1090–1103
24. Neer CS (1990) Shoulder rehabilitation. In: Shoulder reconstruction. Saunders, Philadelphia, pp 487–534
25. Pietu G, Deluzarchers P, Goiun F, Letenneur J (1992) Traumatismes complexes de l'extrémité supérieure de l'humérus traités par prothèse céphalique. A propos de 21 cas revus avec un recul moyen de 4 ans. Acta Orthop Belgica 58:159–169
26. Rietveld ABM, Daanen, HAM, Rezing, PM, Obermann WR (1988) The lever arm in gleno-humeral abduction after hemi-arthroplasty. J Bone Joint Surg Br 70:561–565
27. Siebenrock, Gerber C (1993) The reproducibility of classification fractures of the proximal end of the humerus. J Bone Joint Surg Am 75:1751–1755
28. Sidor ML, Zuckerman JD (1993) The Neer classification system for proximal humerus fractures. J Bone Joint Surg Am 75:1745–1750
29. Sneppen O, Kjaersgaard-Andersen P, Frich LH (1990) Ectopic ossification after total shoulder arthroplasty. A study on 75 Neer total shoulder replacements. In: Post M, Morrey BF, Hawkins RJ (eds) Surgery of the shoulder. Mosby-Year Book, St. Louis, pp 298–301
30. Stableforth PG (1984) Four part fractures of the neck of the humerus. J Bone Joint Surg Br 66:104–108
31. Tanner MW, Cofield RH (1983) Prosthetic arthroplasty for fractures and fracture-dislocations of the proximal humerus. Clin Orthop 179:116–128
32. Walch G, Boileau P (1994) Morphological study of the humeral proximal epiphysis. J Bone Joint Surg Br 74 [Suppl I]14
33. Willems WJ, Lim TEA (1985) Neer arthroplasty for humeral fracture. Acta Orthop Scand 56:394–395

Section XIV:

Complications and Revision

Intra- and Postoperative Complications of Shoulder Arthroplasty

H. Mestdagh, P. Boileau, and G. Walch

Summary

This article addresses the recognition, etiology, treatment and prevention of complications of total shoulder arthroplasty observed in the Aequalis multicenter study. Ten intraoperative humeral fractures were observed: three fractures occurred in the greater tuberosity and seven spiroid fractures occured in the diaphysis and were related to forceful external rotation during exposure of the humeral head. Two late postoperative fractures occurred and were secondary to trauma. Locoregional complications include three hematoma, three deep infections and ten nerve injuries. Anterior instability (five cases) was either traumatic (two cases) or atraumatic (three cases), following previous surgery and was typically associated with disruption of the anterior shoulder repair in all cases. Revision surgery for repair of the subscapularis was performed with simple sutures in three cases but necessitated a pectoralis major transfer in one case and a bone-quadriceps tendon graft in one case. Posterior instability occurred early on three occasions and was related to insufficient correction of excessive glenoid wear with plastic deformation and incompetence of the posterior capsule. Anterosuperior instability occurred in three cases and was related to superior cuff rupture or deltoid loss. Glenoid loosening required revision in four cases. No humeral loosening occurred with the cemented components while eleven humeral loosening and subsidence were observed with the twenty press-fitted components. A glenoid erosion occurred in two cases of hemiarthroplasty, a dissociation of the polyethylene from the metal tray in one case and a persistent stiff shoulder in one case.

Introduction

Complications occurring during total shoulder arthroplasty are not as uncommon as it was thought initially [9, 26, 32, 35, 46]. Unfortunately, little information is available on the recognition or treatment of these complications and most of the information available has been provided by the compilation substantive series [15, 32, 36, 40, 43, 38, 47].

Although the present series has a short follow-up, it has the advantage of representing a multicenter studies with a great number of shoulder replacements performed by different shoulder surgeons using the same unconstrained implant. For this reason, the complications reported here represent the complications that each surgeon can encounter in his daily practice (Table 1).

Intra- and postoperative complications of shoulder arthroplasty are reported here and discussed in all etiologies except for the specific complications in acute fractures cases which are discussed separately (see Chap. 33 and 36).

Table 1. Complications of shoulder arthroplasty

Complications	Number	(%)
Intraoperative perioprosthetic fractures Greater tuberosity = 3 Humeral diaphysis = 7	10	2.5
Late traumatic periprosthetic fractures	2	0.5
Haematoma	3	0.7
Infection	3	0.7
Nerve injuries lower root <C8 = 2 (inter scalene block) axillary = 2 musculocutaneous = 3 axillary + musculocut. = 1 radial = 1 median = 1	10	2.5
Instability anterior = 5 posterior = 3 anterosuperior = 3	11	2.7
Radiological Glenoid Loosening (cemented)	20	10.5
Glenoid loosening revised (cemented)	4	2.1
Loosening and subsidence of uncemented Humeral component	11	55
Glenoid erosion (after hemiarthroplasty)	2	1.3
Polyethylene dissociation from metal-back	1	0.2
Stiff shoulder revised	1	0.2

Intraoperative Periprosthetic Fractures

No glenoid fracture was reported but there were ten intraoperative humeral fractures (2.5 %) which were the only intraoperative complication observed. Three greater tuberosity and seven diaphysis fractures occurred in six total and four hemiarthroplasties in patients with a mean age of 68.5 years (65 to 74). The indications for those procedures were osteoathritis (3 cases), rheumatoid arthritis (1 case), arthritis with massive cuff tear (1 case), sequelae of fractures (4 cases: one of which had avascular necrosis of the head) and one fresh fracture. One of the patients had undergone previous radiotherapy for breast cancer.

Intraoperative Fractures of the Greater Tuberosity

There were three epiphyseal fractures which involved the greater tuberosity; one of which occurred during reaming, one during introduction of the inclination guide and one during impaction of the prosthesis (Fig. 1). There was no correlation with the approach used, as this was a deltopectoral in all the cases, nor with the inclination angle, as the necks used where 125° or 130°. In contrast, the head sizes used where rather large: 39/14 in one, 43/16 in one, 46/17 in two and 48/18 in four. Their treatment consisted of reattaching the tuberosity with sutures (2 cases) or with screws (1 case). The functional results were all poor with failure of the fixation in two cases. In the third, the poor result was attributed to loosening of the glenoid component which had to be revised.

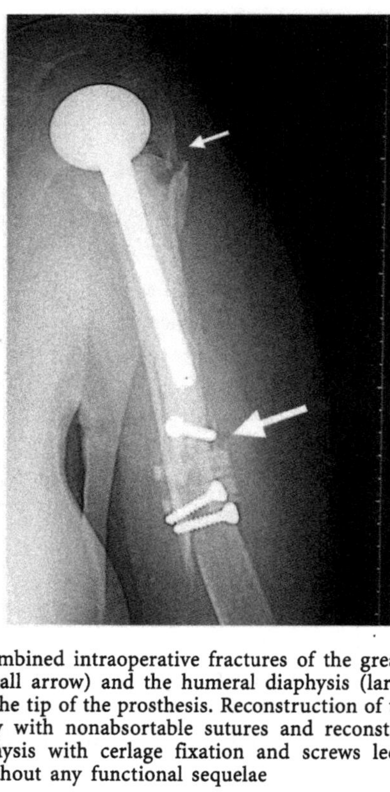

Fig. 1. Combined intraoperative fractures of the greater tuberosity (small arrow) and the humeral diaphysis (large arrow), distal to the tip of the prosthesis. Reconstruction of the greater tuberosity with nonabsortable sutures and reconstruction of the diaphysis with cerlage fixation and screws led to bone union without any functional sequelae

Intraoperative Fractures of the Humeral Diaphysis

There were seven spiral fractures which occurred in the middle third, or junction of the middle and distal thirds. One had a concurrent radial nerve palsy which resolved at follow-up. These fractures occurred during surgical exposure: in five cases while pushing the arm into external rotation, in one case while cementing the humeral component and in the final case the fracture went unnoticed during the operation and was only spotted on the postoperative radiograph by the presence of cement on the medial surface of the humerus. There were no recorded cortical perforations by instruments and the use of oversized stems cannot be held to blame except in the one case where the only size 12 mm stem used was cemented in causing a fracture. However, there did seem to be an overall tendency to use the larger head sizes; 39/14 in one case, 43/16 in two and 48/18 in 4 cases.

Apart from in the undetected fracture, several methods of internal fixation were used at the same time as the arthroplasty (Fig. 1); screw fixation (1 case), circlage wiring plus screws (2 cases) and plate fixation (3 cases). A long stemmed prosthesis was not used to achieve fixation. The results were disparate and could not be correlated with the complexity of the fracture or the type of fixation used because, of the three plate fixations, there was one excellent, one good and one poor result. Similarly for the use of screws, with or without circlage wiring, where there was one excellent, one good result and one failure. The fractures which went unnoticed had a good outcome with a preoperative absolute Constant score of 32 points increasing to 62 points at follow-up.

Overall, the occurrence of a fracture complicating the implantation of the prosthesis and requiring complimentary surgery to fix it, had a prejudicial effect on the final result; especially when the fixation has to be carried out in poor quality bone. In three cases, the Constant score dropped from 15 points preoperatively to 9 points after surgery. The fractures seemed to have little effect on the stability of the humeral implant in that we found no loosening of the components. We did, though, find 3 glenoid lucent lines in the 6 total shoulder replacements.

Intraoperative fractures make-up 20% of the complications in shoulder arthroplasty and have an incidence of 3% [7, 12, 32, 47]. All authors agree that their usual cause is an error in technique. The implicated maneuvers are forced movements in rotation while exposing the head and, especially, the glenoid; reaming with too much force and forced impaction of an oversized component. Wirth and Rockwood add to this list making a false passage in the humerus when the point of entry of the rasp is not aligned with the humeral canal [47]. The use of an uncemented, press-fit humeral component does seem to increase the risk of fracture [47]. Finally, in revision arthroplasties, the significant thinning of the cortical bone increases the risk of fracture.

The treatment for such fractures varies and remains controversial in the literature [7, 11, 23, 32, 47]. Bonutti and Hawkins recommend fixation with a plate and bone graft followed by 6 weeks of immobilization as, in their view, nonoperative treatment carries too great a risk of nonunion [7]. Boyd et al. [11] hold the same attitude for fractures occurring secondarily to hemiarthroplasty. Conversely, Groh et al. achieved fracture consolidation in their 8 cases by using simple circlage wiring [23]. Norris [39] as well as Miller and Bigliani [32] and Wirth and Rockwood [47] prefer to use a long-stemmed cemented prosthesis which confers immediate stability to the fracture and allows rapid rehabilitation.

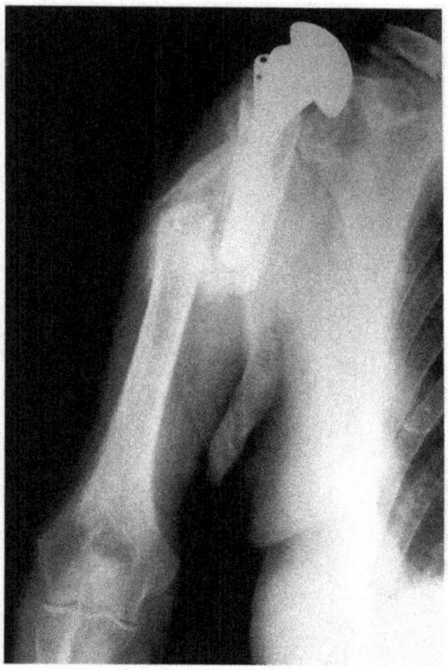

Fig. 2. Late posttraumatic fracture of the humerus distal to the tip of the prosthesis. Nonoperative treatment was decided because of the poor general condition of the patient. Despite bone union, functional result was poor

Late Periprosthetic Traumatic Humeral Fractures

Two patients presented with late traumatic humeral fractures following total shoulder arthroplasty. The first patient sustained a transversal diaphyseal fracture, distal to the tip of the prosthesis when falling down, 3 months after a shoulder replacement for fracture sequelae. A nonoperative treatment was decided, because of the poor general condition of the patient. The fracture healed in 8 weeks, despite an important displacement of the bony fragment but the functional result was poor (Fig. 2). The second patient also felt down and sustained a spiroid fracture, distal to the tip of the stem prosthesis, 3 years after a shoulder replacement for a rheuma-

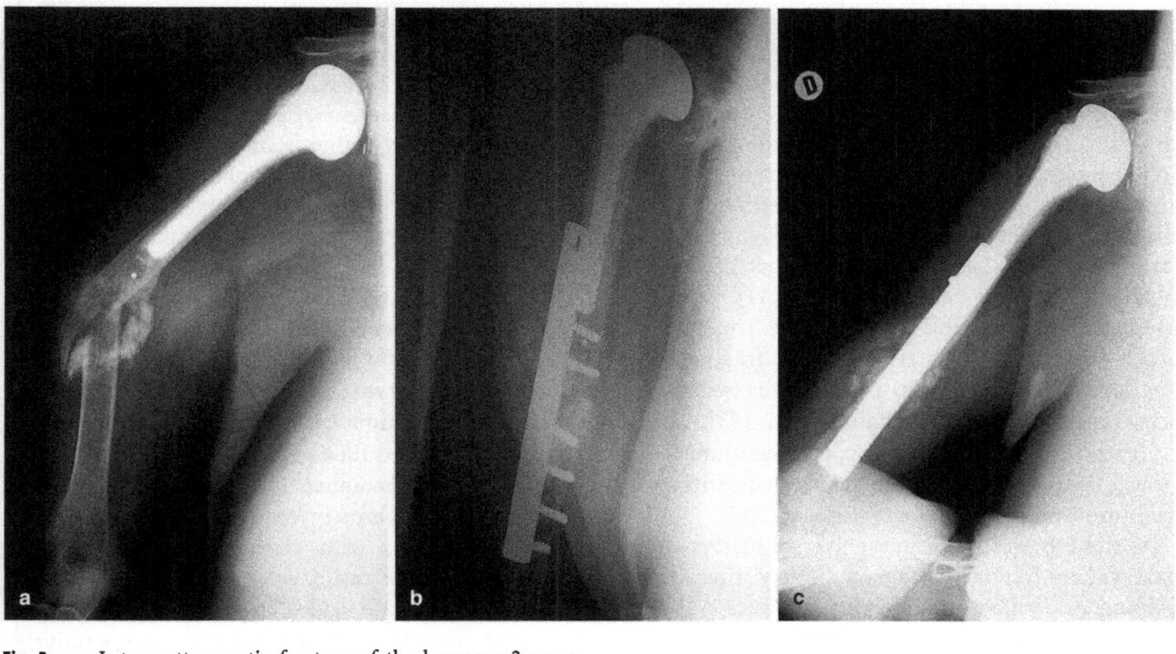

Fig. 3 a–e. Late posttraumatic fracture of the humerus 2 years after shoulder arthroplasty. **a** Initial nonoperative treatment led to nonunion. **b,c** Union was obtained with an AO plate and an autologous bone graft

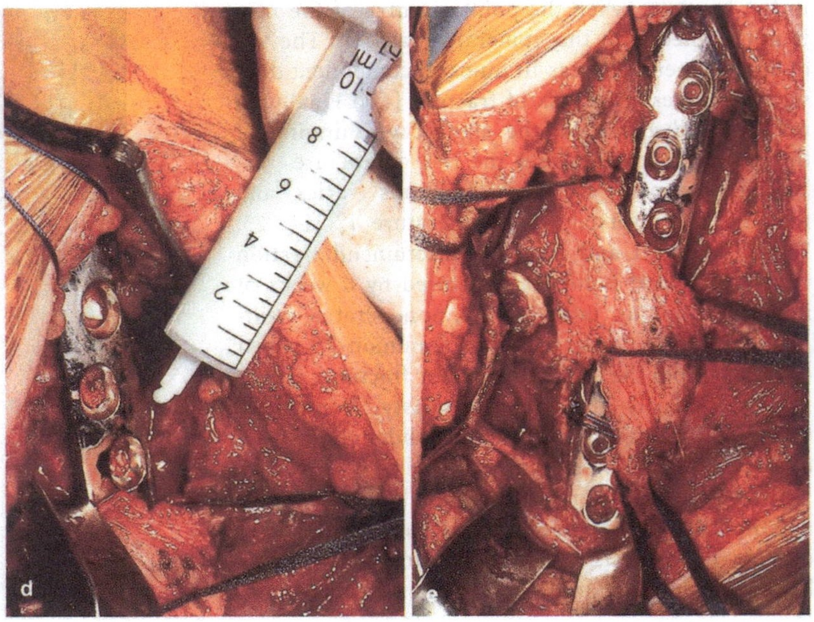

Fig. 3 a–e. (continued) d Intraoperative views show that cement was injected to enhance the screw fixation in the osteoporotic bone. **e** The radial nerve was carefully dissected and protected during all the procedure

toid arthritis. An attempt at treating nonoperatively the patient in another institution with a hanging cast led to a humeral nonunion. The patient was then refered to our institution where we internally fixed the fracture with an AO plate after humeral decortication. Cement was injected in the distal screw holes, because of the osteoporotic quality of the bone (Fig. 3).

The goals of the management of postoperative fractures adjacent to humeral prosthesis should be to obtain union of the fracture but also to preserve glenohumeral motion and shoulder function. Boyd et al. found that immobilization alone was unsatisfactory in most of the patients: they felt that the humeral implant presence may alter the mechanical forces present at the mid-shaft fracture site and this alteration may lead to an increased rate of nonunion [11]. These authors as well as Bonutti and Hawkins believe that the fractures that are treated operatively have a better result [7, 11]. However, Groh et al. recommend nonoperative treatment of such a fracture in their report on 12 fractures that were treated with a brace, isometric exercises, and early range of motion rehabilitation [23]. All of the fractures had progressed to osseous union after 9 weeks and functional results remained satisfactory with an average forward elevation of 120°.

On the basis of our experience, we believe that a conservative treatment should be try first before deciding operative treatment because of the advanced age of many of the patients and the good results classically observed with nonoperative treatment of humeral fractures. However, in case of nonunion after 8 weeks because of severe osteopenia, osteosynthesis and bone grafting should be promptly decided. A long-stem prosthesis is not logical and is overaggressive when the shoulder arthroplasty was functional before the fracture. The treatment of choice, for us, is plating with bone graft after careful dissection and protection of the radial nerve (Fig. 3).

Hematoma

Three hematomas were reported, none of which required surgical evacuation. The first hematoma occurred after insertion of a hemiarthroplasty for avascular necrosis of the humeral head. The concomitant, transient, musculocutaneous nerve paralysis demonstrated the potential effects of an extensive approach and intraoperative manipulations. The functional result here was acceptable with a preoperative Constant score of 39 points (43 % normalized) increasing to 78 points (86 %) after surgery. The second hematoma occurred during revision of a hemiarthroplasty initially implanted for osteoarthritis. The operation was difficult, requiring a humeral osteotomy and iliac graft, and resulted also in a transient musculocutaneous nerve palsy. Nonunion of the greater tuberosity required further intervention at 6 months with circlage wiring and bone grafting. The final result was poor with a Constant score of 9 points (13 %) preoperatively which increased to only 35 points (50 %) postoperatively. The third hematoma case happened after a total arthroplasty in a 72-year-old presenting with a cuff tear arthritis (senile hemorrhagic shoulder). Again the result was poor with a Constant score preoperatively of 14 points (20%) increasing to 45 points (65%) after surgery.

Overall, in our short series, the occurrence of a hematoma caused a disappointing objective result even though the patients were satisfied. The causes of hematoma on shoulder arthroplasty may be related to an extensive dissection. We now systematically ligate the anterior axillary vessels before cutting the inferior part of the subscapularis.

Infection

Three serious infections required reoperation after total shoulder replacement. The first infection appeared early, at 15 days postsurgery, in a 77-year-old male with osteoarthritis. The prosthesis had to be removed after 6 months, which allowed the infection to settle but resulted in a hanging shoulder. The second infection appeared late and presented with a fistula 15 months after surgery on a 63-year-old patient with a chronic posterior dislocation. The prosthesis was removed which allowed the infection to settle and the fistula to heal. The objective result was poor and the Constant score, which had been 31 points (37%) before the intervention, was only 22 points (27%). However the patient was happy because he could do his gardening. In the third case, the prosthesis was also removed due to late infection in a patient who had already undergone two operations to fix a proximal humeral fracture. The infection manifested itself at 18 months with the appearance of a fistula. Two attempts were made to débride the tract but both failed and finally the humeral prosthesis, which was not loose, had to be removed. The patient was left with a resection arthroplasty and the functional result was acceptable.

Although deep infection associated with shoulder arthroplasty is uncommon (0.5% in the literature, 0.7% in our series), surgical management remains difficult. Removal arthroplasty remains one option in failures of infected shoulder arthroplasty with osteomyelitis [42]. However, this dogmatic attitude should be questioned in light of the revision techniques now employed in infection of hip and knee prostheses [8, 14, 30, 31]. The indications are determined by the time of appearance of the sepsis and the potential for surgery which is as dependent on the anesthetic status of the patient as much as the stability of the implant, the nature of the bacteria and their antibiotic sensitivities. An early postoperative fistula is an indication for débridement, irrigation and systemic antibiotic therapy. Where the infection is with a gram-positive bacteria, "nonglycocalyx producing," then the prosthesis may be conserved if it is not loose. However, an early infection with a gram-negative bacteria, and deep wound late presenting infection, require excision of the infected tissues and removal of the prosthesis and all the cement. After a minimum of 6 weeks of antibiotic therapy, Petersen and Hawkins [40] along with Wirth and Rock-

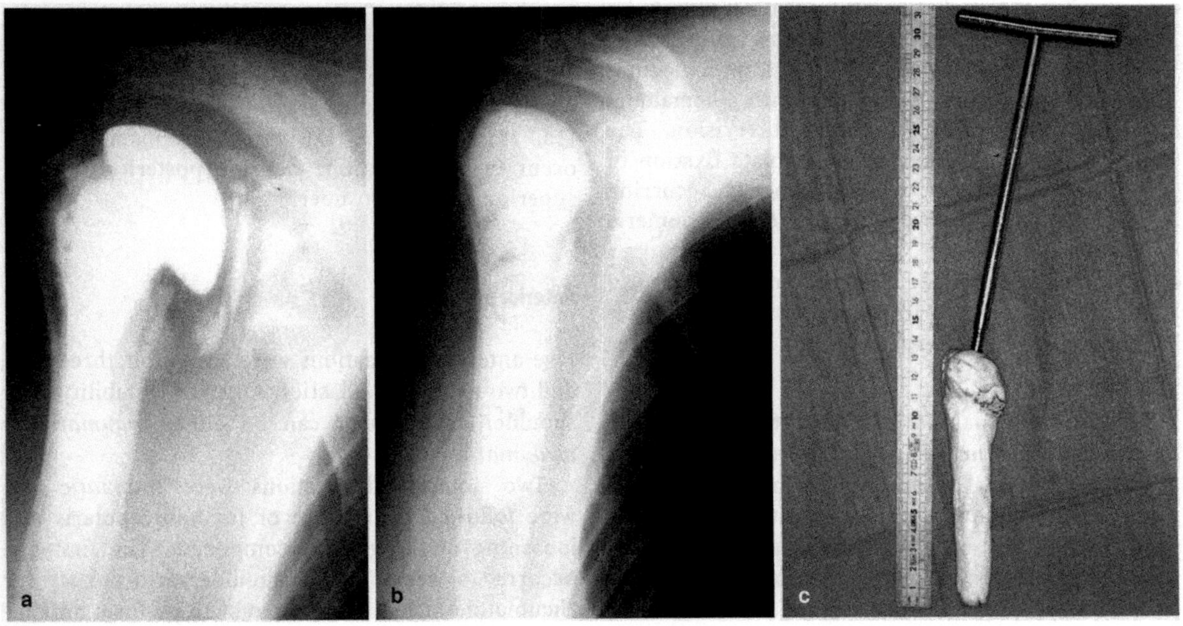

Fig. 4. a Infection after shoulder arthroplasty with humeral and glenoid loosening. **b** A spacer with cement and antibiotics was put in place to maintain the joint space and to distill antibiotics locally. **c** The antibiotic-cement spacer was removed after three months, allowing for implantation of a new shoulder arthroplasty (courtesy of Dr. Molé)

wood [47], suggest that a prosthesis can be reimplanted, providing that the deep infection has been completely irradicated and that there is sufficient bone-stock. Revision arthroplasty may be carried out after insertion of a molded, antibiotic impregnated, cement spacer (Fig. 4). The antibiotic-cement spacer has the advantages of providing local impregnation of antibiotics and to preserve the joint space and humeral length, making revision and reimplantation of the prosthesis more easy.

Nerve Injuries

Apart from a traumatic paralysis of C8 which occurred at the same time as a fracture dislocation of the shoulder which required an arthroplasty, we recorded ten postoperative neurological deficits; lower root involvement in 2 cases and trunk involvement in 8. The axillary (2 cases), musculocutaneous (3 cases), axillary plus musculocutaneous (one case), radial (one case) and median nerves (one case) were involved. These palsies occurred during arthroplasties for osteoarthritis in 3 cases, rheumatoid arthritis in 3 cases, avascular necrosis of the humeral head in 2 cases, traumatic malunion with head necrosis in one case and revision of an arthroplasty for fracture in one case.

Various causes have been implicated:

- *Anesthetic*: Two interscalene blocks resulted in inferior root palsies of C8.
- *Extensive approach or intraoperative manipulation:* an axillary palsy was seen after synovectomy in a rheumatoid patient. Of the 3 musculocutaneous nerve palsies, 2 coexisted with a hematoma and 1 occurred after a difficult revision. The radial palsy was associated with plate fixation of a diaphysis fracture of the humerus occurring during exposure of a malunion of the humeral epiphysis.
- *Extrinsic:* a carpal tunnel syndrome secondary to the arthroplasty and to postoperative immobilization seemed to be responsible for a median nerve palsy.

Seven of the palsies recovered totally with no recurrence. However, the three nonresolving palsies prejudiced the final result because the average Constant score increased from 39 points (50%) preoperatively to only 46 points (65%) after surgery.

All authors mention the particular vulnerability of the axillary and musculocutaneous nerves. In a review of the literature, Silliman and Hawkins estimate the incidence of axillary nerve damage as being from 0.7% to 2% and higher in rheumatoid patients [43]. Cofield mentions that intraoperative manipulations and an extensive approach are particularly dangerous when the tissues are fragile, as in rheumatoid arthritis, and when the anatomical landmarks are altered by trauma or previous anterior surgery [15]. As emphasized by Lynch, in most cases, the presumed mechanism of injury is a traction on the plexus occurring during the operation but fortunately, the prognosis for neurological recovery is good in most cases [29].

Several recommendations may be made from our short series:

- Perform a precise, preoperative, neurological examination to detect any minor deficit unconnected with the surgery but which might be aggravated by it.
- Find and protect the axillary nerve during extensive exposures or revisions at the beginning and the end of the procedure.
- Avoid prolonged or energetic retraction on the conjoint tendon which may damage the musculocutaneous nerve.
- Avoid traction associated with retropulsion on the arm during exposure of the glenoid and use an arm support (see Chap. 15).
- Be wary of ulnar nerve compression caused by the abduction arm holder.

Prosthetic Instability

Owing to the enormous functional range of motion of the joint and its dependence on soft tissues for both stability and motion, prosthetic instability is one of the most frequent cause of complication associated with prosthetic arthroplasty of the shoulder [15, 22, 32, 36, 43, 47]. Prosthetic instability can occur in any direction: anterior, posterior, inferior, superior and anterosuperior.

Anterior Instability

Five anterior dislocations were seen after three total and two hemiarthroplasties. Anterior instability after shoulder replacement can be either *traumatic* or *atraumatic.*

Two anterior dislocations were *traumatic* and were followed by rupture of the subscapularis and loosening of the glenoid component. The first one occurred 6 weeks after a shoulder arthroplasty for rheumatoid arthritis. An attempt to perform an axillary radiograph led to anterior dislocation of the prosthesis with rupture of the subscapularis and dissociation of the polyethylene from the metal tray. A first revision allowed to change the glenoid component and to suture the subscapularis tendon. However, because of the poor quality of the tissue, healing of the tendon failed and a transfer of the pectoralis major on the lesser tuberosity was performed. While the initial functional result was excellent with a complete active elevation, the final result was poor with active elevation at the horizontal level. The second case was due to a fall which occurred 2 years after a total arthroplasty for osteoarthritis which had given an excellent result (Fig. 5). The radiographs showed a distal migration of the humeral component which was initially uncemented and a dislocation and loosening of the glenoid component. An arthrography revealed a rupture of the subscapularis. Both prosthetic components were changed and cemented while the subscapularis tendon was sutured. The final result was satisfactory with a Constant score increasing from 24 points (34 %) preoperatively to 74 points (>100 %) after surgery.

Three anterior dislocations were *atraumatic* and presented between 6 weeks and several months after arthroplasty secondary to previous surgery: a Bristow procedure for recurrent dislocation (two cases) and internal fixation of a 4-part fracture followed by failure of fixation (one case). During arthroplasty, the two patients operated on for instability presented with full thickness tears of supraspinatus. One of the humeral components was retroverted by more than 30°. One patient was operated on at 2 months to repair subscapularis and then at 7 months with a quadriceps graft after failure of that repair. Although he was content with the result, the Constant score was disappointing, increasing from 15 points (21 %) preoperatively to 50 points (71 %) postoperatively. Despite failure of an attempted closed reduction the other patient did not undergo revision. Although he was happy with the outcome, the prosthesis remained subluxed anteriorly with a Constant score improved from 14 points (20 %) preoperatively to 38 points (54 %) after the intervention. In the patient with a fracture of the proximal humerus operated on by a prosthesis after the fixation had failed at 4 months postoperation, the prosthetic head was insufficiently retroverted and the subscapularis was completely torn. The dislocation occurred after several weeks but could not be reduced by closed means and has not been reoperated on. Although the patient is happy and does not want any further surgery, the Constant score is poor, reaching only 24 points (34 %).

In the literature, Neer [35], in a series of 194 cases, reported 2 anterior dislocations occurring 3 weeks after surgery which were reduced closed and 2 anterior subluxations reoperated on because of excessive anteversion of the humeral component. Moeckel [33] reported 10 cases of anterior instability which were reoperated on 9 occasions for subscapularis rupture. Three out of four of the failures with recurrent dislocation required reconstruction using an Achilles tendon graft. Finally, Wirth and Rockwood [47] reported 3 cases of anterior instability with insufficient retroversion of the humeral component, rupture of subscapularis and erosion of the anterior part of the glenoid in one.

Our short series allows us to confirm the frequent association of subscapularis rupture with anterior

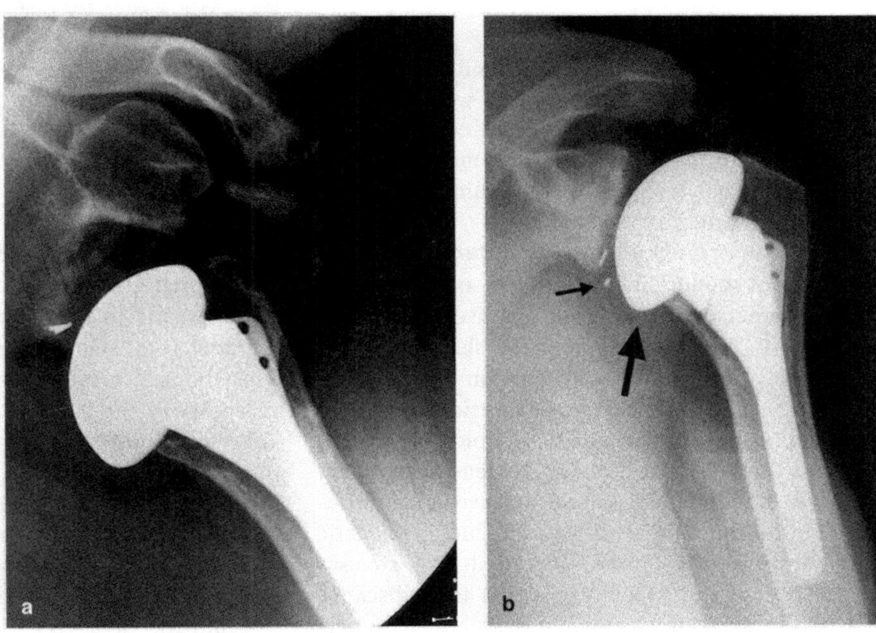

Fig. 5 a–f. a Posttraumatic anterior instability secondary to a fall 2 years after shoulder arthroplasty. **b** After closed reduction, the radiograph demonstrates the glenoid loosening and migration (small arrow) as well as the subsidence of the humeral component, initially non cemented (large arrow). Besides this, a rupture of the subscapularis tendon was found intra-spectively

Fig. 5 a–f. (continued) c Revision surgery was performed to cement new glenoid and humeral components and to repair the subscapularis. **d–f** Excellent functional result after revision

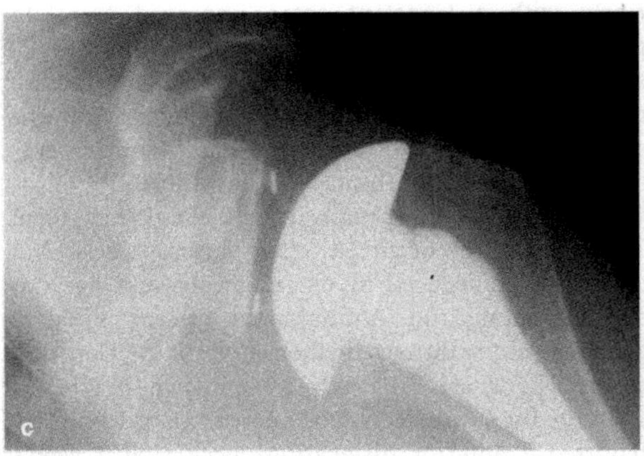

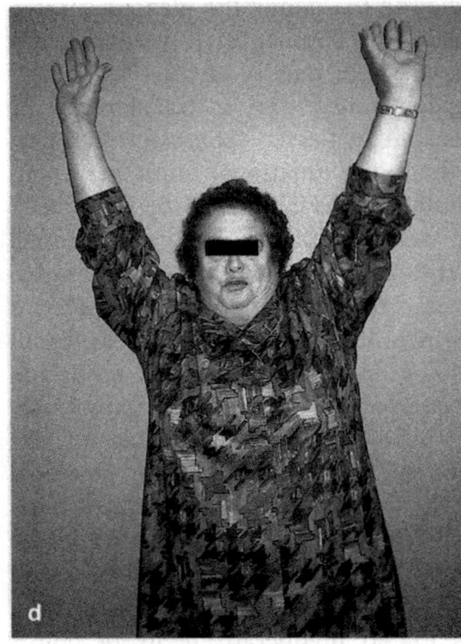

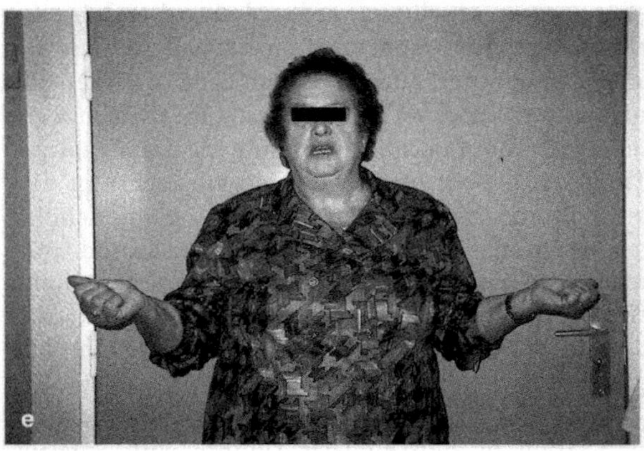

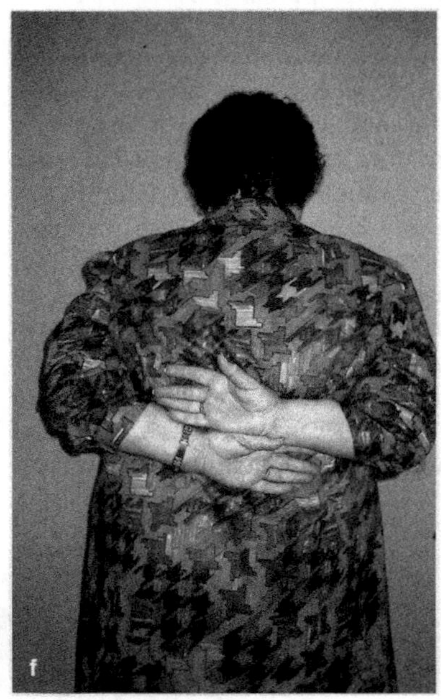

dislocation (four out of five cases) and the prejudicial effect of primary interventions which weaken subscapularis (two cases). Disruption of the subscapularis may be a cause (in atraumatic anterior instability) or a consequence (in traumatic anterior instability) of anterior instability.

Prevention of disruption of the sutured subscapularis tendon should include correct orientation of the prosthetic component, avoid the use of oversized components. Nonabsorbable sutures should be used for suturing the tendon to the tendon and the tendon to the bone. One should be particularly aware when using the metal backed glenoid component which is thicker than the polyethylene component and need more glenoid reaming to avoid lateralization of the joint line. A large and thick prosthetic head may also overtension the joint and stresses the suture line and repair process in the subscapularis. If the anterior tissues are atrophic, it is perhaps better to detach the subscapularis close from the bicipital groove with a peace of bone of the lesser tuberosity to reinforce the tendon. Furthermore, operations to stabilize recurrent anterior dislocations did not prevent the reappearance of anterior instability of the prosthesis.

Revision surgery for repair of the ruptured subscapularis tendon is challenging [15, 33, 36, 47]. The technique depends on the age of the disruption and on the quality of the tendon which is always poor in case of previous operations with an anterior approach (Bankart, Putti-Platt, or Bistow-Latarjet procedures). In a recent tear of the subscapularis with a good quality tendon, a direct repair with tendon to tendon suture is possible. However, in an ancient misdiagnosed subscapularis tear and/or scarred tendon because of previous operations, one should anticipate to perform a muscular or tendon graft. We have used both pectoralis major transfer or bone-tendon graft using the quadriceps tendon with a piece of patella. Otherwise any malposition of the humeral implant must be looked for, especially after arthroplasty for fracture. Finally, anterior instability is often associated with glenoid loosening as demonstrated by our series and reoperation for anterior instability should anticipate change of the glenoid component.

Posterior Instability

Posterior dislocations occurred on three occasions, following shoulder arthroplasty for fracture malunion, rheumatoid arthritis and osteoarthritis (Fig. 6). They all occurred early, with one happening during surgery in a hyperlax patient, one during the anesthetic recovery period and the third early postoperatively in a patient with a massive cuff tear. Two patients presented with posterior glenoid wear which lead to a malpositioning of the glenoid component and the surgeons regretted not carrying out a glenoid graft at the time of operation. The third patient had a stretched tear of the rotator cuff. None of the patients underwent further surgery: the hyperlax patient was immobilized in a simple sling and the two others were reduced closed and immobilized in a neutral rotation splint for 3 weeks. However, one of these recurred. At follow-up, only one shoulder presented with an incomplete and nonprogressive lucent line around the glenoid component. Ultimately, two of the three patients were disappointed with the result. The Constant scores increased respectively from 18 points (26 %) and 22 points (31 %) preoperatively to 31 points (57 %) and 27 points (38 %) after surgery. Only the patient whose posterior dislocation was successfully reduced saw their score increase from 29 points (32 %) preoperatively to 63 points (70 %) after surgery.

A review of the literature allowed Wirth and Rockwood to collect 21 cases of posterior instability after total shoulder replacement [47]. Their seven personal cases, as with the four reported by Moeckel et al. [33], were due to excessive retroversion of the humeral component beyond 45° (5 cases); to excessive retroversion of the glenoid due to posterior wear in 5 cases; to an anteroposterior soft-tissue imbalance (one case); and to a greater tuberosity nonunion (one case). Contrary to Barrett, they recommend revision to reduce the humeral retroversion, reorientate the glenoid by using a graft or rereaming and to balance the soft-tissues by a posterior capsulorraphy at the same time [2].

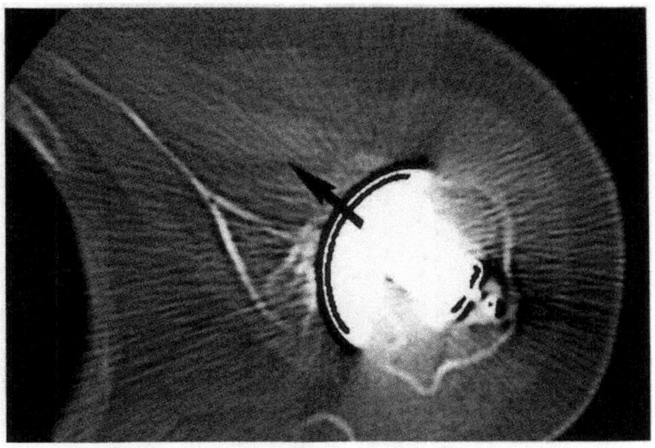

Fig. 6. Posterior instability after shoulder arthroplasty as demonstrated by CT scan. The two main reasons are uncorrected posterior wear of the glenoid surface and uncorrected plastic deformation of the posterior capsule

On the basis of our experience, we believe that the main reason for prosthetic posterior instability is a failure to recognize both the substantial posterior erosion of the glenoid surface and the important plastic deformation of the posterior capsule often associated [12, 34]. This may lead to placement of the glenoid component in excessive retroversion at the time of the operation and a posterior capsular pouch persistence. For this reason, we recommend to always perform a CT scan arthrogram or an MRI to evaluate both posterior glenoid erosion and the posterior capsular laxity. Prevention of posterior instability should include both a correct reorientation of the glenoid surface by anterior reaming to address the asymmetrical bone wear and a posterior capsulorraphy (through the anterior approach) to address the asymmetrical soft-tissue abnormality [15, 34, 43]. One of us (G. W.) has developed a technique of posterior capsulorraply using absorbable sutures passing through the subscapularis in case of large posterior capsular pouch (Fig. 7).

Superior Instability

Superior migration of the humeral head over time is a frequent complication reported in the literature and is usually secondary more to attenuation of the supraspinatus than to a frank rupture of the rotator cuff [28, 38, 47]. Boyd et al. reported 23 % of superior migration in 128 Neer shoulder arthroplasties at an average of 44 months follow-up [10]. The amount of proximal humeral migration was independent of the size of the rotator cuff defect but was positively associated with a torn rotator cuff.

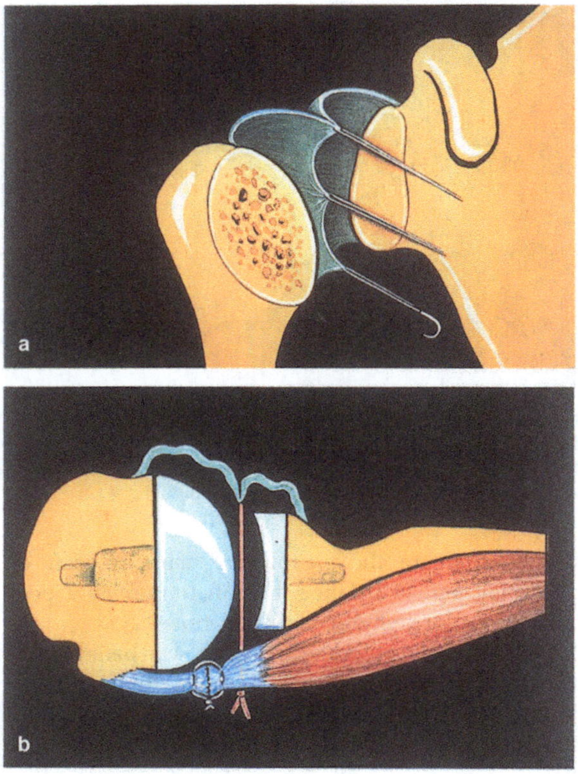

Fig. 7. Walch's technique of posterior capsulorraphy associated with shoulder arthroplasty in case of intra-operative posterior instability. **a** Two large absorbable sutures (no. 5) are passed in the posterior capsular pouch before inserting the definitive prosthesis. **b** The absorbable sutures are passed through the subscapularis before suturing the tendon. The sutures are tied at the end of the operation with the arm in external rotation and will resorbe in 6 weeks

However, postoperative results were good in most of the patients and no increase in pain was observed. Sneppen et al. reported 55% of proximal migration in 51 shoulder replacement in rheumatoid arthritis with a mean follow-up of 92 months [44]. Again, the presence of proximal humeral migration did not significantly influence the average results, neither pain relief, range of motion, abduction force, nor function. Superior migration is commonly associated with patients suffering form rheumatoid arthritis and has been attributed by Kelly to persistence of the disease in the tendons [28]. However, progressive superior migration may lead to potential loosening of the glenoid component as a result of eccentric load on the superior portion of the glenoid component [1, 22].

While we did observed proximal migrations of the humeral component in our previous experience with the Neer prosthesis, we did not observe such superior progressive migrations of the humeral component in the Aequalis series [4]. We believe that, although our follow-up is short, the absence of proximal humeral migration is related to the use of a prosthesis which respects the individual anatomy of each humerus. Precise placement of the prosthetic head allows restoration of the center of rotation and avoids overtensioning of the superior cuff [5, 27].

Anterosuperior Instability

At least three patients presented with an anterosuperior instability in the present series and were always associated with a poor functional result (Fig. 8). Anterosuperior instability is not rare in rheumatoid patients (9% for Hawkins [43]) and can be seen on two circumstances: (a) in patients with thin cuff or massive irreparable rotator cuff tear where a concomitant aggressive decompressive acromioplasty with disruption of the coracoacromial arch was performed and the humeral and/or glenoid prosthetic components were oversized [38]; (b) in patients with loss of the deltoid after shoulder arthroplasty [24]. Prevention should include careful humeral head and glenoid component selection, repair of the rotator cuff, preservation of the coracoacromial arch and of the deltoid because revision is rarely successful.

Inferior Instability

This complication was not observed in our series. Inferior instability after shoulder arthroplasty is less common and is usually observed after treatment of acute fractures of the proximal humerus with severe shortening of the humerus [15, 36, 47]. However, to be diagnosed shortening of the humerus must be severe because it is often compensated by shortening of the deltoid fibbers allowing the prosthesis to face the glenoid. Therefore, we believe that the consequence of shortening of the humerus is not inferior instability but deltoid weakness with poor active elevation.

Glenoid Loosening

Radiological glenoid loosening, with lucent lines superior to one millimetre was observed in 10.8% of the cases. Four cemented loose glenoids were revised. These were painful loosenings and appeared in one case after a traumatic anterior dislocation (Fig. 5). The loosenings occurred after prostheses implanted for osteoarthritis (3 cases) and for fracture malunion with persistent dislocation of the humeral head (1 case). Two glenoid loosenings presented

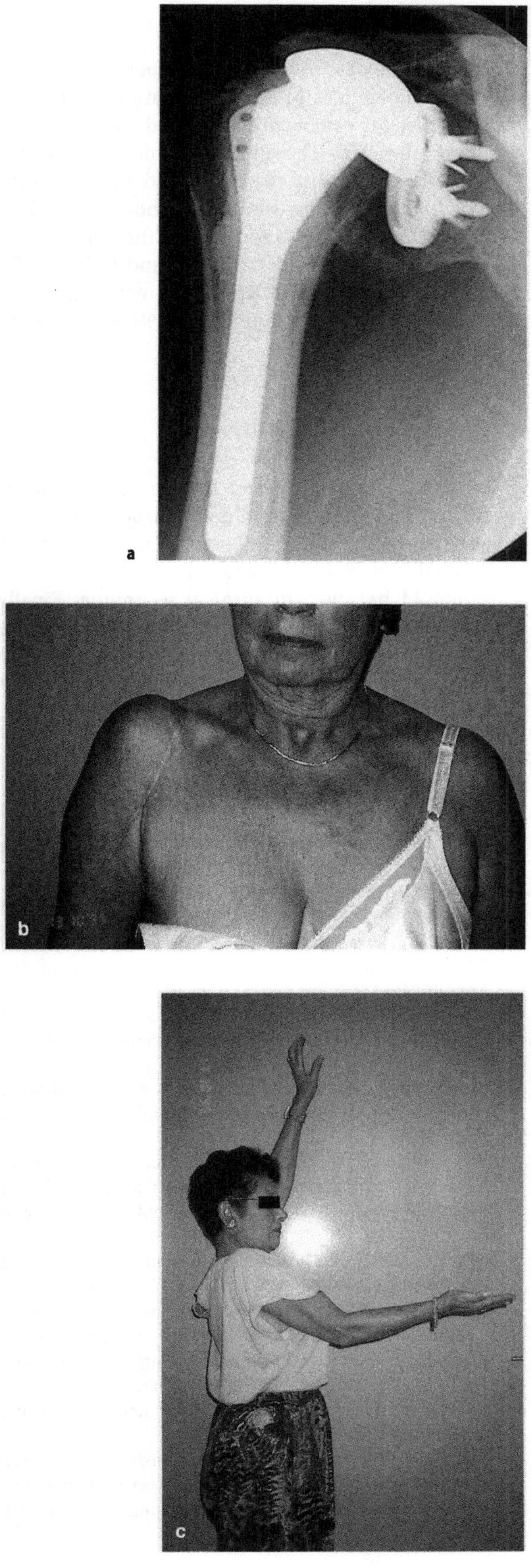

with a rupture of supraspinatus but only one of these have been repaired at the same time as the arthroplasty. The loosenings occurred after a period of 6 weeks and 8 years postoperation. Two presented acutely, one after a traumatic anterior dislocation and the two other for no apparent reason. The glenoids used were of the small size in 3 cases and of the medium size in the other. In the case with the dislocation, the components were recemented and subscapularis repaired. In the other cases, one of which had an irreducible anterior subluxation of the humeral head, the glenoid and cement were simply removed.

Symptomatic glenoid loosening represented one-third of the complications after total shoulder arthroplasty recorded with an incidence of loosening from between 2.6% and 7.8% [6, 15, 22, 26, 32, 43, 47]. The average incidence in the nonrheumatoid population was calculated as 3.5% [43] but was much higher in the rheumatoid patients. This, however, was a very low level in comparison to the high number of lucent lines around the glenoid which varied between 30% [35] and 74% [2] and up to 83% [28] in the rheumatoid patients. The outcome of a lucent line however remains uncertain and the use of uncemented glenoids is seen as the answer by some [16, 17] while others advise a hemiarthroplasty [9]. Torchia and Cofield, analyzing the results of 89 total shoulder arthroplasties with a long follow-up, observed 84% of radiolucent lines and 44% of definitive loosening at an average of 12 years (range, 5–17 years) [45]. They clearly demonstrated that radiographic loosening were increasing with time and that there was an association between radiographic loosening of the glenoid implant and pain.

To prevent glenoid loosening, we optimize the bone-component congruency by using concentric motorized reaming instead of hand burring [18], we use pressurized cement [37] we undersize the slot for the keel and compact the cancellous bone, we favor a mismatch between the humeral and glenoid articular surfaces to decrease loading of the rim and protect the fixation of the glenoid component [25]. Finally, to enhance fixation and durability of the glenoid implant we have introduced a new *uncemented* glenoid design. If revision is needed, change and recementing of the glenoid component has proved to give better results than simple removal of the glenoid component [6, 15, 43, 47].

Fig. 8. Anterosuperior instability after shoulder arthroplasty in a rheumatoid patient is demonstrated radiographically (**a**) and clinically (**b**). The reasons are cuff tear or altenuation, disruption of the coracoacromial arch and/or deltoid loss leading to poor functional result (**c**)

Loosening and Subsidence of uncemented, press-fitted humeral components

Although radiographic evaluation showed some incomplete radiolucent lines around some of the cemented humeral components, no humeral loosening was observed in the cemented humeral prosthesis. By contrast, humeral loosening and subsidence was observed in eleven cases of uncemented, press-fitted components out of 20 cases (55%). Three of them were distally migrated and had to be reoperated to cement the humeral component because of pain and less of active elevation.

Based on our experience, we strongly recommend cement fixation of the Aequalis humeral component and to never use it in a press-fitted manner. The stem is short (105 mm) and has no rough surface to allow biologie fixation. This is concordant with the observations of Cofield who found about 50% of loosening with the uncemented press-fitted Neer humeral components and suggested that surgeons should not continue to use press-fitted humeral components for total shoulder arthroplasty.

Complications Related to the Implants

No complications occurred with the humeral component in our series, contrary to the literature where disassembly of modular humeral prosthesis have been reported [3, 19]. One dissociation of the polyethylene insert from the glenoid metal tray occurred during closed reduction of a traumatic, anterior dislocation 6 weeks after a total shoulder arthroplasty for rheumatoid arthritis. Putting the insert back and repairing subscapularis failed and, finally, a new glenoid was cemented in place and a Pectoralis Major transfer to the lesser tuberosity performed. The final result was satisfactory with the preoperative Constant score of 12 points (17%) increasing to 60 points (85%) after surgery.

In the literature, Burkhead [13], Cofield and Daly [16], Driessnack et al. [20], reported identical cases occurring after anterior dislocation attributed to subscapularis insufficiency. We did not come across any other technical problem such as fracture of the metal tray, the keel or the glenoid fixation screws.

Glenoid Erosion After Hemiarthroplasty

Secondary glenoid erosion were reported in two patients with osteoarthritis treated by a hemiarthroplasty whose pain began immediately after surgery. A glenoid component was inserted with a good result.

Stiff Shoulder

There was one case of marked postoperative stiffness with a complete loss of external rotation after hemiarthroplasty for osteoarthritis carried out by a deltopectoral approach. The appearance of an early rupture of the tendon of the long head of biceps and its combination with a significant shoulder stiffness required surgical revision to release the periarticular adherences, elongate subscapularis and tenodese the biceps tendon. The result was worse, with a Constant score dropping from 44 points (47%) to 39 points (42%) after the revision.

Conclusion

This report stresses the fact that the complications occurring during total shoulder arthroplasty are frequent even early in the following and that some of them could be avoidable suggesting that more attention should be given to surgical technique. Finally, one should remember that the number of complications will probably still increase with longer follow-up. This emphasizes the need to continue to prospectively follow our patients.

References

1. Arntz CT, Jackins S, Matsen FA III (1993) Prosthetic replacement of the shoulder for the treatment of defects in the rotator cuff and the surface of the glenohumeral joint. J Bone Joint Surg Am 75:485–491
2. Barrett WP, Franklin JL, Jackins SE, Wyss CR, Matsen FA III (1987) Total shoulder arthroplasty. J Bone Joint Surg Am 69: 865–872
3. Blevins FT, Deng X, Torzilli PA, Warren RF (1995) Dissociation of modular shoulder arthroplasty components Orthop Trans 18:977
4. Boileau P, Walch G, Liotard JP, Noel E (1994) Neer shoulder prosthesis: results related to the etiology. Rev Rhum 61:539–547
5. Boileau P, Walch G (1997) The three-dimensional geometry of the proximal humerus. Implications for surgical technique and prosthetic design. J Bone Joint Surg Br 79:857–865
6. Brems JJ (1993) The glenoid component in total shoulder arthroplasty J Shoulder Elbow Surg 2 (1):47–54
7. Bonutti PM, Hawkins RJ (1992) Fracture of the humeral shaft associated with total replacement arthroplasty of the shoulder. A case report. J Bone Joint Surg Am 74:617–618
8. Booth RE Jr, Lotke PA (1989) The results of spacer block techique in revision of infected total knee arthroplasty. Clin Orthop 248:57–60
9. Boyd AD Jr, Thomas WH, Scott RD, Sledge CB, Thornhill TS (1990) Total shoulder arthroplasty versus hemiarthroplasty. Indications for glenoid resurfacing. J Arthroplasty 5:329–336

10. Boyd AD Jr, Aliabadi P, Thornhill TS (1991) Postoperative proximal migration in total shoulder arthroplasty. Incidence and significance. J Arthroplasty 6:31–37
11. Boyd AD Jr, Thornhill TS, Barnes CL (1992) Fracture adjacent to humeral prosthesis. J Bone Joint Surg Am 74:1498–1504
12. Brewer BJ, Wubben RC, Carrera GF (1986) Excessive retroversion of the glenoid cavity. A cause of non traumatic posterior instability of the shoulder. J Bone Joint Surg Am 68:724–731
13. Burkhead WZ (1994) Cementless shoulder arthroplasty In: Friedman RJ (ed) Arthroplasty of the shoulder. Thieme, St. Louis, pp 242–253
14. Burger RR, Basch T, Hopson CN (1991) Implant salvage in infected total knee arthroplasty. Clin Orthop 273:105–112
15. Cofield RH, Edgerton BC (1990) Total shoulder arthroplasty. Complications and revision surgery instruction. Course Lect 39:449–462
16. Cofield RH, Daly PS (1992) Total shoulder arthroplasty with a tissue ingrowth glenoid component. J Shoulder Elbow Surg 1:77–85
17. Cofield RH (1994) Uncemented total shoulder arthroplasty. Clin Orthop 307:86–93
18. Collins D, Tencer A, Sidles J, Matsen FA III (1992) Edge displacement and deformation of glenoid components in response to eccentric loading. The effect of preparation of the glenoid bone. J Bone Joint Surg Am 74:501–507
19. Cooper RA, Brems JJ (1991) Recurrent disassembly of a modular humeral prosthesis. A case report. J Arthroplasty 6:375–377
20. Driessnack RP, Ferlic DC, Wiedel JD (1990) Disassociation of the glenoid component in the Macnab/English total shoulder arthroplasty. J Arthroplasty 5:15–18
21. Faludi DD, Weiland AJ (1983) Cementless total shoulder arthroplasty: preliminary experience with thirteen cases. Orthopedics 6:428–438
22. Franklin JL, Barrett WP, Jackins SE, Matsen FA III (1988) Glenoid loosening in total shoulder arthroplasty. Association with rotator cuff deficiency. J Arthroplasty 3:39–46
23. Groh GI, Heckmann MM, Curtis RJ, Rockwood CA Jr (1994) Treatment of fractures adjacent to humeral prosthesis. Orthop Trans 18:1072
24. Groh GI, Simoni M, Rolla P, Rockwood CA Jr (1994) Loss of the deltoid after shoulder operations: an operative disaster. J Shoulder Elbow Surg 3:243–253
25. Harryman DT, Sidles JA, Harris SL, Lippitt SB, Matsen FA III (1995) The effect of articular conformity and the size of the humeral head component on laxity and motion after glenohumeral artroplasty. A study in cadavera. J Bone Joint Surg Am 77:555–563
26. Hawkins RJ, Bell RH, Jallay B (1989) Total shoulder arthroplasty. Clin Orthop 242:188–194
27. Iannotti JP, Gabriel JP, Schneck SL, Evans BG, Misra S (1992) The normal glenohumeral relationships. An anatomical study of one hundred and forty shoulders. J Bone Joint Surg Am 74:491–500
28. Kelly IG, Foster RS, Fisher WD (1987) Neer total shoulder replacement in rheumatoid arthritis. J Bone Joint Surg Br 69:723–726
29. Lynch NM, Cofield RH, Silbert PL, Hermann RC (1996) Neurologic complications after total shoulder arthroplasty J Shoulder Elbow Surg 5 (1):53–61
30. MacDonald DJ, Fitzgerald RH Jr, Ilstrup DM (1988) Two-stage reconstruction of total hip arthroplasty because of infection. J Bone Joint Surg Am 71:828–834
31. Maderazo EG, Judson S, Pasternack H (1988) Late infections of total joint prostheses. A review and recommendations for prevention. Clin Orthop 229:131–142
32. Miller SR, Bigliani LU (1993) Complications of Total Shoulder Replacement, in: Complications of Shoulder Surgery. Bigliani LU (ed) William & Wilkins. Baltimore, p 59–72
33. Moeckel BH, Altchek DW, Warren RF, Wickiewicz TL, Dines DM (1993) Instability of the shoulder after arthoplasty. J Bone Joint Surg Am 75:492–497
34. Namba RS and Tornhill TS (1995) Posterior capsulorraphy in total shoulder arthroplasty Clin Orthop 313:135–139
35. Neer CS, Watson RC, Stanton FJ (1982) Recent experience in total shoulder replacement. J Bone Joint Surg Am 64:319–337
36. Neer CS, Kirby RM (1982) Revision of humeral head shoulder arthroplasties. Clin Orthop 170:189–195
37. Neer CS (1990) Glenohumeral arthroplasty. In: Shoulder reconstruction. Saunders, Philadelphia, pp 181–185
38. Noble JS, Bell RH (1995) Failure of total shoulder arthroplasty: why does it occur? Semin Arthroplasty 6 (4):280–288
39. Norris TR, McElheny E (1990) The role of long stem humeral head prosthesis in treatment of complex humeral fractures and in revision. Semin Arthroplasty 1:138–150
40. Petersen SA, Hawkins RJ (1994) Revision shoulder arthroplasty. In Friedman RJ (ed) Arthroplasty of the shoulder. Thieme, St Louis, pp 234–241
41. Pollock RG, Deliz ED, McIlveen SJ, Flatow EL, Bigliani LU (1992) Prosthetic replacement in rotator cuff-deficient shoulders. J Shoulder Elbow Surg 1:173–186
42. Rockwood CA, Craviotto DF, Williams GF (1991) Resection arthroplasty as a salvage procedure for a failed shoulder prosthesis. Orthop Trans 15:45
43. Silliman JF, Hawkins RJ (1994) Complications following shoulder arthroplasty. In: Friedman RJ (ed) Arthroplasty of the shoulder. Thieme, St Louis, pp 242–253
44. Sneppen O, Fruensgaard S, Johannsen HV, Olsen BS, Sojberg JO and Andersen NH (1996) Total shoulder replacement in rheumatoid arthritis: Proximal migration and loosening. J Shoulder Elbow Surg 5 (1):47–52
45. Torchia ME, Cofield RH (1994) Long-term results of Neer total shoulder arthroplasty. Orthop Trans 18:977
46. Wilde AH, Borden LS, Brems JJ (1984) Experience with the Neer total shoulder replacement. In: Surgery of the shoulder. JE Bateman, RP Welsh (eds) Mosby–St. Louis, pp 224–228
47. Wirth MA, Rockwood CA (1996) Complications of total shoulder-replacement arthroplasty. J Bone Joint Surg Am 78:1174–1181

Reoperation After Shoulder Arthroplasty

H. Mestdagh, G. Walch, and P. Boileau

Summary

The purpose of this paper is to report our experience with revision shoulder arthroplasty failure. The surgical options and principles chosen to affect the best treatment are discussed. Reoperation after shoulder arthroplasty was performed in 23 patients and was always a challenging and technically difficult procedure. The pathogenesis of failed shoulder arthroplasty was directly related to the original shoulder pathology and the type of shoulder arthroplasty performed (hemi- or total arthroplasty). The common causes of failures of shoulder arthroplasties which led to revision surgery were: anterior instability (5 cases), posterior instability (3 cases), glenoid loosening (4 cases), rotator cuff pathologies (3 cases), glenoid erosion after hemiarthoplasty (2 cases), infection (3 cases), failure of tuberosity fixation (3 cases) and limited motion because of stiffness (one case). While pain relief was often obtained after revision shoulder arthroplasty, functional result was less predictable and was sometimes compromised by the condition of the soft tissues.

Introduction

Apart from glenoid lucent lines, relatively little is known about the complications of shoulder arthroplasty. It is clear that many different complications can occur but each has a relatively low incidence. Revisions of unconstrained arthroplasties are also infrequent and few articles have been devoted to this subject [11]. In Cofield's in-depth study [7] of 419 total shoulder replacements, with a follow-up from 21 days to 14 years (mean 4.5 years), the incidence of reoperation was estimated at 1 % per year.

In this chapter we discuss those patients who underwent reoperation after shoulder arthroplasty between 1992 and 1995 either from another prosthesis to an Aequalis or from an Aequalis inserted by one of our group.

Materials and Methods

Between 1992 and 1995, 23 patients with a shoulder arthroplasty underwent reoperation. Fourteen of these had an Aequalis prostheses, seven had a Neer prostheses, one a Cofield and one a Delta (Grammont). There were 14 total shoulder arthroplasties and 8 hemiarthroplasties. The average age was 63 years (40–84) and there were 14 female and 8 male patients. The original conditions leading to the index procedure were osteoarthritis in eight, post-traumatic arthritis in five, rheumatoid arthritis in three, fresh fractures in three and one each for multioperated anterior instability, locked posterior dislocation and avascular necrosis. The preoperative adjusted Constant score was 21 % on average (7 %–32 %).

The complications requiring reoperation were glenoid loosening in four cases, anterior dislocation in five cases, posterior instability in three, nonunion of the tuberosities in three, a cuff problem (rupture) in three, infection in three, glenoid wear in two, dissociation of the polyethylene in one and a prosthesis positioned too low in one case. The average time from the index operation to reoperation was 20 months (1–100).

Results

The overall results were analyzed after an average follow-up of 27 months (19–39) and were encouraging. The mean postoperative adjusted Constant score was 63 % (32 %–74 %). The results varied considerably depending on the complication leading to the reoperation.

Anterior Instability

Five patients were reoperated on for anterior dislocation of the prosthesis:

- On three occasions these were traumatic dislocations occurring between 45 days and 2 years post-operation. In two cases both humeral and glenoid

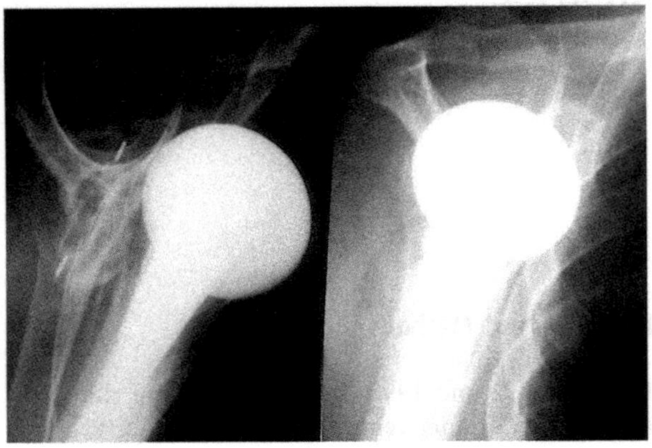

Fig. 1. Recurrent anterior dislocation of a shoulder arthroplasty after disruption of the subscapularis tendon

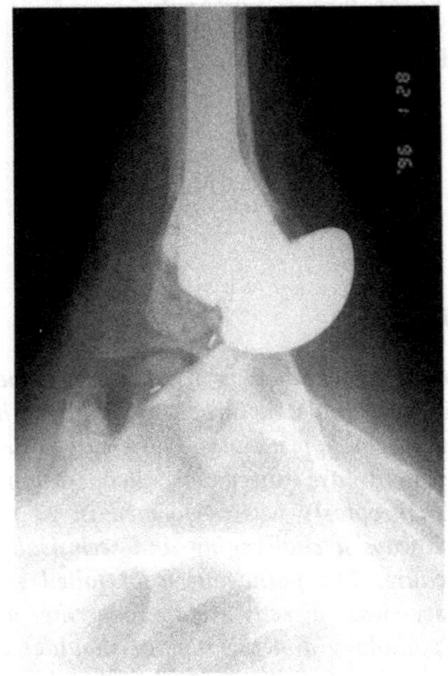

Fig. 2. Posterior dislocation of a shoulder arthroplasty 2 months postoperatively

components were replaced and in the other only the glenoid was replaced. With a follow-up of between 13 and 40 months (average 27) the results in all three were good with an average Constant score of 88 %. All the patients had active anterior elevation greater than 110°.

- One patient presented with a recurrent anterior dislocation (Fig. 1) due to failure of the reattachment of subscapularis after a previous anterior stabilization procedure. An initial attempt to reattach the subscapularis failed and she required a second reoperation using a quadriceps tendon autograft. At 30 months postoperative, the result was good with a Constant score of 70 % and anterior elevation of 130°.
- The last patient in this group had previously undergone a Bristow-Laterjet procedure and developed osteonecrosis with progressive subluxation of the humeral head and significant atrophy of the anterior deltoid. Following arthroplasty the prosthesis continued to sublux anteriorly leading progressively to dislocation. This was revised with the humeral component positioned in over-retroversion. Two years later there was a further anterior dislocation and this patient had a poor result with a Constant score of 40 % and anterior elevation of only 60°.

Posterior Instability

There were three patients with a posterior dislocation. The first was a case of osteoarthritis who had major erosion of the posterior glenoid and posterior instability was noted at the end of the index operation but not treated. The dislocation occurred 2 months postoperation (Fig. 2) and required revision to modify the orientation of both the humeral and the glenoid components. At follow-up, the patient had a disappointing result with a Constant score of 57 % and subluxation of the prosthesis seen on the axillary radiograph.

The second patient had posttraumatic arthritis with a completely absent rotator cuff. The posterior dislocation occurred in the immediate postoperative period and was reduced closed and immobilized for 1 month with the shoulder in neutral rotation. The dislocation recurred but the patient refused revision. The result was poor with a Constant score of 37 %.

The final patient had primary osteoarthritis with posterior subluxation due to uncorrected posterior glenoid wear. The prosthesis dislocated at 3 months and was reduced under general anesthesia and immobilized in neutral rotation for one month. At 20 months follow-up, there was a satisfactory result with a Constant score of 70 % and no recurrence of the posterior instability.

Glenoid Loosening

Four patients underwent revision for loosening of a cemented glenoid which had resulted in migration of the implant (Fig. 3). The loosening occurred between 6 weeks and 8 years after insertion. The reoperations consisted of reconstruction of the bony glenoid in one (satisfactory result with a Constant score of 74 %) and removal of the component and cement in the other three. This led to one good result with a score of 90 % and two poor results with scores of 50 % and 45 %.

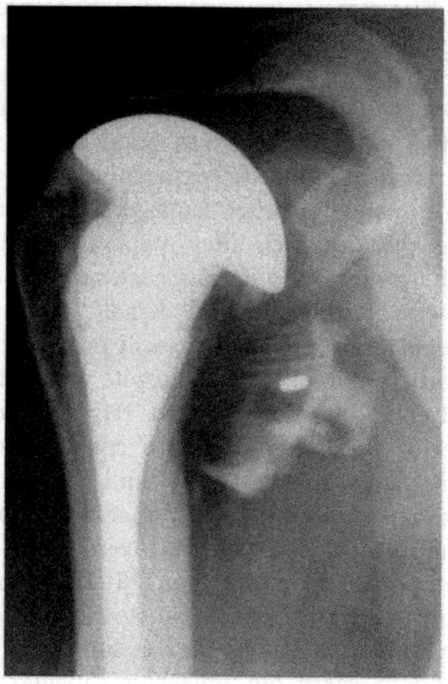

Fig. 3. Glenoid loosening and migration 28 months after implantation

Rotator Cuff Pathologies

Three patients underwent reoperation for rotator cuff pathologies: one patient had cuff pain and two patients had a secondary cuff rupture. There were two hemiarthroplasties and one total shoulder. In the case with cuff impingement a simple acromioplasty was carried out which gave a satisfactory outcome with a Constant score of 66 % and anterior elevation of 140°. However, repair of the cuff in the two cases with rupture, gave poor results with scores of 34 and 57 % and anterior elevation less than 90°.

Glenoid Erosion After Hemiarthroplasty

There were two cases of glenoid wear which occurred one and 2 years respectively after hemiarthroplasty. Due to the modularity of the humeral component it was possible to insert a glenoid implant without having to remove the humeral stem. The results were satisfactory with Constant scores of 60 and 89 % (Fig. 5).

Infection

Three patients were reoperated on at 7 and 15 and 18 months postoperation for infection. Both glenoid and humeral components were removed and the patients left with a hanging shoulder. The functional result was poor in one patient and acceptable in the other one. The last patient died 6 months after the operation.

Failure of Tuberosity Fixation

There were three cases in which the tuberosity fixation had failed (Fig. 4). One patient had been operated on for a fresh, four-part fracture and underwent revision after 18 months to change the humeral

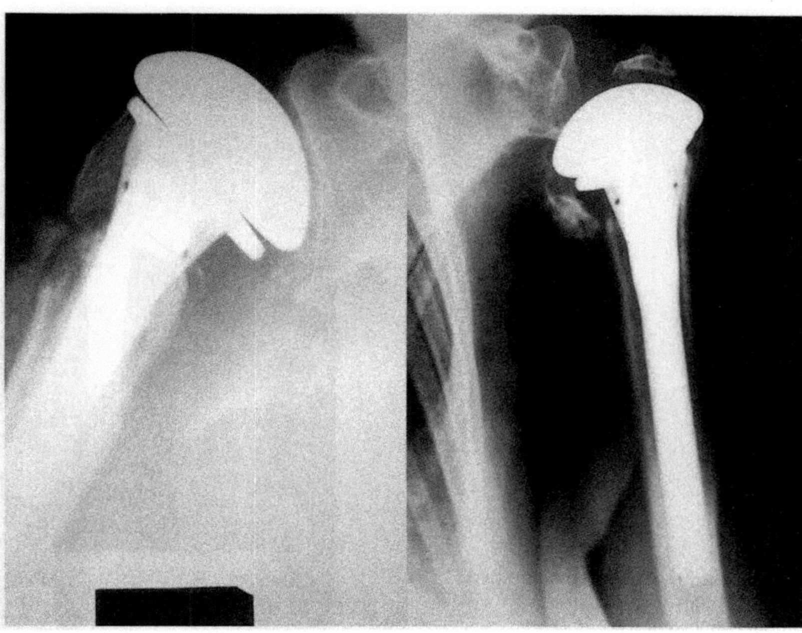

Fig. 4. Nonunion of both tuberosities after hemiarthroplasty for four-part proximal humeral fracture

component which was in excessive retroversion and to reattach the greater tuberosity using a bone graft. This gave a good result with a Constant score of 72 % and good bony consolidation.

The other two patients underwent surgery for the sequelae of fractures with osteonecrosis of the head and nonunion of the tuberosities. In both cases there was nonunion and migration of the greater tuberosity after arthroplasty. They were revised at 75 days and 1 year to reattach the tuberosity plus bone-grafting. The results were poor in both with Constant scores of 38 % and 50 %.

Arthrolysis

One patient was revised for arthrolysis 9 months after hemiarthroplasty for fracture. The result at 19 months was disappointing with a Constant score of 42 %.

Discussion

Anterior instability is the most common complication of total shoulder arthroplasty with a reported incidence of between 0 % and 29 % [14]. The usual causes are subscapularis rupture, malrotation of the humeral component or atrophy of the anterior deltoid. In our short series of five cases we encountered all three factors. Subscapularis repair is usually possible but can lead to repeated rupture as shown by Moeckel et al. [9]. The glenoid component may be damaged during the maneuvers of reduction (Fig. 3). The same is true with excessive anteversion of the humeral component leading to the need for revision to correct the version. The result is satisfactory when the anterior deltoid is functional and four of our five patients recovered good anterior elevation. It is useful to differentiate between anterior prosthetic instability after isolated, *traumatic dislocation* as these do well after reoperation and those cases where there is *progressive atraumatic anterior translation* of the humeral head. In this latter group reoperation does not prevent progressive anterior translation reoccurring despite reinserting the humeral component in excessive retroversion.

Posterior instability is a rare complication after total shoulder arthroplasty [14] and is due to either excessive retroversion of the humeral component by more than 45° or excessive retroversion of the glenoid component by more than 20°. If, after closed reduction, there is recurrent dislocation then revision is required to correct the version of the components and to carry out posterior capsular reefing. It should be noted that one of our patients had a very good result after surgical reduction and immobilization in neutral rotation for one month. Preoperative analysis with an axillary radiograph, or better still, with a CT scan will demonstrate posterior subluxation of the humeral head with posterior glenoid wear in primary osteoarthritis and this situation can then be dealt with during the index procedure to avoid the potential complication of posterior instability of the prosthesis.

Although glenoid lucent lines are the most frequently recorded abnormality after shoulder arthroplasty [4], revision for glenoid loosening is relatively

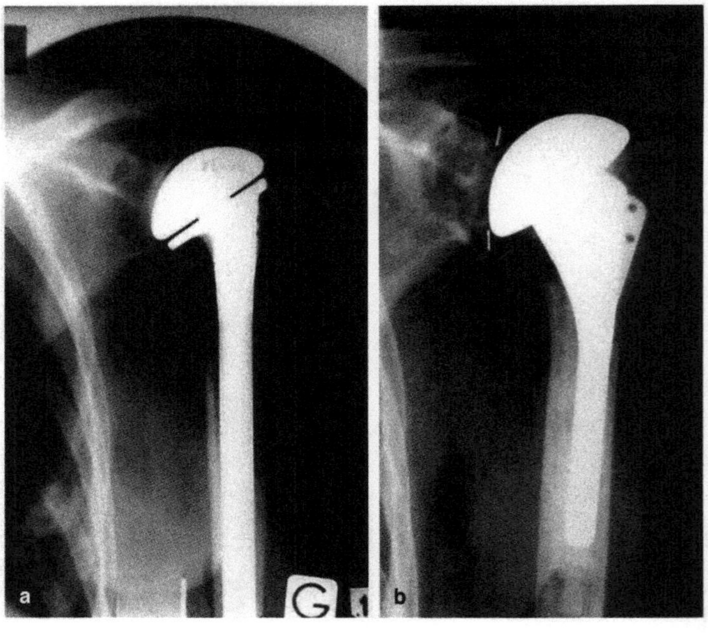

Fig. 5. a Painful glenoid erosion after hemiarthroplasty. **b** Revision with a total shoulder arthroplasty

rare. Cofield reported radiographic glenoid loosening (complete glenoid lucent lines wider than 2 mm) in 12% of a series of 73 Neer prostheses reviewed at between 2 and 6 years [6]. More recently, Cofield and Torchia reported the results in 89 shoulders with an average 12 year follow-up (5–17) and showed radiographic loosening in 44% [13]. It would seem that the incidence of glenoid loosening increases with time. However, in a meta-analysis of the literature by Rodosky there was only a 3.2% revision rate for glenoid loosening [12]. Similarly Brems recorded a 2.9% glenoid revision rate in a meta-analysis of 1400 prostheses [4]. A meta-analysis of 1459 Neer prostheses carried out up to 1992 was analyzed by Cofield and showed a revision rate for glenoid loosening of 1.9% [7]. Cofield, in reviewing the oldest series of total shoulder arthroplasty with an average follow-up of 10 years, reported a glenoid revision rate of 5.3% [7]. Surgical options for glenoid loosening are the simple removal of the implant and cement or reconstruction and replacement of the component. There is no series in the literature to support one treatment over the other. In our series we chose to remove the glenoid implant without reconstruction in three out of four cases and this resulted in a much poorer outcome than that achieved in the one case where the glenoid was reconstructed and a new component inserted.

Wirth considers postoperative cuff tears as being the third most common complication after shoulder arthroplasty occurring in 2% of cases [14]. Usually they are well tolerated and reoperation to carry out a secondary repair does not seem to give satisfactory functional results. In the two cases where we attempted this, the outcome was poor.

Recently Caldwell has reported on seven totalizations of hemiarthroplasties for glenoid erosion [5], although Neer wrote that he had never totalized a hemi [10]. Boyd and Thornhill have reported the highest rate of glenoid erosion in their series with a follow-up greater than 5-year follow-up [2, 3]. Even if the exact incidence of this complication is debatable, the new generation of modular arthroplasties allow insertion of a glenoid implant without the need to remove the humeral stem. Bigliani has reported seven cases which required totalization following glenoid erosion with unsatisfactory results where only half achieved a good outcome [1].

Kozak and Cofield reported a series of 33 shoulder arthroplasties which underwent reoperation for infection [8]. Of those patients who had simple removal of the prosthesis, half had no or little pain and half had moderate pain. The average active anterior elevation was only 40°. On the other hand, all the cases in which the prosthesis was left in place had no or little pain and the active anterior elevation was 98°. Three patients in their series underwent a two-stage revision and none had recurrent infection. It would seem that the worst option is to simply remove the prosthesis as we did in two cases. Two-stage revision after prolonged antibiotic treatment would appear to give the best results both for reinfection and functional outcome.

Bigliani reported ten revision cases for malunion and nonunion of the tuberosities [1] with unsatisfactory results due to persistent nonunion. We found the same in two-thirds of the cases in our series.

Finally, arthrolysis after shoulder arthroplasty is rare with stiffness usually accompanying another problem (malposition of the tuberosities after fracture, progressive glenoid erosion after hemiarthroplasty, etc.). Most of the reoperations included some maneuver of arthrolysis, usually subscapularis lengthening and we have not found any publications on true isolated arthrolysis after shoulder replacement.

Conclusion

The incidence of each complication that can affect a shoulder arthroplasty is small but the overall level of these complications should not be under-estimated. Each reoperation poses specific problems making generalized treatment guidelines difficult [11]. Analysis of each case shows that there are in fact usually at least two or three causes of prosthetic failure leading to the need for revision. Precise analysis of each of these factors allows them to be dealt with intraoperatively and this may perhaps improve the results obtained which, in our series, were not as good as those achieved with the primary operation.

References

1. Bigliani LU, Connor PM, Levine WN et al (1996) The surgical management of shoulder arthroplasties. Presented at the 13th Closed ASES Meeting, Amelia Island, Florida 17–20 October
2. Boyd AD Jr, Thomas WH, Scott RD, Sledge CB, Thornhill TS (1990) Total shoulder arthroplasty versus hemiarthroplasty. Indications for glenoid resurfacing. J Arthroplasty 5:329–336
3. Boyd AD, Thornhill TS (1994) Glenoid resurfacing in shoulder arthroplasty. In: Friedman RJ (ed) Arthroplasty of the shoulder. Thieme, New York, pp 306–316
4. Brems J (1993) The glenoid component in total shoulder arthroplasty. J Shoulder Elbow Surg 2:47–54
5. Caldwell GL, Dines D, Warren R, Altchek D, Wickiewicz T (1993) Revision shoulder arthroplasty. Orthop Trans 17:10
6. Cofield RH (1984) Total shoulder arthroplasty with the Neer prosthesis. J Bone Joint Surg Am 66:899–906

7. Cofield RH (1994) Total shoulder arthroplasty: results, complications and future directions. 8th Meeting of the SECEC, Barcelona, June
8. Kozak TKW, Hanssen AD, Cofield RH (1996) Infected shoulder arthroplasty. Presented at the 12th Open Meeting of the ASES, Atlanta, 25 February
9. Moeckel BH, Altchek DW, Warren RF, Wickiewicz TL, Dines DM (1993) Instability of the shoulder after arthroplasty. J Bone Joint Surg Am 75:492–497
10. Neer CS, Kirby RM (1982) Revision of humeral head and total shoulder arthroplasties. Clin Orthop 170:190–195
11. Neer CS (1990) Glenohumeral arthroplasty. In: Shoulder reconstruction. Saunders, Philadelphia pp 181–185
12. Petersen SA, Hawkins RJ (1994) Revision shoulder arthroplasty. In Friedman RJ (ed) Arthroplasty of the shoulder. Thieme, St Louis, pp 234–241
13. Rodosky MW, Bigliani LU (1996) Indication for glenoid resurfacing in shoulder arthroplasty. J Shoulder Elbow Surg 5 (3):231–248
14. Torchia ME, Cofield RH (1994) Long-term results of Neer total shoulder arthroplasty. Orthop Trans 18:977
15. Wirth MA, Rockwood CA (1996) Complications of total shoulder-replacement arthroplasty. J Bone Joint Surg Am 78:1174–1181

Shoulder Arthroplasty After Failed Surgery for Gleno-humeral Instability or Rotator Cuff Disorders

J. Romero and C. Gerber

Summary

Prosthetic shoulder joint replacement was performed by six experienced shoulder surgeons on 18 patients who had undergone previous surgery for gleno-humeral instability (instability group, ***n****=11) or rotator cuff disorders (rotator cuff group,* ***n****=7). A comparison of the results* **between the two groups** *reveals a better outcome for the rotator cuff group. In addition to subscapularis degeneration, shoulders after failed surgery for instability had more associated cuff lesions and severe weakness of the deltoid muscle giving also rise to a poor functional outcome. Pain was the factor which responded best to prosthetic shoulder replacement: 17 of the 18 patients (94.4%) were satisfied or very satisfied with the result. However, taking the objective results into account, only 12 of 18 patients (66.7%) had a good or satisactory result. The mean active elevation improved from 52° (range 0°–90°) to 107° in the instability group while it improved from 70° (range 20°–90°) to 119° (range 45°–170°) in the rotator cuff group. Nevertheless, prosthetic shoulder replacement was found to be a rewarding procedure for most patients with prior surgery for instability or rotator cuff disorders.*

Introduction

Operative management of rotator cuff disorders and gleno-humeral instability are among the most widely performed surgical procedures on the shoulder, and development of osteoarthritis is a well known long-term complication. The aetiology of disabling degenerative joint disease when associated with severe deficiency of the rotator cuff is not yet clear [1]. Long term radiographic data have shown that shoulders with massive rotator cuff tears progress to degenerative joint disease and ultimately to cranial migration of the humeral head [2]. It has been estimated that 4% of massive rotator cuff defects will progress to cuff-tear arthropathy if left untreated [3]. However, in many cases of rotator cuff tears, the head remains centered in the glenoid cavity, and the need for prosthetic shoulder replacement for disabling osteoarthritis caused by cuff tear is low given the relatively high age-related prevelance of full-thickness rotator cuff lesions [4–6].

The development of degenerative joint disease after surgery for gleno-humeral instability has been referred to as arthritis of dislocation [7]. Numerous aetiological factors may contribute. This includes recurrent subluxation [2], static subluxation in the opposite direction to an excessively tight repair [8], failure to correctly diagnose the direction of instability [9], limited external rotation [10], alterations of gleno-humeral kinematics [11] and loose or incorrectly placed metal implants [12].

Shoulder arthroplasty is a well-accepted treatment for disabling arthritis of the gleno-humeral joint [2]. However, in the absence of a functioning rotator cuff [13] or with ligament imbalance and muscle weakness, as is frequently encountered after operative procedures for instability [14], only limited success can be expected. The purpose of this multicenter study was to analyze the outcome of prosthetic shoulder replacement after failed surgery for instability or rotator cuff pathology.

Material and Methods

Prosthetic shoulder joint replacement was performed by six experienced shoulder surgeons on 18 patients who had undergone previous surgery for gleno-humeral instability (instability group) or rotator cuff disorders (rotator cuff group).

The *instability group* consisted of eleven patients with a mean age at arthroplasty of 55.4 years (range 24–72). Before arthroplasty the supraspinatus tendon was found to have an articular side partial rupture in one case and a full-thickness tear in three cases. An infraspinatus tendon lesion was found in two cases. The subscapularis was severely degenerated in five cases. Eight patients were not able to actively elevate the affected arm over 90°. External rotation was limited to no more than neutral in seven cases. In two cases a biceps tenodesis was performed. At shoulder arthroplasty, rotator cuff repair was performed in one case. A complete mobilization of the subscapularis muscle with juxta-glenoidal capsulotomy was performed in five cases.

Seven patients in the instability group had undergone a single operative procedure to correct the instability: three Bankart repairs, three bony glenoid reconstructions, one coracoid transfer. For one patient the prior procedure was unknown. Four other patients had had multiple procedures. The deltoid muscle was found to be weak in one case, and very weak in two cases.

The *rotator cuff group* consisted of seven patients with a mean age at arthroplasty of 60.8 years (range 54–66). In this group there were also one articular side partial rupture and three full-thickness lesion of the supraspinatus tendon. The infraspinatus was found to be torn in one case. Severe degeneration of the subscapularis was found in two cases. Three patients had less than 90° of active elevation. In one case external rotation was limited to no more than neutral. At shoulder arthroplasty the rotator cuff underwent repair in one case. The subscapularis muscle needed a complete mobilization with juxtaglenoidal capsulotomy in three cases. The deltoid muscle was found to be weak in 4 cases. One patient had sustained a partial injury to the axillary nerve during previous surgery.

An Aequalis prosthesis was implanted via a delto-pectoral approach in each case. The implant options chosen most frequently by the surgeons included: a neck angle of 130° in seven cases, a shaft diameter of 9 mm in nine cases, a head diameter of 50 mm with a thickness of 19 mm in six cases, and an eccentricity of the head at position 8 in six cases. The need for glenoid resurfacing depended on the surgeons' judgement. Table 1 shows the different gleno-humeral pathologies and the frequency distribution of glenoid resurfacing. At arthroplasty, one shoulder in the instability group needed an osseous glenoid reconstruction because of major bone loss.

The mean follow-up time for the *instability group* was 14.5 months (range 9–27) and 17 months (range 10–34) for the *rotator cuff group*. Outcome was analyzed using to the Constant score. Patient self-assessment was also recorded. For objective outcome assessment, a good result required an age and sex adjusted Constant score of at least 75 %, an active elevation of at least 150°, an external rotation of at least +30°, and the fact that the patient was very satisfied with the operation. A satisfactory result required an age and sex adjusted Constant score not below 50 %, an active elevation not below 90°, an external rotation not below +10°, and the fact that the patient was satisfied with the operation. A poor result failed to meet these criteria.

Results

Self-assessment revealed that seven patients were very satisfied, 10 were satisfied and one was disappointed with the result. With objective criteria 5 patients had a good result, 7 a satisfactory and 6 an unsatisfactory result. The results assessed with the Constant score are shown in Table 2.

In the *instability group* (see Figs. 1, 2) the mean pain score improved from 5.4 to 11.3 points (maximum = 15points) of the maximum (gain of 39.3 %). Of the 6 patients who did not undergo glenoid resurfacing, 3 did not reach a Constant pain score of 12 points. The mean active elevation improved from 52° (range 0°–90°) to 107° (range 30°–165°), and the mean external rotation from +3° (range –40° to 45°) to +39° (range 0°–80°). The mean active elevation of the three patients with full-thickness tears of the supraspinatus tendon was 50°, ranging from 30°–70°. Of the two patients with a very weak deltoid muscle one reached 30°

Table 1. Gleno-humeral pathology and glenoid resurfacing

Gleno-humeral pathology	Glenoid resurfacing (n)
Degenerative joint disease (no humeral head migration; n=11)	7
Cuff-tear arthropathy (cranial migration of the humeral head; n=2)	0
Necrosis (n=4)	2
Multidirectional instability (n=1)	0

Table 2. Pre- and postoperative Constant scores (percentage of maximum) in the instability and rotator cuff groups

Constant Score	Instability group			Rotator cuff group		
	Preoperative		Postoperative	Preoperative		Postoperative
Pain (max. 15 points)	5.4	⟶	11.3	4.4	⟶	10.1
Mobility (max. 40 points)	9.4	⟶	20.9	14.7	⟶	26.0
Activity (max. 20 points)	6.4	⟶	11.8	9.0	⟶	12.8
Strength (max. 25 points)	4.6	⟶	7.1	4.3	⟶	5.6
Total (max. 100 points)	25.8	⟶	51.1	32.4	⟶	54.5
Total sex and age adjusted	34.4 %	⟶	56.5 %	43.8 %	⟶	73.0 %

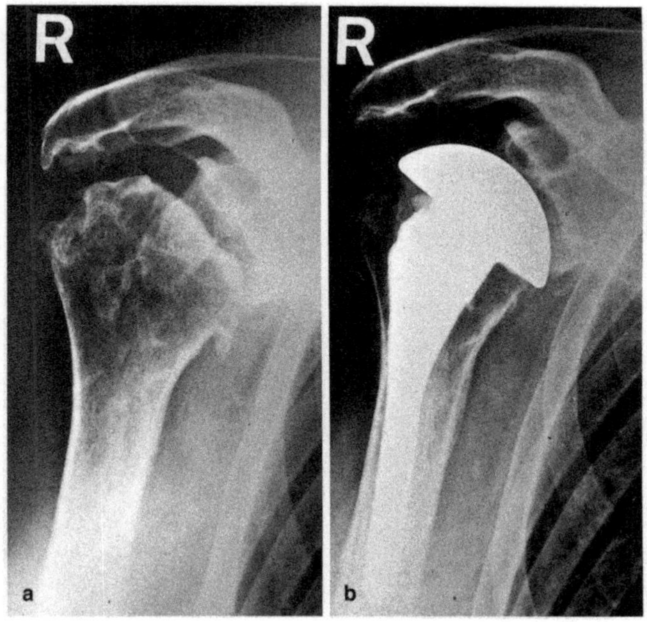

Fig. 1. Shoulder arthroplasty after prior surgery for instability. **a** A 41-year-old woman, allogenous glenoid reconstruction for anterior shoulder instability in 1992: gleno-humeral osteoarthritis, subscapularis degeneration. **b** Total shoulder arthroplasty in 1994: good pain relief, sex and age adjusted Constant score 73%, active forward elevation 160°, external rotation 60°

and another 50° of active elevation. Both had also a full-thickness supraspinatus tear and, in addition, one of them had an infraspinatus defect. The shoulder replacement had no functional effect on abduction strength.

With respect to active internal rotation, three patients reached the 12th thoracic vertebra, another three patients reached the third lumbar vertebra, and another three patients reached the sacrum. Two patients were able to internally rotate their arm to reach only the gluteal muscle. There were two cases with incomplete radiolucent lines around the glenoid component. Radiolucency was complete in one case, but the width of the radiolucent line was less than 2 mm. One patient presented with a locked anterior dislocation of the shoulder prosthesis. He rated himself as satisfactory because pain had decreased dramatically after arthroplasty. His Constant pain score improved from 2–12 points. The total sex and age adjusted Constant score had improved from 20% to 54%. His active elevation was 70°, and therefore rated poorly with respect to objective criteria.

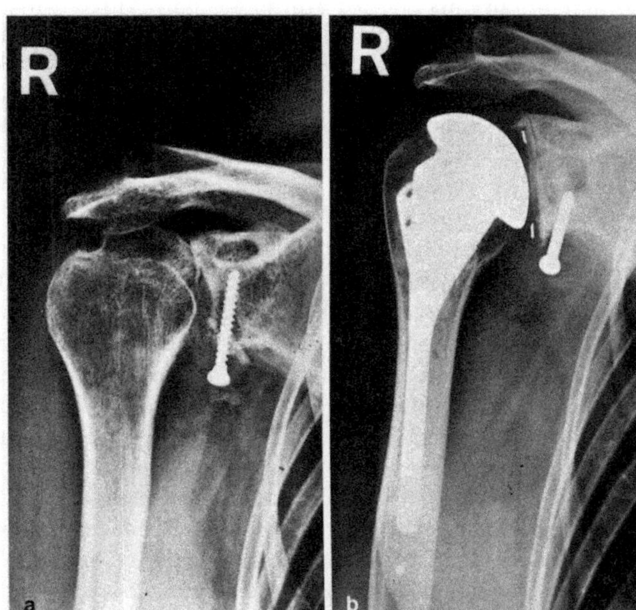

Fig. 2. Shoulder arthroplasty after prior surgey for instability. **a** A 71-year-old woman, coracoid transfer for anterior shoulder instability two decades before, humeral head necrosis, subscapularis and supraspinatus defect. **b** Shoulder arthroplasty in 1994, unsatisfactory pain relief, sex and age adjusted Constant score 54%, active forward elevation 70°, external rotation 80°

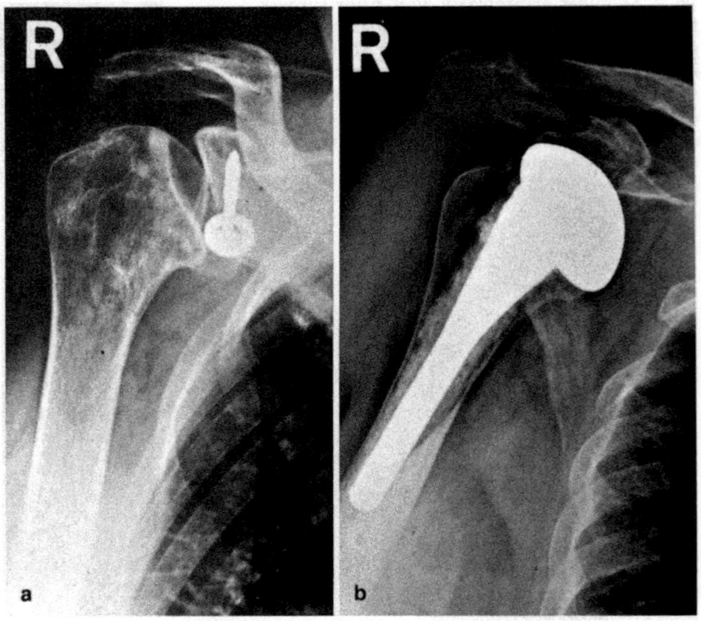

Fig. 3. Shoulder arthroplasty after previous surgery for rotator cuff disorders. **a** A 79-year-old man, rotator cuff repair in 1989, gleno-humeral arthrosis, head centered in the glenoidal cavity. **b** Shoulder hemi-arthroplasty in 1994, moderate pain relief, total sex and age adjusted Constant score 68 %, active forward elevation 170°, external rotation 60°

In the *rotator cuff group* (see Fig. 3), there was an improvement of the mean pain score from 4.4 to 10.1 points (maximum = 15 points). All three patients who did not reach a Constant pain score of 12 points had not undergone glenoid resurfacing. Mean active elevation improved from 70° (range 20°–90°) to 119° (range 45°–170°), and the mean external rotation from 24° (range 10°–35°) to 46° (range 20°–70°), respectively. The mean active elevation of the three patients with full-thickness tear of the supraspinatus tendon was 85° (range 45°–150°). A patient who had sustained an axillary nerve injury was able to raise his affected arm to 45° only. Three patients were able to internally rotate their arm to reach the twelfth thoracic vertebra. Two patients reached the third lumbar vertebra, one patient reached the sacrum, and another reached only the lateral thigh.

Quantitative measurement of abduction strength revealed no improvement. Humeral radiolucencies were found in one case. Radiolucency around the glenoid component was found in two cases, one of them being incomplete, and the other showing radiolucent lines less than 2 mm of width. One patient in the rotator cuff group had recurrent subluxations. His active elevation was 110° and the total sex and age adjusted Constant score was 74 %. The patient was satisfied with the result. He also rated satisfactory with objectve criteria. One patient needed revision surgery 10 months after shoulder replacement because of increased pain and poor function. The prosthesis was found to be in excessive anteversion, a result of a technical error. Revision was performed with a reversed prosthesis (Delta). Initially this patient had an irreparable full-thickness supraspinatus defect and an associated infraspinatus tear. His previous surgery consited of acromioplasty and cuff debridement.

Discussion

Painful disorders of the gleno-humeral joint which do not respond to other treatment methods are best addressed with shoulder arthroplasty. A meta-analysis [3, 15–25] of the results of 918 patients with unconstrained shoulder arthroplasty revealed a mean pain relief in 88.8 % of the cases, a mean active elevation of 108.8° (average gain 40.9°), and a mean external rotation of 38.2° (average gain 23.3°) after a mean follow-up of 3.9 years.

The results of the mean active elevation (107°) and the mean external rotation (39°) in our group after *failed instability surgery* was comparable with the results of the mixed population in the literature. However, the results of the patients after prior surgery for instability in this study are less favorable than those in the literature [14] for the same population group, mainly because of the additional pathology that was found in our patients, in particular subscapularis insufficiency. In Bigliani's series 9 of 17 patients could actively raise their affected arm above horizontal level before the operation. None of our patients was able to do so preoperatively. Two had a very weak deltoid muscle, and another two had a full-thickness supraspinatus lesion, of which one could not be repaired. The unfavorable preoperative conditions of these patients accounted for the inferior results postoperatively.

In the group of patients after *surgery for rotator cuff disorders*, mean active elevation (119°) and mean external rotation (46°) was slightly better than in the mixed population of the literature. The important number of patients with rheumatoid arthritis who have potential large rotator cuff defects may be responsible for the less favorable outcome in those reports. The fact that only one patient in our series had an irreparable supraspinatus tear may be the reason for the slightly better outcome of our patients compared with reports in the literature of shoulder arthroplasty for cuff tear arthropathy [13, 26].

A comparison of the results *between the two groups in this study* reveals a better outcome for the rotator cuff group. In addition to subscapularis degeneration, shoulders after failed surgery for instability had more associated cuff lesions. Severe weakness of the deltoid muscle was more abundant in the instability group, giving also rise to a poor functional outcome.

Deltoid deficency, especially of the anterior portion, can be most disabling [27]. However, in our patients, deltoid weakness was not the sole reason for impairment: all these patients had additional subscapularis or supraspinatius deficiencies.

Pain relief was better if the glenoid was resurfaced. There was, however, a relatively high frequency of radiolucencies around the glenoid component, which did not correlate with the clinical oucome. Glenoid loosening was not found. The follow-up is to short for a conclusive evaluation of this issue. The ",rocking horse" phenomenon, which has been reported to be responsible for glenoid loosening in total shoulder arthroplasty with rotator cuff deficency [28], may also be the cause of eccentric posterior loading of the glenoid component in cases with soft tissue imbalance after instability surgery.

Conclusions

In the patients reviewed in our study, pain was the factor which responded best to prosthetic shoulder replacement. Thus, 17 of 18 patients were satisfied or very satisfied with the result. However, taking the objective results into account, only 12 of 18 patients had a good or satisactory result. Nevertheless, prosthetic shoulder replacement was found to be a rewarding procedure for most patients with previous surgery for instability or rotator cuff disorders. An attempt to restore function by arthroplasty in the described settings is a challenging task. Failure to achieve reasonable results depends on the amount of soft-tissue destroyed by prior surgery. Excessive scarring, adhesions and degeneration of the subscapularis from prior instability surgery is a difficult situation to deal with. Careful mobilization of the subscapularis muscle is mandatory to restore external rotation. The axillary nerve and the vessels are in extreme jeopardy. In irreparable supraspinatus lesions, a less predictable outcome must be expected. Patients after prior instability surgery may also have a supraspinatus tear, giving rise to a disappointing functional result. If the main goal is focused on pain reduction, patient satisfaction can be achieved in a high percentage of the cases.

References

1. McCarty DJ (1989) Robert Adams' rheumatic arthritis of the shoulder - Milwaukee shoulder" revsited. J Rheumatol 16:668–670
2. Hamada K, Fukuda H, Mikasa M, Kobayashi Y (1990) Roentgenographic findings in massive rotator cuff tears - a long term observation. Clin Orthop 254:92–96
3. Neer CS, Craig EV, Fukuda H (1983) Cuff tear arthropathy. J Bone Joint Surg Am 65:1232–1244
4. Grant JCB, Smith GC (1948) Age incidence of rupture of the supraspinatus tendon. Anat Rec 100:666
5. McLaughlin HL (1962) Rupture of the rotator cuff. J Bone Joint Surg Am 44:979–983
6. Cottton RE, Rideout DF (1964) Tears of the humeral rotator cuff. J Bone Joint Surg Br 46:314–328
7. Neer CS, Watson KC, Stanton FJ (1982) Recent experience in total shoulder replacement. J Bone Joint Surg Am 64:319–337
8. Hawkins RJ, Angelo RL (1990) Glenohumeral osteoarthrosis: a late complication of Putti-Platt repair. J Bone Joint Surg Am 72:1193–7
9. Hawkins RJ, Schutte JP (1988) The assesment of glenohumeral translation using manual and fluoroscopic technques. Orthop Trans 12:674
10. Lusardi DA, Wirth MA, Wurtz D, Rockwood CA (1993) Loss of external rotation following anterior capsulorrhaphy of the shoulder. J Bone Joint Surg Am 75:185–92
11. Huber HM (1992) Incidence of recurrence and osteoarthritis after rotational humeral osteotomy according to Weber. J Bone Joint Surg Br 74 [Suppl 1]:7
12. Zuckerman JD, Matsen FA (1984) Complications about the glenohumeral joint related to the use of screws and staples. J Bone Joint Surg 66:175–180
13. Arntz CT, Jackins S, Matsen A (1993) Prosthetic replacement of the shoulder for the treatment of defects in the rotator cuff and the surface of the glenohumeral joint. J Bone Joint Surg Am 75:485–491
14. Bigliani LU, Weinstein DM, Glasgow MT, Pollock RG, Flatow EL (1995) Glenohumeral arthroplasty for arthritis after instability surgery. J Shoulder Elbow Surg 4:87–94
15. Cofield RH (1984) Total shoulder arthroplasty with the Neer prosthesis. J Bone Joint Surg Am 66:899–906

16. Bade HA, Warren RF, Ranawat CS, Inglis CS (1984) Long term results of Neer total shoulder replacement. In: Bateman JE, Welsh RP (ed) Surgery of the shoulder. Mosby, St. Louis, p 294
17. Wilde AH, Borden LS, Brems JJ (1984) Expriences with the Neer total shoulder replacement. In: Bateman JE, Welsh RP (ed) Surgery of the shoulder. Mosby, St. Louis, p 224
18. Barrett WP, Franklin JL, Jackins SE, Wyss CR, Matsen FA (1987) Total shoulder arthroplasty. J Bone Joint Surg Am 69:865–872
19. Frich LH, Moller BN, Sneppen O (1988) Shoulder arthroplasty with the Neer mark-II prosthesis. Arch Orthp Trauma Surg 107:110–113
20. Brenner BC, Ferlic DL, Clayton ML, Dennis DA (1989) Survivorship of unconstrained total shoulder arthroplasty. J Bone Joint Surg Am 71:1289–1296
21. Hawkins RJ, Bell RH, Jallay B (1989) Total shoulder arthoplasty. Clin Orthop 242:188–194
22. Weiss APC, Adams MA, Moore JR, Weiland AJ (1990) Unconstrained shoulder arthroplasty: a 5-year average follow-up study. Clin Orthop 257:86–90
23. Henry JD, Thomas WH, Thornhill TS et al (1992) Total shoulder arthroplasty using the Neer unconstrained implant: Long term results. American Academy of Orthopaedic Surgeons, Washington, 25 February
24. Boileau P, Walch G, Noël E, Liotard JP (1994) La prothèse d'épaule de Neer: résultats en fonction de l'étiologie. Rev Rhum 61:607–618
25. Fenlin JM Jr, Ramsey ML, Allardyce TJ, Frieman BG (1994) Modular total shoulder. replacement: design rational, indications, and results. Clin Orthop 307:37–46
26. Arntz CT, Matsen FA, Jackins S (1991) Surgical management of complex irreparable rotator cuff defciency. J Arthroplasty 6:363–370
27. Groh GI, Simoni M, Rolla P, Rockwood CA (1994) Loss of deltoid after shoulder operations: an operative disaster. J Shoulder Elbow Surg 3:243253
28. Franklin JL, Barrett WP, Jackins SE, Matsen FA (1988) Glenoid loosening in total shoulder arthroplasty: association with rotator cuff deficiency. J Arthroplasty 3:39–46

Section XV: **Synopsis**

Shoulder Arthropathy and Shoulder Arthroplasty: An Overview

G. Walch and P. Boileau

Summary

The large experience gained from the early use of the Neer prosthesis and then the Aequalis clinical multicenter studies together with our basic research concerning anatomical and biomechanical aspects of the glenohumeral joint have led us to improve our knowledge on both shoulder arthropathy and shoulder arthroplasty.

Shoulder Arthroplasty

The Humeral Component

Whenever or wherever shoulder arthroplasty is discussed the reference is always to Neer. It is now over 45 years since his clinical experience began, a long time before Charnley, so when our patients say that shoulder arthroplasty is an untested operation and the follow-up is short we can use his name and experience as reassurance. The first generation of prosthesis, which was modified in 1972 to allow cement fixation, saw few emulators until the end of the 1980s since when there has been a gradual increase in unconstrained, modular prostheses which have variable head sizes to allow them to match the anatomical variations in dimensions encountered. We have also seen a "stem war" (cemented or uncemented) despite the paradox that the complication level with cemented implants was extremely low (0.7 % in a meta-analysis of nearly 1500 cases carried out by Cofield). The wish of the designers was to create stems with the biggest number of diameters possible. For no particular reason cement became «public enemy number one» in the shoulder and a range of partial or fully coated stems appeared covered in hydroxyapatite, plasma-sprayed, porous coated, etc. These were the second, modular, generation of shoulder prosthesis.

We were intrigued by the difficulty in adapting the existing prostheses to the anatomy found in our patients and our work has been directed towards on ever more accurate understanding of the precise anatomy of the upper humeral epiphysis. This made us aware that not only did the head have a variable size but that its spatial orientation with regard to the humeral stem was different to the then recognized belief. The head is positioned slightly medially and posteriorly with a variable angle of inclination and retroversion. Using the anatomical studies carried out between 1988 and 1990 under the direction of Pascal Boileau and with the aid of the engineers from Tornier, we designed a new type of humeral implant: the third generation, which was *adaptable*, allowing it to be constructed to match the individual anatomy of each patient rather than having to alter the patients anatomy to match the prosthesis (Fig. 1). The essential characteristics of this new prosthesis were:

- A short (10.5 cm) stem because the humerus is between 10 and 20 cm shorter than the femur with vastly weaker forces acting on it. Also the humerus has an italic S shape with a curve situated about 10–15 cm from the greater tuberosity. This curvature could cause a diaphyseal fracture during stem introduction, especially if the aim is to go for maximal canal filling with an uncemented stem.

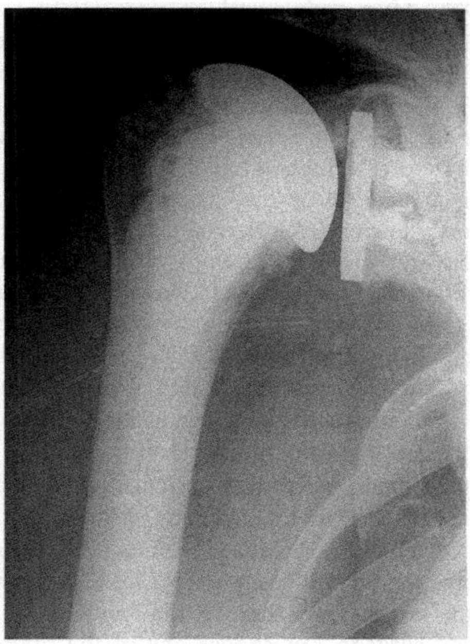

Fig. 1. The Aequalis prosthesis has been designed to reproduce the patient's individual bony anatomy. This concept has been called "bony balancing" and is as important as the "soft tissue balancing"

- The stems are polished and must be cemented to avoid migration as observed by Cofield and Kelly. The polished surface allows for a relatively simple extraction in the rare cases where this is required.
- The inclination is variable due to a range of four neck angles between 125° and 140° which allow adaptation to anatomical variation.
- The humeral head can be translated medially due to the variable medio-lateral offset of the implant. The humeral head can in fact be orientated in all direction of space due to the eccentric dial system situated on its undersurface which allows both posterior/anterior and medial/lateral offset to be reproduced.
- There are two locking screws to hold the three elements together (stem-neck-head) to completely remove the chance of dissociation (which has been reported in the literature on very rare occasions).
- The humeral implant is available in either titanium or cobalt-chrome allowing for surgical preference.
- For revision cases or where there is a diaphyseal extension of a head fracture a 15 cm stem is available.

The Glenoid Component

The glenoid component was not part of Neer's original conception but was initially introduced by him in 1972. After trying various sizes (100 %, 200 %, 600 %) and various constructions (metal-backed or not) he finally opted for a polyethylene component with a keel to be cemented in place. The angle of curvature was the same as that of the humeral head. Despite a high level of lucent lines reported (from 30 % to 90 %) the incidence of revision was extremely low (1 % for Neer and 2 % for Brems) during the first 25 years. Attempts with screw-fixation, uncemented to metal-backed, to plug fixation have been tried by various authors. Some of these were abandoned without the results being published, others failed because of a high complication level while others are still being evaluated. For these reasons we chose to offer our patients the same security as represented by Neer's experience and selected to use an all polyethylene implant with a keel fixed with cement. The Aequalis glenoid component is available in three sizes with a radius of curvature slightly larger than that of the humeral head so that the surgeon can choose any of the three sizes to match any of the humeral heads. In 1992, under the driving force of Dr. Pascal Boileau, we developed an uncemented glenoid component using a system of expanding screws. This works in a similar way to fixations used in cavity walls resulting in primary fixation while bony ingrowth occurs into the hydroxyapatite coated surface. Due to the expanding screw system we were able to avoid too thick an implant which is only 7 mm (3 mm for the metal-back and 4 mm for the polyethylene insert which click-fits onto the tray, Fig. 1).

The Instrumentation

The instrumentation has been designed so that even a surgeon with limited experience can successfully implant the prosthesis.

- *The instrumentation for the humeral side* is relatively simple and because the prosthesis adapts to the original anatomy there is no need for a cutting-guide. The head cut is made by free hand at the level of the anatomical neck after removal of the crown of osteophytes. An angle guide measures the inclination and marks the retroversion which can then be reproduced in the prosthesis.
- *The glenoid instrumentation* is the same for metal-backed and all polyethylene glenoid implants. Two reamers, one large and one small, are used to flatten the glenoid surface to give perfect contact and fit between the bone and implant surfaces.
- *The instrumentation for fracture cases,* i.e., the Aequalis fracture jig, was developed to answer the problem posed in all the published series of matching height and retroversion of the humeral component when the landmark of the tuberosities has been lost. We designed an implant holder which reproduces the anatomical retroversion of 20° related to the transepicondylar axis and the humeral length as measured from the healthy arm.

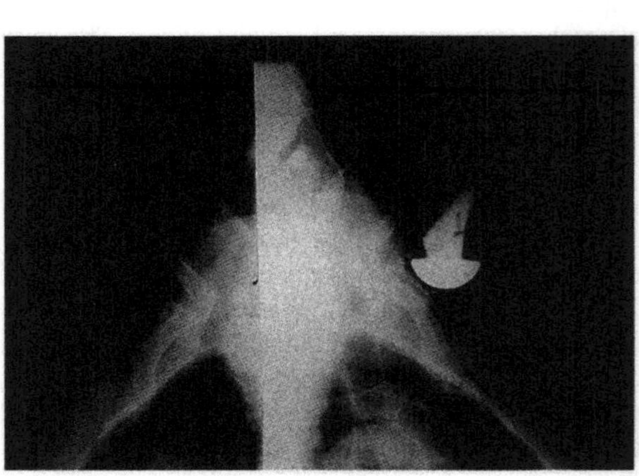

Fig. 2. When there are good muscles an excellent functional result can be obtained because of the "almost normal" kinematics of the shoulder restoration

The first prostheses were inserted in 1991 by the two of us and since 1992 a group of 15 European surgeons have used it with prospective assessment involving evaluation sheets and radiographs pre- and postoperatively. In 1996 the time had come for us to analyze our results eventhough the follow-up was too short to give the results an unquestionable scientific value. The functional result for a prosthesis is established by one year and so we have only included those cases with at least 1 year follow-up.

Shoulder Arthropathy

The prospective analysis and the review of more than 400 patients operated on have bring us much information concerning all etiologies of glenohumeral diseases.

In chronic cases (primary osteoarthritis, rheumatoid arthritis and avascular necrosis) the results for both pain relief and mobility were excellent which supports the validity of the concept of "bony-balancing," i.e., reproducing the bony anatomy without altering either the center of rotation or the moment of action of the intrinsic muscles of the shoulder (rotator cuff and deltoid). Soft-tissue balancing should not rely just on artificially altering the thickness of the humeral head but also on complete release of the contracted soft-tissues: subscapularis, anterior capsule and the posterior and inferior capsule. It seems that, whenever the bone stock permits it, a glenoid implant should be inserted. A wide posterior release is essential not only to recover mobility but to allow proper preparation of the glenoid. The component with a surface encouraging bony ingrowth and using expansion screws clearly results in fewer lucent lines than with a cemented implant but a long-term study will be required to verify this.

In arthritis with massive cuff-tear, a hemiarthroplasty appears to be an attractive alternative in reducing pain but does not result in satisfactory mobility or function. An exact analysis of those patients who had surprisingly good results and the use of new implants should allowe us to improve our results.

In posttraumatic arthritis it is essential to differentiate between cases with solid union of the greater tuberosity in an acceptable position from those which require an osteotomy and fixation of the greater tuberosity to reconstruct the proximal humerus. In the former group the results are good or very good whereas in the latter group the results were unpredictable and often less good than those we obtained in all etiologies together. The greater tuberosity carrying the insertion of the supra and infraspinatus is therefore the final judge of the results that can be expected in posttraumatic arthritis. This may lead onto the development of a different prosthesis or a different surgical approach in cases where the tuberosity-diaphyseal continuity is not in an acceptable alignment.

In fracture cases there still remains the problem of the greater tuberosity which is the limiting factor in the quality of the results now that the problems of humeral length and retroversion have been resolved. The posterior migration that we have observed due to failure of consolidation will lead to new work to develop a prosthesis offering the optimal chance for bony consolidation of the tuberosities.

Analysis of the complications and reoperations in this multicenter study is the most interesting for the surgeon as this makes us aware of any technical or conceptual inadequacies and any errors of indication. The risks and dangers of the surgery can be determined and gives the surgeon essential information on any traps and clarifies the indications for inserting a prosthesis in the best conditions.

Rehabilitation is the twin sister of the surgery in these operations. Although many of the simpler cases only require a few sessions of rehabilitation, there are still many complex cases where the rehabilitation accounts for 50 % of the final outcome.

Finally, the large number of cases analyzed with the multicenter study has made it possible to **classify the different pathologies.** The results of shoulder arthroplasty should be evaluated in the future according to these different classifications to confirm their validity and to make comparison of the results possible.

- *Classification of osteoarthritis:* we described three types of glenoid morphology as seen on the horizontal plane with CT-scan:
  - *Type A* is characterized by a *concentric erosion* (53.5 %).
  - *Type B* has a biconcave appearance with *predominant posterior glenoid erosion* (39.5 %).
  - Type C (5 %) is arbitrarily defined as *glenoid retroversion greater than 25°* (Fig. 3).

This is important to know before planning a shoulder arthroplasty since we have demonstrated that posterior subluxation of the humeral head is associated with a biconcave appearance of the glenoid. Possible persistence of posterior subluxation after shoulder arthroplasty may be responsible for glenoid loosening due to the "rocking horse mechanism" in the horizontal plane and is a concern for the future.

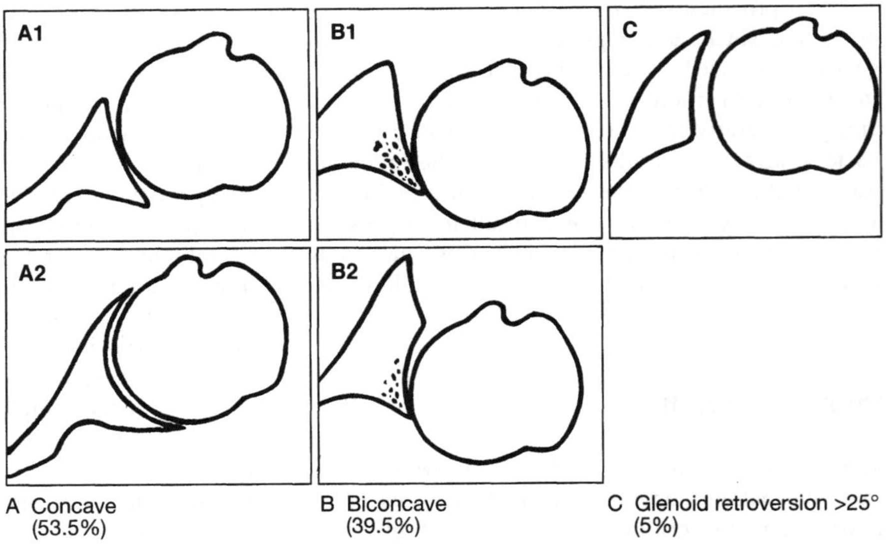

Fig. 3. Classification of the horizontal glenoid shape in osteoarthritis as seen on CT scan: Type A (53.5%) has a concave and central erosion; type B (39.5%) has a biconcave and posterior erosion; type C (5%) is arbitrarily defined as glenoid retroversion greater than 25. Type B (biconcave) is correlated with posterior subluxation of the humeral head

- *Classification of rheumatoid arthritis:* three forms were described based on the radiograhic appearance of the AP-view and are similar to those described by Neer (Fig. 4).
  - *The ascendant (or resorptive) form* (41%) is characterized by upward migration of the humeral head with superior glenoid wear and frequent cuff tear. Implantation of a glenoid component may be technically difficult because of excessive medialization of the joint with retraction of the soft tissues and bone loss.
  - *The centered (or dry) form* (36%) is comparable to classical osteoarthritis with a normal acromio-humeral distance; from a clinical point of view this form is characterized by persistent stiffness even after shoulder replacement.
  - *The destructive (or wet) form* (19%) is characterized by marginal erosion of the humeral head and rapid destruction of the joint. From a clinical point of view this form is characterized by a paradoxical, good functional result after shoulder arthroplasty and recovery of motion beyond the horizontal, despite the worrying destruction of the joint.
- *Classification of osteoarthritis with massive cuff-tear:* three different radiological forms have also been observed leading to different physiopathological hypotheses (Fig. 5). Suprisingly, these three different forms are similar to those descibed in rheumatoid arthritis and can be named in a similar way.
  - In *type 1* (51%), the shoulder looks like the *hip* with femoralization of the humeral head and

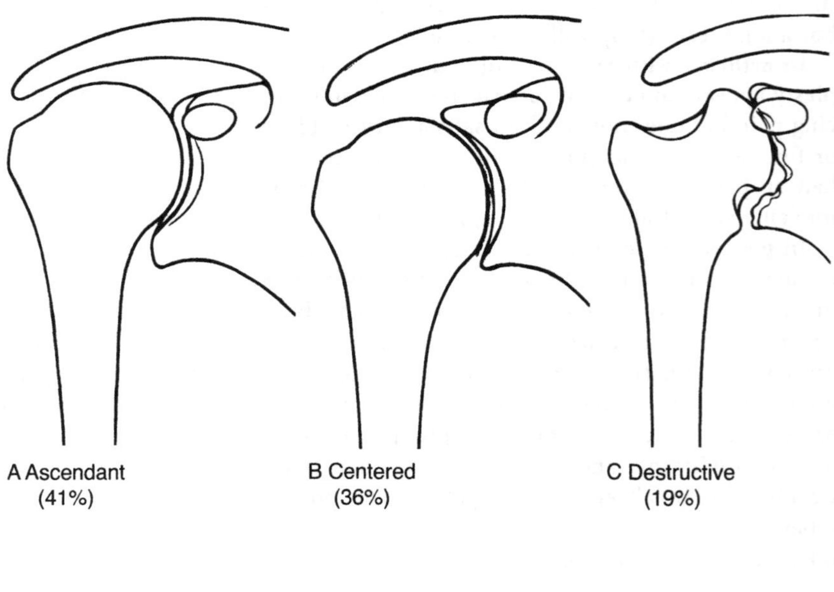

Fig. 4. Classification of rheumatoid arthritis as seen on AP-view: the *ascendant (or resorptive) form (41%)* makes the implantation of a glenoid component difficult because of medialization due to superior bone erosion and cuff tear; *the centered (or dry) form (36%)* is characterized by stiffness; *the destructive (or wet) form (19%)* gives paradoxal good functional result after shoulder arthroplasty

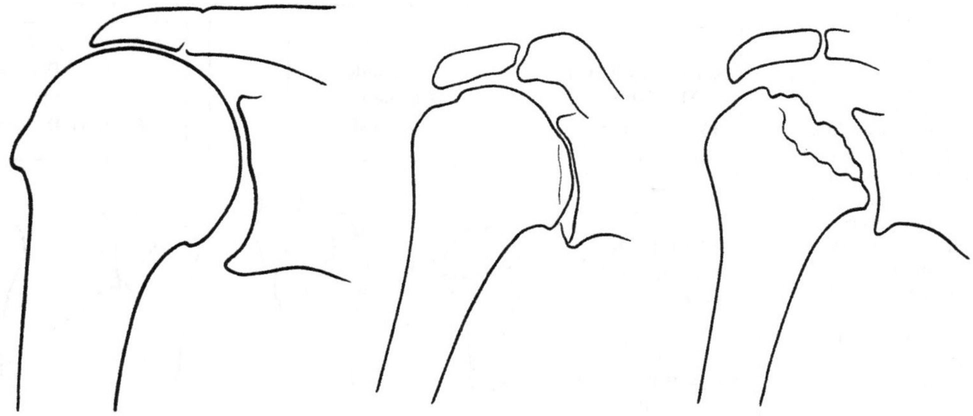

Fig. 5. Classification of osteoarthritis with massive cuff-tear as seen on AP-view: the *ascendant form* (51 %) corresponds to *Neer's cuff-tear arthropathy* with acetabulization of the acromion; *the centered form (19 %)* has little or no alteration in the shape of the acromion without humeral head imprint; the *destructive form* (30 %) is characterized by *lysis* of either the humeral head or the acromion and corresponds to the rheumatological shoulders (*senile haemorrhagic shoulder, Milwaukee shoulder, rapidly destructive arthropathy)*

acetabulization of the glenoid and the acromion: this *ascendant form* corresponds to *Neer's cuff-tear arthropathy* and is the evolution of a long-term rotator cuff tear with predominance of "mechanical factors"; the function is usually conserved for a long time. The shoulder becomes painful either because of subluxation or tenosynovitis of the long head of the biceps, or because of the neoarticulation becoming arthritic or because of bone lysis.

- *Type 2* (19 %) corresponds to osteoarthritis because of the centralized narrowing of the gleno-humeral joint with a massive cuff tear as shown by the narrowing of the acromio-humeral distance. Because of the minor alteration in the shape of the acromion without humeral head imprint, this form can named *the centered form.*
- *Type 3* (30 %) can be named the *destructive form* because of the *lysis* of either the humeral head or the acromion. This group corresponds to the rheumatological shoulders in which "biochemical factors" are predominant and has been described in the literature as "senile hemorrhagic shoulder, Milwaukee shoulder, or rapidly destructive arthropathy".

While a nonconstrained shoulder prosthesis may give a good result in some ascendant or early destructive forms because of the functional adaptation of the shoulder that has found a proximal fulcrum for many years, there is little chance that this type of implant will enable active elevation above the horizontal in most of the osteoarthritis with massive cuff-tear. For this reason, there is probably a place for a constrained shoulder prosthesis in osteoarthritis with massive cuff-tear. We will have to verify these hypotheses in a prospective manner in the future.

- *Classification of post-traumatic arthritis*: two categories of fracture sequelae are evident from a surgical point of view (Fig. 6): *intra-capsular/impacted fractures sequelae* (including necrosis/cephalic collapse and locked luxations and fractures-luxation) *and extra-capsular/desimpacted fracture sequelae* (including nonunions of the surgical neck and severe malunions of the tuberosities). The prognosis is completly different in the two categories: all excellent and good results may be expected in the intra-capsular/impacted group when a greater tuberosity osteotomy is not required. We have observed outcome after arthroplasty requiring an osteotomy of the greater tuberosity is unpredictable, but often poor. Moreover, if prosthetic replacement is possible without an osteotomy, surgeons should accept distorsional anatomy of the proximal humerus and adapt the prosthesis and their technique accordingly. An adaptable prosthesis, like the Aequalis prosthesis, offers here another advantage: to make adaptation of the implant to the distored anatomy of the proximal humerus possible.

Fig. 6. Classification of post-traumatic arthritis: *intra-capsular/impacted fracture sequelae* (including necrosis/cephalic collapse and locked luxations and fractures–luxation) *and extra-capsular/non-impacted fracture sequelae* (including nonunions of the surgical neck and severe malunions of the tuberosities). Osteotomy of the greater tuberosity is needed to implant a shoulder prosthesis in the second group and leads to poor and unpredictable results

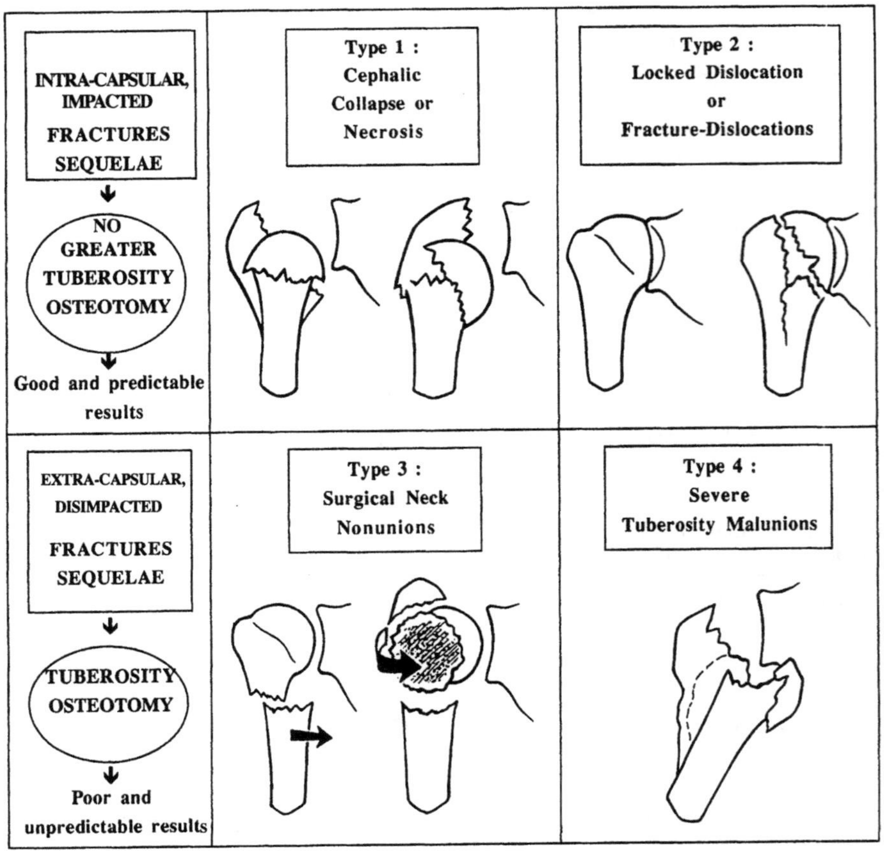

Conclusion

The goal of this book is to pass on to the general orthopedic surgeon and the shoulder specialist the experience of their colleagues who have come across most of the problems that can be encountered in shoulder arthroplasty. We do not pretend to have answered all the questions but we have, at least, asked them in the hope that in the years to come we will obtain even more convincing results for our patients. These results will be again carefully analyzed in the next future.

Subject Index

R

S

T

W

Z

MIX
Papier aus verantwortungsvollen Quellen
Paper from responsible sources
FSC® C105338

If you have any concerns about our products,
you can contact us on
ProductSafety@springernature.com

In case Publisher is established outside the EU,
the EU authorized representative is:
Springer Nature Customer Service Center GmbH
Europaplatz 3, 69115 Heidelberg, Germany

Printed by Libri Plureos GmbH
in Hamburg, Germany